CLINICAL PRACTICE

EXPERIENCE AND EVIDENCE BASED APPROACH

Social Commitment of the Author

The core medical team for whom the author has profound gratitude for the cases presented in the book, consists of some doctors without whom the book would not have come to the reality. In addition to this core team, there are other ancillary supporting team members. There are also many volunteers who help to run a village hospital 'Ranganathananda Gramin Swasthya Seva Kendra' in the Sundarbans of West Bengal. The members of the medical consortium visit the hospital once in a month. Free medicines are distributed on that day among the marginalised people. It is run by the fund contributed by the doctors and the patients. In the western world this kind of service perhaps has little value, but in a developing country like ours any such selfless service does add some value to the society. This organisation also runs a water ambulance which helps to organise clinics in the remote areas of the Sundarbans. The hospital building was erected with donation from respected Sri B. K. Birla and late Smt. Sarala Devi Birla. The organisation has never accepted any fund from any Government and NGO. Anyone interested to join this philanthropic group of medical volunteers may express his/her willingness in the following e-mails:

- Dr. Subrata Maitra: subratamaitra@hotmail.co.uk
- Mrs. Chaitali Maitra: chaitalisubrata@hotmail.com
- Dr. Samarjit Naskar: naskarsamarjit@gmail.com
- Mr. Pranoy Bhattacharjee: pranoybhattacharjee13@gmail.com
- Dr. Subir Kr. Mandal: subir_mallika@yahoo.com
- Dr. Anirban Neogi: draneogi@gmail.com
- Dr. Avirup Chakraborty: avirup.chakraborty18@gmail.com
- Dr. Debkripa Banerjee: devk80@yahoo.com

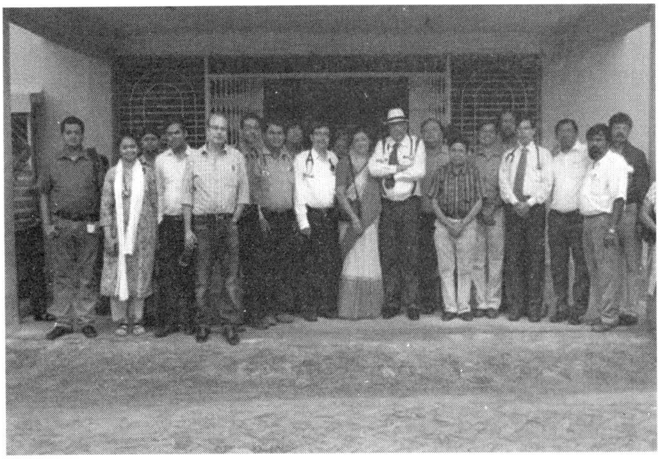

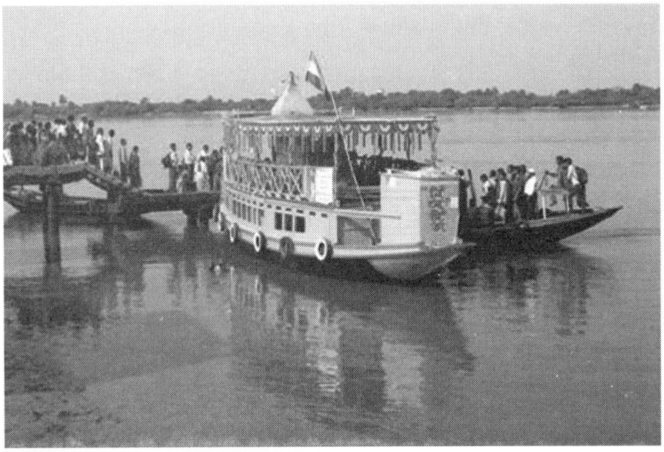

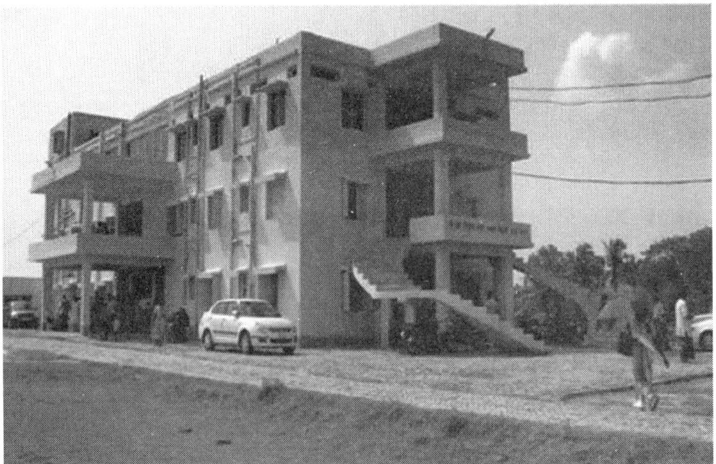

CLINICAL PRACTICE
EXPERIENCE AND EVIDENCE BASED APPROACH

Dr. Subrata Maitra DNB, FRCP (Edin, London, Ire)

Senior Physician
Belle Vue Clinic, B P Poddar Hospital

Member
West Bengal Medical Council

Chairman
Multi Disciplinary Expert Group, Health Reforms, Govt. of West Bengal

Founder President
Ma Sarada Swasthya Seba Parishad

President
Ranganathananda Gramin Swasthya Kendra

Past Chairman
Indian Society of Critical Care Medicine (Kolkata Branch)

Former Consultant Physican in-charge, Critical Care Unit
Woodlands Hospital and Medical Research Centre Ltd

New Central Book Agency (P) Ltd

LONDON

HYDERABAD ERNAKULAM BHUBANESWAR

NEW DELHI KOLKATA PUNE GUWAHATI

NCBA

REGD OFFICE
8/1 Chintamoni Das Lane, Kolkata 700 009, India
email: ncbapvtltd@eth.net

OVERSEAS
NCBA (UK) Ltd, 149 Park Avenue North, Northampton, NN3 2HY, UK
email: ncbauk@yahoo.com

EXPORT
NCBA Exports Pvt. Ltd, 212 Shahpur Jat, New Delhi 110 049
email: ncbaexports@ncbapvtltd.com

BRANCHES

212 Shahpur Jat
New Delhi 110 049
email: ncbadel@ncbapvtltd.com

Shop Nos. 3 & 4, Vinayak Towers
681/B Budhwar Peth, Appa Balwant Chowk
Pune 411 002
email: ncbapune@ncbapvtltd.com

Shop No. 15, Bharati Towers, Ground Floor
Forest Park
Bhubaneswar 751 001
email: ncbabub@ncbapvtltd.com

House No. 3-1-315, 1st Floor
Nimboliadda, Kachiguda, **Hyderabad** 500 027
email: ncbahydb@ncbapvtltd.com

GSS Shopping Complex, 1st Floor
Opposite College Post Office, Convent Road
Ernakulam 682 035
email: ncbaernk@ncbapvtltd.com

Radhamayee Complex (Second Floor)
Opp. SBI, Panbazar, Jaswanta Road
Guwahati 781 001
email: ncbaguwahati@ncbapvtltd.com

Clinical Practice with Experience and Evidence Based Approach • Dr. Subrata Maitra

First Published: July 2015

PUBLISHER AND TYPESETTER
New Central Book Agency (P) Ltd
8/1 Chintamoni Das Lane, Kolkata 700 009

PRINTER
New Central Book Agency (P) Ltd
Web-Offset Division, Dhulagarh, Sankrail, Howrah

COVER DESIGNER
Soumen Paul

COVER PRINTER
Techno Process, Kolkata

PROOF CHECKING
Dr Anirban Neogi, Dr S K Mandol

PROJECT TEAM
Prabhat Jas

ISBN 978 81 7381 973 5

Price: ₹ 750.00

I dedicate this book to my father **Mr. Kashikanta Maitra**, whose idealism, fighting spirit, honesty and uncompromising attitude towards injustice have been the main guiding force throughout my life. It was he who taught me to hold my head high against all provocations.

ACKNOWLEDGEMENT

Before I delve deeper into the actual content of this book, I should remember some people around me who have always been by my side encouraging me to complete this book. Some of them helped me physically, some morally and some intellectually.

I remain deeply indebted to my parents and my family. I must say, this book could not see the light of the day without the perseverance of Mrs. Chaitali Maitra, my wife, who never discouraged me for the time that I had to spend with my work.

Without the help of the doctors of my team, this herculean task could never be completed. I am indeed grateful to these doctors like Dr. Subir Kumar Mandal, Dr. Anirban Neogi, Dr. Debkripa Banerjee, Dr. Abhijnan Maji, Dr.Samarjit Naskar, Dr. Avirup Chakraborty, Dr. Uzma Nafiz and Dr. Kazi Samsuzzaman, whose enthusiasm and encouragement have helped me to complete this uphill task. Copy-editing and proofreading of the entire text they had done themselves. Dr. Gargi De helped in compiling and proofreading. My son Dr. Saurav Maitra also helped me tossing suggestions here and there.

The secretarial staff namely Mr. Saikat Kumar Dutta, Mr. M K Narayana Murthy, Mrs. Iman Banerjee and Miss Sumana Chakraborty helped me profusely in keying-in and other minute editorial emendations. My elder son Mr. Somanka Maitra, although a non-medical person, helped me in typing and many other supportive roles. Mr. Pranoy Bhattacharjee helped me by applying his printing skill and contacts. Photographs are by and large collected by the consortium doctors; a few are taken from Dr. A. K. Sain, radiologist. Some of the pictures are taken from internet as well, and I have gratefully mentioned the sites in the text.

Here I should remember my patients who are like the members of our medical consortium family. We are happy to serve them during their stressful situations. I fondly remember their glowing faces during discharge after getting cured. Without their presence such a vast text of this book was difficult to come to reality. I wholeheartedly pray for their comfort and hassle-free life. I am also grateful to all the RMOs, nurses, doctors-in-charge and doctors of different specialities who enriched me by their loving touch, sincere care and valuable suggestions to cure the patients.

For last few months, I have been particularly ill. All my friends and well-wishers, who helped me sail through amidst turbulence must be thankfully remembered. I would like to thank Mrs. and Mr. Lodha, Mr. Tandon, CEO, Belle Vue Clinic for their wholehearted support. I thank Dr. B. K. Mishra of Hinduja Hospitals for sharing his courage with us while performing the surgery that I had undergone.

Special thanks should go to Dr. R. Jalali of TMC, Mumbai and Dr. R. Achari, for doing a marvellous job by way of curing and cheering me during this time. Prof. R. P. Sen Gupta and Dr. Krishnendu Mukherjee's co-ordination made the entire phase of my treatment smooth and hassle-free. Mr. Arup Kumar Sarkar of ABP, Mr. Anjan Chatterjee of Mainland China and Mr. Pallab Mukherjee of PSAFL, went out of their way to provide the necessary moral and logistic support during this time and to make me smile.

Finally my heartfelt love and pranams to Sri Thakur, Sri Maa, Swamiji and Sister Nivedita, who are the polestars of my life and who continue to inspire me to live meaningfully.My sincere pranams to my gurudev, Srimat Swami Ranganathanandaji, the 13th President of the Ramkrishna Mission, who first gave me the idea of writing a book like this.

Dr. SUBRATA MAITRA

PREFACE

Publication of any book is a memorable event for its author. It holds true for me as well, as I have ventured to publish this book with a lot of enthusiasm. While working on it I often faced the question as to why was I writing a book on medicine, when in the bookstores such books are already aplenty? I found it difficult to explain that medicine is never static, it is always swept with many changes, from root to rhizome. Over the last few decades new guidelines, protocols and information have entered our field, which the busy interns at times find difficult to keep track with. Moreover, symptom-based medicine is vastly different from our day to day clinical practice, where patients present randomly without the label of any specific disease. Naturally an astute clinician has to make a diagnosis and often treat the patient from the presented symptoms, which should not grossly deviate from the guideline-based treatment.

Interestingly, even in the West, the day to day treatment does not follow regular protocol and is often different from the approved track. This is even more evident in a huge country like India. But guidelines and protocols often differ from the clinical experiences; and here lies the conflict. In an era of evidence-based medicine, we cannot ignore evidence-based practice.

In this book, I have made a humble attempt to match evidence with experience. Since I returned from the UK (almost 25 years now), I gathered experiences of all sorts; thanks to my postgraduate training there. Although I could not conduct proper, classical double blind trials, wherever I have practised, including Woodlands Hospital, Belle Vue Clinic and B.P. Poddar Hospital, I have mentioned some of the observational trials, which the reader might find useful.

Here, I must say that this is not merely a textbook. Rather, it is a concept-oriented book with information gathered from the contemporary journals and texts. Let me re-emphasise that my target audience consists of interns, house-staff, medical consultants and of course PG students. My apologies for any mistake in the text, statistical or otherwise.

I would consider myself extremely privileged, even if a single doctor finds the book useful and is able to save a single life.

DR. SUBRATA MAITRA

CONTENTS

CONTENTS

CONTENTS

CONTENTS

01

A PATIENT WITH CHEST PAIN DUE TO ACUTE AORTIC DISSECTION

CASE: *A 74-years-old lady presented with a history of collapse preceded by chest discomfort. On examination, she was haemodynamically stable. She complained of vague chest discomfort, dizziness and neck pain. Repeated ECGs were normal except for sinus bradycardia, cardiac enzymes normal, Troponin-T negative, X-ray cervical spine-spondylosis and CT brain scan showed degeneration of cerebral cortex. A provisional diagnosis of TIA due to cervical spondylosis was made. She was discharged on request in next 72 hours of admission. She was readmitted with similar complaints of dizziness, vague chest discomfort, abdominal pain and diarrhea and before admission she had a momentary collapse. Cardiac evaluation did not reveal anything specific except for echo which suggested aneurysm of ascending aorta. X-ray chest this time showed widened mediastinum and a positive calcium sign (the distance between the calcification of aortic notch and the outer border of aortic shadow > 1 cm). An immediate CT scan of the thorax was done which confirmed the presence of aortic dissection from ascending aorta right upto the abdominal aorta. Surgical opinion was taken and in view of her age and the nature of the disease, the high risk of surgical intervention was explained to the relatives and conservative line of management was pursued.*

She was treated with nitroglycerine infusion to keep her BP around 120/80 mmHg. Unfortunately, within next 24 hours she developed sudden chest pain and had a cardiac arrest possibly due to proximal extension of the dissection and could not be resuscitated. The cause of her death was due to dissection of ascending and descending aorta.

DIAGNOSIS: Acute aortic dissection.

DISCUSSION:

This is a fairly uncommon condition in the Indian setting. In last 13 years in my hospital practice, I have come across only two cases of diagnosed aortic dissection. However, the clinician should be aware of this situation before thrombolysing for suspected myocardial infarction. Points in favour of acute aortic dissection are-

a) History of hypertension

b) Elderly

c) No definite ECG evidence of MI (although there may be ECG evidence of MI if coronary ostia is involved by the flap).

d) The initial pain is very severe and so intense that the patient collapses. It is sharp and stabbing in nature which finally degenerates into a constant dull ache and can be radiate to the back.

e) There may be pulse deficit because of the pressure from the false lumen on the aortic conduit.

f) Differential BP in two arms.

g) There may be a neurodeficit if the dissection involves the carotid arteries.

h) Abdominal pain- if involvement of mesenteric arteries (as possibly in this case).

i) Paraplegia- due to involvement of the spinal arteries.

j) Presence of aortic regurgitation.

k) On X-ray- widened mediastinum, positive calcium sign.

l) Echo showing effusion or aortic flap.

Other diagnostic tests are

1. Aortogram (advantage: coronary anatomy can be demonstrated)
2. Contrast CT (as used in this case)
3. Contrast MRI (better than CT)
4. Trans-oesophageal echo

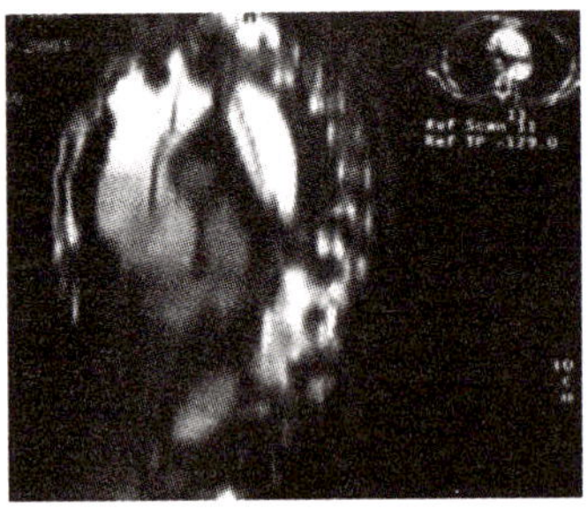

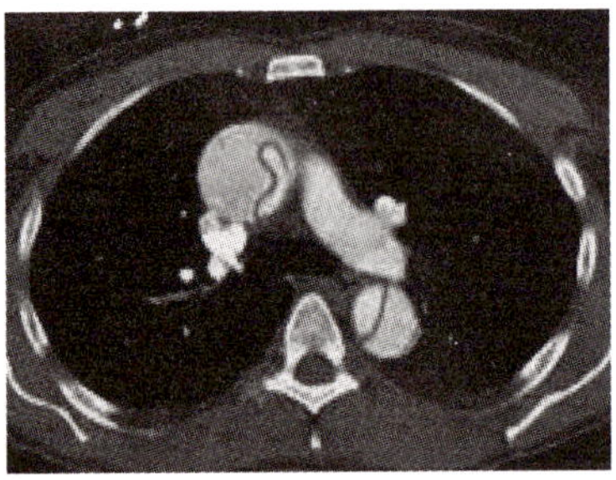

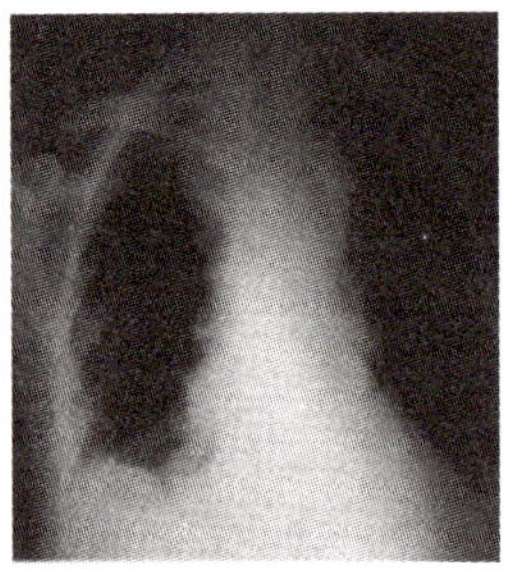

MANAGEMENT:

Dissection is classified into:

Stanford Type A – All dissections involving the ascending aorta (managed surgically).

Stanford Type B – All dissections not involving the ascending aorta (managed medically).

[De Bakey - **Type I** - ascending aorta may extend beyond it.

Type II - continued to descending aorta

Type III - originates in the descending aorta and extends distally.]

Left untreated acute dissection has a high mortality. Initial management is medical however. This involves pain relief, control of cardiac failure and strict control of BP and the drugs commonly used are:

1) Nitroglycerine Infusion
2) Nitroprusside Infusion
3) Labetalol infusion (not generally available in India)
4) Beta blocker like esmolol infusion.
5) Sublingual nifedipine may also be used if betablockers are contra indicated.

However, the definite treatment for acute dissection is surgical repair particularly dissection involving the proximal aorta. Surgical intervention is also indicated in distal dissection if there is compromise of the vital organs and when it occurs in patients with Marfan's syndrome.

Medical management is preferred in patients with uncomplicated distal dissection and stable chronic dissection (uncomplicated dissection presenting 2 weeks or later after the onset).

This patient had Type-A aortic dissection and in view of her age the extent of the dissection and high risk surgical procedure, it was decided to take a conservative approach with control of her BP, pain relief and the maintenance of the haemodynamic status at least for the initial period of time. Unfortunately within 24 hours of the diagnosis, she had a cardiac arrest and died.

CASE: *A 63 yrs old male presented with severe left sided chest pain of two hours duration. The pain was constant in nature and increased with cough and breathing. Recently he had a febrile episode. Examination revealed a pleuritic rub and few crepitations at the left base. X-Ray chest revealed a left basal pneumonia with mild pleural reaction.*

DIAGNOSIS: Pneumonia with pleuritic chest pain.

CASE: *A 32 years old lady presented with left sided chest pain which was continuous in nature. She was having breathlessness along with drowsiness. She was haemodynamically stable. X-Ray Chest and ECG were normal. Blood gas showed normal PaO_2 and $PaCO_2$ levels with respiratory alkalosis. Clinically there was no evidence of deep vein thrombosis.*

DIAGNOSIS: Functional chest pain with hyperventilation.
(Caveat – possibility of pulmonary embolism should always be thought of).

CASE: *A 56 years old male presented with intermittent left sided chest pain of two days duration. The pain was sharp in nature and could not be localized properly. ECG, X-Ray Chest and Echo were normal. Troponin-T, CPK, CPK-MB were also normal. The patient was admitted and given treatment in the line of unstable angina. However 48 hours later he developed classical rash of Herpes zoster in the left upper intercostal nerve segment and the diagnosis was revised as intercostal neuralgia due to Herpes zoster.*

DIAGNOSIS: Neuralgic pain due to Herpes zoster.

DISCUSSION: Chest pain is one of the commonest causes of presentation in the emergency department with myriad of causes ranging from a psychosomatic illness to life threatening conditions like heart attack, pulmonary embolism, aortic dissection etc.

Frequently, clinical examination and investigations may be elusive and a thorough history taking which is almost a forgotten art in the era of technology oriented modern medicine, may help in clinching a proper diagnosis.

Causes of chest pain:

- **Cardiac**: Myocardial Infarction, IHD, acute aortic dissection, pericarditis, aortic stenosis
- **Gastrointestinal**: Peptic ulcer, oesophageal reflux, oesophageal spasm, acute cholecystitis
- **Pulmonary:** Pneumonia, pneumothorax, pulmonary embolism, lung cancer
- **Musculoskeletal**: Acute cervical disc prolapse, costochondritis, vertebral collapse due to any cause like osteoporosis etc
- **Neuropsychiatric**: Intercostal neuralgia may be functional. However since myocardial infarction and ischaemia are common conditions presenting in emergency department with frequently normal ECG initially history may give useful clues to make a proper diagnosis.

Symptoms favouring MI/ IHD:

- Usually retrosternal in location.
- Usually radiation towards left arm, jaw and left shoulder some times to the right side, exertion related, compressive type.
- Associated nausea, vomiting and perspiration relieved by sublingual nitroglycerine.
- Associated with sweating.
- Males and post menopausal women with presence of risk factors.

Symptoms suggesting other causes than IHD:

- Infra-mammary location, sharp in nature
- Reproducible by palpation (tender spot)
- Changes with position, cough and respiratory movement

Other causes which symptom-wise closely resembling angina:

Oesophageal reflux-

Burning, retrosternal, postprandial

[Relieved by antacids]

Oesophageal spasm-

Retrosternal, may be relieved by nitroglycerine

[Sometimes very difficult to differentiate from IHD]

Pulmonary embolism- On the side of the embolism

Pericarditis- Sharp, retrosternal, may be relieved by stooping forward, may radiate towards the left shoulder

Pneumonia- Pleuritic in nature, lateralized, varies with respiration

Gall Stone Peptic Ulcer- Substernal or epigastric [burning in nature]

Aortic dissection- Acute, severe, radiates towards the back with differential BP on both hands

Herpes Zoster- Sharp, lateralized, dermatomal distribution

INVESTIGATIONS IN EMERGENCY DEPARTMENT:

- ECG
- X-Ray Chest (PA)
- Cardiac markers like Troponin T and Troponin I

If the clinical features and tests are inconclusive it is always preferable to admit the patient and do serial ECG and blood tests, Echocardiography, skeletal X-Rays like cervical spine, dorsal spine, ultrasound of abdomen and if still the diagnosis is not forthcoming, the patient should be offered to undergo conventional coronary angiography (in high risk patients) or a CT Coronary angiogram (in low risk patients). Once cardiac causes are excluded, one may investigate the gastrointestinal tract on outpatient basis. Missing an appropriate cause for chest pain is a common medicolegal issue in the western country, which is also becoming a problem in India as well.

Sometimes the patients, mainly middle aged female, present with classical chest pain with ECG changes and subsequent coronary angiogram show normal pattern. Thallium Scan also shows positivity for ischaemia. This condition is known as Syndrome 'X' which is thought to be either due to small vessel disease or diminished coronary reserve. Nicorandil or trimetazidine may be tried as therapeutic options.

CASE: *A 26 years old lean and thin male patient attended the emergency with a recurrent history of cough and cold. The reason of presentation was sudden onset of sharp pleuritic chest pain on the left side. Initial X-Ray Chest and ECG in the clinic did not reveal anything specific. The patient refused admission and was prescribed a course of antibiotic. The next day the patient developed shortness of breath and presented to another hospital where he was finally admitted. Repeat X-Ray and a C.T. Scan showed a moderate sized pneumothorax on the same side. He was put on a chest drain with symptomatic relief. On retrospective analysis it was noticed that he had a small chink of pneumothorax on the very first day which was missed in the emergency department and finally the pneumothorax increased with symptoms of breathlessness which was detected easily in the subsequent chest films. The patient was subsequently diagnosed to have Marfan's syndrome and had repeated pneumothorax on the same side which later led to surgical intervention for the pneumothorax.*

DIAGNOSIS: Pneumothorax in a patient with Marfan's syndrome.

: KEY POINTS :

- Chest pain is a common problem in clinical practice.
- Cause may vary from trivial causes to life threatening condition.
- A proper clinical history and basic investigation will clinch the diagnosis in majority of cases.
- Acute aortic dissection is an uncommon cause of acute chest pain.
- Initial diagnostic work up may be normal.
- High index of suspicion should be present in patient with Marfan's syndrome. (hypertensive and elderly patients presenting with intense chest pain and non diagnostic ECG)
- Clinical examination, X-ray Chest and echo can give some diagnostic clues.
- Before discharging the patient with acute chest pain or thrombolysing for clinical suspicion of MI, dissection should be excluded.

REFERENCE: Harrison's Principles of Internal Medicine, 17th edition.

02 A PATIENT HERPES ZOSTER INFECTION

CASE: *A 64 year old lady suffering from rheumatoid arthritis on disease modifying drugs complained of shooting pain over the left thigh and leg. Initially she took NSAID which was not very helpful. A telephonic opinion from the doctor suggested possible sciatica. However, she was perturbed when she found few crops of rash over the thigh region. She thought it to be due to either allergy to one of the medications or an insect bite. The next day the rash started spreading and she consulted our medical team. Examination revealed vesicular rash over the left thigh which was excruciatingly painful. There was no neurological deficit and the straight leg raising test was normal.*

DIAGNOSIS: Herpes zoster infection of L_3 L_4 segment.

DISCUSSION:

Herpes zoster infection is a common clinical condition encountered in clinical practice. Sometimes it is misdiagnosed as allergic reaction, insect bite etc. by an inexperienced clinician leading to delay in commencing specific treatment.

Varicella zoster (VZV) causes two distinct clinical entities – chicken pox and herpes zoster. Chicken pox is a common condition in childhood characterized by vesicular rash while herpes zoster usually presents in the middle or old age with painful vesicular rash unilaterally restricted to specific dermatomal distribution of VZV virus resulting in Herpes zoster in later years. The exact mechanism is unknown; however it is presumed that following chicken pox, the virus may remain latent in the dorsal root ganglion from where it may reactivate later on.

FEATURES:

1. Classically it is distributed over a particular dermatomal segment. However, dermatomal overlap, although uncommon, may occur.
2. The lesions are vesicular initially with scab formation later on.
3. In immune competent patients, it does not cross the mid line. If the lesions are bilateral, one should consider immuno-compromised state like –
   a) Diabetes mellitus
   b) Underlying malignancy like leukaemia, lymphoma, chronic lymphatic leukaemia
   c) Long term steroid therapy
   d) HIV infection

Any dermatome can be involved. Involvement of ophthalmic division of trigeminal nerve is a potentially serious condition as there is 50% chance of involvement of the eyes.

Herpes zoster should be considered in any painful unilaterally distributed vesicular lesion involving a particular dermatome.

DIFFERENTIAL DIAGNOSIS OF VESICULAR RASH:

- Herpes zoster – usually unilateral
- Chicken pox
- Disseminated Herpes simplex in atopic patients
- Coxsackie virus infection
- Echo virus infection
- Atypical measles
- *Rickettsial pox* – There is a herald spot at the site of mite bite.

TREATMENT:

Treatment instituted within 72 hours of vesicle formation may reduce the severity of pain and duration of the illness. Specific treatment beyond 72 hours may not be of much help unless there is development of fresh crops of vesicles indicating ongoing infection. Timely intervention may also reduce post herpetic neuralgia.

Antivirals:

The specific antiviral medication is acyclovir (800 mg 5 times a day for 7 days). Other antivirals that can be used are famciclovir (500 mg thrice daily × 7 days) or valacyclovir (1000 mg twice daily × 7 days). They are all equipotent but the newer drugs have better user friendly dose schedules. There is no role of topical anti-viral agents in the treatment. Drugs must be used as soon as possible in Herpes zoster ophthalmicus as it reduces the chance of sight threatening eye involvement from 50% to 20%. Similarly all immune compromised patients should be treated with antiviral as soon as possible.

Steroids:

Steroids can reduce the duration of pain and unwell being. It has no role in reduction of post herpetic neuralgia. It should be used in conjunction with antivirals. It should be avoided on its own and in patients with immune compromised state.

Pain relief may be needed with analgesics and tricyclic antidepressants (Amitriptyline). Antibiotics should be used to prevent secondary infection.

Vaccine is available for the prevention of VZV infection which is effective in prevention of chicken pox and herpes zoster infection which is effective and safe.

In high risk patients like immuno-compromised transplant recipients varicella-zoster immunoglobulin may be considered within the first 3-4 days of exposure to an infected person.

Anti-viral prophylaxis (7 days course) may be considered in a high risk exposed person who is ineligible for vaccination.

POST HERPETIC NEURALGIA:

It is difficult to treat and can be a chronic problem leading to severe depression. The principles of management are:

1. Analgesics
2. Tricyclic antidepressants
3. Gabapentin or carbamazepine
4. Local application of – Lignocaine ointment, Capsaicin ointment

In study of patients with intractable post herpetic neuralgia intrathecal injection of methyl prednisolone acetate once weekly for four weeks resulted in a significant reduction in pain. However this is still investigational.

Patients should be referred to the pain clinic for further evaluation and consideration for nerve blockage.

This patient was promptly treated with acyclovir and steroid with quick resolution of her symptoms. Till now she has not complained of any post herpetic neuralgia.

CASE: *A 59 years old patient presented with features of Herpes zoster involving the right trigeminal nerve. There was significant involvement of the ophthalmic division. He was treated with valacyclovir, steroids and other supportive therapy. However, the anti-viral treatment was started late because of delayed presentation to the hospital. One week following discharge, the patient presented with drowsiness and weakness of the left side of the body. He was readmitted and MRI scan demonstrated a right sided stroke on the right thalamic region.*

DIAGNOSIS: Post Herpes zoster CVA.

DISCUSSION:

Herpes zoster vasculopathy is increasingly described now-a-days presenting with cerebrovascular accident, myocardial infarction or giant cell arteritis. Both extra cranial and intra cranial arteries may be involved and the symptoms may appear after disappearance of the rash. The exact mechanism is unknown. However it is postulated that probably there is endothelial dysfunction and associated vasculopathy which leads to vascular damage. Involvement of the ophthalmic branch of trigeminal nerve is the strongest association. Although not conclusively proved, early antiviral therapy may reduce the incidence of vasculopathy. Since herpes zoster is a common presentation in clinical practice, internists should be aware of this newly described association.

: KEY POINTS :

- In any unilateral painful vesicular rash, Herpes zoster should be considered.
- Bilateral or disseminated Herpes zoster can occur in immunocompromised state.
- Antiviral drug should be started within 72 hrs of onset of rash.
- There is no role of topical antiviral drugs.
- Steroids used in conjunction to antiviral medication can reduce the duration of pain and swelling. It should be used with caution in immunocompromised patients.
- Except for appropriately timed used of antiviral, no other measures reduce the incidence and severity of post herpetic neuralgia.

FURTHER REFERENCES:

- John W Giann, Richard J Whitley, *Herpes Zoster*, NEJM Vol. 347 No. 5, August 2002.
- *Harrison's Principal of Internal Medicine* – 17th edition.
- M.Nagel et al – *Varicella zoster viral infection – Clinical Infections Disease* – June 2014 Vol 58, No-11, Page – 1504-1506
- S.M. Langan et al – *Risk of stroke following Herpes zoster - Clinical Infections Disease* – 1 June 2014:58 – no – 11, P-1493-1503.

CASE: *A 36-years-old lady presented with a history of severe unilateral throbbing headache along with vomiting. The pain was excruciating and she also had mild* *photophobia. Examination revealed no neurodeficit, no local tenderness of the sinus or cervical spine. There was no scalp tenderness. She was admitted to the hospital and underwent routine blood tests which were normal except for presence of mild maxillary sinusitis.*

DIAGNOSIS: Migraine without aura.

DISCUSSION:

Headache is a common presentation both in outpatients clinic and as well as in the emergency department. Most of the acute onset headache presents in the emergency and the main concern is the possibility of subarachnoid haemorrhage although migraine may sometimes present in emergency. Usually patients with chronic intermittent headache present in the outpatients clinic and there is a long list of differential diagnosis.

COMMON CAUSES OF HEADACHE:

Subarachnoid haemorrhage: Severe, sudden, thunder clasp type headache, causes momentary fainting attack. There may be warning headache particularly in a case of expanding aneurysm. Features are:

Neck stiffness

Positive Kernig's sign

Bilateral up going plantars

With this background, urgent admission and neuro-imaging will be required. *CT brain scan is the preferred investigation as it can detect presence of blood much earlier than MRI scan which may be negative initially.*

Migraine (with aura, without aura): Diagnostic features are:

- Unilateral pain
- Pulsating in nature
- Common in young females
- Nausea vomiting and light sensitivity
- Reversible brain stem and cortical dysfunction (with aura).
- Visual aura is classical (with aura).

Cluster headache:

- Male preponderance

- Usually nocturnal
- Usually unilateral
- Usually periodic with features of autonomic disturbance like nasal stuffiness and congested eyes.

Acute attack should be treated with *sumatriptan* 6 mg sc, maximum upto twice/day. High flow oxygen therapy should also be instituted during the acute attack.

For preventive purpose:

Short term: Tapering dose of steroid for a period of 10-15 days may be used. Similarly methysergide with a maximum dose of 9 mg (starting with 1 mg) may be used maximum upto 6 months [restricted use upto 6 months]

Long term: *Lithium* with a starting dose 30 mg may be used. *Verapamil* is a slow acting drug which can be used upto 80 g twice daily.

Tension headache:

- Bilateral
- Non-pulsating
- No aggravation by simple physical activity
- No nausea, vomiting
- A band like sensation over the head
- Usually chronic

It is a very common presentation in daily practice. Acute attack should be treated with NSAID and sumatriptan. For preventive purpose amitriptyline may be used.

Headache due to be brain tumour:

- Progressively worse
- Associated with vomiting
- Increased with exertion, cough
- Other associated neurological signs

  (Like cerebellar sign, facial weakness in case of acoustic neuroma).

Menstrual Migraine:

Transdermal oestrogen 100 ml used from 2-3 days prior to menstruation may be of additional value.

Giant cell arthritis:

- Elderly male
- Unilateral
- Scalp tenderness
- High ESR
- Visual problems

Not so common in India. However diagnosis is important as steroid improves the condition and prevents visual loss. I have come across only 4 cases of cranial arteritis who responded to steroid. Any patient presenting with proximal muscle weakness and pain along with headache, one should strongly consider polymyalgia rheumatica along with giant cell arteritis (Common association).

Other causes of headaches – commonly encountered:

1. Sinusitis
2. Cervical spondylosis
3. Acute glaucoma (this diagnosis will be missed if not thought of – features: headache, eye pain and vomiting).
4. Another common and challenging differential diagnosis is medication overuse headache (MOH). *This typically complicates migraine which is transformed into chronic daily headache. Regular use of ergots leads to MOH.*

This patient had features of migraine without aura. CT brain was done to rule out subarachnoid haemorrhage. She responded to the usual line of management and discharged home on prophylactic medication.

MANAGEMENT OF MIGRAINE:

Analgesics:

The first important thing is to relieve the symptoms of headache, nausea and vomiting. Drugs commonly used are:

a) Aspirin

b) NSAID

c) Combination analgesic and antiemetic, paracetamol + metoclopramide. Opiates should be avoided because of its abuse potential especially in the genesis of MOH.

Triptans:

This has revolutionised the treatment of migraine since early 90's. Of five types of triptans so far available sumatriptan is commonly used in India. It can be used orally or is subcutaneous injection. Sumatriptan 50 mg or 100 mg is the drug of choice. It can also be given by subcutaneous route.

Other triptans (naratriptans, zolmotriptan, almotriptan) are not generally available in India. They are almost equipotent.

Triptans should be used with caution in patients with cardiac problem. Triptans are better than analgesics in acute migraine. However daily use must be avoided as it may cause MOH. Although more effective than ergots, these are more expensive.

Ergots:

This is still a very popular drug in India. It is cheap and effective. It should be used with caution in patients with cardiac problem. Abuse potentiality with resultant MOH is there.

Although there is a genetic predisposition for migraine, certain exogenous factors like dietary factors and stress may trigger migraine and manipulation of these factors may help in the management of migraine. Such factors are: 1) Coffee, 2) Tea, 3) Cola, 4) Alcohol.

TREATMENT OF ACUTE AFFECT: Specific treatment with triptans and doses:

TRIPTANS	DOSES
Almotriptan	12.5 mg upto 25 mg
Eletriptan	40 mg upto 80 mg
Frovatriptan	2.5 mg upto 5 mg
Naratriptan	2.5 mg upto 5 mg
Rizatriptan	5 mg upto 20 mg
Sumatriptan (oral)	50 mg upto 300 mg
Zolmitriptan	2.5 mg upto 10 mg

PREVENTIVE TREATMENT:

Prevention of recurrence:

One third of the patients with migraine will have recurrence. Use of prophylactic medication will reduce the incidence of recurrence. The drugs commonly used for this purposes are:

1. **Beta-blocker (Propranolol)** – Drug of choice in the presence of co-morbid condition like hypertension.
2. **Amitriptyline (25 mg – 75 mg)** – Particularly in patients with depression and insomnia. It can cause *drowsiness.*
3. **Sodium valproate (400 mg – 600 mg)** thrice daily, can cause *liver problem.*
4. **Pizotifen (0.5 mg – 3 mg)** – can cause *drowsiness, weight gain.*
5. **Methysergide (1 mg – 6 mg)** – it should be used with caution, causes *retroperitoneal fibrosis* in prolonged use.
6. **Flunarizine (5 mg – 15 mg)** – Most commonly used drug in India. Long term use may cause *weight gain, depression and Parkinsonism.*
7. **Topiramate** – It is also used to prevent migraine headaches. It works by affecting several chemicals in the brain that help to reduce seizure activity and prevent migraine headaches from occurring.

OTHER FACTS OF MANAGEMENT:

Life style modification like avoidance of stress, sleep irregularity and relative hypoglycaemia but intake of regular fibre containing diet etc. may be helpful. International travel is a frequent trigger for migraine and appropriate precautionary measures should be taken.

Migraine with aura is a risk factor (*albeit minor*) for cerebral stroke. So it is preferable to avoid oestrogen containing oral contraceptive pills (OCP) and other forms of contraceptive devices are preferable in patients with migraine.

Certain foods may trigger migraine headaches, so try to avoid these. The most common are: wine, processed and fermented foods, pickle, marinated foods, much chocolate, nuts and dairy products, cured meats, chicken liver etc.

Avoid certain odors or perfumes, loud noises or bright lights, and smoking may also trigger a migraine. Drink plenty of water and place a cool cloth on your head and forehead.

Additional cases of migraine

CASE: *A 30-years-old lady from Bangladesh attended the clinic with history of 6-8 months of headache. Of late, her vision in the left eye was deteriorating and she had episodic vomiting. Examination revealed normal BP, there was 6th nerve palsy on the left side. Fundoscopy revealed grade IV papilloedema in both eyes.*

DIAGNOSIS:

Raised intracranial tension probably due to space occupying lesion in the brain. She underwent urgent MRI Scan of the brain which revealed a left sided big cerebellar tumour with evidence of gadolinium enhancement. She underwent operative intervention with symptomatic relief. However, her vision still remained poor on discharge. Biopsy revealed haemangioblastoma of the cerebellum.

Early morning headache, associated with effortless vomiting is a feature of SOL of brain. In case of posterior fossa tumour, papilloedema appears early because of obstruction of CSF drainage.

CASE: *A 28-years-old obese, mildly hypertensive lady had been complaining of severe headache following a recent pregnancy. Initial investigations were all satisfactory. CT scan of brain was normal. MRI angiogram of cerebral vessels did not reveal any aneurysm. Ophthalmological examination which was initially missed during her 1st consultation revealed gross papilloedema both eyes. A diagnosis of benign intracranial hypertension was made and she responded to repeated lumbar puncture, diuretic and a short course of steroid therapy.*

DIAGNOSIS: Benign Intracranial hypertension in an obese hypertensive lady.

Causes of benign intracranial hypertension:

- Steroid in the long term
- Tetracycline
- Vitamin A intoxication
- Oestrogen
- During pregnancy or post partum period

This condition is frequently associated with obesity and hypertension. Ophthalmoscopic examination is essential during routine examination in a patient with headache which can give useful clues to the diagnosis.

***Case**: A 36-years-old lady presented with a severe headache and unconsciousness. She was found to have subarachnoid haemorrhage and after a stormy course in the hospital was finally discharged from the hospital in a stable state. During the course of treatment she was formed to have an arterio-venous malformation which bled to give rise to her current complication. In the past she was treated by many physicians for her chronic headache, CT scan on couple of occasion was normal and she recommend migraine prophylaxis without much help.*

DIAGNOSIS: Cerebral bleed due to AV malformation.

DISCUSSION:

In case of persistent headache with negative CT scan, one should suspect vascular anomalies like aneurysm or AV and request for either CT or MRI angiogram of cerebral vessels or conventional digital subtraction angiography as plain CT scan may be elusive. Clinical judgment is important in this regard.

: KEY POINTS :

- Migraine is a common cause of acute and chronic headache in clinical practice.
- In patients presenting with unilateral, throbbing, headache and vomiting– particularly in young females – migraine should be considered first.
- In acute headache, CT brain scan is preferable to MRI scan, as it detects blood early.
- In acute attack triptans are the drug of choice, although ergots are also effective and cheap.
- Very frequent use of ergots can cause medication over use headache.
- If the attack of migraine is frequent, prophylactic medication should be used and the selection should depend upon other co-morbid condition.

FURTHER REFERENCE:

Dr. Batra. BJHM – Headache and Migraine.

04 A PATIENT WITH DEPRESSION

CASE: *A 46-years-old gentleman presented in the outpatient clinic with a 6 months history of generalized unwell being, weakness and lethargy, loss of weight, poor appetite, insomnia and extreme tiredness. He lost his wife 2 years back and did not have any children and also suffered from diabetes mellitus. He has consulted many physicians and underwent a battery of tests without any conclusive diagnosis. His diabetic status was well under control with oral hypoglycaemic drugs. Routine biochemical parameters (LFT, thyroid function test, auto immune screening, cortisol, electrolytes, CRP) haematological parameters (Hb, TC, DC, platelet, ESR), virological screening (Hepatitis B, Hepatitis C, HIV) were all satisfactory. X-ray and ECG were normal. CT brain was normal.*

DIAGNOSIS: Depressive illness.

DISCUSSION:

Depression is a major problem in primary care. At least 30% of patients attending clinic have major depression. However, majority of them are unrecognized or inappropriately treated leading to loss of productivity, functional decline and increased mortality. Diagnosing depression can be difficult as patients rarely present with symptoms that fit neatly into diagnostic taxonomies. Patients in medical settings usually present with physical, social and psychological problems along with somatic symptoms and the consulting doctor has to find out depressive illness from the above mentioned presenting problems. Consulting styles also influence whether depression is recognized. It has been found that doctors who ask open question initially (like enquiring about sleep pattern, mood etc.), give more time, are more empathetic, make more eye contact and interrupt less, are more likely to detect depression.

When to consider depression in the differential diagnosis?

The patients usually complain of depressed mood, diminished interest or pleasure in all activities, unintentional weight loss or weight gain, insomnia or hypersomnia nearly every day, early morning waking or interrupted sleep, feeling of guilt, worthlessness, loss of energy, lack of concentration and in severe cases, thoughts of death and suicide. In addition, there are certain co-morbid medical conditions, where depression is common and the clinician should positively look for evidence of depression if suggestive symptoms are present in such cases. These conditions are –

- Cancer
- Parkinson disease
- Cerebrovascular accidents
- Old MI, chronic pain
- Diabetes mellitus
- Old age

Anxiety disorder like phobia, panic disorder, obsessive compulsive state, generalized severe anxiety are quite common presentations in general practice. These patients are also more vulnerable to depression and the clinician should be aware of this. Somatization is also an integral part of the presentation in depression. As the psychiatric definition of depression does not take into account somatic presentation, an astute clinician should be aware of this fact and try to find out whether depression is theunderlying cause for the somatization.

TREATMENT:

Majority of the depressive illness can be treated at primary care level (if the clinician is willing). However some alarm signs should prompt the physicians for a prompt psychiatric referral.

DRUG THERAPY:

If used appropriately, drugs are successful in more than 70% of cases. However, selection of medication is important. It was recognized in the 50's that the depression was mediated mainly by the deficiency of monoamine neurotransmitter like serotonin, nor-adrenaline and dopamine. The major pharmacological maneuver involves increasing the level of these monoamines in the brain by either inhibiting the enzyme monoamine oxidase, blockage of auto receptors that generate negative feedback on the release of neurotransmitters and blockage of the reuptake of the transmitter back into the nerve cell.

Monoamine oxidase inhibitors:

The initial drugs were monoamine oxidase inhibitors. However because of their side effect profile and drug interactions they are not used at least at the primary care level.

Nonselective serotonin and nor-adrenaline reuptake inhibitors:

The second group of drugs to come was tricyclic anti-depressant (non selective serotonin and nor-adrenaline uptake inhibitors) which is being still used very commonly in the clinical practice. The problem with them is the non-selective nature of their receptor blockage and the resultant side effect profile. Commonly used drugs are:

1. Amitriptyline - special indication if there is associated insomnia, chronic pain, migraine, post herpetic neuralgia.

2. Imipramine - Enuresis, insomnia, panic disorder, post traumatic stress disorder, obsessive, compulsive state.

These drugs have adverse effect on cardiac function and should be avoided in patients with cardiac problems. They have prominent anti-cholinergic side effects.

Selective serotonin and noradrenalin uptake inhibitors:

Venlafaxine: This is a comparatively new class of drug - devoid of cardiac side effects and has quick onset of action. This is also emerging as an effective treatment for anxiety disorder (so commonly associated with depression).

Special indications: Anxiety, neuropathic pain, obsessive compulsive disorder. It can cause sedation and anti-cholinergic side effects but are less common.

Selective serotonin re-uptake inhibitors (SSRI):

1. ***Citalopram*** - particularly helpful in post CVA depression, diabetic neuropathy panic disorder, obsessive compulsive disorders.
2. ***Escitalopram*** - It is a comparatively new drug (isomer of citalopram) and has a very quick onset of action (compared to citalopram).
3. ***Fluoxetine***
4. ***Paroxetine*** - Post traumatic stress disorder, panic disorder.
5. ***Sertraline***

They usually do not cause sedation. This group of drugs can cause both weight loss and weight gain. These are cardiac friendly drugs and can be safely prescribed in cardiac patients.

Serotonin antagonists:

Mirtazapine - This is particularly helpful in anxiety and insomnia. It can also cause weight gain. It has got sedative potential.

Noradrenaline and dopamine reuptake inhibitors:

Bupropion - Particularly helpful in smoking cessation and post traumatic stress disorder.

Serotonin antagonist and re-uptake inhibitors:

Nefazodone - Panic disorder

Trazodone - Post-traumatic stress disorder, insomnia.

Common side effects of antidepressants:

TCA - anticholinergic symptoms, weight gain, G.I. symptoms, sedation.

SSRI - insomnia, G.I. symptoms, Anorgasmia, SIADH.

Trazodone - sedation, weight gain.

Mirtazapine - sedation.

Duloxetine - insomnia, G.I symptoms.

Bupropion - insomnia.

Sedative Properties of mirtazapine and trazodone may be used therapeutically in patients with insomnia while bupropion may be used additionally in patients with anorgasmia.

The use of antidepressants (SSRI) is controversial and their use should be individualized in patients with depression, the risk for suicide should be assessed and in risk patients, urgent referral to psychiatrist should be done.

Few points to remember:

- Antidepressants will be effective in approximately 70% of cases.
- It may take 4-6 weeks before it may be fully effective.
- If within 6 weeks therapy there is no appreciable change, one drug can be substituted for another.
  (Failure of one drug does not necessarily mean that the other drug of the same group may not be effective).
- Wash out period is not necessary while changing from SSRI to another drug like venlafaxine or mirtazapine. (However abrupt withdrawal of SSRI may cause symptoms).
- SSRI should not be co-prescribed with sibutramine (appetite suppressants).
- All anti-depressants should be used with caution in hepatic disorders.
- If no appreciable change is noted with the 2nd drug, psychiatric opinion will be needed. In anxiety disorders, although benzodiazepines are the most effective drugs, they should only be used for a very brief period because of dependence potential. One of the antidepressants with prominent anti anxiety effect should therefore be chosen for long term treatment of primary anxiety disorders.

When to refer to a Psychiatrist?

1. If the patient needs specific therapy like prolonged counseling, conditioned behavior therapy then opinion of a psychiatrist should be taken.
2. If the patient is not responding to the use of two successive antidepressants over a period of 2-3 months.
3. If the patients have evidence of **psychosis like hearing voice or visual hallucination, have manic symptoms** or **judged to have high risk for suicide.**

Once the treatment has been successfully instituted, it should be carried out for at least 6 months. If the patient has a high risk of relapse (i.e., past history of recurrent depression), the treatment should be continued for at least 2 years.

Risk factor for suicide:

Old age	Alcoholism
Male	Unemployed
Living Alone	Associated co-morbid condition
Divorced	Previous attempts of suicides

CASE: *A 33 years old lady was admitted on three occasions with three different symptoms each time. The first with severe chest pain and investigation ruled out any specific organic cause. On second occasion, she presented with headache and again no organic cause was forth coming. During her third admission she presented with severe abdominal pain. This time also any organic cause was not detected. She was referred to a psychiatrist and at present she is on a SSRI and counseling with stabilization of her symptoms.*

DIAGNOSIS: Multiple Somatic Symptoms in a patient with anxiety disorder.

DISCUSSION:

Stress anxiety and depression are major manifestation in clinical practice and may present with multiple bodily symptoms and are variedly called multiple somatic disorder, medically unexplained symptoms or functional disorder. This may present with various forms of symptoms involving different systems –

Respiratory	: Hyperventilation syndrome
Cardiac	: Non cardiac chest pain (De Costas syndrome)
Rheumatological	: Fibromyalgia

Gastrointestinal	: Irritable Bowel Syndrome
CNS	: Tension headache
ENT	: Globus hystericus
Maxillofacial	: Atypical facial pain

These symptoms should be differentiated from malingering which is deliberately and consciously done for some gainful purpose.

In my clinical practice, I found multiple somatic symptoms are very common clinical presentation in outpatient practice and clinician should take a thorough history to make a diagnosis. A sympathetic and empathetic approach is essential for the treatment. They frequently need to refer to psychiatry colleague.

The condition is treated with prolonged conversation and rational explanation, understanding the symptoms rather than ignoring them and reassurance should be given affirmatively.

They frequently require SSRIs to treat the underlying anxiety. Cognitive behaviour therapy has been found to be helpful in similar conditions in the category of medically unexplained symptoms.

Hypochondriasis

Simple somatoform disorders

Somatisation disorder (Briquet's syndrome)

Conversion reaction (loss of function of any part of the body)

While matching a diagnosis of somatoform disorder no stone should be unturned to rule out organic diseases, as many organic disorders may be initially present with non specific symptoms and early investigation may be elusive. In my experience, I have come across some-

Mitotic lesions like – Cholangiocarcinoma, pancreatic cancer, brain tumor,

Infections like – Tuberculosis, infective endocarditis,

Autoimmune disorders like – SLE, vasculitis,

Miscellaneous disorders like – Pheochromocytoma, cardiac arrhythmias and porphyria presenting like symptoms apparently suggestive of somatic disorder.

: KEY POINTS:

- Depression is a common presentation in clinical practice.
- A positive approach and leading question from the clinician will help in diagnosing depression.
- Most of the illnesses may be treated at primary care level.
- Choosing the right drug will depend on the clinical circumstances and the presence of other associated conditions like anxiety disorders, presence of cardiac problem and sleep disturbance.
- In high risk patients, the patients should be referred to psychiatrists.
- Somatoform disorder and medically unexplained symptoms are common presentation in clinical practice.
- In elderly patients depression is common and occasionally associated with cognitive dysfunction.
- Higher risk of brain stroke has been noticed with the use of SSRI.
- Second line psychotropic drug like olanzapine and aripiprazole has been increasingly used in resistant cases in the treatment of nonpsychotic depression.
- Donepezil but not memantine has been shown to have some benefit in patients with mild cognitive impairment.
- Cognitive behaviour therapy, by focussing reframing negative and dysfunctional thoughts and encouraging participation in pleasurable and social activities, may have positive role in the treatment of depression.
- Electro convulsive therapy is the most effective therapy for resistant depression however it needs to be used with caution in patients with cardiovascular and neurological disorders.

FURTHER REFERENCES:

- *Managing Depression in Medical Outpatients,* M.A. Whodey et al, NEJM Vol 343 Dec 28, 2000, No. 26 P 1942-1950.
- *Depression - Editorial Hospital Medicine* - Vo. 63, No. 10, Oct 2002, P 580-581.
- *Venlafaxine - A new class of antidepressant* - Julia Hardy et al, Hospital medicine Vol- 63, N-9, Sep 2002 P 549-552.
- Oxford Text Book of Medicine. 5th edition.
- Caren G. solomon depression in elderly, NEJM 2014, 371; 1228-1236.

05 A PATIENT WITH PULMONARY EMBOLISM

CASE: *A 32-years old body builder was admitted with a history of shortness of breath for 4 days duration. Initially, he consulted a cardiologist who could not detect any cardiac problem and referred him to our medical unit. Examination showed sinus tachycardia (pulse rate 110/m). Chest was clear. ECG showed RV strain pattern with inverted T waves in V_1-V_4, X-ray chest– normal, Blood gas PO_2– 64 mm/Hg, O_2 sat 90%, PCO_2– 28 mmHg, echo- dilated RV. Biochemical and hematological parameters were normal. Ventilation perfusion scan showed high probability of pulmonary embolism.*

Blood test for D-dimers, protein C, protein S and antithrombin III were sent and he was started on IV heparin infusion. Compression ultrasonography and duplex venous Doppler study of both legs did not reveal any venous thrombosis. Next day he underwent CT scan of thorax with CT angiogram which showed evidence of bilateral pulmonary embolism. He did not have any history of any substance abuse or any high risk behavior. He used to take regular durabolin injection (anabolic steroid) as a part of muscle build up exercise. Coagulation profile, protein C, protein S and antithrombin III came back to be within the normal range. D-dimer test received later on was positive.

DIAGNOSIS: Pulmonary embolism.

DISCUSSION:

Although estimated 600,000 episodes of pulmonary embolism occur each year in the United States, the exact incidence in India is unknown. It is generally agreed however that both the incidence of pulmonary embolism and deep vein thrombosis is much less common compared to the western countries. Most cases of pulmonary embolism develop in high risk bed ridden hospitalized patients although occasional patients presenting with shortness of breath are found to be due to pulmonary embolism.

DIAGNOSIS OF PULMONARY EMBOLISM:

In any patient with acute onset breathlessness, tachycardia and relative paucity of findings in chest auscultation, pulmonary embolism should be strongly suspected. In addition, one should look for evidence of DVT or presence of any risk factors for development of DVT.

CASE: *A 19-years-old college girl was admitted with severe respiratory distress, sweating, chest pain and tingling in the hands. Examination showed pulse rate- 110/min, BP- 106/70 mmHg, clear chest, normal heart sounds, ECG normal, X-ray chest normal, echo normal, PO_2– 96 mmHg, PCO_2– 22 mmHg, pH- 7.51, serum Na and K normal, serum calcium low, while checking her BP, she developed carpopedal spasm.*

DIAGNOSIS: Hyperventilation syndrome with respiratory alkalosis.

She was treated with anxiolytics, sedatives and anti depressants and with calcium gluconate injection. She was also encouraged to breath in a paper bag. The family members were reassured and she was discharged within 72 hours.

The reason of presenting this case is to emphasize that psychological hyperventilation syndrome is getting increasingly common and may be confused with other serious organic causes of respiratory distress. Young females with paucity of chest findings, presence of carpopedal spasm and normal investigations (except for respiratory alkalosis) will point towards a functional cause.

SYMPTOMS:

Shortness of breath, pleuritic chest pain and haemoptysis is the event of pulmonary infraction, paucity of clinical findings in the chest in spite of symptoms and hypoxemia. ECG shows sinus tachycardia, RV strain, new onset RBBB and right axis, prominent R in V_1, V2 rarely $S_1Q_3T_3$ pattern in case of a major thromboembolism. Bed side echo also shows dilated RV.

Risk factors for venous thrombosis:

- Obesity, congestive cardiac failure
- Prolonged immobility
- Paraplegia, hemiplegia
- Post operative bed ridden patients
- Pelvic fracture, fracture tibia fibula
- Spinal operation
- Knee replacement
- Genetically determined
- Deficiency of Protein C
- Deficiency of Protein S
- Deficiency of Anti-thrombin III
- Deficiency of Factor V Leiden
- Anticardiolipin antibody syndrome
- Drugs like oral contraceptives

INVESTIGATIONS:

D-dimer test: This is a highly sensitive test but lacks specificity. Other causes that may give rise to positive D-Dimer tests are:

- Trauma
- Infection
- Vasculitis
- After surgery, in an association with incisions
- Pregnancy
- Malignancy

Thus these tests have a strong negative predictive value (negative test makes the diagnosis of DVT very unlikely, while a positive test does not always confirm the diagnosis). This test is not routinely available in most of the hospitals in our country and I strongly feel that this should be made available more easily in the general hospitals all over the country.

The most sensitive and accurate test for diagnosis of DVT is venogram which is cumbersome to perform in an acutely ill patient. Moreover it is an invasive test with attendant risk attached to it.

B-mode venous compression ultrasonography has a high sensitivity and specificity to diagnose proximal venous thrombosis. However it is not so sensitive in diagnosing calf vein thrombosis. Other methods of detecting DVT are Doppler ultrasonography, impedance Plethysmography and iodine 125-labelled fibrinogen scanning. (Apart from Doppler study, these techniques are not routinely available in most of the settings and they are less sensitive than venous compression ultrasonography in diagnosing proximal calf vein thromboembolism).

Ventilation perfusion scanning:

A normal scan rules out pulmonary embolism while a high probability scan is strongly associated with pulmonary embolism. Care should be taken in interpreting the test result in the presence of COPD which make the interpretation of the result difficult.

CT scan – CT pulmonary angiogram:

This has a high specificity and sensitivity particularly if the emboli involve the main and lobar pulmonary arteries. In a recent study of sensitivity of helical CT from detection of embolism in sub-segmental arteries ranged from 71-84%.

Conventional Pulmonary angiography:

This is the gold standard test. However, its role is limited in the Indian setting. In spite of the availability of a number of sophisticated tests, sometimes the clinician is at a loss and the final decision making depends upon the clinical judgment. A low clinical probability for DVT or pulmonary embolism along with a negative D-Dimer test rules out pulmonary embolism whereas a patient with high clinical probability for DVT or pulmonary embolism should undergo ancillary test like CT, VQ scan tests described above depending upon the availability in that particular set up.

Predicting probability:

Risk factors:

Clinical signs and symptoms of DVT	3.0
An alternative diagnosis seemed less likely Than pulmonary embolism	3.0
Heart rate more than 100 beats/m	1.5
Immobilization or surgery in the previous 4 weeks	1.5
Previous DVT or pulmonary embolism	1.5
Haemoptysis	1.0
Cancer (Receiving treatment, treated in the past 6 months for palliative care)	1.0

Clinical probability

Low	< 2.0
Intermediate	2.0-6.0
High	> 6.0

This patient had an intermediate probability of pulmonary embolism. He had a positive D-Dimer test and CT scan and ventilation scan were highly suggestive of pulmonary embolism.

He was treated with IV heparin for 7 days followed by oral anticoagulant. His symptoms improved over next 7 days and he was subsequently discharged. He remains on long term oral anticoagulant. The cause of embolism remains enigmatic.

DVT prophylaxis should be routinely incorporated in the management plan of any acutely ill, postoperative bed ridden patients. Even in community practice the primary care physician should be aware in dealing with patients with bed ridden stroke patients, terminally ill cancer patients and trauma patients lying in bed. The physician should also advice high risk patients scheduled for long air travel to use special stockings, drink plenty of water and move about during the flight.

Side effects of heparin or LMWH heparin are negligible if proper prophylactic dose is being used. Occasionally bleeding may be a problem. Prolonged use of heparin can cause osteoporosis and thrombocytopenia. Low mol wt. heparin has significantly less incidence of such problem but they are costly. Elastic stocking by producing a pressure gradient between ankle and knee, prevents DVT. It should be used with caution in patients with ischemic legs. Such prophylactic measures will save many lives by preventing DVT, fatal and non-fatal pulmonary embolism. In very high risk cases, combination of anticoagulant and elastic stocking should be provided.

Advantages of low molecular weight heparin over heparin:

- Can be given subcutaneously.
- No monitoring of coagulation profile is generally needed.
- Heparin induced osteoporosis and thrombocytopenia is much less common.
- Less protein bound so bioavailability is more predictable.

However, they are more expensive worldwide. LMWH is gradually replacing heparin for the prophylaxis of DVT.

A patient with unilateral swelling of leg:

CASE: *A 56-years-old gentleman was admitted with sepsis with multi organ failure needing dialysis through a catheter introduced through right femoral vein. On the 5th day of admission he developed painful swelling of the right leg. A clinical diagnosis of DVT upto the right femoral vein was made which was confirmed by a venous Doppler test. The catheter was removed and he was treated with Heparin followed by dabigatran which was continued for 3 month following discharge.*

DIAGNOSIS: Deep Vein Thrombosis on right leg.

DISCUSSION: Deep vein thrombosis is a common problem in clinical practice. Although it is not as common as clinical problem encountered in the western world, it is becoming increasingly recognized in India particularly in the field of critical care medicine. Although pulmonary embolism and DVT encompass the same disease spectrum, DVT is three times common than pulmonary embolism. The predisposing factors are related to any alteration of three factors known as Virchow's triad which ensures smooth blood flow in the venous system like- stasis, alteration of the vessel wall and change in the coagulability of blood.

CASE: *A 34-years-old male suffering from quadriparesis with bulbar palsy needing mechanical ventilator support through tracheostomy was making a steady progress over couple of week's period to the extent that he was successfully weaned off from the ventilator and started moving his upper extremities following IV gamma globulin therapy and intensive physiotherapy. The relatives were given an optimistic prognosis in view of his favorable progress. Unfortunately one morning he suddenly became breathless with tachycardia and cyanosis, with ECG showing sinus tachycardia, blood gas showing hypoxia and hypocarbia. X-ray chest- NAD, chest auscultation clear, cardiac enzymes normal. A presumptive diagnosis of massive pulmonary embolism was made and thrombolysis was carried out. Unfortunately, the patient expired in spite of full resuscitative measures.*

PRESUMPTIVE DIAGNOSIS: Acute massive pulmonary embolism in a bed ridden quadriplegic patient.

DISCUSSION:

This case illustrates well the importance of DVT prophylaxis in prevention of DVT and pulmonary embolism in high risk cases. This was a high risk case DVT (prolonged immobilization) in appropriate prophylactic measures could have avoided this condition.

As evidenced in this case, DVT may be clinically silent and can strike suddenly with catastrophic results. In critical care or any high risk patients, it is very important to check for any leg swelling during daily ward rounds. Clinically DVT may be silent and it may strike suddenly with pulmonary embolism. It is not practical to do screening ultrasound tests to detect silent DVT and certainly is not cost effective. The approach should be to use prophylactic measures which will prevent DVT in high risk cases.

The measures are:

- Use of elastic stocking
- Use of s/c heparin or low molecular weight heparin

In very high risk cases to combine both these measures will significantly reduce the incidence of DVT and fatal and non fatal pulmonary embolism. Since 1996, protocol driven DVT prophylaxis was routinely started in our ITU particularly in high risk cases. Since that time the incidence of sudden death or death due to acute pulmonary thromboembolism in acutely ill bed-ridden patients has decreased considerably.

DIFFERENTIAL DIAGNOSIS: DVT should always be kept in mind if there is unilateral leg pains and swelling. Other causes of unilateral swelling of leg are:

- DVT
- Cellulitis
- Ruptured Baker's cyst
- Lymphangitis
- Superficial thrombophlebitis

DIAGNOSIS: Venous ultrasonography with Doppler test gives the confirmatory clues to the diagnosis of DVT. The classical features in ultrasonography are:

- Lack of vein compressibility
- Visualization of thrombus
- Flow blunted rather than augmented as in normal cases with calf compression

TREATMENT:

The standard treatment is either use of s/c or IV heparin titrated to an APTT level of 1.5 to 2.5 times the normal value or use of subcutaneous low molecular weight heparin either in the form enoxaparin, fraxiparine or tinzaparin in two divided doses. Alternatively short acting synthetic polysaccharide fondaparinux; may be used subcutaneously in the dose of 2.5 mg once daily. Both the low molecular weight heparin and fondaparinux do not need any laboratory monitoring. The dose of these drugs should be adjusted if the creatinine clearance is less than 30 ml/minute. The duration is usually for 5 to 7 days and the anticoagulation should be continued with oral agents like Warfarin or which is a vitamin-K antagonist. Since it takes 48 hrs to achieve the required the level of INR of 2 to 3, it should be commenced at least 48 hrs of continuation of heparin or low molecular weight heparin. Alternatively, newer oral anticoagulants like direct thrombin inhibitor dabigatran may be used which has a quicker onset of action of 2-3 hours and can be started immediately following discontinuation of heparin. The advantages and disadvantages of dabigatran and warfarin have been discussed later on in this chapter.

DURATION OF ANTI-COAGULATION:

- Usually 3 months in cases of reversible cause for the DVT.
- Usually 6-12 months if the DVT is idiopathic.
- Usually for 12 months and may be extended for indefinite period in case of thrombophilic disorder and anticardiolipin antibody syndrome.

All of these above mentioned criteria also apply for patients with pulmonary embolism. Prophylaxis for prevention of DVT has already been discussed.

ORAL DIRECT INHIBITOR OF COAGULATION:

These are the new group of drugs that are recently available as an alternative to traditional warfarin. They are 1) Dabigatran – a direct thrombin inhibitor, 2) Apixaban and rivaroxaban– inhibitors of activated factor Xa. These new group of drugs have been found to be equipotent with warfarin in the treatment of DVT and prevention of thromboembolism in atrial fibrillation.

Advantages	Disadvantages
• Rapid onset of action • Few drug interaction • Routine monitoring of coagulation in not needed • Fixed dosing	• Lack of specific antidotes • High cost

Dabigatran is contraindicated in patients with creatinine clearance of less than 30 ml/min; where as Rivaroxaban and Apixaban are contraindicated if creatinine clearance is less than 15 ml/min. These drugs are contraindicated in severe liver failure and should be used with extreme caution if liver enzymes are more than thrice the normal value.

Anticoagulants and antifibrinolytics in clinical practice:

Since arterial and venous thrombosis is quite common in clinical practice, these agents are commonly used by the physician in day to day practice. Although the mechanism of thrombosis is quite similar in the both the cases, in arterial system the platelets form major problem while in the venous system the fibrin is the primary contributor thereby making the antiplatelets the drugs of choice for the treatment of arterial disorders while the anticoagulants are the sheet anchor for the venous disorders.

ANTIPLATELETS DRUGS:

Aspirin:

Mechanism of action: Cox_1 inhibitor in higher doses Cox_2 inhibitor.

Indications: Prevention of MI, CVA, and Peripheral Vascular disease.

Primary prevention: In patients with estimated annual risk of M.I. >1%.

Dose: 75-325 mg per day.

Side effects: Gastro intestinal bleeding, aspirin allergy, problem on aspirin resistance.

Thienopyridines: Ticlopidine, Clopidogrel, Prasugrel.

Mechanism of action: ADP induced platelet inhibitor.

Indications: Primary and secondary prevention of cardiovascular death. Combination of clopidogrel and aspirin is better than aspirin alone in reducing cardiovascular death.

Dosage: Ticlopidine– 250 mg twice per day.
Clopidogrel – 600 mg, maintenance dose 75 mg per day.

Side effects: Ticlopidine– GI hemorrhages, neutropenia, thrombocytopenia, TTP.
Clopidogrel – side effects are much less compared to ticlopidine. Similar to aspirin, clopidogrel resistance may be an issue.

Dipyridamole:

Mechanism of action: It blocks the breakdown of CAMP which in term prevents platelet activation.

Indications: Combination of dipyridamole (200 mg) and aspirin (75 mg) has been formed to reduce the recurrence of ischaemic stroke.

Side effects: Headache, flushing.

Newer antiplatelets: Prasugrel, Ticagrelor.

GPIIb IIIa inhibitors:

These agents are useful in the management of ischemic coronary syndromes as well as an adjunct therapy for PCI. These agents are commonly used in clinical practice e.g. Abciximab, Eptifibatide, Tirofiban.

Mechanism of action: they form adhesive molecules like fibrinogen and Von- Willebrand factor.

Side effects: Thrombocytopenia in 5% of cases which is immune mediated.

ANTICOAGULANTS: Heparin, Low molecular weight heparin.

Heparin:

Mechanism of action: By activating antithrombin.

Monitoring of action: By measuring a PTT level.

Side effects:

- Bleeding
- Thrombocytopenia which is immune mediated (HIT) and it can cause both arterial and venous thrombosis. It occurs usually 5-10 days after its commencement.
- Osteoporosis
- Liver enzymes derangement

Low molecular weight heparin: It consists of small fragments of heparin with molecular wt of less than one third of that of heparin.

Mechanism of action: By activating antithrombin.

Advantages of low molecular weight heparin over heparin:

1) Better bioavailability(less protein bound)
2) Low osteoporosis
3) Lower risk of HIT
4) Predictable pharmacological action

Commonly used low molecular weight heparins are Enoxaparin, Fraxiparine, Tinzaparin.

Fibrinolytic agents:

Indications:

- Reperfusion therapy for Myocardial interaction
- Dissolution of arterial and venous thrombolysis
- Ischaemic stroke

1st Generation	2nd Generation	3rd Generation
➢ Streptokinase ➢ Urokinase ➢ APSAC	➢ rtpA	➢ Reteplase ➢ Tenecteplase

Mechanism of action: All of them work by converting fibrinogen to fibrin

Oral anti-coagulant – Warfarin:

Side effects:

- Bleeding
- Drug interaction
- Skin necrosis in patients with inherited Protein C and Protein S deficiency.

Monitoring: By measuring P. Time (INR) level.

Antidote: Vitamin-K

Direct thrombin inhibitors:

- Dabigatran (Direct thrombin inhibitor)
- Apixaban (Factor Xa inhibitor)
- Rivaroxaban (Factor Xa inhibitor)

Surgical procedures in patients without anticoagulants:

For minor surgery like dental extraction or cataract surgery, oral anticoagulants can be continued if INR is kept within the therapeutic range. Similar consideration may be undertaken for the newer anticoagulants on steady dose (INR is not helpful with these drugs). For major surgery Warfarin needs to be discontinued for 5 days prior to surgery and replaced by low molecular weight heparin which should be stopped 12-24 hrs prior to surgery. If Heparin is used instead, it can be discontinued 6 hrs prior to surgery. Commencement of anticoagulants should be done in a similar fashion. However it needs to be individualized depending on the bleeding risks and necessity of using anticoagulants for the original problem for which it has been prescribed.

During 1st and 3rd trimester of pregnancy, Warfarin must be avoided as it is teratogenic and crosses the placental barrier. Heparin can be used instead, although there is a risk of Osteoporosis from its prolonged used.

CASE: *A 51 years old diabetic patient, who underwent cardiac bypass surgery (CABG) and eventually extubated, was reported to have increasing amount of blood loss through thoracotomy drainage tube. His coagulation profile was normal. He was on aspirin which was stopped 24 hours before the surgery. Before going for the reopening procedure it was decided to go for conservative measures first. With this view in mind, the medical team was consulted and it was decided to commence him on IV aprotinin infusion. 24 hours after commencement of aprotinin, his bleeding eventually stopped and thus another invasive surgical procedure was avoided.*

DIAGNOSIS: Post CABG bleeding responding to aprotinin.

DISCUSSION:

Increased bleeding is a common problem encountered in hospital practice. Majority of the patients are post surgical. However acute medical cases are also equally frequently encountered like bleeding in uremia, chronic liver disease, DIC and other coagulation abnormalities, cerebral hemorrhage etc.

While blood transfusion is the initial treatment of choice, it is fraught with dangers like transfusion reaction, mismatched transfusion, transmission of diseases and sometimes non-availability.

In these situations, there drugs which can be helpful to reduce the bleeding by their haemostatic action may circumvent the necessity of re-exploration of surgical procedure.

Drugs commonly evaluated are–

1) Aprotinin
2) Antifibrinolytics
3) Desmopressin
4) Recombinant factor VII

Aprotinin has been evaluated in randomized controlled trials and was found to be helpful in controlling post surgical bleeding. This was particularly noticeable in post CABG patients where its use has been associated with significantly reduced use of blood transfusion.

Doses: Tranexamic acid (dose 3-10 g) and epsilon aminocaproic acid (does 10-30 g) has also been found to be useful albeit to a lesser degree.

Problems: Aprotinin may cause a) post operative renal dysfunction, b) increases the risk of stroke and other cerebrovascular events. Side effect profiles are less with the other two fibrinolytics.

Clinical use: Aprotinin is used in post CABG and other post operative building, particularly those who have been on aspirin. However risk-benefit ratio needs to be judged before its use.

Recombinant factor VII- Initially licensed for use in haemophilia with antibodies to factor VIII or IX, this drug is increasingly finding its place in the other conditions with success. The condition where it has been found to reduce bleeding significantly, are-

1) Major hemorrhage from surgery
2) Following open prostatectomy
3) Trauma
4) Intracerebral hemorrhage (if used early)
5) Following the liver transplant

Dosage: 80 -100 μg/kg of body wt. In trauma the dose may be increased.

Like other haemostatic agents, it can also increase the risk of thromboembolic events like stroke and myocardial infarction. In clinical practice, jury is still out regarding its beneficial role in the treatment of bleeding.

Desmopressin- This acts by way of releasing Von Willebrand factors the endothelium and associated factor VIII may be a useful haemostatic agent in certain clinical situations:

1) Mild Hemophilia A.
2) Von Willebrand disease.
3) Bleeding in cirrhosis.
4) Inherited platelet disorders.
5) Uremic bleeding.

[Although, since the advent of erythropoietin which improves homeostasis by increasing red cell mass, its role as haemostatic in uremia has declined.]

Dose: 0.3 μg/kg IV/SC or 300 μg for body wt > 50 kg (1 spray in each nostril).

Side effects: Flushing and hyponatraemia.

In conclusion, haemostatic drugs if carefully chosen can reduce bleeding and reduce the necessity of blood transfusion in many clinical situations. However, there is no panacea and other basic principle of homeostasis should be taken care of in order to stop bleeding.

What is Von Willebrand factor (VWF)?

VWF is a complex multimeric glycoprotein with two important roles in haemostasis. It binds to the platelet receptors bridging them to other platelets and sub endothelial tissue. It also acts as carrier protein for factor VIII, thus preventing its proteolytic inactivation in plasma. The absence of these multimers leads to defect in platelet adhesion thereby leading to increased bleeding. Ristocetin, an antibiotic increases the interaction between VWF and platelet, on the basis of which ristocetin co-factor activity test is used as a surrogate marker of the functional activity of the VWF. The absence of VWF leads to Von Willebrand disease, a coagulation disorder characterized by bleeding. Type-I Von Willebrand disease is the most common form of inherited coagulation disorder affecting 1% of the general population. Desmopressin is effective in this condition in type-III Von Willebrand disease, there is near total absence of VWF and Desmopressin will not be effective. In type-II Von Willebrand disease where there is qualitative defect of VWF, Desmopressin would probably also not effective in this condition.

: KEY POINTS :

- Pulmonary embolism in India is not as common as it is found in western countries although it is being detected more frequently in recent times.
- It is usually seen in hospital settings in bed ridden, immobile, moribund and post operative patients.
- One should consider the diagnosis in a patient with a high probability score for DVT or PE who develops breathlessness with a relatively clear chest on auscultation and evidence of hypoxia.
- D-Dimer test has a very good negative predictive value.
- Prophylactic heparin low mol wt. heparin and elastic stocking are the best preventive measures for DVT and PE in high risk cases.
- Primary care physicians should be aware of it as many of their patients are immobile and bed bound in the community.

Further references:

- Managing Pulmonary Embolism – Karin Janata BMJ Vol. 19, No. 7 Sep. 2003, P-590-591.
- D. Dimer in venous thromboembolism – P Bockenstedt- NEJM Vol 349- N-13 Sept. 25 2003, P 1247-1256.
- The evaluation of suspected pulmonary embolism – PF Fedullo *et al*. NEJM Vol. 344 – N 13,
  Sept. 25, 2003, P 1203 - 1207.
- HG Watson, oral direct inhibitors of Coagulation – J. R Coll Physician Edinb, 2014:44 46-49.
- Harrison's Principle of Internal Medicine 17th edition.
- Oxford Book of Medicine 5th edition.
- Ref- Pior. M. Mannucci et. al. Prevention and treatment of major blood loss. NEJM-2007 the: 356-2301-II.

06

A PATIENT WITH ATRIAL FIBRILLATION

CASE: *A 71-years-old man suffering from IHD, diabetes mellitus, and COPD, had a history of fever, cough and cold for few days. The reason for his admission in ICCU was increasing palpitation along with shortness of breath. Examination revealed pulse rate of 150-160/min irregular, BP- 130/80 mmHg, chest-scattered rhonchi and crepitations. ECG-atrial fibrillation with non-specific ST changes in lateral leads X-ray chest- left basal pneumonitis, WBC count- 15,000, cardiac enzymes and Troponin-T normal, random glucose- 225 mg%, urea/creatinine slightly raised, urine- no ketone bodies, blood gas: PO_2- 56 mmHg, PCO_2- 39 mmHg.*

DIAGNOSIS: Atrial fibrillation.

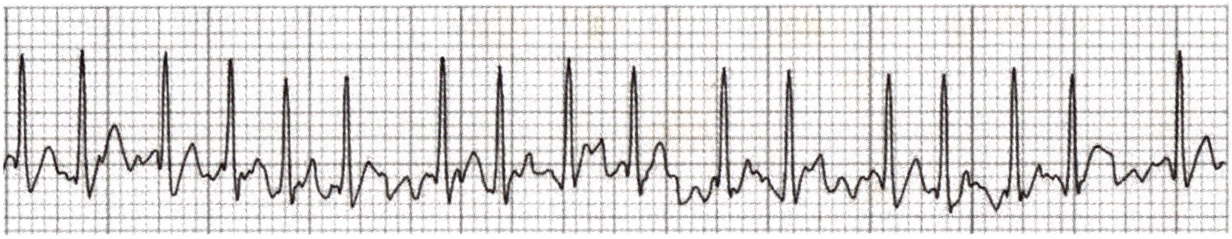

DISCUSSION:

Atrial fibrillation is a common condition encountered in acute medical practice needing frequent ICU admission.

Common causes encountered:

- IHD, HTN, DM, age > 75 years.
- Rheumatic heart disease
- Cardiomyopathy and myocarditis, Pericardial disease
- Prior transient ischemic attack
- Medical conditions like pneumonia, hypoxia and electrolyte imbalance
- Post operative following cardiac and non-cardiac surgery
- Congenital heart disease
- As a part of sick sinus syndrome
- Thyrotoxicosis

CASE: *A 68 year old patient presented with recurrent attacks of palpitation and syncope. However while in hospital his ECG was non contributory. His echocardiogram was normal however on discharge he was put on event loop recorder. After 7 days the developed similar symptoms and the event recorder showed evidence of recurrent attack of atrial fibrillation and occasional long pauses of more than 2.5 m sec duration.*

DIAGNOSIS:

Paroxysmal attack of atrial fibrillation along with recurrent long sinus pauses in a patient with sick sinus syndrome. He was put on permanent pacemaker and commenced on amiodarone and oral anticoagulant therapy.

CLASSIFICATION:

- Paroxysmal AF
- Persistent AF (lasting for more than 7 days)
- Permanent AF
- Silent AF
- Secondary AF
- Valvular AF

CLINICAL FEATURES:

Due to AF pulse	Due to Complication
1. Palpitation	1. Stroke
2. Breathlessness	2. Thromboembolism
3. Angina	3. Heart failure
4. Syncope	4. Tachy-cardiomyopathy

The most common causes that an acute care physician encounters in India are:
IHD, MI, acute medical condition like chest infection, hypoxia due to any cause like COPD, electrolyte imbalance, sick sinus syndrome and rheumatic valvular heart disease.

Diagnosis is fairly straight forward with ECG which shows irregular rhythm with occasional fibrillary waves. Sometimes it is difficult to differentiate from VT if the atrial fibrillation is associated with aberrant condition like RBBB or LBBB and atrial fibrillation in WPW syndrome [This will be discussed in wide complex tachycardia chapter]. Clinically the pulse rate is irregular with a pulse deficient of more than 10/min.

MANAGEMENT:

Initiating causes should be treated promptly with oxygen, antibiotics, correction of electrolyte imbalance. If the rhythm persists in spite of the correction of underlining problem, urgent action has to be taken to either convert it to sinus rhythm or control of rate. ***Rhythm control is always preferable to rate control*** but there are situations where one has to be happy with rate control only. (However, recent studies are indicating that this may not be so and patients with rhythm control may have increased incidence of adverse outcome.)

IV Ibutilide is another drug which can be used in this situation. The drug is mainly used in United States and at present not generally available in India.

Once cardioverted, they usually do not require long term anti-arrhythmic or anticoagulant therapy. If the patient fails to be converted into sinus rhythm oral antiarrhythmics alone or in combination may be carried out. The drugs commonly used in this situation in addition to **amiodarone** are- **Beta blockers, calcium channel blocker (diltiazem)** and **digoxin** in various combinations depending upon the medical situation (beta blockers, diltiazem cautiously in cardiac dysfunction, beta-blocker with caution in COPD *etc.*). In a young patient cardioversion should still be attempted with a 4-week course of oral anticoagulation with another 2 weeks of oral anticoagulation afterwards. This is important as the risk of thromboembolism persists even after successful cardioversion because of the atrial standstill. Suitably chosen oral antiarrhythmics may be continued for indefinite period following the conversion into sinus rhythm.

In patients with chronic atrial fibrillation (more than 3 months duration) or patients with failed DC cardioversion, rate control is the only way forward. In India, most of the patients fall in this category like chronic ischaemic heart disease, rheumatic heart disease, cardiomyopathy *etc.* The ***predictors of unsuccessful cardioversion are- AF of long duration, left atrial size > 4 cm, poor LV function*** *etc.* So one should not attempt for cardioversion if these conditions exist as the failure rate is high and in this situation, rate control should be the target by drugs like amiodarone, β-blocker, diltiazem and digoxin.

Commonly used drugs in AF	
Amiodarone	Rate and rhythm control
Digoxin	Rate control
Diltiazem	Rate control
Dofetilide	Rate and rhythm control
Sotalol	Rate control
Verapamil	Rate control
Atenolol/ metoprolol	Rate control
Contraindicated structural heart disease	
Propafenon (class1c)	Rate and rhythm control
Flecanide (class1c)	Rate and rhythm control

Atrial fibrillation in different clinical situations:

- **Drugs in cardiomyopathy: Amiodarone** may prevent sudden cardiac death. **Digoxin** may improve symptoms of heart failure. **β-blockers** with carefully selected dose will prolong survival.
- **Drugs in COPD: Calcium channel blocker *or* amiodarone** may be preferred (**Digoxin** has increased side effect in COPD).
- **Drugs in Thyrotoxicosis: β-blocker** may be referred.
- **Drugs in valvular heart disease with cardiac failure: Digoxin** is the drug of choice.
- In chronic atrial fibrillation in patients with valvular heart disease and cardiomyopathy and big left atrium rate control may be the only option.

Role of anticoagulants:

Atrial fibrillation imposes an increased risk of thromboembolism (5% risk each year) and oral anticoagulation is essential to prevent this. Few clinical studies have addressed on this issue and the consensus is that oral anticoagulants are much superior to aspirin in prevention of thromboembolytic event (aspirin may be used where anticoagulant is contraindicated or at risk of thromboembolism). If the patient is less than 55 years of age without any obvious cardiac risk factor, anticoagulants may be avoided. However if other associated risk factors like history of CVA, heart failure, valvular heart disease and history of valve surgery, ischaemic heart disease *etc.* are present, they should be anticoagulated.

Occasionally patients present with paroxysmal atrial fibrillation, the drugs most effective in this condition are:

a) Flecainide- (caution-cardiac failure)
b) Sotalol (caution-cardiac failure)
c) Dofetilide (if available)
d) However, amiodarone is the most commonly used drug because of the safety profile in cardiac dysfunction.
e) If the patient has had more than 2 recurrent attacks, they should be anticoagulated as well (If age > 65 or in the presence of risk factors).
f) In clinical practice, we find many patients with sick sinus syndrome present with atrial fibrillation. Great caution has to be exercised in prescribing antiarrhythmics as they may aggravate bradyarrhythmia with serious consequences. Prophylactic pacing may be required before prescribing antiarrhythmics in these patients.

g) Many of the patients present in CCU with thromboembolic stroke. As the immediate risk of recurrence is low in the first two weeks, anticoagulants may be deferred for the first 2 weeks as they may increase the incidence of haemorrhage in the infarct area. The situation should be reviewed after 2 weeks with a follow up CT brain scan and anticoagulation should be started only if there is no evidence of haemorrhagic transformation. (I have seen patients where hasty anticoagulation has resulted in haemorrhagic transformation with adverse effects.) It should be remembered that primary prevention is much better and every effort should be anticoagulated high risk AF patients in order to prevent cerebrovascular accident.

Surgical therapy:

Surgical ablation therapy (maze procedure) designed to interrupt the macro-reentrant pathway may be contemplated in centres with appropriate facilities., further to the traditional procedure (MAZE procedure) newer modes of ablation therapy have been recently developed and the clinician should discuss the available facilities during the process of consultation.

There are different risk assessment tools like CHADS Score calculator to evaluate the risk of thromboembolism in AF.

High Risk: Previous stroke, age more than 75 years, hypertension, diabetes mellitus, Valvular heart disease, cardiac failure.

Moderate risk: Age between 65 and 75 years with hypertension, diabetes mellitus, valvular heart disease and cardiac failure.

Low Risk: Age less than 65 years with no associated hypertension, diabetes or valvular heart disease.

CASE: *A 76 years old lady with diabetes mellitus ischemic heart disease, mitral stenosis and atrial fibrillation was admitted with severe pain left leg. Her house physician prescribed some analgesic over telephone without any effect. She was admitted and found to have cold left leg, and absence of pulse in arteria dorsalis pedis and posterior tibial artery. A diagnosis of acute thromboembolism of left leg was made. She underwent embolectomy (with Fogarty catheter) with relief of her symptoms. Fortunately her peripheral circulation was restored with symptomatic relief therapy. She was discharged with the advice of lifelong anticoagulation with warfarin.*

DIAGNOSIS: Peripheral thromboembolism in a patient with chronic atrial fibrillation.

A recent study comparing rate control with adequate anticoagulation (drugs used in rate control group digoxin, verapamil, Beta-blocker) and rhythm control with **defibrillation** (drugs used in rhythm control group- amiodarone, sotalol) showed that the former may be equally effective [Rhythm control group had slightly increased mortality at 5 years]. So the debate still continues. **(From Annuals of Internal medicine, 2nd march 2004 issue.)**

Stroke risk evaluation for AF: CHADS2 score		
Condition	**Points**	**Score**
C	Congestive heart failure	**1**
H	Hypertension: BP consistently >140/90 mmHg (or treated hypertension on medication)	**1**
A	Age ≥75 years	**1**
D	Diabetes mellitus	**1**
S_2	Prior Stroke or TIA or Thromboembolism	**2**
Score < 0 : low risk; Score < 1 : moderate risk; Score > 2 : high risk		

: KEY POINTS :

- Haemodynamically unstable atrial fibrillation should be treated with D.C. cardioversion.
- Rhythm control is preferable to rate control (although most recent studies indicate otherwise- close follow up of the literature will be needed to make a final comment).
- In chronic atrial fibrillation with a big left atrium, rhythm control is not an achievable target.
- Patients over 65 years old with or without associated risk factors should be anticoagulated.
- In patients below 65 years, anticoagulation may be deferred if there are no associated risk factors.
- In an embolic stroke, anticoagulation should be withheld for initial two weeks as the incidence of haemorrhage is high.

FURTHER REFERENCES:

Present Treatment Option for Atrial Fibrillation- S.K.S. Lairikyengbam *et al.*

Post Graduate Medical Journal 2003: Vol-79, page 67-73.

K. Vargava- A trial fibrillation, Clinical and epidemiological aspect, Journal of clinical and preventive cardiology, Vol-31, No- 2, April 2014. P-55-60.

Harrison's Principle of Internal Medicine- 17th edition.

Oxford Text Book of Medicine- 5th edition.

07

A PATIENT WITH MENOPAUSAL SYNDROME

CASE: *A 48-years-old lady presented with symptoms of headache insomnia, mood swings, bodyache and a sense of unwellbeing. She also complained of occasional chest pain, fluctuating BP and a warm sensation around her head. Numerous investigations including CT scan of brain and symptomatic treatment came to nothing. The symptoms were interfering with her day to day activities. Examination revealed normal haemodynamic status BP 150/100 mmHg rest of the examination NAD.*

Investigations were essentially normal, Thyroid function was normal. FSH was markedly elevated, LFT and bone biochemistry were normal. ECG and X-ray chest was normal. USG whole abdomen was NAD [she had history of hysterectomy with intact ovaries for fibroid uterus 5 years back]. Bilateral mammography was normal.

DIAGNOSIS: Menopausal syndrome.

DISCUSSION:

This is a common presentation to the internists where middle-aged women present with vague, non-specific symptoms of generalized unwell being with headache, flushing, chest pain, bodyache and symptoms of insomnia and irritability. They usually undergo numerous investigations without any fruitful results. A diagnosis can be obtained by taking proper history of oligomenorrhoea of recent onset. Many times there is history of oophorectomy along with hysterectomy. The diagnosis is further substantiated by the presence of elevated level of FSH. Many of the symptoms are quickly relieved by judicious use of HRT, antihypertensive, short course of anti depressants and counselling. Diagnosis is clinical; however elevated FSH may provide some clue.

SYMPTOMS:

- Hot flushes
- Episodic sweating
- Insomnia
- Depression
- Mood swings
- Vaginal Dryness
- Somatic symptoms
- Loss of memory
- Impaired memory
- Sexual Dysfunction

MANAGEMENT:

Until recently, HRT was very popular as they are quick in relieving postmenopausal symptoms.

Conjugated oestrogen (Premarin 0.625 mg daily) is commonly used for this purpose. In addition to quick symptom relief it also has a bone conserving effect and helpful in prevention of osteoporosis in late ages. However, unopposed effect of oestrogen has a carcinogenic effect on uterus. So it should be used with progesterone while using in patients with intact uterus. Moreover it increases the incidence of breast cancer, regular follow up with yearly mammography is essential. It is always prudent to get a thorough gynaecological check up including cervical smear and mammography before commencing HRT.

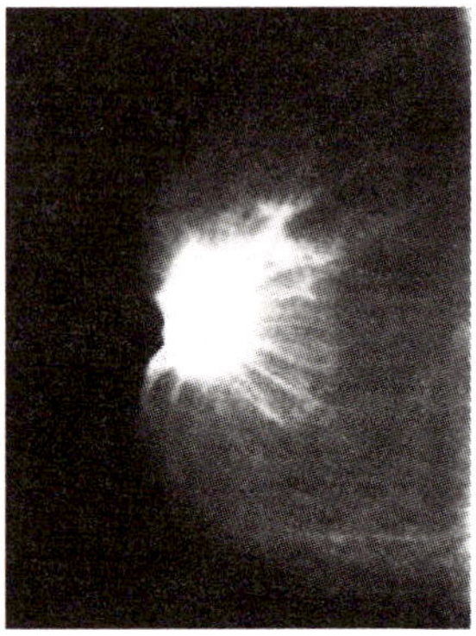

Typical schedule of HRT:

- **Oestrogen (0.625 mg)** – daily **: in patients with hysterectomy.**
- **Oestrogen (0.625 mg)** – day 1 to day 21 + **Medroxyprogesterone (2.5 mg)** day 14 to day 21 **: in patients with intact uterus.** This regime will cause cyclical bleeding.

However following the publication of HERS study where oestrogen was shown to increase cardiac mortality in the 1st year in patients with angina, as well as other side effects like hypertension, increased incidence of DVT, this regime has fallen into disrepute.

Problems of HRT:

Although HRT was Popular and considered to be cardio-protective few decades ago in publication of the report of HERS study as well as other observational studies, have indicated many adverse effects of HRT and subsequently the use has declined considerably.

Problems found with HRT with Oestrogen:

- Endometrial carcinoma in case of unopposed use of oestrogen in patients with intact uterus [increased by 3 folds if used in short term for 1-5 years] sequential use of progesterone offsets this risk, although increases the risk of breast carcinoma.
- Deep Vein thrombosis
- Breast cancer, if used for more than 5 years. Addition of progesterone increases the risk.
- Increased risk of coronary artery disease.

Problems encountered in patients on oestrogen containing HRT:

- Breast carcinoma
- Increased DVT
- Increased IHD
- Increased pulmonary embolism
- Increased hypertension

Other contraindications of oestrogen:

- Active liver disease
- Unexplained vaginal bleeding
- Gall bladder disease
- Severe hypertriglyceridemia

Those who are severely affected by post menopausal flushing it can be used as short term (2-3 months) without much of a problem (In selected cases it can still be used as long term).

Other drugs:

- **Tibolone** is a newly available synthetic hormone which can be used as substitute. It does not have any adverse effect on the breast or uterus.
- **SERM** (Selective Estrogen Receptor Modulator): **Raloxifene** (60 mg daily) can be used as a substitute for HRT. It has estrogenic actions on bone and anti-estrogenic actions on the uterus and breast. So it does not have any adverse effect on breast or uterus. It is partially effective for prevention of osteoporosis. Unfortunately it does not help to reduce the post menopausal symptom of flushing.

- Other drugs for flushing: When hormones cannot be used, one should look for other drugs. Few drugs can be tried e.g. **Clonidine** (100 microgram daily). It can cause dryness of mouth and abrupt withdrawal may cause problems. **Anti-depressant drugs** particularly SSRI (Fluoxetine) may be tried with mixed results. Of late, newer group of antidepressants like *venlafaxine* has also been used with partial success.

GENERAL MANAGEMENT:

Good nutritious diet containing calcium is essential. Control of blood pressure with appropriate medication will also be required. *While treating with HRT, migraine may be aggravated and HRT should be discontinued.* With appropriate management and counseling most of the patients will go back to normal life within 5-6 months.

PRACTICAL APPROACH:

How to use if:

- In postmenopausal local symptoms like vaginal dryness, local oestrogen may be used.
- In severe symptomatic post menopausal symptoms like flushing, sweating etc, very short term oestrogen may be used without any concern. However if the symptoms present and HRT needed for more than 1 year, gynecological opinion will be needed.
- If the patient has hysterectomy, oestrogen may be continued for a longer period. In patients with intact uterus, cyclical oestrogen and progesterone may be considered for some time (although long term use may increases the risk of breast cancer).
- Longer term use of oestrogen particularly in combination of progesterone increases the risk of breast cancer specifically in patients with family history of breast cancer, BRCA1 & BRCA2 gene positivity.

From clinician point of view very short term use in symptomatic patients may be considered, longer term use that is beyond 6 months should be contempt only after consultation with gynecologists. Other ways of combating the post menopausal symptoms need to be considered as well.

For flushing:

- Venlafaxine
- Gabapentin
- Clonidine

For osteoporosis:

- Bisphosphonates
- Raloxifene (SERM)
- Smoking cessation
- Adequate calcium intake

: KEY POINTS :

- ➢ Any non-specific symptoms of unwell being along with insomnia, flushing, depression and irritability in a middle-aged woman, menopausal syndrome should be thought of.
- ➢ Good history taking along with estimation of FSH, will obviate the need of many unnecessary expensive tests.
- ➢ HRT quickly improves the menopausal symptoms and can be used for a short term.
- ➢ Long term HRT should be used with caution.
- ➢ Tibolone and raloxifene does not have adverse effect on breast and uterus.
- ➢ Raloxifene helps in prevention of osteoporosis but not in post menopausal flushing.
- ➢ Clonidine, fluoxetine and venlafaxine sometimes help alleviate some of the post menopausal symptoms.

FURTHER REFERENCES:

- Graendale G.A. *et al.* (1999). The Menopause Lancet. 353: 571 -580.
- Gruber C.J. *et al.* (2002). Production and action of oestrogens. NEJM 346: 340-352.
- Harison's Principle of Internal Medicine 17th edition.

08 A PATIENT WITH ABDOMINAL ABSCESS

CASE: *A 32-years-old male presented with 2 weeks history of vague abdominal discomfort associated hectic rise of temperature. The temperature was coming every day with chill and rigor. Examination did not reveal any abnormality. Investigations revealed Hb- 10.5 g%, WBC- 21 000, poly- 90%, bilirubin- 1.6 mg%, alkaline phosphatase more than double the normal value, AST and ALT slightly elevated, X-ray chest- normal, stool examination- NAD, urine exam- NAD, amylase & lipase- normal, blood culture- no growth, malaria not detected on several occasions. Echo- no vegetation, USG whole abdomen- presence of 3 cm × 4 cm hypo dense shadow in the right upper posterior quadrant – consistent with an abscess.*

DIAGNOSIS: Liver abscess, ?Amoebic.

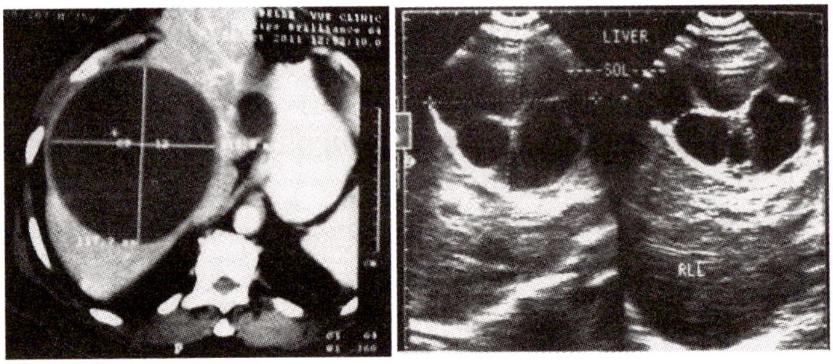

CASE: *A 57-years-old gentleman presented with fever and back pain along with left loin pain. His ESR and CRP was high, X-ray L-S spine and routine urine examination did not reveal anything specific. On examination his left leg was found to be flexed and internally rotated. CT scan and subsequently MRI scan of the spine demonstrated left sided psoas abscess along with involvement of $D_{12}L_1L_2$ vertebrae, characteristic of tuberculosis. The abscess was surgically drained and the patient was subsequently started on antitubercular medication.*

DIAGNOSIS: Psoas abscess of tubercular origin.

DISCUSSION:

Psoas abscess is occasionally encountered in clinical practice where the patients usually present with abdominal pain, back pain and fever. Additionally the patient may have symptoms of psoas muscle spasm leading to flexed position of the leg. Tuberculosis is a common cause; however staphylococcal osteomyelitis may be responsible for it as well. In patients on oral anticoagulant, local haematoma will also come into the differential diagnosis.

CASE: *A 21-years-old young man presented with a history of fever of 3 weeks duration. He was on irregular antibiotic therapy, ultrasound examination and later on CT scan of abdomen showed multiple splenic abscesses. Blood culture later on grew Salmonella typhi.*

DIAGNOSIS: Fever due to *Salmonella* species with multiple splenic abscesses.

DISCUSSION:

Causes of splenic abscess:

1. Infective endocarditis
2. *Salmonella*
3. Tuberculosis

CASE: *A 47 years old patient presented with fever of 3 weeks duration along with abdominal pain. Her WBC count was 21 000, bilirubin- 2.1 mg%. Alkaline phosphatase was 484 (high). The reason for admission was breathlessness. X-ray chest showed right plural effusion and ultrasound of abdomen showed a big abscess in right upper lobe segment of liver, he was started on metronidazole and broad spectrum antibiotic. Unfortunately he become very toxic and was reported to have haemoptysis which was later on found to be anchovy-sauce like pus, he underwent urgent surgical evaluation of the abscess and intercostal drainage of the pus, which was extended into the right plural cavity. After a stormy post operative course he made a full recovery.*

DIAGNOSIS: Amoebic liver abscess extending into the pleural cavity and lung parenchyma.

DISCUSSION:

Amoebic liver abscess is a common cause of fever of unknown origin in India. Classically patients have fever with chill and rigor along with right hypochondrial discomfort, although very occasionally they do not have any abdominal symptom altogether. Pleuritic chest pain and cough (if the abscess irritates the diaphragm) may be present. Associated gastro intestinal symptoms like nausea, vomiting, diarrhoea may be present in 10-33% of cases. In a typical case there may be point tenderness of the right rib cage and hepatomegaly (however hepatomegaly may be absent).

Investigation reveals moderate leukocytosis with polymorph preponderance, bilirubin may be mildly elevated, alkaline phosphatise is characteristically raised with mild to moderate alteration of liver enzymes. X-ray chest may show elevated right hemidiaphragm.

Stool examinations frequently do not show any abnormality. The diagnosis is confirmed by USG abdomen or CT scan of abdomen. Other tests that available are stool for *Entamoeba histolytica* antigen (positive in 50% of cases) and anti-amoebic antibodies (70-80%). These tests are generally not available in day to day clinical practice in India.

Complications of liver abscess:

- Pleuropulmonary involvement
- Rupture into the pericardium and peritoneum

ORGANISMS:

Apart from amoebic liver abscesses, pyogenic abscesses are also commonly encountered in clinical practice. These patients are more toxic and organisms vary depending upon the source whether it is biliary, pelvic or any other intraperitoneal source. Usually the organisms are gram negative enteric and *Streptococcus* or *Staphylococcus* if the spread is haematogenous. The flora is usually mixed or anaerobic if the source is pelvic. *Candida* infection can also cause liver abscess particularly in the case of disseminated candidaemia.

Differential Diagnosis of amoebic liver Abscess:

Occasionally ultrasound examination reveals space occupying lesion in the liver poising a diagnostic dilemma. Examination of stool, immunological tests like serology to detect amoeba hydatid cyst tumour markers and radiological tests like CT scan or MRI Scan will clinch the issues.

Personal experience:

In the unit I used to work, we have treated 54 cases of amoebic liver abscess in last 6 years. On 40% of occasions, the symptoms were only fever with chill and rigor without any localizing symptom. 4 patients were on long term steroids as was immuno-suppressive for renal transplant. Leukocytes of more than 16,000 were present in all of them. Mild hyperbilirubinaemia (up to 2.5 mg %) and high rise of alkaline phosphatase were present in 70% of the cases. In our opinion, in patients presenting with prolonged fever with aforementioned biochemical and haematological features, routine USG screening of abdomen would help in diagnosis of amoebic liver abscess at an early date.

Once detected, it should be differentiated from –

- Pyogenic liver abscess where the patients are usually more toxic, the abscess is usually multiple.
- Necrotic hepatoma (raised alpha fetoprotein)
- Hydatid cyst (usually incidental finding – not associated with abdominal pain) – USG and CT scan show characteristic septation.

INVESTIGATIONS:

- Ultrasound
- CT scan
- MRI scan

Contrast enhanced CT scan and MRI scan are particularly helpful in differentiating between metastatic liver diseases, primary hepatoma, haemangioma of liver and simple hepatic cyst where ultrasound examination may fail to provide the exact diagnosis.

MANAGEMENT:

The initial management is medical and the commonly used drugs are either metronidazole or tinidazole for a minimum period of 10 days (initially intravenous followed by oral). It is judicious, also to use broad spectrum antibiotics along with anti amoebic therapy. In recalcitrant cases, CT or USG guided percutaneous drainage of the abscess may be required. Drainage is essential in case of impending rupture of the abscess (lesion more than 5 cm or presence in the left lobe).

In our experience, we have found that early drainage of the abscess combined with anti-amoebic therapy ever in the absence of impending rupture, causes quicker defervescence of the symptoms and we routinely perform it while dealing with such cases. In patients with fulminant colitis with rupture of liver abscess, dehydroemetine (1-1.5 mg/kg/day for 5 days) may be added to metronidazole. It can cause cardio toxicity (needs ECG follow up) and muscle weakness. In spite of the treatment with metronidazole, luminal cyst persists in 40-60% of cases so the treatment should be followed by a course of diloxanide furoate for 7-10 days. Iodoquinol- 650 mg three times daily for 20 days may also be used to treat luminal cyst. It can rarely cause neurotoxicity.

: KEY POINTS :

- Amoebic liver abscess is a common cause of prolonged fever with chills and rigor not responding to conventional antibiotics and empirical anti-malarial.
- Localized liver tenderness may be absent.
- Characteristic laboratory tests that points towards the diagnosis are, increased WBC with high polymorph nuclear count, mildly raised bilirubin and markedly raised alkaline phosphatase.
- Aspiration should be done if there is evidence of impending rupture.
- Defervescence is quicker with aspiration.
- Ultrasound examination should be incorporated in the diagnostic work up of fever with chills and rigor.
- Intra-abdominal abscess like splenic abscess, perinephric abscess, psoas abscess and subphrenic abscess should be considered in the differential diagnosis of fever with abdominal pain.

FURTHER REFERENCES:

- R. Haque *et al.* - Current Concepts in Amoebiasis – NEJM Vol- 348, No. 16, P- 1565-1573.
- Harrison's Principle of Internal Medicine – 17th edition.
- Oxford Book of Medicine 5th edition.

09

A PATIENT PRESENTED WITH MICROSCOPIC HAEMATURIA

CASE: *A 61 years old gentleman came for consultation because his routine urinary examination showed presence of persistent RBC- 15-20/field. He was asymptomatic however; he was mildly hypertensive and was on Calcium Channel Blocker for his BP. General examination was satisfactory. Biochemical and haematological parameters were normal. He was non-diabetic. He received several courses of antibiotics but to no avail. His PSA was normal and USG of abdomen did not reveal anything apart from mildly enlarged prostate gland. He was very anxious to know whether anything serious was going on.*

DIAGNOSIS: Microscopic haematuria ?cause.

DISCUSSION:

This is not an uncommon problem encountered in clinical practice and very often extensive investigation does not reveal anything specific. It is important to know that frequently some common physiological causes may give rise to isolated haematuria (microscopic and macroscopic) and proper history taking is very much important. Such conditions are:

- Urine examination during menstrual period
- Heavy exercise
- Sexual activity
- Drugs like warfarin or anti-platelet agents

Repeat examination is sometimes necessary. Once the persistence of microscopic haematuria was confirmed one should differentiate between haematuria of glomerular or non-glomerular origin.

Haematuria of glomerular origin:

- Presence of RBC cast
- Presence of dysmorphic RBC
- Presence of acanthocytes (particular form of abnormal RBC)

If there is suspicion of haematuria of glomerular origin-following clinical conditions should be considered.

- Glomerulonephritis due to any cause including vasculitis
- IgA nephropathy
- Hereditary nephritis

CASE: *A 9 years old girl with history of impetigo presented with a history of fever, oliguria and swelling of the face. Her BP was 140/90 mmHg, facial puffiness present, urine showed RBC- 40-50/field, RBC cast, protein++, ASO titer- 450 units.*

DIAGNOSIS: Classical case of acute post streptococcal glomerulonephritis.

In absence of other accompanying classical finding in the urine, non-glomerular causes should be considered. Common causes encountered in clinical practice are:

- Upper urinary tract causes:
  - Stones
  - Pyelonephritis
  - Trauma
  - Renal tumours
  - Renal infarction
  - Papillary necrosis particularly in patients with diabetes mellitus and prolonged intake of NSAID's.
  - Polycystic kidney disease
  - Renal tuberculosis (particularly in our country)
  - Interstitial nephritis
- Lower urinary tract causes:
  - Cystitis, prostatitis, urethritis
  - Bladder tumours (benign and malignant)
  - BPH and prostate cancer

Haematuria due to glomerular cause should be referred to a renal physician for further work up.

For non-glomerular haematuria, the initial investigation should be an ultrasound examination which should detect most of the causes like stone, tumour, enlarged prostrate. However, the sensitivity of this test is less for tiny stones or tumour less than 3 cm diameter. The next choice of investigation is between IVU and CT scan. Now-a-days, CT scan is preferred as in addition to picking up of tiny stones, it can also detect mass lesion like a tumour. Moreover IVU may not be possible in patients with renal failure. Initially the CT scan should be done without contrast in multiple cuts which is a very sensitive test to diagnose small stone (sensitivity is more than that of IVU). After stone has been excluded, IV contrast should be given (if not contrast indicated) for the detection of any tumour.

If no cause is detected, the next step should be referred to an urologist for cystoscopic examination. One should remember that the diagnostic yield like finding a bladder cancer is much more common in men than women. In addition to cystoscopy, other routine tests like blood for PSA, urine for AFB and urine for cytology (first morning specimen) might be helpful. Urinary cytology has got good sensitivity in patients with bladder cancer than in renal cancer.

On many occasions, no cause can be found and the patients should be kept under regular surveillance. In our country genitourinary tuberculosis should be strongly suspected in patients with persistent haematuria with negative test results. There is a caveat in testing urine for AFB as on many occasions positive AFB in the urine is due to presence of saprophytic organism (which is only acid fast but no alcohol fast). Culture of AFB should resolve the haematuria and prolonged antibiotic therapy may be indicated.

In this particular patient all the tests were negative. He was found to be on aspirin for primary prevention of heart disease. Although, though to be unlikely, his aspirin was discontinued with eventual disappearance of his haematuria.

CASE: *An 81 years old lady presented with haematuria. Ultrasound examination was suggestive of an SOL of urinary bladder which was confirmed by CT-scan of abdomen. Cystoscopy revealed a mass in the anterior wall of urinary bladder which was removed cystoscopically, biopsy revealed high grade invasive carcinoma. In view of her age various options of treatment like urinary bladder resection with ureteric diversion, chemo therapy and intravesical infiltration of BCG vaccination (as a second option, as the tumour was already invasive) were discussed. In view of her age the relatives opted for palliative care only.*

DIAGNOSIS: Haematuria due to carcinoma of urinary bladder.

CASE: *A 52 years old male was referred by an urologist for persistent haematuria following TURP. No surgical cause or any underlying cause was apparent. His prothrombin time, platelet count were normal while APTT was slightly prolonged which was not checked pre-operatively. Subsequently he was found to be partially deficient in factor VIII he was referred to the haematologists and was treated with factor VIII replacement. On retrospective analysis he was reported to have increased bleeding tendency following minor trauma which did not need any medical attention.*

DIAGNOSIS: Mild Haemophilia leading to increased postoperative bleeding.

DISCUSSION: The moral of this case history is that patients undergoing surgery like TURP should undergo coagulation profile check up including prothrombin time and APTT in addition to bleeding time and clotting time as I have encountered these cases of severe post operative bleeding following TURP. Multiple blood and FFP transfusion were given and who finally was diagnosed to have mild haemophilia.

PROTEINURIA: Proteinuria is a common condition encountered in clinical practice although conventional dipsticks methods detects albumin of more than 300 mg/dl, microalbuminaemia (protein level 30-300 mg/dl) is clinically important as it may indicate early nephropathy in patients with diabetes mellitus. In this regard urinary protein creatinine ratio may be a better indicator of early kidney damage. Proteinuria more than 3.5 g/day is classically associated with nephrotic syndrome with characteristic features of hypoalbuminaemia, hyperlipidaemia and oedema.

CAUSES:

Microalbuminuria

- Diabetes mellitus
- Hypertension

Physiological proteinuria

- Exercise
- Fever
- postural
- Congestive heart failure

Nephrotic syndrome

- Diabetes
- Amyloidosis
- Membranous glomerulonephritis
- Minimal change disease
- Mesangioproliferative glomerulopathy

In addition to conventional proteinuria which is of glomerular in origin there may be tubular proteinuria like Tamm-Horsfall protein or β_2 microglobulin or light chain protein as found in plasma cells dyscrasias which can be detected by special tests.

: KEY POINTS :

- Microscopic haematuria is common in clinical practice
- One should first exclude normal physiological causes of haematuria
- Glomerular causes should be differentiated from non-glomerular causes
- During investigation, CT scan is preferred to IVU
- Genitourinary tuberculosis should be excluded in persistent microscopic haematuria with negative results.

REFERENCE:

- Microscopic Haematuria- A Robert *et al.*, NEJM 2003, 348 page-2330-8.
- Oxford Book of Medicine – 5th edition.
- Harrison's Principal of Internal Medicine – 17th edition.
- Oxford Book of Medicine 5th edition.

10 A PATIENT PRESENTING WITH CARPAL TUNNEL SYNDROME

CASE: *A 56-years-old obese lady presented in the clinic with a history of tingling and numbness of both hands more on the right side. The symptoms were increasing in severity and interfering with her day to day activities. There was also associated pain which was worse at night. The pain radiated towards her elbows as well. She also had pain in her neck along with dizziness. Her BP was 156/90 mmHg. Neurological examination was satisfactory. Tinel's sign was positive so was the Phalen's sign. Neck movement was painful. Locomotor– NAD. Her TSH was elevated at a level of 20. Rest of the blood tests were normal. X-ray cervical spine showed spondylotic changes in C_5, C_6 and C_7 vertebrae. X-ray chest was normal.*

PROVISIONAL DIAGNOSIS: Carpal tunnel syndrome.

DIFFERENTIAL DIAGNOSIS: Cervical radiculopathy, Peripheral neuropathy.

NCV study of both upper extremities was carried out which showed classical evidence of median nerve compression in the carpal tunnel, right more than the left.

DISCUSSION:

Carpal tunnel syndrome usually presents with tingling and numbness mainly of the lateral three and a half fingers. There may be associated pain which may radiate towards the elbow. The symptoms are worse at night and the symptoms are partially relieved if the hands are held upwards to reduce the oedema. The diagnosis should always be kept in mind if the patient is a –

a) middle aged female
b) has obesity or hypothyroidism
c) has history of osteoarthritis
d) during pregnancy

Other associated conditions are acromegaly, amyloidosis. There may be a history of trauma in the past. As cervical spondylosis is a common accompaniment, it is frequently misdiagnosed as cervical radiculopathy. Early NCV study will settle the issue.

Examination reveals positive **Tinel's sign** (tapping of the volar aspect of the wrist with a hammer causes tingling in the lateral 3½ fingers) and a positive **Phalen's sign** (forced flexion of the wrist for 60 seconds will reproduce the symptoms of carpal tunnel compression). In long standing cases, there may be wasting of the thenar eminence muscles. There may also be sensory impairment of the lateral 3½ fingers. Thumb abduction may be impaired.

DIAGNOSIS: It is confirmed by nerve conduction velocity study which differentiates from other causes like cervical radiculopathy or polyneuropathy.

MANAGEMENT:

In mild cases simple wrist splint or hand brace during working might provide symptomatic benefit. **NSAID** and **diuretics** also help in relieving symptoms but **oral steroids** are more effective. Even more effective is local injection of steroid (1cm proximal to the distal flexion crease of the wrist between palmaris longus and flexor carpi radialis). However the process is blind and exact location of the target is not guaranteed. It is usually given where CTS is transient as in pregnancy. Short acting steroids (e.g. hydrocortisone) are now-a-days preferred to long acting ones (triamcinolone) to avoid long term side effects.

The treatment of choice in persistent CTS **is surgical decompression** with a success rate of 95% in expert hands. Now-a-days in certain centres endoscopic decompression is being practiced. The success rate is more or less same but the procedure is less painful and return to work is earlier. Whichever procedure is chosen, it should be properly timed as permanent damage to the nerves would render the operation a failure. In bilateral involvement the operation should be done sequentially with a gap of few months to ensure good recovery from the first procedure.

The patient mentioned above underwent surgical decompression (sequential) of her CTS. She was also treated with thyroxin and at one year follow up she was doing very well.

Causes of Carpal tunnel syndrome-

- Osteoarthritis
- Hypothyroidism
- Obesity
- Amyloidosis
- Inflammatory arthropathy

CASE: *A 49 years old lady presented with history of vague pain around her left wrist was unable to carry out her daily activities. Anti-inflammatory analgesics gave her only partial relief of her symptoms. Examination revealed Finkelstein's test (the thumb flexed and placed in the clench of the hand grip with the patient actively deviating the hand downwards with ulnar deviation). Her fasting blood glucose was 193 mg% with a uric acid level of 7.2 mg%. She was diagnosed to be suffering from De Quervains' tenosynovitis and injected with local hydrocortisone injection with relief of her symptoms.*

DIAGNOSIS: Re De Quervains' tenosynovitis in a hyperuricaemia and diabetic patient.

Hand pain and shoulder pain are a very common presentation in clinical practice and in majority of cases they present to the internists who with careful clinical examination may make a definitive diagnosis and offer successful treatment.

Common causes of hand pain:

- Trauma
- Infection
- Osteoarthritis – distal PIP joints and commonly involved 1st MCP joints
- Uric acid related problems
- Inflammatory arthropathy – MCP joints commonly involved
- Carpal tunnel syndrome – discussed

Tenosynovitis of different tendons around the wrist joints (main associated causes are-over use, diabetic mellitus, high uric acid, gonococcal infection.

: KEY POINTS :

- CTS is a common presentation in clinical practice.
- It is frequently misdiagnosed as osteoarthritis or cervical spondylosis.
- Careful history taking clinical examination and early NCV test will detect the condition earlier.
- Surgical decompression is the treatment of choice with adequate symptomatic relief.
- Underlying causes like hypothyroidism should be ruled out.

Further references (Selected articles and chapters from):

- NEJM
- Post Grad Med Journal
- Oxford hand book of Rheumatology
- The journal of Royal college of physicians of London
- Patten – Neurological differential diagnosis.
- Harrison's Principle of Internal Medicine – 17th edition

11 A PATIENT WITH NON-ALCOHOLIC HEPATIC STEATOSIS

CASE: *A 53-year-old obese lady with Type II diabetes mellitus and hyperlipidaemia came for consultation because of her routine liver function test showed high AST and ALT levels on two consecutive occasions. She never had any history of jaundice or alcohol intake. Apart from oral hypoglycaemic and ACE inhibitors she was not on any medication. She did not complain of any specific symptoms. Examination revealed an obese lady with a BP of 160/90 mmHg, LFT showed AST– 88, ALT– 109, bilirubin– 0.9 mg%, Albumin-globulin ratio normal, alkaline phosphatase level within normal range. Hepatitis B surface antigen and HCV antibody were negative. ANF, smooth muscle antibody and anti-mitochondrial antibody negative, USG abdomen showed evidence of fatty infiltration of liver.*

PROVISIONAL DIAGNOSIS: Non alcoholic hepatic steatosis.

DISCUSSION:

Asymptomatic elevation of liver enzyme is a common condition for medical consultation. Common conditions leading to abnormal liver function tests are:

- Alcohol intake (MCV and gamma GT will be high)
- Non alcoholic hepatic steatosis
- Infections like Hepatitis B and Hepatitis C
- Drugs
    - Antitubercular (INH)
    - Anti-epileptic (valproate)
    - Statins– simvastatin
    - Oral contraceptive
    - Antiarrhythmics
    - Anti-neoplastic (methotrexate) for rheumatoid arthritis
    - Anti-HIV therapy
- Auto immune hepatitis and primary biliary cirrhosis
- Metabolic disorders (rare)

Enzymes inducing antiepileptic drugs like phenytoin, carbamazepine, and phenobarbitone can cause elevation of gamma GT which does not need detailed follow up.

Components of liver function test:

➢ Bilirubin

- *Un-conjugated more:* Jaundice due to haemolytic anaemia, congenital defect of bilirubin metabolism.
- *Conjugated more:* Obstructive jaundice due to CBD or tumour or stricture of CBD.
- *Both conjugated and unconjugated:* Hepatitis (A, B, C, E), alcoholic liver disease, non-alcoholic liver disease.

➢ Elevated Alkaline phosphatise

In intra hepatic and extra hepatic obstruction due to any cause

Infiltrative disorders of liver

➢ ALT and AST

ALT > AST in acute hepatitis

AST > ALT in alcoholic hepatitis

➢ Albumin

Decreased in chronic liver disease (alcoholic, non-alcoholic)

➢ Prothrombin time

Prolonged in chronic liver disease

Causes of un-conjugated hyperbilirubinaemia:

- Haemolysis
- Ineffective erythropoiesis
- Decreased bilirubin clearance due to impaired conjugation
- Physiologic neonatal jaundice (impaired conjugation)
- Crigler-Najjar syndrome type I and type II (impaired conjugation)
- Gilbert's syndrome

Hyperbilirubinaemia due to impaired hepatic excretion:

- Dubin-Johnson syndrome
- Rotor syndrome
- Benign intrahepatic cholestasis

CASE: *A 21-years-old college student presented with recurrent history of mild jaundice over last 4 years. Examination did not reveal anything specific. Investigations revealed bilirubin of 2.6 mg, AST normal, ALT normal, P. Time normal, albumin, globulin normal, HBsAg -ve, HCV antibody -ve, ANF negative, Hb electrophoresis– normal, reticulocyte normal, Coomb's test -ve, G-6-PD normal, USG-abdomen– normal. He was reassured that probably this was a cause of Gilbert's syndrome and he need not have to worry about it.*

DIAGNOSIS: Mild recurrent unconjugated hyperbilirubinaemia due to Gilbert's syndrome.

DISCUSSION:

This is a common cause of consultation in the clinic. Although the diagnosis is usually quite apparent from the LFT itself, one needs to rule out other causes of hyperbilirubinaemia as was done in this case.

It is mandatory to routinely check for hepatitis B and hepatitis C profile, autoimmune screening and take a meticulous drug history. In selected cases with appropriate associated clinical findings, metabolic screening for Wilson's disease, haemochromatosis should also be done. In a sizable proportion of cases all investigations may be negative and one should think of the diagnosis of non-alcoholic fatty liver or non- alcoholic steatohepatitis (NASH). This is the most common cause of abnormal liver function test in USA. One should think of this diagnosis in patient with obesity, Type II diabetes mellitus and hyperlipidaemia.

Other causes of fatty liver:

- Protein Calorie Malnutrition
- Drugs- steroids, oestrogen, Amiodarone, tetracycline, valproate, methotrexate, Zidovudine.
- Fatty liver of pregnancy
- Inflammatory bowel disease
- Environmental hepatotoxins

The condition is usually asymptomatic and detected only on routine blood tests. However, occasionally there may be abdominal pain and fullness. Investigations reveal elevated AST and ALT. In latter stages it might progress to cirrhosis with full blown biochemical picture of jaundice, altered albumin-globulin ratio and increased prothrombin time. Many of the cryptogenic cirrhosis may actually be due to NASH. USG abdomen shows fatty infiltration of liver and CT scan shows low-density liver parenchyma, liver biopsy findings are similar to that of alcoholic liver disease. The presence of fibrosis suggests more advanced liver disease.

The condition is managed by meticulous control of blood sugar and lipid levels. Weight reduction improves liver function test. Drugs like gemfibrozil, Vitamin E, metformin have shown promising results. Ursodeoxycholic acid in the dose of 10-15mg/kg body wt for 12 months has been shown to improve the abnormal LFT along with regression of hepatic steatosis. However the long term effect on the disease outcome is not known yet. Once the patient progresses towards cirrhosis, the treatment should be identical to that of end stage chronic liver disease. Meticulous follow up is needed.

The index patient was treated in the similar line as above. Her blood glucose and lipid were controlled meticulously. She was instructed to reduce her weight and she was put on ursodeoxycholic acid. She is under regular follow up and her LFT has improved considerably.

CASE: *A 48-years-old patient presented with jaundice anorexia, abdominal pain and joint pain. His bilirubin was 5.6 mg%, AST (more than ALT), high GGT, high uric acid, ANF negative, HBsAg negative, HCV antibody negative. Ultrasound examination showed hepatomegaly with fatty changes; gastroscopy- antral gastritis but no varix.*

DIAGNOSIS: Alcoholic liver disease.

Alcohol is hepatotoxic and prolonged exposure to alcohol predisposes to chronic liver disease.

Predisposing factors:

- Gender – female are more susceptible
- Amount– Ingestion of 60-80 g/day of alcohols in males, 20-40 g/day of alcohol in females.

1 pint of beer	4 ounce of wine	1 ounce of 80% spirit

- Malnutrition
- Concomitant HCV infection.

Spectrum of illness:

- Fatty liver is reversible if abstinence is followed
- Alcoholic hepatitis may still be reversible
- Cirrhosis of liver is irreversible

Treatment:

- Abstinence.
- Nutritional support.
- Since damage in alcoholic hepatitis is cytokine mediated, glucocorticoid 40 mg/day for 4 wks may be helpful.
- Alternately Pentoxifylline in the dose of 400 mg daily for 4 weeks may also be tried.
- In chronic liver disease, supportive therapy is the only option available.

: KEY POINTS :

- Asymptomatic abnormal LFT is a very common finding in clinical practice.
- Hepatitis B, hepatitis C profile should be checked routinely.
- In selected cases autoimmune screening should also be done.
- A thorough drug history and history of alcohol intake is mandatory.
- NASH is being diagnosed with increasing frequency in our country.
- NASH may progress to cirrhosis.
- Weight reduction, control of diabetes and lipids are the treatment of choice.
- Ursodeoxycholic acid can improve the biochemical parameters.
- NASH can lead to chronic liver disease and even hepatocellular carcinoma.
- Steroids may be helpful in alcoholic hepatitis.

FURTHER REFERENCES:

- Non alcoholic hepatic steatosis- Seminars in liver disease - Paul Angelo *et al*. Vol-21, No 1 2001, Page 81-86.
- Non alcoholic fatty liver disease - Paul Angelo *et al.* NEJM Vol-346, No-16, April 18, 2002, Page 1221-1231.
- Harrison's Principle of Internal Medicine– 17th Edition.

12 A PATIENT WITH FIBROSING ALVEOLITIS

CASE: *A 59-years-old lady presented with persistent cough for last 2 months. She also complained of shortness of breath on exertion along with joint pain. Recently she has been noticing swelling of her legs and increasing tiredness. There was no history of asthma, family history of asthma or any relevant occupational exposure. She was treated with different kinds of antibiotics, diuretics without much improvement. Examination revealed basal crepitations with occasional rhonchi, pulse rate 96/min, BP 140/80 mmHg, pedal oedema present. Liver palpable, JVP slightly elevated. Haematological and biochemical parameters within normal range, ESR was high, LFT normal, ECG snowed sinus bradycardia, echo– LVH with normal systolic function, X-ray chest slightly enlarged heart with bibasilar reticulonodular shadowing, O_2 saturation 96% on room air, resting blood gas showed normal PO_2 and PCO_2. HRCT scan of thorax showed reticulonodular shadowing at both bases with no hilar lymphadenopathy, lung function test showed restrictive pattern of defect. Sputum for AFB for 3 days- negative, auto immune screening- ANF, rheumatoid factor, ANCA all negative.*

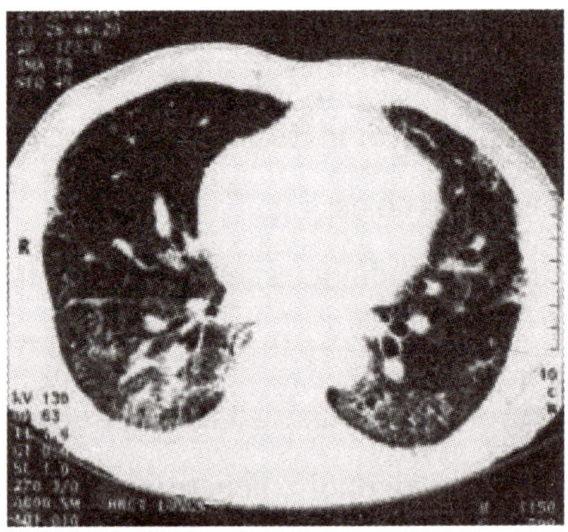

PROVISIONAL DIAGNOSIS: Interstitial fibrosis of the lungs.

DISCUSSION:

The initial presentation of fibrosing alveolitis may be perplexing and the diagnosis is very often not considered in the initial work up. Most of the time cough is considered to be due to chest infection. However, the patient does not respond to antibiotics. Late onset asthma is a common diagnosis made; again they show partial response to inhaler therapy. Cardiac failure is also a common diagnosis made, but they fail to respond to diuretics. Although clubbing is characteristically present in fibrosing alveolitis, in 50% of cases it is absent. Moreover the initial X-ray chest (PA) looks apparently normal.

Common causes of cough which persists in spite of conventional treatment are-

- Post nasal drip because of different nasal conditions
- Allergic asthma and rhinitis
- Gastro oesophageal reflux
- Chronic bronchitis
- Drug induced – ACE inhibitor
- Pulmonary eosinophilia (Common in Indian background)

In viral rhino-sinusitis (common cold) the symptoms respond to 1st generation antihistaminic (with anticholinergic properties) and local ipratropium spray. They usually do not respond well to the newer generation antihistamines as they are devoid of anti cholinergic properties. Post infection persistent cough may need short course of steroid therapy. X-ray of PNS should be done to exclude bacterial sinusitis and if present a course of antibiotics along with local decongestant drop should be given. Cough due to chronic bronchitis should respond to inhaled and oral steroids (In tropical eosinophilia specific anti-filarial therapy should be given for 3 weeks). In allergic rhinitis and asthma, avoidance of specific allergens should also be advised. Gastroesophageal reflux should be treated with proper dietary advice and proton pump inhibitor.

In allergic rhinitis and asthma, the symptoms respond reasonably well to newer generation anti-histaminic and local steroid spray.

Although vast majority of patients will fall in the aforementioned category and will eventually respond, the rest may have persistent symptoms and will need further diagnostic work up. Causes of such cases are-

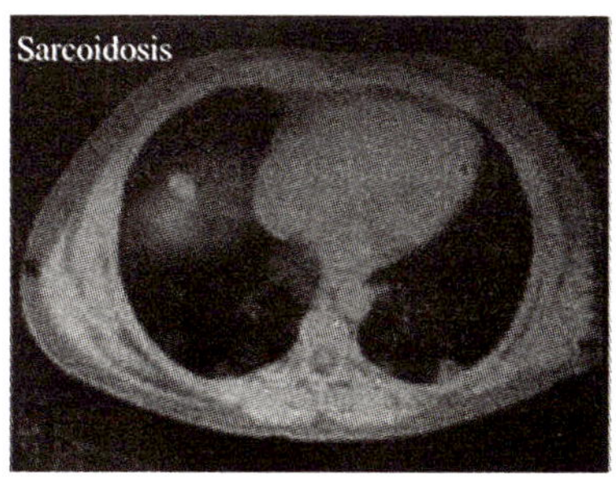

- Interstitial fibrosis of lung
- Bronchogenic carcinoma
- Psychogenic
- Sarcoidosis
- Tubercular infection should always be excluded.

Clinical suspicion of interstitial fibrosis of lung:

- Persistent cough and shortness of breath in a middle aged patient not responding to the above mentioned therapy.
- Generalised symptoms of low-grade fever, myalgia, arthralgia, clubbing (50% of cases).
- Increased CRP, ESR.
- Occasional presence of positive ANF, rheumatoid factor (30%) even in the absence of such conditions.
- Restrictive pattern of defect (with reduction of lung volume) in pulmonary function test. There will be decrease in carbon monoxide diffusing capacity.
- X-ray chest shows bilateral reticular opacities most prominent in the periphery and basal region. Later on there may be honey-combing pattern. Pleural effusion and hilar adenopathy suggest an alternative diagnosis.
- HRCT shows patchy peripheral reticular abnormalities with interlobular linear opacities, septal thickening, and honey combing and traction bronchiectasis.
- Evidence of hypoxemia during graded exercise.
- Final proof by lung biopsy.

Common differential diagnosis:

- Connective tissue disease
- Drugs : gold, carmustine, amiodarone, radiation
- Occupational
- Sarcoidosis
- Eosinophilic granuloma

X-RAY CHEST MIGHT BE HELPFUL IN DIFFERENTIATING SOME OF THE CAUSES:

Predominant upper lobe involvement in X-ray chest.

Connective tissue disorders: Rheumatoid arthritis, ankylosing spondylitis affect the upper lobes.

Occupational lung disease: Silicosis, berylliosis predominantly affect upper lobes.

Sarcoidosis: hilar lymphadenopathy present.

Eosinophilic granuloma: strong history of smoking.

Drugs

LUNG FUNCTION TEST MIGHT BE HELPFUL IN DIFFERENTIAL DIAGNOSIS:

Interstitial lung disease with preservation of lung volume-

- Lymphangioleiomyomatosis
- Sarcoidosis
- Tuberous sclerosis
- Chronic hypersensitivity pneumonitis
- Neurofibromatosis

Many of these causes are rare and the diagnosis will usually be made by a speciality unit rather than the primary care physician.

CAUSES OF DIFFUSE ISOLATED GROUND GLASS OPACITIES:

Opportunistic infections:

- Pneumocystis pneumonia
- CMV pneumonia
- Herpes simplex viral pneumonia
- RSV bronchiolitis

Interstitial lung disease:

- Desquamative interstitial pneumonia
- Respiratory bronchiolitis – associated interstitial lung disease
- Non-specific interstitial pneumonia
- Acute interstitial pneumonia
- Hypersensitivity pneumonitis
- Cryptogenic organizing pneumonia

Alveolar disease:

- Pulmonary oedema
- Diffuse alveolar haemorrhage
- ARDS

Drug toxicity

- Sulphasalazine
- Methotrexate
- Gold
- Busulfan

TREATMENTS:

1. ***Steroids*** – Approximately 40% of the patient will respond to steroid therapy, CT scan findings might indicate whether the patient is going to respond to steroid. It is said that presence of ground glass opacity predicts initial good response whereas presence of honey combing does not. However steroid does not prevent the ultimate progression to irreversible honey comb fibrosis. A trial of steroid for initial 6 months may be given to see the response.

2. ***Cytotoxic drugs*** – Azathioprine may be used as an adjuvant, however they also have limiting side effects like myelo-suppression, secondary cancer and drug induced interstitial pneumonitis.

3. ***Anti-fibrotic agents*** – Drugs like colchicines and penicillamine have been used without much success.

4. ***Other drugs on trial*** – Pirfenidone (an inhibitor of collagen synthesis and fibroblast proliferation). Interferon gamma-1b (immune modulator).

5. ***Lung transplantation*** may be a viable option for a small number of patients under the age of 55 yrs without other complicating illness.

Overall the prognosis is poor for this condition and the median survival for this condition following diagnosis is approximately 3 years.

The patient described above was started on oral steroid (60 mg/day) along with respiratory adjuvant therapy. She had quick symptomatic relief of her cough breathlessness and general unwell being. However the family members were told about the ultimate prognosis of the condition. She is under regular follow up.

Newer treatment option:

Recently 3 trial up INPULSIS-1 and INPULSIS-2, ASCEND and PANTHER-1 PE trials have accessed the role of nintedanib (an antifibrotic agent working through tyrosine kinase inhibitor), pirfenidone (an antifibrotic agent) and N-acetylcysteine along with azathioprine and prednisolone respectively have been accessed in the treatment of idiopathic fibrosis of lungs. Both nintedanib and pirfenidone have been shown to ↓ the fall of FVC and ↑ in excess tolerance if used in the initial stages of the disease. However, N-acetylcysteine failed to show any significant improvement in patients with idiopathic fibrosis of the lungs. It is now clear that idiopathic fibrosis of lungs is due to aberration of wound healing rather than primarily perpetration of ongoing lung inflammation.

: KEY POINTS :

- Cough is a common presentation in clinical practice.
- Common cold responds better with 1st generation antihistaminic because of their anticholinergic properties, whereas allergic cough responds better to the newer generation antihistaminic.
- Differential diagnosis of persistent cough is long and one should take a thorough history of allergy, drug intake, smoking, occupational exposure etc.
- Fibrosing alveolitis is an uncommon cause of persistent cough.
- Fibrosing alveolitis should be considered in the differential diagnosis of persistent cough, breathlessness, clubbing and apparently normal looking X-ray chest. Steroid may be helpful initially but the ultimate prognosis of fibrosing alveolitis is poor.

FURTHER REFERENCES:

- T J Gross et al, Idiopathic pulmonary fibrosis – NEJM Vol 345 No. 7, August 16-2001, P 517 - 525.
- J Rajgopal, A 58 year old man with interstitial pulmonary disease – NEJM Vol 347 No. 16 Oct 17 2002, P 1262 – 1265.
- R. S. Eridin, The diagnosis and treatment of cough – NEJM Vol 343 No. 23, Dec 2000, 1715 – 1721.
- Gary M: Hunning Hake NEJM- May 2014:370:2142-2143.
- NEJM June 2014 – 370: 25 21 – 25 30 – Case records – A 65 years old man with dyspnoea and progressed lung disease.
- Harrison's Principle of Internal Medicine – 17th edition.
- Oxford Text Book of Medicine – 5th edition.

13 A PATIENT WITH SEPTIC SHOCK

CASE: *A 58-years-old diabetic female was admitted with fever, abdominal pain and jaundice (investigation revealed obstructive jaundice). ERCP confirmed presence of stone in CBD with dilated CBD, however stone extraction was technically difficult and eventually the patient underwent open cholecystectomy with exploration of CBD. The operation was lengthy but uneventful. In the second post operative day, her BP was found to be low and the urine output was less. She had one episode of fever with shivering on the previous night (1st post operative day). Since the fluid challenge produced suboptimal result and the patient had a tachycardia (130/min) the ITU team was called in and the patient was transferred to the ITU.*

Investigations revealed: WBC- 25,000, 90% poly, creatinine- 2.4 mg%, urea- 116 mg%, glucose- 416 mg%, bilirubin- 3.4 mg%, SGPT- 240, lactic acid- 4.2 mg%, PO_2- 78 mmHg, CO_2- 31 mmHg, base excess– 10.6, pH- 7.2, urine- trace of ketones, SVO_2- 64%, CVP- 1 mmHg, X-ray chest (PA) normal, USG abdomen- no obvious collection.

PROVISIONAL DIAGNOSIS: Septic shock.

DISCUSSION:

Although clinical features of sepsis in general is quite well known like fever, tachycardia, increased respiratory rate, falling urine output, leucocytosis or leukopenia, it was not associated with any infection. These features occur as an immune mechanism to any insult to the body and was called **"systemic inflammatory response syndrome" (SIRS).** SIRS caused by any infection is called ***sepsis.***

Sepsis and septic shock are common causes of morbidity and mortality in hospital practice. Each year 750,000 patients develop sepsis related complication in the USA and is the most common cause of non-cardiac deaths in ITU. Many times the diagnosis is delayed so prompt resuscitative measures are not taken in appropriate time which could have been life saving. In post operative cases which are mainly treated in the general ward, lack of awareness amongst the junior medical and nursing staff are one of the reasons of delayed diagnosis of sepsis and septic related complication and when the diagnosis is eventually made, organ dysfunction, starts setting in. Prompt diagnosis with the help of early warning sign in general wards is the way forward to detect the condition early.

Early warning system (EWS):

By measuring simple ward based parameters like heart rate, respiratory rate, BP, temperature and CNS status, one can reliably predict who are the patients at risk of deterioration and prompt intervention can be called for.

[Heart rate < 40 or >130 per minute, systolic BP less than 70 or more than 200 mmHg, respiratory rate less than 8 per minute or more than 30 per minute, temperature less than 35.0°C or more than 37.7°C, deteriorating sensorium – are the warning signs of impending decompensation]. Although not validated as yet, may still be used in day to day clinical practice.

Initial resuscitation (1st 6 Hours)

CVP – 8-12 mmHg

Mean arterial pressure MAP ≥ 65 mmHg

Urine output ≥ 0.5 ml/kg – 1 Hr

S.V.C or Mixed venous oxygen saturation - > 70% or ≥ 65% respectively.

DEFINITIONS:

Systemic Inflammatory response syndrome (SIRS)

- Temperature >38°C or <36°C
- Heart rate > 90/min
- Respiratory rate > 20/min or $PaCO_2$ < 32 mm/Hg
- WBC > 12,000 or < 4000
- Immature band forms

Systemic inflammatory response syndrome may be due to various causes like:

a) Pancreatitis

b) Ischemia

c) Multiple trauma

d) Haemorrhagic shock

e) Infections

Sepsis – When SIRS is due to an infection we call it sepsis.

Severe Sepsis – Defined as sepsis associated with hypotension or organ dysfunction. It is usually associated with oliguria, lactic acidosis and alteration of mental state.

Sepsis induced hypotension – Defined by the presence of BP of less than 5th percentile of normal for age or its reduction of 30% or more from the baseline in the absence of other causes for hypotension (e.g. cardiogenic shock).

Septic Shock – Defined as sepsis induced severe hypotension resistant to fluid resuscitation along with presence of hypo perfusion abnormalities or organ dysfunctions.

Multiple organ dysfunction syndromes (MODS) – Different scoring systems are available to detect failing organ systems (cardiac, respiratory, haematological, gastrointestinal, hepatobiliary and renal).

The prognosis worsens with the increase in number of organ-failure.

Although in its full blown form, it is quite easy to diagnose, the real challenge is to detect in the early phase where quick corrective measure can prevent further degeneration to full blown sepsis and MODS which has a very high mortality rate. Since many of the evolutionary sepsis would occur in the general wards following an operative intervention or any intervention like (urinary catheterisation, CVP line insertion), there should be certain guidelines in the ward which would facilitate early detection of sepsis.

GENERAL PRINCIPLE OF MANAGEMENT:

Although prognosis of septic shock remains poor, over the past few years certain interventions have shown to improve the outcome to certain extent. Some of the interventions will be mentioned over here.

1. Fluid therapy – early goal direct therapy:

It has been shown that early resuscitative measures in the first 6 hours of sepsis may alter the prognosis. This includes vigorous fluid resuscitation with colloids / crystalloids, early inotropic and vasoconstrictor therapy and blood transfusion if necessary. Enteral nutrition rather than TPN is suggested as the verified method of choice which may be supplemented by IV Glucose or TPN if needed. The end point of resuscitation is not merely the clinical parameters like BP, pulse, CVP, urinary output but other physiological indicators of tissue perfusion like lactate level (high level indicates tissue hypoxia) and mixed venous O_2 saturation (blood drawn from central venous line for O_2 saturation. More than 70% indicates adequate tissue oxygenation and low SVO_2 indicates increased O_2 extraction in the peripheral tissues with subsequent low SVO_2 in the venous return). This again indicates the importance of strict vigilance of at-risk patients in the general wards.

Which fluid?

The debate regarding the correct choice of fluid still continues. Crystalloids have to be used for initial fluid resuscitation. However, the general opinion is in favour of crystalloids than colloids. Colloids with high molecular weight must be avoided. Albumin may be used in selected cases.

2. Choosing of right antibiotics:

In many occasions the initial antibiotics is chosen on empirical basis pending the culture reports from different body fluids. If the initial choice of antibiotic is right, the outcome of patient is better compared to those patients where antibiotics need changing following the receipt of the culture sensitivity report. The clinician should be aware of probable site of sepsis and most likely causative organism. The antibiotic sensitivity pattern of that hospital has also to be taken into account. To commence one or two antibiotic therapy as soon as possible is important as each hour delay in institution of therapy will cause increase in mortality.

Procalcitonin may be used to assess regarding the discontinuation of antibiotic therapy. Common organisms detected in different site of infection are:

a) **Urosepsis** - **Gram negative organisms**

b) **Billiary Sepsis** - **Gram negative, anaerobes.**

c) **Intra abdominal sepsis** - **Gram negative, anaerobes.**

d) **Chest infection** - **Community acquired (*H influenza*, *Pneumococcus*, *Moraxella***

- **Hospital acquired (Gram negative, MRSA)**

e) **Soft tissue infection** - ***Staphylococcus, Streptococcus***

f) **Central line infection** - ***Staphylococcus, Pseudomonas, Candida.***

Combination of antibiotics may be needed with aminoglycosides, quinolones *etc.* depending upon the culture, sensitivity report and severity of the case.

While treating, blood culture is mandatory. We have isolated 15 cases of Candida septicaemia in patients with severe sepsis with intermittent fever who finally responded to antifungal therapy (5 patients died, 6 patients responded to IV fluconazole, 4 patients responded to IV Amphotericin). At risk patients for fungal septicaemia need ***prolonged ITU stay, multiple antibiotics for prolonged period and long term catheterization.***

3. Controlling blood glucose:

Intensive control of blood glucose at a level of 80-120 mg% has been shown to improve the outcome. This is a difficult task because of insulin resistance in infected patients. Moreover, other manoeuvres like parenteral nutrition, inotropes, steroid therapy sometimes make this task unachievable. The recommendation was based on the "Van den Berg" study performed in a surgical ITU. However, since then many other studies like

NICE-SUGAR Study and two meta-analysis have shown that intensive control of blood glucose may be more harmful in view of increased incidence of hypoglycaemia and at present the recommended target of blood glucose is less than 180 mg% (SSC guidelines 2008).

The practical goal should be to control the glucose as meticulous as possible without risking severe hypoglycaemia. The target of blood glucose should be around 180 mg% rather than 110 mg% as proposed earlier.

4. Steroid therapy:

Low dose steroid therapy (physiological supplement) – 50 mg four times daily 7 days particularly in those patients with relative adrenal insufficiency has been shown to decrease the dose of vasopressor requirement and improve the outcome. Since the benefit is only observed in patients with adrenal insufficiency, adrenal function test should be performed prior to the commencement of steroid. A baseline cortisol level less than 14 microgram/dl and increase of cortisol one hour following IM synacthen 250 microgram, less than 9 microgram/dl may be an indication of commencement of steroid. Practical problem in India is frequent non-availability of synacthen (Synacthen ACTH). In these instances baseline random cortisol may be used for decision regarding steroid therapy. Steroids put blood glucose out of gear and very high doses of insulin (to the tune of 120-150 units/day) may be required to maintain blood glucose at optimal level. This recommendation was based on the ANNANE study. However other studies including CORTICUS study have shown that steroid may be more harmful than beneficial and at present the guideline is to use steroid only in patients of vasopressor resistant hypotension (SSC guideline 2008).

5. Lung protective ventilation:

Many of these patients develop acute lung injury and ARDS as a part of multi-organ dysfunction syndrome and need ventilator support. The ***criteria for ALI/ARDS are:***

a) Bilateral Pulmonary infiltrates

b) PaO_2/FiO_2 < **300 in ALI** (Acute lung injury)

< **200 in ARDS** (Acute respiratory distress syndrome)

c) Pulmonary artery occlusion pressure < 18 mmHg (thereby excluding LV failure).

ARDS has a uniformly bad prognosis with a high mortality rate. Recently adopted newer ventilatory strategies have shown to improve the outcome. These are:

- ***Low tidal volume ventilation** – The traditional high tidal volume ventilation (Tidal volume 10-12 ml/kg)* has been shown to be associated with volume associated lung injury due to repeated opening and closing of the alveoli at high volume and thereby liberation of cytokines which perpetrates the cascade of sepsis. Recent study has shown that ventilating at a *low tidal volume (5-6 ml/kg)* was associated with significantly better outcome.
- ***PEEP*** – Addition of PEEP, titrating according to the hemodynamic response and oxygenation alters the prognosis of ARDS. It acts by opening up of collapsed alveoli thereby preventing liberation of cytokines.
- ***Lung recruitment manoeuvres*** – Also help in prevention of alveolar collapse and improvement of tissue oxygenation.

6. Blood transfusion:

Restrictive vs. Liberal blood transfusion: Although traditional approach is to keep Hb above 10 g%, recent studies have shown that restrictive transfusion approach to keep the Hb level at around 8 g% is better than to aim at Hb of > 10 g%. Patients with active bleeding and with ischaemic heart disease are two exceptions to this restrictive approach.

7. Renal replacement therapy:

About 5% of the patient will need renal replacement therapy. [Option includes intermittent dialysis and continuous renal replacement therapy (CRRT). The latter offers number of theoretical advantages including better fluid management, less haemodynamic variability and more stable metabolic control].

8. Specific therapy:

Use of activated protein C (APC)

The treatment described so far, is mainly supportive and has nothing to do with the basic mechanism and pathogenesis of the disease. Inflammatory cytokines activate procoagulant activators and initiate fibrinolysis. Endogenous activated protein C is a regulator of inflammation, coagulation and fibrinolysis and its production may be impaired in sepsis. Administration of APC in septic patients inhibits inflammation, coagulation and fibrinolysis. In PROWESS study, recombinant human activated protein C was shown to a) reduce mortality, b) decrease in vasopressor requirement and c) improvement in ventilator free days. The mortality benefit was observed from day 4 and becomes statistically significant from day 14.

This is the only fruitful treatment available aiming at the basic pathological mechanism of the disease. Main deterrent to its use is its prohibitive cost in an already heavily burdened critically ill patient.

Main problem encountered is bleeding. Contraindications to APC are low platelet counts, major surgery within 12 hours, recent gastro intestinal bleeding, pregnancy and breast feeding. Patients with sepsis and MODS should be accessed for APC therapy and this treatment option should be discussed with the relatives. Since the publication of PROWESS study further studies published later on fail to show any beneficial effect of APC, on the contrary it was shown to be rather harmful. As a result APC therapy has been withdrawn from 2008 Surviving Sepsis guideline-2008, as a method of treatment in the management of sepsis.

9. Haemodynamic management:

Haemodynamically sepsis is characterised by reduced peripheral vascular resistance and low cardiac index (initially the cardiac index may be high) and frequently vasopressor and inotropes are needed for resuscitation.

- Dobutamine (β stimulation) is commonly used to increase stroke volume.
- Noradrenaline (alpha stimulation) is a very effective vasopressor in sepsis. It also increases the urinary output by maintaining the mean arterial pressure.
- Combination of dobutamine (to increase stroke volume) and noradrenaline (as a vasopressor) is very useful in septic patients.
- Dopamine – can be used as vasopressor. It is cheap compared to other drugs which are an added advantage in India. Low dose dopamine commonly used to increase urinary output is not generally practised any more. No doubt it increases urinary output, but does not alter renal function. Moreover it has other adverse immunological effects.
- Adrenaline (alpha and beta stimulant) – can also be used as vasopressor and inotropes. It can cause lactic acidosis.
- Recently vasopressin in low dose has been used as a vasopressor in septic patients.

In clinical practice combination of dobutamine and noradrenaline are the most frequently used drugs that are used in septic shock.

10. Nutrition:

Enteral nutrition is the preferred route in septic patients as it maintains the gut mucosal integrity and thus prevents bacterial translocation from gut mucosa to portal circulation. However in many cases it is not possible to pursue with enteral nutrition because of intestinal obstruction, fistula or peritonitis. In those cases parenteral nutrition should be used with particular attention given to:

- Calorie requirement– 30-35 kcal/kg in septic patients.
- Appropriate protein supplementation – as there is catabolism of muscle protein at an early stage.
- Immuno-nutrition– It has been suggested that addition of certain immuno-nutrients like glutamine, arginine, fish oil might improve prognosis by maintaining mucosal integrity. Debate is still on about their utility.
- Supplementation of trace elements is important as in prolonged sepsis deficiency of certain trace elements may cause serious problems.
- Prokinetics like mosapride and erythromycin are frequently required in case of gut hypomotility, a common accompaniment in an enterally fed septic patient.

11. Stress ulcer prophylaxis:

Acute G.I. bleeding is common in septic patients. Routinely these patients should be given stress ulcer prophylaxis with either mucosal protective agent like sucralfate or H_2 blocker like ranitidine or proton-pump inhibitors like pantoprazole. Theoretically sucralfate is preferred as the other two agents cause gastric acid suppression and enhanced proliferation of endogenous gastric micro flora which may ultimately colonise in the oropharynx and cause nosocomial pneumonia by way of aspiration. GI bleeding is more common with sucralfate than the other two agents; however, clinical judgement is needed regarding the choice of the appropriate agents.

12. DVT prophylaxis:

Asymptomatic DVT is common in severely ill septic patients who are bed bound for prolonged period. The real danger is that of fatal pulmonary embolism which might strike suddenly without any warning sign. Prophylactic measures must be taken in the form of –

- Elastic stocking
- Thromboprophylaxis with either heparin or low molecular weight heparin.

In high risk patients combination of both will be required. Since many of the patients have sepsis induced coagulopathy, thromboprophylaxis has to be used with caution.

The index patient was immediately transferred to ITU. Fluid resuscitation under CVP guidance was done with crystalloids. She received dobutamine and noradrenaline. Her glucose was controlled with continuous IV insulin infusion. She was started empirically with meropenem (her blood culture report subsequently showed growth of ESBL producing *E. coli* sensitive to meropenem). Her base line cortisol level was normal so she was not given hydrocortisone. Her Hb was 7 g% and she was given 2 units of blood. She was assessed for consideration of APC but because of her financial constraints it was not given. Fortunately she responded to the supportive therapy and finally transferred out of the ITU after 7th day.

With the advent of new therapeutic modulations in ITU with invasive gadgets, the mortality of critically ill patients is definitely decreasing over the decades. However, it is leaving one problem in its trail that is sepsis. The incidence of sepsis is increasing in critically ill patients with a high mortality if not detected in the nick of time. To increase the awareness "The Surviving Sepsis Guideline" was initiated by a group of experts representing II organizations to make an early diagnosis in order to reduce mortality. The first guideline was published in 2004, revised in 2008 with the last revision in 2012. The initial discussion is based on the 2004 guidelines with the excerpts of the recommendation in 2012 later on.

13. Vasopressors, Inotropes & Steroid.

- **Vasopressors**
  - Nor epinephrine is the drug of choice. Epinephrine may be used as single agent or as an additional agent.
  - Vasopressin (0.03 units/minute) can also be added or substituted.
  - Dopamine should not be used as a renal protective agent (it may be used as vasopressor).

- **Inotropes therapy**

Dobutamine may be added to the vasopressor in the presence of myocardial dysfunction. Achievement for supra normal cardiac index is not indicated.

- **Corticosteroid**

Should only be used in the dose of 200-300 mg/day if vasopressor and fluid therapy fail to maintain BP (septic shock).

13. Mechanical ventilation

To use low tidal volume ventilator i.e. 6 ml/kg.

14. Sedation, analgesic and neuromuscular blockade (NMBA)

To use sedation either as interrupted infusion (with wakeup call) or continuous infusion with daily wakeup calls. Agents used: - 1) Midazolam, 2) Propofol, 3) α_2-agonist dexmedetomidine.

Neuromuscular blocking agents should be avoided as much as possible. In ARDS, NMBA may be used for not more than 48 Hrs.

15. Other recommendations

- Blood product administration

  Erythropoietin, Antithrombin III - not recommend

  Platelet transfusion- If platelet count is less than 5000 or the count is between 10000-30000 and where the bleeding risk is high. FFP should not be routinely transfused.

- Source control
- DVT prophylaxis
- Stress ulcer prophylaxis
- Consideration after limitation of life support

It will be noticed that in the current recommendation there have been some important changes like:

- APC is fallen out of vogue in further studies did not corroborate the findings of previous study that showed mortality benefit.
- Colloids need to be avoided as the initial resuscitation fluid
- Steroids should only be used in septic shock
- The target of glucose control will be around 180 mg% rather than 110 mg%
- Duration of antibiotic therapy should be monitored by inflammatory markers like procalcitonin.

The concept of bundle therapy

In order to monitor the compliance of the recommendation, for comparative study, audit and to measurement of outcome, it has been proposed to divide the guideline into two bundles:

1) Resuscitation bundle (within 6 hrs) composed of
   - Blood tests like lactate
   - Antibiotic administration
   - Fluid management with CVP, SvO_2 measurement
   - Using vasopressors, inotropes
2) Management bundle
   - Administration of steroid
   - Maintenance of Glucose
   - Maintaining plateau pressure of less than 30 cm of H_2O

Studies have already shown that compliance with each bundle improves survival of patients with sepsis significantly in western countries.

However a study in 17 Asian countries (which also included some centres from India) (MOSIAC) has shown that compliance in the majority of the Asian countries is poor and it has been suggested that in the poor countries the most important parameters that should be paid attention to are - 1) Blood culture, 2) Appropriate fluid management and 3) Appropriate antibiotics as soon as possible.

PERSONAL EXPERIENCE:

On behalf of the medical consortium (a group of medical practitioner practising independently of which the author is a member) a one day point prevalence study along with an audit regarding the compliance of 'BUNDLE' in 10 tertiary ITUs in Kolkata [9 of them corporate sector hospitals and 1 Govt Hospital] was conducted on 18th December 2012.

Total number of patients studies on that day (18.12.2012) – 197

Sepsis diagnosed – 66

Source of sepsis:

Chest – 60%, UTI – 20%, skin/ soft tissue – 7%, device/ blood stream – 7%, others – 6%.

Compliance with 6 hr Bundle

Blood culture within 2 hr –71%

Lactate measurement – 33%

Antibiotic within 1 Hr – 93%

Fluid treatment – 100%

SvO_2 measurement – 21%

CVP measures – 63%

Blood transfusion needed – 30%

Vasopressor needed – 45%

Urine output measured – 80%

Compliance with 24 hr Bundle

Steroid therapy given – 70%

Glucose controlled appropriately – 82%

Ventilated appropriately – 90%

It is evident that the tertiary hospitals of Kolkata are doing well as far as the compliance to the bundles is concerned. However this kind of audit is needed to see how the secondary tier ITU's are doing, in order to translate the therapy into actual mortality benefit.

In my opinion each ITU must have a chart of the bundles and all staff should be geared to audit it regularly in the day to day practice.

CASE: *A 39-years-old gentleman was transferred from another medical facility with a history of persistent fever following an episode of acute pancreatitis. He had received imipenem and linezolid along with TPN for the last few days. His WBC count was 23,000 with poly of 91%, urea & creatinine raised, liver enzymes were altered, CRP high, procalcitonin high. In view of high risk factors for invasive fungal infection, he was started on caspofungin. Blood culture report received after 72 hours showed growth of Candida albicans. Within another 48 hours, his temperature remitted and finally went home uneventfully.*

DIAGNOSIS: Invasive fungal infection with sepsis in a high risk patient.

DISCUSSION:

Fungal infections are now-a-days increasingly detected in clinical practice particularly in high risk patients. Common invasive fungal infections commonly encountered in clinical practice are *Candida* species (Yeast) and *Aspergillus* species (mould). However other fungal infections like mucormycosis, cryptococcosis, *Fusarium* species and *Scedosporium* species are occasionally encountered in clinical practice in high risk susceptible hosts. As far as the *Candida* infection is concerned, approximately 50% of infections are due to *Candida* non-albicans group of organisms like *C. tropicalis, C. glabrata, C. krusei, C. lusitaniae, C. guilliermondii, C. parapsilosis etc.* and many of which are resistant to fluconazole.

The common risk factors for *Candida* infections are-

- ICU stay
- immunosuppression
- chronic liver disease and renal failure
- central venous catheter
- neutropenia, acute pancreatitis
- recent GI surgery *etc.*

Risk factors for Aspergillosis are-

- neutropenia
- bone marrow transplantation
- COPD
- steroid therapy

DIAGNOSIS:

- Blood culture
- Radiological test like CT scan of thorax [Halo sign in case of Aspergillosis]

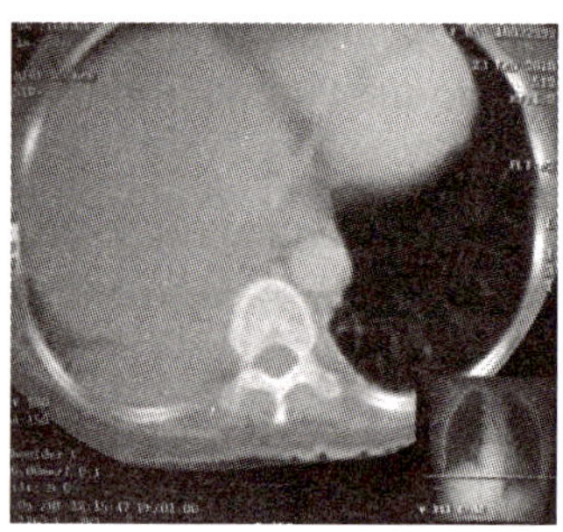

- Serological tests like:
    - D-Glucan test in Candida, Aspergillosis
    - Galactomannan test – in Aspergillosis only
        - Has good negative predictive value
        - May be false positive in patients on piperacillin-tazobactam

Clinical suspicion is the sheet anchor in the diagnosis of *Candida* infection.

This is based on Candida Score with the following criteria like:

TPN -1
Surgery -1
Multifocal colonization – 1
Severe sepsis – 2

A cut off valve of more than 2.5 will help the clinician to highly suspect *Candida* infection.

DRUG THERAPY FOR EMPIRIC TREATMENT FOR CANDIDAEMIA IN ITU:

- **Fluconazole** – 800 mg loading followed by 400 mg daily (in fluconazole susceptive patients)
- **Echinocandin** – received in patients with severe sepsis, known resistance to fluconazole and for the patients who received fluconazole in the recent past.

The treatment should be carried out at least 14 days following the blood culture becoming negative. In blood culture negative patients, the treatment should be carried out until there is defervescence.

For invasive Aspergillosis:

Voriconazole or liposomal amphotericin may be used. Other second line agents that can be used are caspofungin, micafungin, posaconazole, itraconazole.

- In case of *Zygomycosis*, *Mucor mycosis* amphotericin is the drug of choice whereas posaconazole may be used as an alternative salvage therapy.
- In fusariosis, voriconazole is the drug of choice.
- In *Scedosporium*, voriconazole has been used successfully.

Risk factors for *Mucor*

- IDDM
- Renal failure
- Nephrotic syndrome
- Steroid therapy

Drug interaction of voriconazole:

Voriconazole has many drug interactions with some antiepileptics and antitubercular drugs and clinicians should be aware of it.

The index patient was a high risk patient for Candida infection as judged by the Candida score which was corroborated by +ve blood culture report which came later on.

Fortunately, empirical antifungal therapy was instituted early in view of presence of high risk factor to which the patient responded favourably.

: KEY POINTS :

- Sepsis is a common condition in hospital practice.
- Diagnosis is often delayed in the general ward.
- Fever, hypotension and decreased urinary output in a post operative patient should point to the diagnosis of sepsis.
- Early warning scoring in the general ward might help detect sepsis early.
- Prompt resuscitation might improve the prognosis.
- Surviving sepsis campaign guideline has been updated in 2012.
- Adherence to specific bundles of SSC improves survival.
- Fungal infection is emerging as an important cause of sepsis in high risk patients.

FURTHER REFERENCES:

- Hotchkiss RS, Karlle: The Pathophysiology and Treatment of Sepsis – NEJM 348; 138, 2003.
- Rivers et al.: Early goal directed therapy in the treatment of severe sepsis and Septic shock – NEJM 345; 1368, 2003.
- Harrison's Principle of Internal Medicine 17th edition
- Oxford Book of Medicine 5th edition
- Surviving sepsis guideline 2008.

14 THREE CASES OF THROMBOCYTOPENIA

CASE: *A 53 years old gentleman presented with history of purpuric spots in the body and he was also complaining of headache and vomiting. Investigations revealed platelet count of 14,000, CT Brain scan revealed cerebellar haematoma, autoimmune screening was negative. Bone marrow examination was consistent with idiopathic thrombocytopenic purpura.*

DIAGNOSIS: ITP with cerebral bleeding.

He was urgently treated in ITU with IV gamma globulin, IV methyl prednisolone (both for five days), followed by high dose of oral prednisolone. He also needed platelet infusion for first few days. His cerebral lesion was treated conservatively and after prolonged hospital stay, he was discharged home and at present is on remission without any steroid therapy.

CASE: *A 56 years old gentleman, husband of one of our staff nurses presented in the clinic with one week history of headache. He was known hypertensive. There were other associated symptoms, although clinically a diagnosis of migraine was made, a CT scan was requested for to exclude any intracranial pathology.*
To our surprise, CT scan showed multiple interlobar haematomas. He was urgently admitted in ITU for further management.

[Multiple interlobar haemorrhages are unusual in case of hypertensive bleeding. It usually indicates: a) trauma b) coagulation abnormalities c) amyloid angiopathy etc.

We were even more surprised when our haematologist rang up with the report of Hb- 7 g%, WBC- 36,000 with immature white cells, (promyelocytes) and a platelet count of 11,000 & coagulation profile showed raised FDPs, prothrombin time and APTT. An urgent bone marrow examination revealed the diagnosis of acute myeloid leukaemia M_3 variety.

DIAGNOSIS:

- Cerebral bleeding due to thrombocytopenia due to M3 variety of acute myeloid leukaemia.
- DIC.

He was treated with blood transfusion. Haematologist started him on ATRA (tretinoin), a retinoic acid derivative; in combination with daunorubicin & dexamethasone and supportive therapy with platelet and FFP infusion. M_3 variety of AML is a biologically distinct disease with typical clinical and morphological features. DIC is a characteristic feature and patients usually respond favourably with ATRA. This patient likewise showed a good initial haematological response but finally succumbed to the cerebral injury.

CASE: *An 11 years old girl was transferred from another district hospital where she presented with weakness, mild jaundice and progressively increasing renal impairment. Before transfer she also developed purpuric spots. Investigation revealed Hb- 7 g%, WBC- 16,000, platelet- 16,000, LDH- high, bilirubin- 4.2 mg% (mostly unconjugated), Coomb's test negative with high reticulocyte count, high urea and creatinine. Blood film showed microangiopathic picture. Coagulation profile showed slightly prolonged PT, APTT, TT and some increase in FDPs.*

DIAGNOSIS: Haemolytic uraemic syndrome.

She was treated with blood and platelet transfusion, regular fresh frozen plasma infusion, steroids and received several cycles of peritoneal dialysis. After a prolonged stay, she recovered completely and was discharged in a stable state. [This case will be discussed in detail later on]

CASE: *A 13 years old boy was admitted with a 5 days history of fever, joint pain, abdominal pain and purpuric rash mainly in his lower extremities. Blood tests showed normal Hb, WBC and platelet count. ASO titre, rheumatoid factor, ANF was negative. Urine test showed few RBCs (5-6 /field).*

DIAGNOSIS: Henoch Schonlein purpura (Non thrombocytopenic purpura)

He was treated with antibiotics, non steroidal anti inflammatory drugs and a short course of steroid with prompt improvement. Follow up reports did not reveal any microscopic haematuria.

[Purpuric rash may be present with normal platelet count, like in this case and in some cases of vasculitis or drug related side effects. In elderly, vitamin C deficiency and steroid therapy should also be considered. The clinician should be aware of it and do appropriate tests].

Common cause of thrombocytopenia (encountered in clinical practice)

- Infective causes - Viral fever, Dengue fever, Malaria.
- Auto Immune - ITP
- Drugs - Thiazide, quinine, heparin, leflunomide, frusemide, antibiotic like linezolid, anti-neoplastic drugs, *via* bone marrow suppression.

- Bone marrow suppression - Myelodysplastic syndrome, Lymphoproliferative disorders, Leukaemia, Anti neoplastic drugs.
- Hypersplenism - Chronic liver disease with portal Hypertension, Felty's syndrome.
- Due to increased consumption - D.I.C mainly seen in ITU patients with septicaemia,

  * Obstetric emergencies like HELLP syndrome,

  * Microangiopathic anaemia like HUS, TTP.

Management Scheme for ITP:

If the patient presents with a platelet count of less than 20,000, it is a life threatening condition and emergency management should be instituted.

Drugs commonly used are: -

- IV gamma globulin (400 g/kg/day for 3-5 days)
- IV methyl prednisolone (maximum 1 g/day for 3-5 days)
- Anti D immunoglobulin
- Inj. Vincristine IV may be added to the regime
- Platelet transfusion may also be needed in desperate emergency situations.

Newer drugs:

Platelet stimulators-

Romiplostim is a fusion protein analog of thrombopoietin, a hormone that regulates platelet production.

Eltrombopag is an agonist of the c-mpl receptor, which is the physiological target of the hormone thrombopoietin.

If the platelet count is between 20,000 and 30,000 oral prednisolone (1 - 1.5 mg/kg) may be used. Clinical judgement will be necessary regarding the use of IV gamma globulin or methyl prednisolone in this situation. If the platelet count is more than 50,000, then oral prednisolone will be sufficient to treat the condition. In children, since the disease is self limiting in most of the cases, watchful waiting is all that is required. However, if the platelet count is less than 20,000 IV gamma globulin or anti D-immunoglobulin may be used. Short term oral steroids can also be used keeping in mind the side effects of steroid in the children population.

Once the platelet counts goes above 50,000 the dose of steroid can be tapered off and finally discontinued.

In spite of successful treatment a sizable number of patients will relapse. In these patients additional therapy like danazol or dapsone may be tried. However, splenectomy is the most appropriate step in the event of relapse and should be discussed with the patients.

Approximately 30-40% of adults does not have a response to splenectomy or have a relapse after the surgery. These patients are generally treated with prednisolone with addition of danazol or dapsone. Anti D-immunoglobulin should not be used in these patients.

Immunosuppressive therapy should be reserved for those patients whose platelets count remains as low as 20,000 or the patients are intolerant to the other regime. The drugs common used are:

- Azathioprine: 1-4 mg/kg or cyclophosphamide – orally (1-2 mg/kg/day or IV).
- Cyclophosphamide pulsed therapy every 4 weeks (1-1.5 mg/square meter of the body surface area). These drugs are toxic and regular haematological and biochemical follow up will be necessary.
- Cyclosporine.
- Immunomodulator – Interferon, Colchicine.

In pregnancy complicated with life threatening thrombocytopenia, IV gamma globulin can be safely used. One has to be watchful of the adverse effects of steroids during pregnancy. Other causes of thrombocytopenia like HELLP syndrome should be borne in mind. Epidural anaesthesia should be avoided if the platelet count is less than 100,000. New born babies should be checked for low platelet count as 10% of the babies will be affected with thrombocytopenia.

TREATMENT:

Reticuloendothelial blockade with high dose intravenous immunoglobulin (1 g/kg over 6 hours) in two consecutive days or anti D in rhesus positive patients (75 g/kg) will work very rapidly with those steroids in 80% of cases. The peak action is within 7 days which may last for 4-8 weeks.

Second line therapies like danazol, vincristine or vinblastine as well as azathioprine may be used in recalcitrant cases.

Other agents that may be considered in refractory cases are thrombopoietin stimulating agents like romiplostim and eltrombopag as well as monoclonal anti-CD20 antibody that targets B cells like rituximab may also be considered.

CASE: *A 68 years old male hypertensive and friable patient presented with anorexia, nausea and presence of purpuric spots in the body. Investigations revealed normal platelet count along with normal coagulation profile. His urea was 140 mg% with a creatinine of 5.2 mg%, ANF and ANCA was -ve. His Hb was 8.1 g% with a WBC count of 7,800/min.*

DIAGNOSIS: Chronic renal failure with qualitative functional platelet defect.

DISCUSSION:

Abnormalities in platelet function is occasionally encountered in clinical practice where there is evidence of easy bruising, epistaxis and other bleeding episodes presenting with normal platelet count and normal coagulation profile. Platelet function tests will help making a diagnosis.

: KEY POINTS :

- Purpuric spots are common presentation in clinical practice and thrombocytopenia needs to be excluded.
- In thrombocytopenia infection, autoimmune, drugs and bone marrow suppression should be considered.
- If platelet counts are normal then drug, rash, vasculitis and senile purpura are the possible causes.
- In multiple interlobar haematomas of brain coagulation abnormalities should be excluded.

FURTHER REFERENCES:

- Guidelines for the investigation and management of idiopathic thrombocytopenic purpura in adult, children and pregnancy – Br. Journal of Haematology, 120-574, 2003.
- Harrison's Principle of Internal Medicine 17th edition.
- Oxford Book of Medicine 5th edition.

15 FOUR PATIENTS PRESENTING WITH ASCITES

CASE: *A 38 years old female presented with abdominal pain and low grade intermittent fever for last 6 months. She also had menstrual irregularities. Examination revealed mild ascites. Investigations showed Hb- 8 g%, ESR-110, CA125- raised, LFT normal, ascitic fluid analysis - high protein content, LDH-raised, AFB and gram stain negative, cells 50/field - mostly lymphocytes. No malignant cells seen in ascitic fluid CA-125 was raised as well. USG and CT abdomen revealed left sided ovarian mass, gastroscopy, colonoscopy and barium follow through did not reveal any abnormality. Mantoux test (1:10,000) moderately positive, gynaecological review suggested a left sided TO mass.*

DIAGNOSIS: Exudative ascites with left sided ovarian mass with raised CA-125 level. Tubercular in origin? Ovarian malignancy with peritoneal carcinomatosis.

Because of diagnostic dilemma, she underwent laparotomy which revealed tubercular tubo-ovarian mass. There was severe adhesion of small intestine along with plastic peritonitis; left sided salpingo-oophorectomy was done along with intestinal adhesiolysis. Her post operative recovery was uneventful. She was discharged on 4 drug anti-tubercular regime. On follow up she has been keeping well.

FINAL DIAGNOSIS: Tubercular salpingo-oophoritis with exudative ascites.

CASE: *A 57 years old lady presented with low grade fever along with gradual increase in abdominal girth. Examination revealed moderate ascites. Hematological and biochemical parameters were within normal range. CA-125 was raised. CT and USG abdomen did not reveal anything specific except for thickened peritoneum. Gynaecological consultation failed to reveal any major problem. Ascites was exudative in nature with a protein content of 4.8 g/dl. Cell count less than 100, predominantly lymphocytes. LDH and CA-125 were raised, AFB, gram stain and PAP smear were all negative. Mantoux test was equivocal.*

DIAGNOSIS: Exudative ascites - ?Tubercular

She was treated with a course of steroid and 4 drugs anti TB regime with an initial good response. During her next follow up at 8 weeks time, she was again symptomatic and was found to have re-accumulation of ascites. Repeat ascitic fluid analysis on two successive occasions showed malignant cells. Repeat CT pelvis showed a cystic lesion in the left ovary (which was not evident in the previous scan).

FINAL DIAGNOSIS: Malignant ascites due to peritoneal carcinomatosis due to ovarian malignancy. She was referred to an oncological centre for further management.

CASE: *A 42 years old gentleman, with past history of childhood Koch's, was admitted with history of fever for last 6 months with abdominal pain along with swelling and weight loss. The reason of his admission was increasing swelling of his abdomen along with high grade temperature for last 10 days. He looked cachexic with an Hb of 7 g%, ESR-120, low albumin level, USG showing moderate ascites, with normal hepatobiliary system. The ascitic fluid was greenish in colour with a protein level of 3.4 g%, LDH was high and pH was low, cell count was 450, 80% neutrophil, culture grew Pseudomonas.*

DIAGNOSIS: Secondary bacterial peritonitis probably super imposed on tubercular peritonitis.

He was treated with a course of piperacillin-tazobactam with resolution of his symptoms. Before discharge, he was symptom free although a small amount of residual ascites was present. Follow up at 1 month showed further fall of his Hb and re-accumulation of ascites (exudative). CT abdomen revealed thickened omentum and intestinal wall. Mantoux test was strongly positive. He was treated with antitubercular 4 drugs regime with a course of steroid along with supportive care. Over the last one year he has been keeping well.

CASE: *A 62 years old lady was suffering from chronic liver disease. She was diagnosed to have NASH many years back and recently progressed to cirrhosis with evidence of mild decompensation. Her bilirubin was hovering around 3-4 mg% with an AST and ALT level of about 200-300 units. She also had grade II oesophageal varices (for which she underwent banding) and mild grade ascites.*

The reason for her recent consultation was sudden increase in her jaundice and ascites. Her hepatitis B and C status were negative. Ascitic fluid albumin 3.6 g%, cells less than 50, predominantly lymphocytes. Gram stain, AFB stain negative, PAP stain repeatedly was found to be negative. Her alpha fetoprotein level was raised at a very high level. CT scan consistent with chronic liver disease but no space occupying lesion was detected. MRI and MRI angiogram however revealed a space occupying lesion in the left lobe of the liver and there was extensive thrombosis of the portal vein.

DIAGNOSIS: Hepatoma complicated with portal vein thrombosis in a patient with chronic liver disease.

Shortly after diagnosis she decompensated rapidly and following a bout of massive gastro intestinal bleeding she went into hepatic coma from which she did not recover.

DISCUSSION:

Ascites is a common clinical presentation although the differentiation between the causes is traditionally made by examining the fluid to find out whether it is exudative or transudative (protein level 3.5 g/dl as a demarcating figure), type of cells present in the fluid, presence of malignant cells and the level of different tumour markers, it is sometimes difficult to pinpoint the diagnosis solely on the basis of fluid analysis as evidenced by four different cases described above.

Although the concept of transudate and exudates still holds true, there are clinical conditions where this is not helpful. As for example in congestive cardiac failure, the protein content of the fluid may be high, in spite of its being a transudate while in some cases of infective ascites, the protein content may be low.

There is a suggestion that serum ascitic albumin gradient (SAAG) may be a better discriminator in the differential diagnosis of ascites. SAAG is defined as the serum albumin concentration minus the ascitic fluid albumin concentration. It is claimed that SAAG correlates directly with the portal pressure. It has been found that the patients with SAAG of > 11 g/litre have portal hypertension whereas no patient with **SAAG** < 11 g/litre has this disorder.

SAAG:

Wide > 11 g / litre	**Narrow < 11 g / litre**
• Chronic liver disease • Veno-occlusive disorder • Massive hepatic metastasis • Congestive cardiac failure • Spontaneous bacterial peritonitis.	• Peritoneal carcinomatosis • Reduced plasma oncotic pressure (Nephrotic syndrome) • Tubercular peritonitis • Secondary peritonitis • Nephrotic Syndrome

In some cases, conditions that produce low SAAG may supervene in patient with portal hypertension (which causes high SAAG). In such cases, SAAG will remain wide and further differentiation should be made by other parameters like cell count, cell type, glucose, pH, LDH which might point towards an inflammatory process (e.g. spontaneous bacterial peritonitis supervening on cirrhosis of liver). For accuracy, the blood albumin level and ascitic fluid albumin level should be checked simultaneously without much of a time gap.

Infections:

Spontaneous bacterial peritonitis usually occurs in cirrhotic patients and it usually occurs in patients with low protein content in the ascitic fluid. Thus the SAAG is wide. The cell count will be high (more than 250/field).

Secondary bacterial infection is due to heavier bacterial load. This is usually due to perforated viscus. The resultant growth of bacteria causes low pH, high LDH and high protein content leading to low SAAG. The glucose content of fluid will also be low.

Malignancy:

In case of peritoneal carcinomatosis, the ascitic fluid protein content is high leading to low SAAG and the chances of positivity for PAP stain is very high. While in hepatoma or massive hepatic metastasis the ascitic fluid protein is low (wide SAAG). They also have negative ascitic fluid cytology. Elevated alkaline phosphatase, alpha fetoprotein etc. may help in the differential diagnosis. In cases of chylous ascites, ascitic fluid triglyceride level will be much higher than serum triglyceride level.

The ascitic fluid can be mobilized with diuretics in hepatoma or hepatic metastasis but not in peritoneal carcinomatosis or chylous ascites.

Tumour markers in ascitic fluid:

CA-125 may be elevated in ascitic fluid in cases other than ovarian malignancy and may not have a discriminating value. Similar limitations are also applicable to other tumour markers like CEA, CA-19.9 and HCG.

Cytology:

Usually it is positive in peritoneal carcinomatosis while negative in hepatoma and massive hepatic metastasis.

Other discriminating tests:

- Cell count more than 250, with predominant polymorphs usually indicative of bacterial infection.
- Lymphocyte count is high in tubercular, fungal and lymphomas.
- Indication of inflammatory ascites: in addition to low SAAG, low pH, high lactate, low glucose, usually indicates inflammation.
- Adenine deaminase (ADA): High ADA level in peritoneal fluid strongly suggests tuberculosis.

Bacteriological culture and Gram staining sometimes gives diagnostic clue. Although the list is long, majority of patients presenting with ascites in outpatients clinic are due to:

Cirrhosis of liver - features of chronic liver disease along with wide SAAG gradient.

Tubercular infection - inflammatory exudates with low SAAG, other ancillary tests may be suggestive.

Malignancy e.g. Lymphoma - narrow SAAG, high triglyceride level.

Peritoneal carcinomatosis - low SAAG, positive PAP. In gynaecological malignancy tumour markers may be helpful.

Hepatoma and hepatic metastasis (High SAAG, negative PAP) - other discriminating tests may be helpful. Careful analysis of ascitic fluid may help in making the final diagnosis.

Pancreatic Ascites - Acute Pancreatitis, pancreatic pseudo cyst or a mass may give rise to ascites. Measurement of pancreatic fluid amylase level, which will be very high, will help in making diagnosis.

Other Causes of Ascites:

- Constrictive pericarditis
- Acute pancreatitis
- Nephrotic Syndrome
- Protein loosing enteropathy
- Budd-Chiari syndrome

Causes of Polyserositis:

- Malnutrition
- Nephrotic Syndrome
- Connective Tissue Disorder like SLE
- Viral Infection
- Tuberculosis
- Lymphoma
- Chronic Liver Disease
- Any other Causes of low albumin

CASE: *A 67 years old businessman presented with shortness of breath. Investigation revealed pericardial effusion, right pleural effusion, ascites, and oedema, relevant investigation with CT scan of thorax, MRI Scan of thorax and echocardiogram revealed evidence of constrictive pericarditis, malignancy was excluded by appropriate tests. A clinical diagnosis of constrictive pericarditis due to tuberculosis was made. The patient received 1 year course of anti TB medication along with six weeks of steroid in the initial period with improvement.*

DIAGNOSIS: Constrictive pericarditis of tubercular origin.

Although constrictive pericarditis is rare, it needs to be considered in patients with recurrent congestive cardiac failure along with pericardial effusion in appropriate background.

Other complication of Ascites:

- Mechanical- respiratory disorders
- Hepatorenal syndrome
- Plural effusion
- Umbilical Hernia
- Spontaneous bacterial peritonitis

MANAGEMENT OF ASCITES:

- Sodium and water restriction.
- Judicious use of diuretics like frusemide in combination with either spironolactone or amiloride.
- Paracentesis along with IV albumin infusion or colloid replacement may be tried in moderate to severe ascites. Albumin or colloid replacement is important, failure of which may lead to acute oliguria.
- Vasopressin antagonist tolvaptan may be used to deal with persistent hyponatraemia.
- In refractory ascites, specialist's opinion needs to be taken regarding peritoneovenous shunt or transjugular intrahepatic portosystemic shunt (TIPPS).

CASE: *An alcoholic patient with known chronic liver disease was admitted with abdominal pain, fever and tense ascites. Diagnostic paracentesis revealed very high protein level, cell count was more than 5000/cumm with 90% polymorphonuclear neutrophils, culture grew streptococcus pneumonia. He was treated with IV ceftriaxone and vancomycin along with repeated paracentesis with improvement.*

DIAGNOSIS: Spontaneous bacterial peritonitis.

Spontaneous bacterial peritonitis in a patient with cirrhosis of liver should be considered in patients with sudden increase in ascites with abdominal pain and features of infection and other features of hepatic decompensation like encephalopathy.

: KEY POINTS :

- Ascites is a common clinical presentation
- Tuberculosis is a common cause of ascites in India.
- High ADA level in peritoneal fluid strongly suggests tuberculosis.
- Traditional approach of transudative and exudative ascites has limitation in differential diagnosis.
- SAAG is relatively newer concept that may have a better diagnostic role in ascites.
- Low glucose, low pH, high LDH and high neutrophil count in ascitic fluid indicate infection.
- Ascitic fluid tumour markers have their limitations in diagnosing malignancy.
- PAP stain is usually negative in hepatomas and hepatic metastasis whereas usually positive in peritoneal carcinomatosis.

FURTHER REFERENCES:

- Harrison's Principle of Internal Medicine - 17th Edition.
- J. Jeffery *et al*. Ascitic fluid analysis- the role of biochemistry and Haematology- Hospital Medicine May 2001, Vol- 62: No. 5: P 282- 286.
- Oxford Text Book of Medicine – 5th Edition.

16 A PATIENT WITH HAEMOLYTIC URAEMIC SYNDROME (H.U.S.)

CASE: *An 11 years old young girl was transferred from another medical facility with the history of fever followed by mild jaundice, anaemia and progressive renal failure. Examination revealed mild jaundice and anaemia. Her Hb level was 7 g% WBC- 16,000, platelet- 16,000, LDH- 1120 (high), bilirubin- 4.2 mg%, mostly unconjugated, reticulocyte count 6%, creatinine- 4.2 mg%, urea- 188 mg%, urine shows few RBC and protein++, blood film showed crenated and fragmented RBC, schistocytes were also present in the blood film, Coomb's test negative. Coagulation profile showed PT, APTT slightly prolonged, FDP- slightly raised.*

DIAGNOSIS: Micro-angiopathic anaemia due to haemolytic uraemic syndrome.

This is an uncommon presentation in clinical practice and if the blood film is not interpreted properly can easily be misdiagnosed as sepsis with multi-organ failure. Thrombotic thrombocytopenic purpura is an allied condition with similar pathological features. However CNS manifestations predominate in this condition.

CASE: *A 38 years old lady was transferred from a district hospital with 2 weeks history of fever, jaundice, bleeding manifestation and renal failure. On admission, she was unconscious, her CT brain scan was normal. Investigations revealed negative MP on several occasions, very high urea & creatinine, LDH moderately high, unconjugated hyperbilirubinaemia, very low platelet count. Initially septicaemia with DIC, cerebral malaria and viral haemorrhagic fever were the differential diagnosis. On admission, blood film showed classical evidence of micro angiopathic anaemia and the* ***final diagnosis was thrombotic thrombocytopenic purpura.***

DISCUSSION: Thrombotic microangiopathies are rather uncommon presentation in clinical practice. Nevertheless they do present in acute medical care and if the blood film is not interpreted properly, may be misdiagnosed as septicaemia with DIC, viral infection with multi-organ failure and malaria with multi-organ failure. The basic features are:

☞ Fever, thrombocytopenia, progressive renal impairment, jaundice.

In thrombotic thrombocytopenic purpura, in addition, CNS manifestations predominate. Biochemical tests show high urea, creatinine, high bilirubin, high LDH (due to tissue necrosis rather than haemolysis). Blood film is very characteristic with presence of fragmented and misshaped RBCs which is due to the passage of blood through the obstructed circulation (by platelet aggregates).

Haemolytic uraemic syndrome:

- Predominant renal failure.
- Often preceded by gastroenteritis caused by verocytotoxin producing *E. coli* 0157: H7 and exposure to shigella toxin.
- Similar kind of feature may be found in patients receiving mitomycin, cyclosporin, tacrolimus, quinine, metronidazole post bowel surgery.

MECHANISM:

The bacterial toxins stimulate the endothelial cells to secrete unusually large multimers of Von Willebrand factor. This in turn leads to platelet aggregation in the peripheral circulation leading to microthrombi.

In familial haemolytic uraemic syndrome, there is also deficiency of factor H, a plasma protein which prevents the normal host cells from accidental damage of the endothelial cells by the activation of alternate complement pathway. In deficiency of factor H, there is activation of alternate complement pathway thereby leading to host cell damage; aggregation of platelets and formation of platelet microthrombi.

In haemolytic uraemic syndrome, plasma exchange or plasma infusion may be tried with equivocal results. Anti motility agents will increase production of bacterial toxins and should be avoided. Supportive therapy like renal replacement therapy should be instituted as per the requirement of the patient.

Thrombotic thrombocytopenic purpura:

- Predominant CNS manifestation
- There may be familial, chronic relapsing variety
- Ticlopidine and clopidogrel can rarely cause TTP.

MECHANISM:

Multimers of Von Willebrand factor are cleaved into monomeric subunits by an enzyme called ADMTS13. TTP may be acquired or hereditary (relapsing) also called Upshaw-Schulman syndrome is usually due to ADAMTS 13 mutation while acquired. TTP is due to auto antibody mediated inhibition of ADMTS activity. In TTP, the enzyme ADMTS13 is deficient. Infusion of fresh plasma may replace the deficient enzyme. There may be antibody formation against ADMTS13.

In some cases, if the antibody titre is high immunosuppressive therapy with steroids and splenectomy may be needed. Platelet transfusion should be avoided. It will aggravate formation of platelet microthrombi. However, if there is obvious bleeding, it will be unavoidable. The role of aspirin in the face of bleeding is controversial. Other drugs used in refractory cases are vincristine, rituximab (experimental).

Any patient presenting with features of microangiopathic haemolytic anaemia features (either TTP or HUS) should be presumed to have TTP and treated with plasma exchange.

The first patient described above had daily plasma infusions, needed regular blood and platelet transfusion, (she had gastrointestinal bleeding) and received peritoneal dialysis

After a long stay in the hospital, she was discharged home and 6 months at follow up her renal function had returned back to normal.

The second patient had a delayed presentation. Although she received plasma infusion, steroids, renal replacement therapy with haemodialysis, she progressively deteriorated and finally expired.

Common differential diagnosis in patients with thrombocytopenia, bleeding and altered LFT:

	Platelet	Smear	PT	LDH	ALT
T.T.P	low	Schistocytes	N	⇑⇑	N
D.I.C (due to septicaemia)	low	Schistocytes	⇑⇑	N	N or ⇑
I.T.P	low	Normal RBCs	N	N	N
HELLP Syndrome (in pregnancy)	low	Schistocytes	N Or ⇑	⇑	⇑

It is of note that although low platelet along with schistocytes may be present in many conditions, in TTP the unique feature is very high - LDH.

Conditions presenting with combination of thrombocytopenia, schistocytes, altered LFT and increased LDH:

HUS/TTP :	Clinical features, altered renal function and very high LDH normal prothrombin time.
I.T.P :	Absence of schistocytes, normal LFT, normal LDH.
HELLP Syndrome :	Raised AST and ALT, LDH may be normal, prothrombin time may be raised.
Septicaemia with DIC :	Raised prothrombin time, LDH is usually normal.

Common disorder associated with microangiopathic haemolytic anaemia and thrombocytopenia.

- Systemic infection
- Systemic Cancer
- HELLP syndrome
- Severe Hypertension
- Autoimmune disorder
- SLE
- Systemic Sclerosis
- Haemopoietic Stem Cell or organ transplantation.

Thrombotic angiopathic syndrome may be complement mediated, toxin mediated, drug mediated, which may be immune or toxic dose related, metabolism related like cobalamin C deficiency, a hereditary disorder of vitamin B_{12} metabolism or coagulation mediated as in genetic abnormalities of thrombomodulin or plasminogen.

Drugs Causing thrombotic microangiopathy (immune or toxic dose related):

- Cyclosporine
- Tacrolimus
- Quinine
- Clopidogrel

CASE: *A 31 years old female presented with low grade fever along with normal WBC and low platelet count. Investigation ruled out common causes like dengue, malaria, and enteric fever. Her urine shows 15-20 RBC/field, and ultrasonography was suggestive of pyelonephritis. A presumptive diagnosis of pyelonephritis was made and broad spectrum antibiotic was commenced. However her platelet count remained persistently low with a normal WBC count. Blood film showed normocytic normochromic picture with no abnormal cell. Her vitamin B_{12} level was found to be low and bone marrow picture showed megaloblastic picture and although not characteristics the possibility of ITP could not be excluded altogether her bilirubin was 1.4 μg% and reticulocyte count was 4%. Coomb's test was negative.*

She was communed with vitamin B_{12} injection but platelet count did not increase. Her LDH level was high which was thought to be due to vitamin B_{12} deficiency on replacement with vitamin B_{12} injection. After discussing with the haematologist, IV gamma-globulin was given with no improvement. Later in her developed convulsion and psychotic behaviour and the subsequent blood film started showing schistocytes along with other pictures of microangiopathy. A revised diagnosis of TTP was made and the patient had a full recovery following plasmapheresis.

DIAGNOSIS: Typical presentation of TTP along with presence of concomitant vitamin B_{12} deficiency.

MANAGEMENT:

The principle of treatment of TTP is by replacement of plasma. A randomized trial in 1991 showed the use of plasma exchange had improved the survival rate from 10% to 78%. Glucocorticoid and rituximab may be indicated in complicated cases.

Complement mediated angiopathies may be additionally treated with eculizumab which is currently the only available anticomplement agent. Parenteral vitamin B_{12} is the principle treatment in micro angiopathy related to cobalamin metabolism.

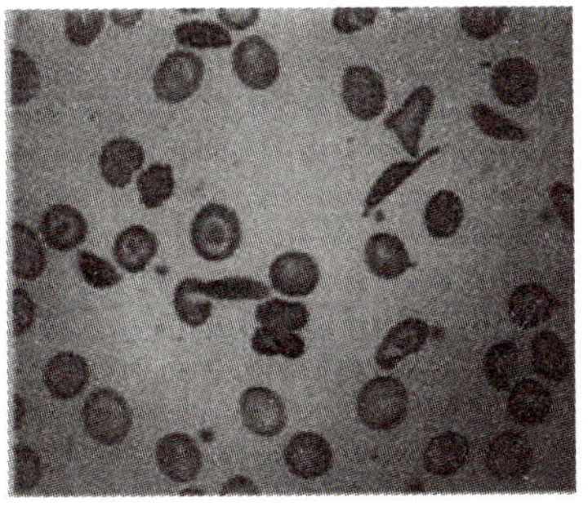

: KEY POINTS :

- Micro angiopathic haemolytic anaemias are uncommon presentation in clinical practice.
- HUS has prominent renal involvement whereas TTP has predominant neurological involvement.
- Presence of thrombocytopenia, micro angiopathic blood picture, renal impairment and very high LDH, should prompt the diagnosis of HUS or TTP.
- Specific diagnosis is important as plasma infusion with or without plasmapheresis is an effective treatment for these conditions.

FURTHER REFERENCE:

- Jamer .N. Gorge *et al.* NEJM 2014, 371: 654-666.

17 A PATIENT WITH SYNCOPE

CASE: *A 64-years old male was admitted in the hospital for evaluation of spell of sudden unconsciousness. He was otherwise mobile and active. Apart from history of neck pain and dizziness, he did not have any significant medical problem. Neurological examination was satisfactory. He was slightly hypertensive. ECG showed normal sinus rhythm, CT brain scan was normal. X-ray cervical spine– spondylotic changes, in echo and carotid Doppler NAD.*

DIAGNOSIS: Syncope ?cause.

Syncope is a very common cause of clinical presentation needing urgent hospitalization for evaluation. Frequently, they are admitted to ITU or ICU and undergo a battery of tests for identification of cause which frequently come out to be inconclusive.

Before approaching such patients, the clinician should at first differentiate between a syncope and seizure.

Points in favour of syncope:

- Usually precipitated by pain, exercise, micturition, defecation– vasovagal syncope.
- May be preceded by nausea and sweating.

Points in favour of seizure:

- Presence of aura
- Disorientation after the event
- Unconsciousness lasting for more than 5 minutes.
- Abnormal jerking movement of the body or biting of tongue.

Common causes:

- Neurogenic or vasovagal syncope is the most common cause, this includes micturition syncope, cough syncope, syncope associated with defecation, carotid sinus syncope etc. History will be helpful in making the diagnosis.
- Orthostatic hypotension is also a common cause in elderly with autonomic failure, volume depletion and intake of anti-hypertensive medication. Postural check up of BP is important.
- Cardiac Syncope: Both bradyarrhythmias and tachyarrhythmias can cause syncope. The ECG on admission may show evidence of heart block of precursors for heart block like bifascicular block. Patient with poor ejection fraction are more prone to

have ventricular arrhythmias. ECG might show long QT interval indicating the cause of syncope is ventricular fibrillation.

Patients with aortic stenosis and pulmonary hypertension are more prone to have syncopal attack.

- Psychiatric illness: Patients with anxiety state or conversion disorder present with recurrent attacks of syncope with negative investigation. One needs to consider such conditions in young females presenting with recurrent syncopal attacks.

Causes of Syncope:

1. **Cardiovascular**

    a. Vasovagal
    - Cough Syncope
    - Micturition Syncope

    b. Orthostatic Hypotension

    c. Cardiac
    - Bradyarrhythmia
    - Tachyarrhythmia

    d. Structural Cardiac
    - Aortic Stenosis
    - Hypertrophic obstructive Cardiomyopathy (HOCM)
    - Arrhythmogenic right ventricular dysplasia
    - Atrial myxoma

    e. Drugs
    - Anti hypertension
    - Sublingual nitroglycerin

2. **Cerebrovascular**

    a. TIA, CVA
    b. Seizure

3. **Psychogenic**

TIA is a common cause presenting as syncope. Usually there is a history of vertigo, dysarthria or diplopia. There may be history of cervical spondylosis in patients presenting with vertebrobasilar TIA. **We have found it to the second most common cause of admission for assessment of syncope in our ITU/ICCU (Vasovagal – most common).**

In spite of a thorough investigation, no apparent cause is found in approximately 30% of cases.

Diagnostic work up:

In addition to thorough medical checkup, detailed history of sequence of events, drug history and check of postural BP, one should also check for routine biochemical and haematological parameters – other tests that should be done are:

1. **ECG** – to look for bundle branch block, MI, Q-T interval, ventricular ectopics. It is usually positive in less than 5% of cases.
2. **Echo** – to evaluate LV function, valvular heart disease.
3. **24 hours Holter monitoring** – It is helpful in diagnosing arrhythmic syncope [In 4% of patients symptoms are found in conjunction with arrhythmias, in 17% cases symptoms occur without arrhythmias ruling out arrhythmic syncope and in 79% of cases no arrhythmia is noted thereby necessitating further tests as arrhythmia can be episodic. Continuous event loop monitoring may be helpful for long term monitoring (weeks and months). The patients may activate the system in the event of symptoms.
4. **Electrophysiological study** – In patients with history of MI or LV dysfunction, electrophysiological study sometimes detects inducible ventricular arrhythmias (approximately 21%). Although 34% of patients show brady-arrhythmias, EPS has got poor sensitivity and specificity for brady-arrhythmias. Due to lack of widespread availability this test is not commonly done in India.

Vasovagal Syncope:

- Tilt testing provokes vasovagal syncope in susceptible persons. This test is usually done with some provocative agents like nitroglycerine. The specificity of the tilt test with provocative agents approaches around 90%.
- In carotid sinus hypersensitivity, carotid sinus massage yields diagnostic results. While conducting this test one has to be cautious regarding carotid artery atherosclerosis as it might dislodge clot to cause stroke.

OTHER INVESTIGATIONS:

Cardiac Tilt Table Test:

During this test, the patient is tilted upto 60° to 80° for 30 to 40 minutes which may provoke vagal stimulation with either bradycardia (Cardio inhibitory response) or hypotension (Vasodepressor response). The specificity of this test is approximately 90°. The test duration may be shortened by administering medication like nitroglycerine although the specificity declines.

Event loop recorder:

The recorder may be kept in situ for prolonged period of time which can capture intermittent arrhythmias hitherto undiagnosed by 24 hr. Holter monitoring.

Neural Imaging:

- CT brain scan may show infarct.
- EEG – It is positive in 2% of patients presenting with syncope.

MANAGEMENT:

In cases of vasovagal syncope, atenolol has been shown to reduce symptoms at one month. In patients with recurrent vasovagal syncope with tilt test showing significant bradycardia pacemaker may be considered. In cases of significant postural drop of BP, fludrocortisone and midodrine (alpha-stimulant) may be considered. Cardiac syncope should be treated appropriately (antiarrhythmics like amiodarone or by ICD implantation).

The patient's drop attack was considered to be due to vertebrobasilar insufficiency with associated cervical spondylosis. On discharge, he was treated with soft cervical collar and aspirin prophylaxis.

CASE: *A 71 years old lady presented with recurrent syncope. Repeated ECGs did not reveal anything specific. 24 Hrs. holter monitoring was also noncontributory except for showing occasional bradycardia. Echocardiography was normal. Neurological evaluation was satisfactory. Subsequently an event loop recorder study revealed recurrent 2:1 heart block with a heart rate of 34/min. She was symptomatic. She was implanted with a dual chamber pacemaker with abetment of her symptoms.*

DIAGNOSIS: Intermittent heart block leading to recurrent syncope, diagnosed by event loop recorder.

: KEY POINTS :

- Syncope is a common presentation in clinical practice.
- Clinician should differentiate syncope from seizure.
- Vasovagal syncope is the most common cause of syncope.
- Tilt testing with provocative agents will establish nerve mediated syncope.
- Atenolol may be helpful in treatment of vasovagal syncope.
- In recurrent vasovagal syncope with bradycardia, pacemaker may be needed.

FURTHER REFERENCES:

- Syncope – W. N. Kapoor, NEJM Vol-343, N-25, Dec-21 2000, P 1856-1862.
- Harrison's Principle of Internal Medicine – 17th edition.

18 AN OBESE PATIENT WITH TYPE-II DM

CASE: *A 49-years-old obese male presented with generalised unwell being and pain in the knee joints. Examination revealed BP of 160/100 mmHg with no other abnormality. Investigation revealed fasting glucose of 211 mg% postprandial glucose 286 mg%, LDL cholesterol 166 mg%, triglyceride 302 mg%, HDL 32 mg%, uric Acid 7.4 mg%. Urine for routine examination showed glucose++ with trace of protein. ECG normal, X-ray chest normal. T3, T4, TSH normal. He gave a family history of diabetes mellitus.*

DIAGNOSIS: Type II diabetes mellitus, hyperlipidaemia, hyperuricaemia

DISCUSSION:

The incidence of diabetes mellitus is increasing at an alarming proportion and majority of them are Type II diabetes mellitus. Prompt diagnosis and treatment of diabetes mellitus can reduce the mortality and morbidity. Unfortunately the individuals may have undetected diabetes for many years before they come into limelight following routine examination and many of them will already be having involvement of at least one organ. Since this disease is taking an epidemic proportion in India, the primary care physician will have to bear much of the burden for diabetes management in the years ahead.

It is a well known fact that tight control of blood glucose reduces diabetes related complication. UKPDS study has shown that 1% reduction of HbA_1C will cause:-

- 21% risk reduction in any diabetic related end point.
- 21% reduction in diabetes related death.
- 14% risk reduction in MI.
- 37% risk reduction in micro vascular complication.

So physicians should strive for meticulous glycaemic control.

The first step in that direction will be *advice regarding life style modification* which include dietary alternations, regular physical exercise, and reduction of weight and reduced alcohol intake.

If with the aforementioned measures the target HbA_1C level is not achieved then one should go for oral hypoglycaemic agent as monotherapy.

CAVEATS OF UKPDS STUDY:

Despite the positive data regarding the benefit of tight control of blood glucose, from UKPDS Study, recent studies like ACCORD failed to show any lowering of risk of cardiovascular events or death. Moreover in ACCORD, the study with most stringent criteria for glycaemic control was stopped early because of major adverse effect of hypoglycaemia in patients above 70 yrs. From these afore mentioned facts, from practical point of view it would be reasonable to conclude that-

a) Once advanced micro vascular and macro vascular have established. While improvement of strict diabetic control may be beneficial, aiming for a tight control is unlikely to be so and the targets should be individualized.

b) If patients with age above 70 years, the benefits of tight control is limited.

c) The benefits of tight control must always be balanced against the risk of hypoglycaemia.

WHICH AGENT?

In the presence of obesity (BMI >23 kg/m^2) metformin should be used first. This drug is *contraindicated in renal and hepatic impairment*. Moreover some of the patients are intolerant to this drug (nausea, diarrhoea etc.) an *alternative agent like sulphonylureas should be chosen. In patients with erratic life style or anticipated risk of hypoglycaemia or weight gain, a rapid acting secretagogue* ***(repaglinide, nateglinide)*** should be used instead.

Metformin- It has been shown to reduce diabetic related deaths (32%), all cause mortality (36%) and myocardial infarction (39%).

Sulphonylureas- Act by triggering insulin release from the pancreatic beta cell.

Pioglitazone- It has been found to reduce all cause of mortality of 31-39% when used alone or in combination. However it can cause weight gain or exacerbation of heart failure by way of fluid retention. There have also been concerns regarding the possible link with the development of bladder cancer and the increased risk of fracture of distal radius in women. Glitazones can cause *fluid retention and oedema* and therefore should be used with *caution in patients with cardiac failure*; Liver function should also be monitored. Rosiglitazone was linked with increased risk of myocardial infarct and was temporarily withdrawn. One should remember that glitazones take a while to exert their maximum effect (8-12 weeks).

If the desired effect is not achieved with single drug, then combination therapy should be considered. The following combination may be tried –

- **Metformin + Sulphonylurea** (risk of hypoglycaemia should be considered).
- **Metformin + Nateglinide or repaglinide** (they can control PP glucose well).
- **Metformin + Glitazone** (Pioglitazone, rosiglitazone)
- **Sulphonylurea + Glitazone**

Triple therapy: sulphonylurea + metformin + glitazone

In day to day clinical practice triple therapy combination is a very helpful and effective combination to achieve adequate glycaemic control.

Occasionally glucosidase inhibitors (Acarbose) may be added to control the post prandial surge. However its use is limited by its *very embarrassing side effects of flatulence.*

Insulin- *If combination therapy fails to achieve the goal within 6 months; drug therapy should be combined with insulin.*

Initially once daily medium acting insulin (**Neutral Protamine Hagedorn Insulin**) at bed time may be tried with a starting does of 10 units with the dose gradually titrated upwards. However, it can cause nocturnal hypoglycaemia. Newer varieties of long acting insulin – like **glargine insulin** may be used instead. The advantage is that it is long acting basal insulin, thus the nocturnal hypoglycaemia is rarely a problem.

If single daily insulin is not sufficient enough to achieve adequate glycaemic control, then twice daily NPH insulin should be tried. Metformin can still be continued for synergistic effect. The other oral hypoglycaemics should be withdrawn. Another common practice in India is the combination of insulin with glitazone which is very effective.

In spite of these measures, HbA_1C is still out of range and the blood glucose fluctuates considerably, one should consider basal-bolus insulin (NPH insulin twice daily or glargine insulin once daily with rapidly acting regular insulin as bolus). **Lispro insulin** or **aspart insulin** may also be used as a bolus with lesser risk of post prandial hypoglycaemia.

Sometimes the patients are unwilling to take multiple injections. In that event, premixed insulin in twice daily dosage is an alternative (Huminsulin 30/70 or Huminsulin 50/50).

Insulin was used along with metformin and sulphonylureas to obtain tight glycaemic control in the Steno-Z-study achieved more than 50% reduction in cardiovascular and micro vascular end points. Weight gain is an important problem encountered with insulin therapy.

NEWER THERAPY:

Dipeptidyl peptidase-4 inhibitors- Commonly known as '*gliptin*' are newer groups of agents which work through inhibition of (DPP-4) which ordinarily inactivates incretin. The net effect is inhibition of glucagon release and increased insulin secretion. Four drugs are currently available e.g.

1. Sitagliptin (Januvia)
2. Vildagliptin (Galvus)
3. Saxagliptin (Onglyza)
4. Linagliptin (Tradjenta)

Apart from gastrointestinal side effects, the main problem is the risk of development of pancreatitis. They are weight neutral and may cause loss of wt. Except for linagliptin, they need dose adjustment in renal impairment.

Glucagon like peptide-1 (GLP-1) analogues- They lower glucose level through the combined stimulation of insulin production and suppression of glucagon. The activity of GLP-1 is promoted via inhibitor of DPP-4, an enzyme responsible for the degradation of incretin. Exenatide (Byetta) and Liraglutide (Victoza) are GLP-1 analogues currently available in clinical practice. They are given subcutaneously as once or twice daily dose. Recently once weekly formulation of exenatide has been approved for clinical use. These drugs cause weight loss and lesser chance of hypoglycaemia.

Insulin or GLP-1 analogous as 2nd line agent		
Points	**Glucagon like peptide agonist**	**Basal Insulin**
Mortality	No effect	Reduces
Hypoglycaemia	Rare	Common
Effect on weight	Reduce	Gain
Side effects	Gastrointestinal	Lipodystrophy
Cost	More expensive	Cheaper

From the aforementioned discussion it will be evident that while considering 2nd line treatment both Insulin and GLP-1 analogous may be considered and since no definite guideline is available till date, the use will depend upon clinician's judgement.

Role of bariatric Surgery in treatment of diabetes modality Type II:

Remission of diabetes was significantly higher in those undergoing adjustable laparoscopic banding compared to conventional therapy. Although there is initial high cost outlay, in the long run it is cost effective. NICE (2006) guidance recommends that bariatric surgery to be considered for obese patients with body mass index between 30 and 35 kg/m^2, with failure of conventional treatment. Bariatric surgery falls under 3 categories- *restriction, malabsorption* and *combination procedures*.

Complications of bariatric surgery:

Sepsis, thromboembolic events and anastomotic leaks, nutritional deficiency, gastric dumping, depression, cosmetic surgery may be required to remove excess skin. However, these risks need to be balanced against the long term benefit that will be derived from the control of diabetes.

Newer agents just available in the pipeline:

1. **Sodium glucose lithium co-transporter-2 inhibitors:** Dapagliflozin reduces glucose by regularising glucose transport through renal tubules. This drug is just available in the UK. It should not be used with frusemide.

2. **Bile acid sequestrants (Colesevelam):** It is listened in USA since 2009. It reduces endogenous glucose production and it also increases incretin hormones GLP-1.

3. **Aniline analogues:** It is a neuroendocrine hormone secreted in conjunction with insulin in response to insulin from islet of Langerhans beta cells.
   Pramlintide has been approved for use in USA in type II diabetes mellitus. It is seen by subcutaneous injection and it can cause weight loss.

4. **Dopamine 2 receptor agonists:** Bromocriptine has been proposed for use in diabetes mellitus (type II) in USA at a 2 to 6 fold lower dose used in Parkinson's disease. It improves insulin resistance through dopaminergic and serotonergic pathways.

5. **11β hydroxysteroid dehydrogenase inhibitors:** One such product, carbenoxolone reduces the rate of glucose production in diabetic patients.

6. **Glucokinase activators:** Piragliatin is in the developmental stage. It works by interfering with the enzymes in the neoglucogenesis cascade.

7. **Pancreatic G-protein receptor agonists:** These agents may also prove to be useful in the management of diabetes mellitus by way of modulating glucose homeostasis through enhanced glucose induced insulin secretion.

: KEY POINTS :

- In India, primary care physicians have to share the burden of treating diabetes mellitus.
- Metformin is the drug of choice in obese diabetics.
- Judicious use of combination therapy will help control the blood glucose.
- If combination therapy fails single dose long or medium acting insulin may be added.
- Twice daily insulin can be effectively combined with metformin.
- Combination of lispro insulin (bolus) and glargine insulin (basal) may be used in difficult cases.
- It is equally important to take care of hypertension and hyperlipidaemia as they adversely affect the outcome of the patients with diabetes mellitus particularly with regard to the macro vascular complications.

FURTHER REFERENCES:

- Campbell I.W. et al, Scottish intercollegiate guidelines Network: management of diabetes- (SIGN 55) Br J Diabetes Vasc, Disease 2002: 2: 50-2.
- Cambell I- Management of diabetes, Scottish Intercollegiate guidelines, Network (SIGN 55). Journal RCP edin 32, 2002: 3: 162.
- T.C. Handman et al BJHM – New therapies in the management of type II Diabetes Mellitus, April 2013 Vol-74. No 4,202-207.
- CMB Edwards – Sweagon like peptide-1 agonists in the treatment of type II diabetes – BJHM-April 2013 Vol-74. No-4, 198-201.
- Harrison's Principle of Internal Medicine 17th Edition
- Oxford Book of Medicine 5th Edition

19 A PATIENT WITH GUILLAIN BARRE (G.B.) SYNDROME

CASE: *A 32-years-old gentleman presented with a history of breathlessness. He had a past history of bronchiectasis. Examination revealed left sided coarse crepitations. He was cyanosed with a pulse rate of 130/min. Blood gas showed PO_2 of 56 mmHg and PCO_2 of 68 mm of Hg, pH – 7.2. After a brief trial of non invasive ventilation, he was intubated and started on mechanical ventilation. He was also on broad spectrum antibiotics and respiratory adjuvant therapy. Next day, as his condition was stable, after a successful trial of T-piece for 1 hour, he was extubated. During the visiting hours in the evening, while chatting with his relatives, he suddenly became severely breathless and cyanosed and was reintubated and ventilated. Following extubation after 24 hours, he had another episode of respiratory failure needing reintubation and ventilation. His blood for T3, T4, TSH and CPK were checked urgently which were found to be within normal range. On the 5th day, on careful examination, he was found to have weakness of his upper and lower extremities. On the 6th day, he also developed bilateral facial weakness. A neurological consultation was made and on the 7th day a lumbar puncture revealed raised CSF protein (102 mg%) with normal cell count. MRI brain and cervical spine were normal and NCV study was consistent with acute demyelinating polyneuropathy.*

DIAGNOSIS: Acute inflammatory demyelinating poly-neuropathy (G.B. Syndrome).

He received 5 days course of IV gammaglobulin. In the course, he developed bulbar palsy and needed percutaneous tracheostomy. After 6 weeks stay in the hospital he was discharged. During discharge, he was still bed bound although he had started moving his extremities with the help of physiotherapy. After 3 months his tracheostomy was withdrawn and he was managing to walk with zimmer frame with the help of a physiotherapist.

Interestingly, his elder brother was admitted under our care 6 years back with features of bilateral facial palsy followed by quadriparesis. He also received IV gammaglobulin and made a good recovery. Fortunately, he did not need any respiratory assistance with intubation or ventilation. The link between these two cases in the same family could not be established.

DISCUSSION:

Although not so common in primary care practice, critical care physicians frequently confront with Guillain-Barre syndrome. Although easy to detect when it presents with typical features, diagnosis may be delayed if the classical features are absent during initial presentation.

Clinico-Pathological types:

- Acute inflammatory demyelinating polyneuropathy
- Acute motor axonal neuropathy
- Acute motor sensory neuropathy

About half of the patients with GB Syndrome will have antibodies to various gangliosides *e.g.*

GM1	Pure motor G.B. Syndrome
GD1α	Acute motor axonal neuropathy
GM1ß	Pure motor G.B. Syndrome
GD1ß	Ataxia in G.B. Syndrome
GQ1 ß	Miller Fisher Syndrome
GT1α	Bulbar palsy in GB Syndrome

Although these tests are not available in routine clinical practice, some other tests such as antibodies to EB Virus, CMV Virus, HIV, *Campylobacter jejuni, Herpes simplex, Mycoplasma pneumonia* may be carried out in specialized centres to find out the triggering factors for the G.B Syndrome.

CLASSICAL PRESENTING FEATURES:

- Usually there is an antecedent history of upper respiratory tract infection or diarrhea.
- Numbness, tingling, pain and weakness.
- Weakness worse in legs than arms.
- Usually symmetrical.
- Reflexes are lost.
- Objective sensory signs may not be present.
- Half will have cranial nerve and bulbar nerve involvement.
- Weakness increases to its maximum 1-2 weeks from onset and 20% will require mechanical ventilation.

- Pain may be a prominent feature.
- Autonomic disturbances like sudden changes in BP and heart rate are common.
- Sometimes the patient may present with respiratory failure because of respiratory muscle weakness.
- Bilateral facial palsy can also be a presenting feature.

Although unilateral facial palsy is easy to diagnose, inexperienced clinicians may miss the diagnosis of bilateral facial nerve palsy because of symmetric involvement. Careful examination of eye-closure, blowing and whistling test will make it obvious.

3% of Guillain Barre Syndrome present with features of ophthalmoplegia, areflexia and ataxia (Miller-Fisher syndrome)]. There may not be motor weakness.

Common causes of bilateral facial nerve palsy:

1. Guillain Barre Syndrome
2. Sarcoidosis – with bilateral parotid gland enlargement

DIFFERENTIAL DIAGNOSIS:

In the setting of acute neuromuscular paralysis, the diagnosis of GB syndrome is largely clinical. However, it has to be differentiated from some other conditions like:

1. **Poliomyelitis**	Asymmetrical, pure motor, CSF pleocytosis
2. **Transverse myelitis**	Acute, lower extremities, symmetrical Predominant sensory findings.
3. **Myasthenia gravis**	Pure motor, tests like EMG
4. **Polymyositis**	Muscle pain and raised CPK
5. **Motor neurone disease**	Chronic disease, mixed upper motor Neurone and lower motor neurone signs, EMG
6. **Hypokalaemia**	Serum potassium level.
7. **Botulism**	Typical history
8. **Critical care myopathy**	Typically in long stay ITU patients on steroids, high CPK.

DIAGNOSIS:

1. LP shows raised protein with normal cells (may be normal in first 2 weeks).
2. NCV study – shows spectrum of motor and sensory involvement. (18% pure motor involvement). Predominantly there is demyelinating neuropathy although axonal involvement with minimal demyelination can also occur.
3. Pure motor variety is usually associated with Campylobacter and anti gM1 antibodies and severe sensory variety with Cytomegalovirus and anti gM2 antibodies.

Predicting prognosis:

Following factors are associated with high probability of poor outcome.

1. Preceding history of diarrhoea.
2. Rapid onset-bed bound within 2 days.
3. Requirement of artificial ventilation.
4. Reduced or excitable motor action potential amplitude.

MANAGEMENT:

The most important part of the management is to recognize impending respiratory failure and intubate and ventilate in appropriate time. The patient should be managed in ITU and oxygen saturation, respiratory and abdominal muscle movement should be watched carefully (increased abdominal muscle movement is a warning sign). Increased secretion and swallowing problem should also be noticed. Their vital capacity and peak flow should be observed regularly. Any other suggestive sign should prompt the clinician to prophylactic intubate and ventilate. [Most of the deaths occur due to delayed intubation in the event of a cardiorespiratory arrest with a very poor outcome].

Other aspects of general care:

1. Physiotherapy
2. Urinary catheterization
3. Nutrition
4. Deep vein thrombosis prophylaxis (very important)
5. Monitoring automatic function

Sudden bradycardia and cardiac arrest is a common cause of death. One has to be careful about this while doing suction. Prophylactic atropine and even pacemaker insertion may be needed.

Specific therapy:

Two forms of therapy are effective:

1. **IV gammaglobulin (0.4 g/kg IV daily × 5 days)**- It can be useful even after 2 weeks of onset of weakness. Headaches, meningism and eczema of the hands are uncommon side effects. Anaphylaxis is rare.
2. **Plasma exchange** is cqually helpful. However it is more hazardous and inconvenient. Moreover the chance of viral transmission is there. Therefore it is preferable to use IV gammaglobulin in most of the clinical situations.

There is no role of **steroid** in the management of G B Syndrome. Other general managements are-

- Supportive care
- Airway and breathing
- Circulation
- Autonomic dysfunction which is present in 70% of cases should be managed meticulously. It usually presents with arrhythmias, orthostatic hypotension and hypertension.
- Bowel and bladder care
- Pain control
- Anticoagulation

OUR EXPERIENCE:

In last 10 years, we have treated 63 patients presenting with GB syndrome. All of them received IV gammaglobulin. 26 patients made an uneventful recovery. 10 patients needed only intubation for tracheal toileting. 27 patients needed mechanical ventilation, 10 patients died – 3 of them due to sudden cardiac arrest and 5 of them due to sepsis related problems. 5 of the patients had only cranial nerves palsy (bulbar, seventh and ocular) one of them died because of aspiration pneumonia.

CASE: *A 56-years-old lady presented with swallowing problem with choking sensation. She had a loss of gag reflex. Initially there was a diagnostic dilemma. Later on during her stay, she developed bilateral seventh nerve palsy as well as ophthalmoplegia. She eventually needed tracheostomy. LP and NCV studies were non-diagnostic. Although she received IV gammaglobulin, it did not shorten the course of her illness. She was in ITU for nearly six weeks. At present she is off tracheostomy tube.*

CASE: *A 29-years-old lady presented with diplopia. Clinical examination revealed ophthalmoplegia due to bilateral 3rd and 6th nerve palsy. She also developed right sided 7th nerve palsy. MRI brain was normal. Lumbar puncture and NCV studies were non-contributory. With a provisional diagnosis of a typical GB syndrome, she was given IV gammaglobulin. She made a complete recovery within next 10 days.*

CASE: *A 62-year-old gentleman was admitted with profound weakness of all extremities. He gave a history of diarrhoea for 3 days before admission. Examination revealed quadriparesis without any bladder involvement. Clinical diagnosis of G.B. syndrome was made. Blood reports showed* K^+ *of 2.1 mg%. He was started on* K^+ *replacement and IV gammaglobulin. The weakness started improving within 24 hours and his* K^+ *level became normal within 48 hours. He also completed the course of IV gammaglobulin for 5 days. He underwent lumbar puncture which was normal. He also underwent NCV study which was normal. Before discharge, he was also given glucose challenge [to exclude hypokalaemic periodic paralysis) without any subsequent fall of serum* K^+ *level. He was discharged on the 6th day with absolutely normal muscle power.*

DIAGNOSIS: Diarrhoea induced severe hypokalaemic paralysis simulating GB Syndrome.

CASE: *A 40-years-old lady presented with acute generalized weakness of all extremities. Examination revealed muscle power of O/5. All the deep reflexes were brisk and the cranial nerves were well preserved. Her LP and NCV tests were normal. Because of inconsistencies in clinical findings, she was referred to a psychiatrist and later a diagnosis of hysterical conversion reaction was made.*

CASE: *A 30-years-old lady (wife of a doctor) presented with weakness of extremities. Examination: Motor and sensory – normal, ankle jerks lost, walked with ataxic gait, LP – non contributory. Initially it was thought to be functional. Later on she developed bilateral ptosis. NCV showed evidence of demyelinating. She was diagnosed to have Miller-Fisher syndrome. She responded well to IV gamma globulin.*

CASE: *A 42-years-old gentleman was admitted in the clinic for treatment of seropositive rheumatoid arthritis with severe pain in the joints. On the first day he received methyl prednisolone pulsing (1 g) and he felt much better as far as the pain was concerned. However he complained of some weakness in the body. Following the 2nd dose next day, his pain improved further but during the evening round he distinctly complained of weakness of his upper extremities. At night, the nurse had to rescue him from the toilet as he fell and could not lift himself up. A detailed clinical examination revealed weakness of upper and lower limbs (power grade 1/5). Blood tests for CPK, electrolytes, TSH were sent urgently and his K^+ was found to be 1.9 mg%. He was given urgent K^+ replacement and methyl prednisolone was not given any further. Within next 48 hours, he regained his muscle power and his K^+ level rose to normal limits. Although initially scared and grumbling (as he thought that his paralysis was iatrogenic) he left the hospital happy and contended.*

DIAGNOSIS: Pulsed methyl prednisolone induced severe hypokalaemia with quadriparesis.

(Pulsed methyl prednisolone can also give rise to hypertensive crisis, acute gastric perforation and severe hypokalaemia. The patients should be monitored closely during the therapy).

CASE: *A 56-years-old gentleman who was admitted with fracture neck femur undergoing surgical fixation developed post operative deep vein thrombosis of right leg needing a medical consultation from our team. He was treated appropriately and before discharge he was complaining of tingling and numbness for more than 3 months of upper and lower extremities which lead to his fall. Neurological opinion was taken and detailed neurological examinations done, which showed loss of deep reflexes indicating evidences of peripheral neuropathy. Following this opinion, lumbar puncture was done which showed increased protein with normal cell count. Nerve conduction studies done later on showed chronic inflammatory demyelinating polyneuropathy (CIDP).*

He was treated with IV steroids, followed by oral steroids for 3 months with substantial improvement of symptoms.

DIAGNOSIS: Chronic inflammatory demyelinating polyneuropathy (CIDP).

2 years later he presented with sudden onset of weakness of both legs while he was returning from his holiday. Examination revealed power of legs was 0/5 and that of upper extremities was 2/5 with loss of reflexes. Lumbar puncture showed increased protein with normal cell count and nerve conduction study was consistent with CIDP.

DIAGNOSIS: Relapsing CIDP.

This time after neurological consultation he was treated with IV gammaglobulin, which showed dramatic improvement of muscle power within a week's time. Following discharge he received monthly IV gammaglobulin 400 mg/kg one dose every month for 6 months. At present he is doing well. It can take a relapsing course. Once diagnosed, it should be treated with the help of a neurologist.

DISCUSSION: CIDP can sometimes be confused with GB syndrome but symptoms are usually present for 3 months duration as opposed to GB syndrome, which is of acute onset.

TREATMENT: Treatment of CIDP is with steroid and immunoglobulin with variable result.

CASE: *A 45 years old gentleman presented with acute onset of weakness of both legs following an episode of upper respiratory infection. Examination revealed flaccid paraplegia with a sensory level at D10. He had retention of urine for which he was catheterized. MRI screening of the entire spine and brain did not reveal any specific abnormality. Lumbar puncture revealed CSF protein 88 mg%, cell count 12 and predominantly lymphocyte.*

DIAGNOSIS: Acute transverse myelitis.

PROGRESS: He was treated with IV methyl prednisolone 1g daily for 5 days along with intensive physiotherapy. 3 months following discharge, his muscle power had improved significantly although he was still wheel chair bound.

Acute transverse myelitis usually presents with similar clinical picture to that of G.B Syndrome. However cranial nerve palsies are very rare and upper extremity involvement is also rare. There is associated pain along the distribution of the involved nerve. Bladder and bowel involvement are common. It is usually precipitated by an autoimmune process or as a sequelae of vaccination.

PRECIPITATING FACTORS:

Infection- Bacterial, Viral

Autoimmune- SLE, Vasculitis

Vaccination

Gadolinium enhanced MRI Scan would differentiate it from multiple sclerosis which may present such similar clinical picture. A variant, acute disseminated encephalomyelitis may present with similar picture to that of multiple sclerosis with widespread involvement of central nervous system. Again MRI Scan may be helpful to make a proper diagnosis.

TREATMENT:

Corticosteroid given in the dose of methylprednisolone 1 g. daily for 3 to 5 days, in the acute phase is effective. Plasma exchange may also be of benefit in patients not responding to steroids. A small trial has suggested that cyclophosphamide may be of some help.

CASE: *A 49 years old school teacher presented with back pain and progressive paraparesis which progressed over a few days' time preceding to this history he had a minor back injury while playing football and the weakness was attributed to the trauma. He subsequently developed bladder and bowel involvement. MRI Scan showed compression D_{12}-L_1 vertebra level. Surgical decompression was carried out but the improvement was tardy. 7 days hence, biopsy revealed metastatic deposits in the vertebral body. PSA was sent which was very high. (He did not have any definite urinary symptoms prior to this illness). Prostatic biopsy, later on confirmed the diagnosis of prostatic carcinoma and at present is on hormonal chemotherapy. 6 months following this incidence, he is now just been able to stand without assistance.*

DIAGNOSIS: Paraparesis due to metastasis of the vertebral body.

: KEY POINTS :

- Transverse myelitis, multiple sclerosis and metastatic disease should be considered in the differential diagnosis of GB Syndrome.
- Steroids may be helpful in transverse myelitis while it is not in G.B Syndrome.

REFERENCE:

K. Stephenson *et al,* Traumatic Neurological Emergencies, BJHM – Vol.72, No.5, May 2011.

K. Das *et al* – Guillain Barre Syndrome, a review, BJHM – Vol 71, No.9, Sept 2010.

20 A PATIENT WITH BACK PAIN

CASE: *A 48-years-old gentleman presented with history of low back pain radiating towards right leg for last 6 months. The pain was interfering with his day to day activity. Initially he tried with pain killers which gave only temporary relief. For last one month he has been off work. Examination revealed tenderness over lumbosacral area. Straight leg raising was restricted to 50°, the right ankle jerk was selectively absent on the right, right foot dorsiflexion was slightly weak and there was some sensory diminution on the lateral aspect of the right foot and the sole.*

X-ray lumbosacral spine showed mild degree degenerative changes, haematological and biochemical parameters were satisfactory.

DIAGNOSIS: Sciatica.

DISCUSSIONS:

Back pain is a common problem encountered in clinical practice and is one of the most common causes of outpatient presentation.

Most of the time, no specific cause is found and the diagnosis is ascribed to muscular or postural pain. It is very common in middle aged obese woman and in most of the times detailed investigations do not reveal anything specific. Postural care, physiotherapy, analgesics and calcium supplementations are usually advised. Hyperuricaemia and lumbar spondylosis are other common conditions associated with back pain. In young patients, presenting with back pain one needs to exclude trauma, some forms of spinal cord tumour and ankylosing spondylitis. In middle aged patients, osteoarthritis, herniation of intervertebral disc and spinal canal stenosis are the causes. Claudication of spinal cord is a classical symptom of spinal canal stenosis. The patient complains of pain and numbness of the legs on walking which immediately gets better on rest. The symptoms are also relieved by forward bending. In elderly patients additional causes like osteoporotic fracture, metastatic bone disease and multiple myeloma are the causes to be considered. Infection, particularly tuberculosis, spinal cord tumours can occur at any age. Associated symptoms and clinical features along with investigations are helpful in making a diagnosis. In females, referred pain due to gynaecological problems should also be excluded.

Causes of back pain:

- Muscular
- Fibromyalgia
- Herniated intervertebral disc
- Spinal canal stenosis

- Inflammatory spondyloarthropathies
- Infection with paravertebral abscess (tuberculosis is common in India)
- Osteoporotic fractures (in elderly)
- Metastatic bone disease and multiple myeloma
- Gynaecological problems like endometriosis
- Other rare causes like (Paget's disease – rare in India)

INVESTIGATIONS:

Routine tests including full blood count, ESR, bone profile, uric acid, rheumatoid factor, creatinine, X-ray – lumbosacral spine are the usual initial investigations. In young patients careful assessment of sacroiliac joint has to be done to look for evidence of sacroiliitis (frequently missed in early involvement). Other ancillary examination like local tenderness of S.I. joint, forward and lateral bending of the spine has to be done carefully.

MRI or CT scan is not indicated in the initial management. However, these are indicated if following warning symptoms are present:

- Pain is constant and not relieved by rest.
- Associated symptoms of weight loss, fever and high ESR.
- Cauda equina symptoms with involvement of bowel and bladder.
- In case of sciatica and spinal canal stenosis, persistence of hard neurological signs (like loss of reflexes, weakness of muscle or sensory loss) not improving with conservative treatment.
- In patients with suspected malignancy or past history of malignancy e.g. breast, prostate etc.

MRI or CT or myelography:

Now-a-days myelography is rarely done. MRI and CT are equally useful. However MRI has certain advantage in diagnosing.

- Infarction
- Metastatic cancer
- Neural tumour

I have seen few cases of tubercular spine where CT scan gave equivocal results. MRI scan was particularly effective in detecting tubercular paravertebral abscess in such cases.

MANAGEMENT:

For lumbar sprain, strain and spondylosis, simple analgesic, NSAIDS, muscle relaxants and physical therapy will help reduce the pain. Bed rest for few days may also be required. In some cases orthopaedic manipulation and epidural steroid injection may sometimes be needed. In addition to NSAIDS, antidepressants (particularly tricyclic antidepressants rather than SSRI's) may be required. In case of herniated disc and spinal stenosis, pelvic traction and lumbar corset are frequently prescribed (although hard evidence of their beneficial effect is lacking, prolonged bed rest is not recommended).

Management of Sciatica: The most common site of involvement in sciatica is L_4L_5 and L_5S_1 lesion.

Features of Sciatica:

- Restricted straight leg raising to 60°.
- Restricted crossed straight leg raising (elevation of one leg causing pain in the other leg). This is a more specific sign.
- Loss of ankle jerk (S_1).
- Reduced plantar flexion ($L_5 - S_1$).
- Loss of sensation over the lateral aspect of the foot (L_5) and the sole (S_1).

This has to be differentiated from nerve lesion mainly lateral popliteal nerve damage. Common causes -

a) trauma

b) vasculitis due to various causes

c) diabetes mellitus

Peripheral neuropathy can also give rise to similar features but it is usually bilateral and has a glove and stocking distribution.

The initial management is by conservative measures. If the symptoms persist beyond 3 months with persistence of hard neurological sign, MRI scan is indicated and the patient should be referred to neurosurgeon for consideration of surgical intervention, like lumbar discectomy for herniated disc.

It should be remembered that the best way to prevent recurrence of low back pain is by doing regular muscle strengthening exercise of the back.

The patient described underwent MRI scan of lumbosacral spine which showed L_5S_1 disc lesion. Since his symptoms persisted for >3 months, he underwent discectomy and made an uneventful recovery. 3 months at follow up he was reported to be symptom free.

CASE: *A 36-years old gentleman presented with back pain for 1 month duration. X-Ray lumbosacral spine did not show any significant lesion. His SLR was restricted on both sides. Initial bio-chemical and haematological parameters were normal. He was diagnosed to have sciatica and referred to the physiotherapist. Unfortunately his symptoms started getting progressively worse with increasing pain at night. He underwent MRI scan of LS spine which showed destruction of vertebral bodies of L1 and L4. There was no paravertebral abscess, however. Possibility of tuberculosis and metastatic bone disease was considered. Isotope bone scan showed multiple hot spots all over the skeletal symptom favouring the diagnosis of metastatic bone disease. He was urgently referred to the oncologist for further diagnostic workup.*

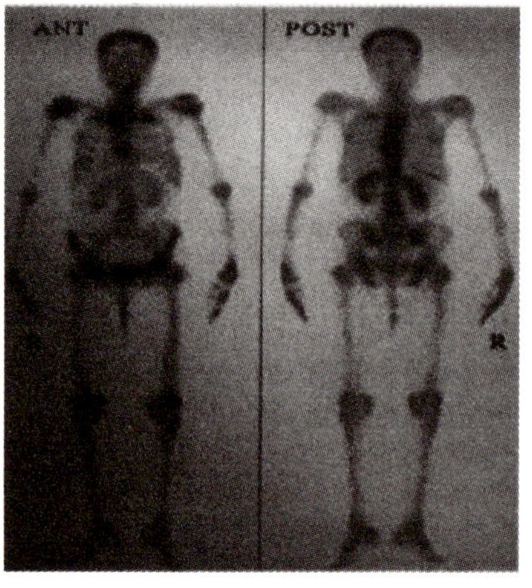

DIAGNOSIS: Metastatic bone disease.

CASE: *A 46 years old lady presented with pain around the left hip region. X-ray pelvis and lumbosacral spine did not reveal anything. Specific clinical examination revealed tenderness over the lateral aspect of the hip joint region. A diagnosis of subtrochanteric bursitis was made and steroid was injected locally with relief of her symptoms.*

DIAGNOSIS: Trochanteric bursitis.

CASE: *A 39 year old gentleman presented with pain around the right groin over last 6 months preventing him from cycling. Examination revealed tenderness over the anterior pubic rami. A diagnosis of Osteitis pubis was made and injected with local injection of steroid with relief of her symptoms.*

DIAGNOSIS: Osteitis pubis.

Different modes of investigations in back pain	**Indications**
Ultrasound Examination	Synovial cysts Rotator Cuff lesion
Isotope Scan	Metastatic bone disease Paget's disease Osteomyelitis
C.T. Scan	Intervertebral disc disease Spinal trauma
MRI Scan	Avascular necrosis Muscular or soft tissue lesions Intervertebral disc disease Osteomyelitis Synovial disorders of joints Derangement of axial skeletons

Pain around the hip joint is a common clinical presentation confronted by the internists. Common causes are –

- Sacroiliac pain due to involvement of the joint from any cause
- trochanteric bursitis on the lateral side of hip joint
- Ischiogluteal bursitis – over the gluteal region
- Iliopsoas bursitis – Antero lateral aspect of hip joint
- Osteitis pubis – lateral to symphysis pubis
- Meralgia paraesthesia – lateral aspect of thigh
- Pain over the anterior superior iliac crest due to enthesitis

In addition, sciatica and other causes of back pain discussed previously will also be common in the differential diagnosis.

A thorough clinical examination will clinch the issue and local injection of steroid will provide symptomatic relief in majority of cases and many unnecessary expensive investigations may be avoided.

: KEY POINTS :

- Low back pain is a common presentation in clinical practice.
- In most of the cases no specific cause is found and treated symptomatically with analgesic and physiotherapy and postural care.
- Antidepressant drugs may be needed in chronic non-specific back pain
- Warning signs for CT or MRI scanning include –
    - Constant pain
    - Elderly patients
    - Fever, weight loss and high ESR
    - Hard neurological signs like loss of jerk, reduced motor power and sensory loss, bladder and bowel involvement.
    - MRI scanning has an advantage over CT scanning.
    - In sciatica, persistence of symptoms for > 3 months along with presence of neurodeficit is an indication for surgical intervention.

REFERENCES:

- Low back pain – R A Deyo *et al*, NEJM Vol 344, No.5, Feb 2001, P 363 – 370.
- Neurological Differential Diagnosis – John Patten.
- Harrison's Principle of Internal Medicine, 17th edition.

21 A PATIENT WITH DEMENTIA

CASE: *A 64-years-old diabetic patient with history of IHD and past history of CABG 5 years back presented with gradually increasing behavioral problems. He was getting forgetful particularly for recent events. His sleep pattern changed with insomnia at night and day time sleepiness. On numerous occasions, he was found to wander around, unable to locate his own house with his neighbors rescuing him back. His family members were finding him difficult to cope.*

Examination did not reveal any local neurological sign. Investigations revealed reasonably controlled blood glucose, normal haematological and biochemical parameters, normal thyroid function test and liver function test negative, VDRL normal, autoimmune screening, cardiac investigations were satisfactory. CT scan brain revealed prominent cortical atrophy with multiple infarcts bilaterally.

DIAGNOSIS: Dementia– multi infarct.

DIFFERENTIAL DIAGNOSIS: Alzheimer's disease.

DISCUSSIONS:

Degenerative brain disease is a common problem in clinical practice. The patients present with disruptive symptoms causing a great deal of problem for the relatives and medical care givers.

Three common conditions causing dementia are:

i) Multi infarct
ii) Alzheimer's disease
iii) Dementia with Lewy body (abnormal aggregates of proteins inside the nerve cells)

In multi-infarct and Alzheimer's disease delusional ideas are common whereas visual hallucination and Parkinsonian features are common in dementia with Lewy bodies.

Clinical features of dementia:

- Progressive loss of memory particularly for recent events with preservation of old memories.
- Loss of interest, social withdrawal.
- Acalculia, agnosia, apraxia
- Confabulation
- Behavioral problems
- Loss of normal sleep pattern/Altered sleep pattern
- Urinary incontinence

Many of these symptoms overlap with depression which is a treatable condition and appropriate evaluation is needed in this regard.

Usually there is no focal neurological sign but the deep reflexes may be brisk with positive Hoffmann's sign and presence of ankle and patellar clonus.

During assessment of mental status, mini mental test scoring may be helpful in this regard.

Salient questions in mini mental test scoring [Total Score – 30]

- **Orientation**- Name, date, time, year
- **Registration**- Give the names and ask to repeat
- **Attention and calculation**– Serial 7 subtraction from 100
- **Recall**- Name three objects present earlier
- **Language**- Show pencil or watch and tell to
    - Name them
    - Ask to write
    - Ask to copy

Differential Diagnosis of dementia:

Irreversible causes of dementia	Reversible causes of dementia
Vasculitis	Hypothyroidism
Lewy body dementia	Hyperparathyroidism
Dementia with Parkinson's disease	Thiamin deficiency
Creutzfeldt Jakob disease	Vit B_{12} deficiency
End stage multiple sclerosis	Normal pressure hydrocephalus
Drug reaction	Subdural haematoma
Hepatic encephalopathy	Brain tumour
Kidney failure	Alcoholism
Neurosyphilis	Depression

Psychiatric conditions that may masquerade as dementia:

Depression

Schizophrenia

Conversion reaction

Since there are many reversible causes of dementia, proper investigation is important to find out those treatable causes.

Hb, TC, DC Platelet PCV
Urea Creatinine, LFT, Glucose
Na, K, Calcium, T3, T4, TSH, PTH level
Vitamin B_{12} level
VDRL, HIV antibody
CT or MRI Scan of Brain
EEG
CSF Study
X-Ray Chest

TREATMENT:

In severe aggressive behavior, following drugs may be used-

Risperidone (0.25–1 mg) twice daily

Olanzapine (2.5–5 mg) twice daily

Carbamazepine – 100 mg twice daily

In Insomnia and restlessness-

Trazodone – 25–100 mg at bed time

Zolpidem – 5 at bed time

However these drug therapies should be monitored carefully as they can paradoxically cause excitement and day time drowsiness.

Other modalities of treatment:

Domiciliary nursing care, rehabilitation therapy, occupational therapy and social care are very important in the management of dementia.

While dealing with the disruptive symptoms in dementia, traditional antipsychotic drugs are still in common use e.g.

a) **Chlorpromazine and haloperidol**

Extra pyramidal problems are common with long term use. Prophylactic anticholinergic drugs may exacerbate confusional state and thus are contraindicated. These drugs should be avoided in dementia with Lewy body as they may precipitate Parkinsonism.

b) **Atypical Antipsychotics**

Like risperidone (1-2 mg) or olanzapine (5-10 mg) has been shown to reduce disruptive aggressive and agitated behavior. Extra-pyramidal symptoms are much less common. The dose should be titrated according to the response as over dosing may cause drowsiness. Quetiapine is also effective and has the least chance of causing Parkinsonian side effects.

c) **Cholinesterase inhibitors:**

Donepezil (5-10 mg)

Rivastigmine (3-12 mg)

Galantamine

d) **Memantine** (NMDA receptor antagonist which may be combined with cholinesterase inhibitors).

These drugs have been shown to improve the cognitive scores, performance and daily activity scores, when used long term. Memantine (works on NMDA receptors) is the latest drug approved for the use in moderate to severe dementia. These drugs are given in patients with mini mental score of less than 24 (total score 30). However, in patients with score less than 12 (severe dementia), their use is perhaps not justified. Again, these are not very suitable for aggressive behavior and the confusional state. In any case their use is justified in view of the long term beneficial effects. Diarrhoea is a common side effect.

e) **Anti-depressants:**

Frequently these patients are depressed and use of anti-depressants particularly one of the SSRIs may be helpful. Tricyclics should be avoided as the anticholinergic effect may be detrimental.

f) **Carbamazepine and Valproate:**

Carbamazepine has been shown to reduce aggressive behavior. Drowsiness may be a side effect of carbamazepine. If clinically indicated carbamazepine may be combined with the other antipsychotics. Valproate has been found to have no effect on aggressive behavior.

g) **Anxiolytics and hypnotics:**
Insomnia and anxiety are common in dementia. When indicated, anxiolytics and hypnotics should be used only on short term basis.

In conclusion, behavioural abnormalities in dementia are sometimes difficult to manage. Atypical antipsychotics are the agents of choice. If indicated, antidepressants like SSRI and anxiolytics or hypnotic (as short term) may be added. Carbamazepine may reduce aggressive behaviour.

Anticholinesterase drugs produce improvement in cognitive scores and daily living score in long term but their role in behavioral abnormality is not well known as yet.

CASE: *A 65 years old gentleman with stable IHD was admitted with fracture of right femur of his right leg following a road traffic accident. 2 days following surgical fixation, he became very agitated and confused with paranoid ideas. He also developed acute insomnia. Electrolytes, ECG, blood gas, routine urine tests were normal. He was diagnosed to have acute post operative delirium and was successfully treated with haloperidol and risperidone. On discharge, he did not have any residual symptom.*

DIAGNOSIS: Acute post operative delirium.

This is a rather common condition in hospital practice mainly occurring in patients who are actually ill with electrolyte imbalance, infection, trauma etc. It is also common in post operative patients particularly those undergoing orthopaedic procedures. It is particularly common in ITU surroundings (ITU psychosis). It is treated with antipsychotics (haloperidol, risperidone, olanzapine and quetiapine). Benzodiazepines are indicated if the symptoms are due to alcohol withdrawal. These patients usually respond favourably and rarely need brain imaging like C.T. Scan.

Differentiation between delirium and dementia:

Sometimes it becomes difficult to differentiate delirium from acute aggressive behaviour due to dementia. In delirium, the onset is acute, with clouding of consciousness and pronounced hallucination while in dementia consciousness is clear, the problem is usually a long standing one and hallucination is not as prominent.

CASE: *A 63 years old gentleman with chronic renal failure presented with drowsiness apathy, forgetfulness for last few weeks. Investigations revealed Creatinine of 7.2 mg%, Urea 143 mg%, TSH normal, Na^+ normal, K^+ 5.3 mg%, LFT normal, MRI Scan of brain showed mild cerebral atrophy. Although his urinary output was satisfactory, it was thought that his deteriorating mental status was a reflection of uraemia. He underwent haemodialysis on 3 successive days with immediate improvement of his mental condition.*

CASE: *A 47 years old alcoholic patient was admitted with confusional state along with behavioural problem. His LFT was altered but other biochemical parameters were satisfactory. He was admitted to the hospital and started with 5% Dextrose infusion. His symptoms deteriorated in next 24 hours with acute agitation. 5% Dextrose was supplemented with thiamine with reversal of the acute behavioral symptoms. Later on he was diagnosed to have chronic hepatic encephalopathy. Gastroscopy showed Grade II varices. He was treated with low protein diet, high bowel wash along with other supportive measures for hepatic encephalopathy with gradual improvement of his symptoms.*

DIAGNOSIS:

1. Chronic Hepatic encephalopathy presenting with features of dementia.
2. Precipitation of acute Wernicke's encephalopathy due to thiamine deficiency which was aggravated by 5% dextrose infusion which further depleted the thiamine resource of the body.

CASE: *A 49 years old engineer, presented with rapidly developing symptoms of dementia. Initially it was thought to be due to depression. However anti depressants did not help. He was admitted and examination did not reveal anything specific apart from mild degeneration and demyelization in the MRI brain scan and slow wave activity in the frontal lobe area in the EEG. CSF study was normal. VEP was normal. Multiple neurological and psychiatric consultations were done and the consensus was that probably he was suffering from a slow virus disease of the brain and referred to a higher neurological centre for further assessment.*

DIAGNOSIS: Dementia due to slow virus disease.

: KEY POINTS :

- Dementia is a common clinical problem.
- Memory loss, cognitive impairment, loss of orientation, language problems are the initial presentation.
- Multi infarct dementia, Alzheimer's, Lewy body dementia are the most frequent causes.
- Biochemical screening like T_3, T_4, TSH, VDRL, vitamin B_{12}, folate levels should be checked.
- Atypical antipsychotics are the treatment of choice for aggressive behaviour.
- Anticholinesterase drugs improve cognitive scores (in mild to moderate dementia).
- Delirium is common in hospital practice and they are mainly due to reversible causes.
- Antipsychotics are treatment of choice for delirium while in alcohol withdrawal, benzodiazepines should be used.

FURTHER REFERENCES:

- Oxford Text Book of Medicine
- Harrison's Principle of Internal Medicine – 17th edition.
- The 5 minute clinical consult – 20th edition

22 A PATIENT WITH PROSTATIC HYPERTROPHY

CASE: *A 56 years old gentleman presented with urinary frequency, diminishing urinary flow and incomplete voiding. He also complained of increased nocturnal frequency. He was non diabetic and normotensive. Routine haematological and biochemical parameters were within normal range. His PSA was normal, urine for routine test was normal. USG of abdomen revealed increased prostate size with a residual urinary volume of approximately 60 ml.*

DIAGNOSIS: Symptomatic benign prostatic hypertrophy.

DISCUSSION:

Lower urinary tract symptoms are quite common in men over 50 years and the commonest cause is benign prostatic hypertrophy. However other causes like urinary tract infection, cerebrovascular accident (urinary bladder is under inhibitory control from higher centres), heart failure (by redistribution of body fluid while recumbent) should also be excluded. Lower urinary symptoms are a very common problem encountered by an internist or primary care physician.

Causes of lower urinary tract symptoms:

- Benign prostate hyperplasia
- Prostatitis
- Urethral stricture
- Bladder or ureteric stones
- Urinary tract infection
- Over-active bladder
- Detrusor under activity
- Bladder tumour

While assessing such a patient one has to differentiate uncomplicated from complicated lower urinary tract symptoms. Presence of dysuria, haematuria, palpable urinary bladder, recurrent urinary tract infection, high urea, creatinine, high PSA, usually indicate complicated urinary tract problem and should be referred to an urologist.

While treating such patients, self-management techniques should be encouraged. These include-

- Avoidance of caffeine containing drink.
- Avoid diuretics in the evening.
- Fluid restriction towards evening.
- Double voiding of the bladder.

SYMPTOMS: The symptoms may be classified as –

- Storage symptoms like urgency, nocturia, frequency.
- Voiding symptoms like hesitancy, poor flow, straining.
- Post micturition like feeling of incomplete voiding.

DRUGS:

Alpha Blockers reduce the tone within the prostrate and bladder neck. They have no effect on prostate size. Commonly used alpha blockers are *prazosin, terazosin* and *doxazosin* and recently introduced more **selective alpha blocker** are *tamsulosin* and *alfuzosin*. They are equipotent in reducing symptoms of prostatism by around 30-45% and increasing flow rates by around 15-30%.

Postural hypotension is a common side effect and the dose titration should be done cautiously with the first dose taken at the bed time to prevent postural hypotension.

Side effects of α-1 blockers:

- Postural hypotension
- Retrograde ejaculation

5 Alpha reductase inhibitors (Finasteride):

- These inhibit conversion of testosterone to dehydrotestosterone leading to reduction of prostatic volume.
- These drugs reduce lower urinary tract symptoms and reduce the rate of TURP and acute retention of urine. However they may take at least 6 months to produce symptomatic improvement. Usual dose of finasteride is 5 mg or dutasteride 0.5 mg daily. These drugs should be used if the prostatic volume is more than 40 ml. One should remember that these groups of drugs reduce the PSA level by half and while on these drugs, PSA level should be interpreted accordingly.
- These drugs may be added if the prostate volume is more than 30 cm^2, secure symptoms are depressed peak flow rate and PSA more than 1.4 mg/ml. It works by preventing conversion of testosterone to dehydrotestosterone. Combination therapy reduces relative risk of disease progression, reduces incidence of retention and need for surgery. It causes loss of libido, precipitate impotence and Gynaecomastia.

Antimuscarinic drugs:

Commonly used drugs are oxybutynin, solifenacin and tolterodine. These drugs are particularly helpful in urge incontinence resulting from detrusor instability in patients with CVA. In patients with BPH these drugs may be used although there is theoretical risk of urinary retention. They are contraindicated in patients with significant outflow tract obstruction.

For troublesome micturition, afternoon dose of furosemide or nocturnal desmopressin may also be tried.

Catheterization: Intermittent self-catheterization may be tried. However the risk of infection is high.

Surgery:

Transurethral resection of prostate is the gold standard of treatment. Side effects include retrograde ejaculation (75%), bleeding (5%) and urinary incontinence (2-3%).

Holmium Laser Enucleation of Prostate (HOLEP) is particularly good for larger prostate gland. The incidence of bleeding and hospital stay is reduced.

Bladder neck resection is a method used for tight neck with small prostate gland. Injection of botulinum toxin may also be tried with some risk of paralysis of destrusor muscle. The patient must be taught about self catheterization techniques. Alternatively cystoplasty may be contemplated which is a major procedure.

Role of PSA assessment: Nearly a third of patient with benign hyperplasia will have PSA level of more than 4.0 mg/ml. PSA of >1.4 mg/ml is associated with higher risk of urinary retention and high risk for requirement for surgery.

Special tests:

- Uroflowmetry is the electronic recording of urinary flow rate throughout the course of micturition and may indicate bladder outflow obstruction.
- Post void residual urine by ultrasound examination can also through some light regarding impending obstruction.
- Flexible cystoscopy may be needed in patients with recurrent infection, pyuria or haematuria.
- Urodynamic Study or pressure study may be performed to confirm presence of obstruction, particularly for those patients considered for surgery.

CASE: *A 62 years old gentleman presented with history of dull perineal pain, dysuria followed by urinary retention. He was admitted and catheterized and started on IV antibiotics for UTI. USG showed evidence of enlarged prostate. In next 5 days time, the urinary catheter was withdrawn successfully. However, the family members were very concerned because of a very high PSA level (44 units, normal 0-4 units). He was given 4 weeks course of ofloxacin and a repeat PSA after 6 weeks was absolutely normal. This patient has prostatitis and UTI which caused his PSA to go high.*

Cause of high PSA – other than carcinoma.

- Urinary tract infection
- Prostatitis
- Urinary tract instrumentation
- Prostatic massage but not rectal examination

If there is persistent evaluation of PSA, one should go for prostatic biopsy and refer to an urologist.

: KEY POINTS :

- Lower urinary tract symptoms are very common in middle aged and elderly population.
- BPH is the most common cause of such problem.
- Patients with complicated symptoms should be referred to an urologist.
- Alpha blockers improve symptoms without affecting the prostatic size.
- 5 alpha-reductase inhibitors reduce prostatic size but takes 6 months for symptomatic improvement.
- 5 alpha-reductase inhibitors reduce the PSA level by half and the PSA value has to be interpreted accordingly.
- There are some non-malignant causes of raised PSA and PSA should be repeated after appropriately treating those conditions.
- Persistently raised PSA needs an urgent urological referral for a prostatic biopsy.

FURTHER REFERENCES:

- Klahr, S, Urinary tract obstruction – disease of kidney – 7th ed., Boston, Little Brown 2001, 751-787.
- Mr. Mathew Jafferien – Management of lower urinary tract symptoms in men. BJHM Sept 2013 Vol. 74-no 9 p- 5148-522.
- Harrison's Principle of Internal Medicine 17th edition.
- Oxford Text Book of Medicine 5th edition.

23 A PATIENT WITH SYSTEMIC LUPUS ERYTHEMATOSUS (S.L.E.)

CASE: *A 34 years old lady presented with joint pain muscle pain, oral ulceration, skin rash over the face (butterfly rash) and fever. She also complained of tingling and numbness of her extremities. Examination revealed BP of 170/100 mmHg, butterfly rash over the face. Deep reflexes were diminished in the extremities. Hb- 9.8 g%, ESR-120, urea, creatinine high normal, urine showed protein++, few RBCs, ANF and antibody to dsDNA strongly positive. Rheumatoid factor negative, CPK normal, X-Ray chest normal, Echo showed LVH.*

DIAGNOSIS: Systemic Lupus Erythematosus (SLE).

DISCUSSION:

Systemic Lupus Erythematosus is an autoimmune disorder with multisystem involvement. With the easy availability of routine screening tests like ANF and antibody to dsDNA, it is not uncommon to get SLE in the day to day clinical practice. The main brunt is in the immune system leading to easy susceptibility to different kinds of infections. Genetic and hormonal factors have a contributory role.

DIAGNOSTIC TESTS:

Initial routine blood tests may show anaemia, leucopenia and thrombocytopenia along with elevation of ESR, Liver and Kidney functions may be deranged and urine examination may show proteinuria. X-Ray Chest showed reduced volume (vanishing lung syndrome) and echocardiography may show pericardial effusion. However the hallmark of diagnosis is auto antibody screening which usually clinches the diagnosis.

Auto antibodies that are usually positive are:

Antinuclear factor	98% positive – may be positive in other conditions
Anti-dsDNA	70% more specific correlation with disease activity
Anti Sm & Anti RNP	More common in overlap syndrome
Anti La and Anti Ro	Also associated with Sicca (Sjogren) syndrome & congenital heart block
Antihistone antibodies	Usually associated with drug induced lupus
Antiphospholipids antibodies	Usually associated with recurrent abortion, low platelet, DVT
Coomb's test	Associated with haemolytic anaemia

DIAGNOSTIC CRITERIA:

- Malar rash
- Discoid rash
- Photosensitivity
- Oral ulcers
- Arthritis – usually non erosive
- Serositis – Pericardial pleural
- Renal disorder – proteinuria
- Neurological disorder – Seizure, Psychosis
- Haematologic disorder – Haemolytic anaemia
- Immunological disorder
- ANF positivity

CLASSIFICATION OF LUPUS NEPHRITIS:

- Stage I (minimal mesangial) disease
- Stage II disease (mesangial proliferative)
- Stage III disease (Focal lupus nephritis)
- Stage IV lupus nephritis (diffuse proliferative)
- Stage V (membranous lupus nephritis)
- Stage VI (advanced sclerosing lupus nephritis)

GENERAL MANAGEMENT:

Since the skin rash gets exacerbated in the sunlight, use of protective sun screen cream over the exposed area is helpful in preventing the skin flares. Although vaccination is not contraindicated, one has to be cautious, while using live vaccination in patients on long term steroid. Oral contraceptives containing oestrogen should be avoided if possible as it can cause disease flare up.

DRUGS COMMONLY USED IN SLE:

- NSAID
- Hydroxychloroquine
- Steroids
- Immunosuppressives

For arthralgia or myalgia drug of choice is either NSAID or hydroxychloroquine (HCO). Hydroxychloroquine is particularly helpful in **arthralgia, myalgia, fatigue and malar rash**. Fatigue, myalgia and malar rash are particularly responsive to HCO. 6 monthly eye check up is needed for long term hydroxychloroquine therapy. Usual dose is 400 mg daily.

Long term NSAID use precipitate dangers like gastrointestinal ulcers and renal impairment.

Steroid is indicated in the event of organ involvement like **heart, lungs, kidneys and CNS**. The common protocol is to start with methyl prednisolone 1 g IV daily for 3 days followed by prednisolone 60-80 mg daily in a tapering manner. For long term steroid therapy, Osteoporosis prophylaxis with either alendronate (10 mg daily) or risedronate (5 mg daily) should be considered as well.

In case of kidney involvement, immunosuppressive drugs should be started simultaneously. In mild involvement (proteinuria <1.5 g/24 hr) azathioprine (2–3 mg/kg) daily can be used. However in moderate to severe involvement (proteinuria > 1.5 g/24 hr monthly pulsed cyclophosphamide IV (500–750 mg) for 6 months followed by 3 monthly for 3 years produce better results than azathioprine. The choice should be guided by renal biopsy if possible.

Recently daily mycophenolate mofetil with steroid has been found to be equally effective compared to steroid and pulsed cyclophosphamide with much less toxicity. This combination may soon become the treatment of choice in SLE with renal involvement.

Although methotrexate is used quite extensively in rheumatoid arthritis, it has not been shown to be particularly effective in SLE.

IV gamma globulin can be used in specific problems like thrombocytopenia, or immune-haemolytic anaemia.

Treatment of concomitant hypertension with either single or multiple drugs is very important in order to halt the progression of kidney disease.

In spite of treatment if the kidney function continues to deteriorate nephrological consultation for renal replacement therapy or renal transplantation should be done.

Since there is increased incidence of atherosclerotic heart disease, risk factor modification like treating hyperlipidaemia should be a worthwhile move.

Treating SLE during pregnancy is a difficult problem. Many of the drugs are contraindicated during pregnancy– like cyclophosphamide, hydroxychloroquine and NSAID should be avoided if possible. Steroid can be used during pregnancy. If clinically indicated, one can cautiously use azathioprine. Mycophenolate mofetil should be avoided during pregnancy.

In case of antiphospholipid syndrome with high incidence of spontaneous abortion, anticoagulants like low molecular heparin and aspirin should be used.

The list of drugs causing SLE is getting increasingly big. Classically following drugs are known to cause SLE (drug induced SLE).

- INH
- Phenytoin
- Penicillin
- Hydralazine
- Procainamide

Kidney involvement is uncommon. Anti-histone antibody is characteristically present in drug induced SLE. Treatment is withdrawal of the offending agent.

Use of infliximab in rheumatoid arthritis causes antibody to dsDNA to become positive without any clinical features of SLE. Simply the presence of antibody to dsDNA is not an indication of withdrawal of infliximab.

Infection is common in SLE and it has to be differentiated from disease flare up as both may have identical symptoms like fever. Flare up of SLE classically causes high ESR with normal CRP whereas infection would cause rise of both ESR and CRP. This is important as disease flare up needs high dose of steroid while infection needs appropriate antibiotics.

CASE: *A 21 years old girl presented with fever, bilateral pleural effusion and pericardial effusion. The pleural effusion was exudative in nature. Her mantoux test was positive. Her ESR was high and CRP high normal. She was started on empirical anti TB medication. Unfortunately on the 10th day, she developed high fever and status epilepticus needing transfer to ITU. CT brain and LP were normal. Her ANF and antibody to dsDNA reports came back as strongly positive. She was treated with IV methyl prednisolone and anticonvulsants. She was successfully weaned off from ventilator and 2 months at follow up, doing extremely well. She is on oral steroid and pulsed cyclophosphamide.*

CLINICAL MANIFESTATION:

It has got a female preponderance and oral contraceptives may flare the symptoms up. Although any organ may be involved the most common symptoms are related to musculoskeletal system with arthralgia and myalgia as well as dermatological symptoms of rash and photosensitivity. SLE should always be considered in the differential diagnosis in patients presenting with recurrent plural effusion, pericarditis, nephritic syndrome and seizure disorder, haematological problems like thrombocytopenia, haemolytic anaemia, psychosis, Raynaud's phenomenon or vasculitis.

CASE: *A 58 years old lady presented with 3 months history of intermittent fever, depression and decreasing mobility. She was also having intermittent confusional state. Her Hb was low, normal WBC Count, altered LFT (NAST, NALT, Low albumin high globulin, normal bilirubin, (high AST and ALT), USG– hepatosplenomegaly with few retroperitoneal lymph nodes. CPK normal, Mantoux test positive with 10 mm induration, TB gold (gamma-interferon) was negative. Gastroscopy showed antral gastritis but no varix. Colonoscopy was normal, MRI screening of spine – no evidence of compressive myelopathy, NCV test – demyelinating neuropathy both legs. ANF tests from two sources (immunofluorescence and ELISA method) were both positive. In view of her progressive weakness of legs along with retention of urine, she underwent MRI screening of her spine which did not reveal any compression. Similarly CSF Study to rule out TB Meningitis was grossly normal except for mildly elevated protein. She was commenced on steroid with improvement of her symptoms*

DIAGNOSIS: SLE with early demyelinating polyneuropathy and possible autoimmune chronic active hepatitis.

Follow-up: She became apyrexic, her mobility started improving and later on her anti liver kidney microsomal antibody came as positive.

CASE: *A 69 years old lady presented with high grade fever and joint pain. Clinically she had oedema of her legs. Her blood culture was positive for Klebsiella with the probable source being the urinary tract as her urine showed pus cells+++, RBC++, protein++. Her Creatinine was 1.8 mg% (high) and ANF was strongly positive. She was treated with IV antibiotics for 10 days along with supportive therapy.*

DIAGNOSIS: SLE, with UTI and probable involvement of Kidneys (Nephritis).

Follow-up: Following antibiotic therapy, repeat urine test did not show any pus cell, protein trace, 24 hr protein, no gross proteinuria and creatinine was normal (1 mg%) thereby excluding active nephritis. She was put on steroids along with prophylactic antibiotics for her UTI for 6 weeks. She has been reported to be doing well.

CASE: *A patient with SLE, later on presenting as haemolytic anaemia, has been described in the chapter of haemolytic anaemia. While writing of this chapter, 15 years on follow up, he is doing well on steroid 5 mg. every alternate day, without having any further relapse of his symptoms.*

: KEY POINTS :

- SLE is an autoimmune disorder with multi-system involvement.
- In a young female it should be in the differential diagnosis of fever of unknown origin, polyserositis, nephrotic syndrome, neuropsychiatric problems, and skin rash particularly facial with butterfly distribution, recurrent abortion, haemolytic anaemia etc.
- Disease flare up should be differentiated from infection.
- Arthralgia, skin rash and fatigue respond well to hydroxychloroquine.
- Organ involvement demands use of steroid along with cytotoxic medication.

FURTHER REFERENCES:

- Current concepts for the management of SLE in adults a therapeutic challenge – Y. Loannov *et al.*, Post Grad Med Journal, Vol. 78 – No. 924, P 599 – 605.
- The Systemic Lupus international collaborating – Clinics group – origins and outcome – Isenberg DA *et al.* Lupus 2001 10 275 – 277.
- Harrison's Principle of Internal Medicine – 17th edition
- Oxford Text Book of Medicine – 5th edition.

24 A PATIENT WITH RESTLESS LEG SYNDROME

CASE: *A 64 years female presented with aches and pain in the legs. The pain got worse at night. She had a peculiar burning sensation in her feet and frequently got up at night needing rubbing the legs and walking for few minutes. It caused her sleep disturbance. She took vitamins without much help.*

DIFFERENTIAL DIAGNOSIS:

- Burning feet syndrome
- Peripheral neuropathy
- Nocturnal muscle cramp
- Restless leg syndrome

Routine tests like TFT, LFT, FBC, urea, electrolytes, blood glucose, were normal. Nerve conduction study did not reveal anything. She was diagnosed to have restless leg syndrome.

DISCUSSION: Burning feet is a very common problem in clinical practice and very frustrating for the patients and the doctors because of suboptimal therapeutic response.

While dealing with this condition one should rule out different causes of peripheral neuropathy like diabetes, thyroid problems, alcoholism, vitamin B_1, vitamin B_6, and vitamin B_{12} deficiency by appropriate tests. Multivitamin tablets (injection vitamin B_1-B_6-B_{12}) may be prescribed. Restless leg syndrome (Ekbom Syndrome) is an uncommon condition mainly found in western population and occasionally in our practice, characterized by peculiar burning sensation in the feet along with pain mainly at night time and irresistible desire to move the legs to find a suitable posture. This is a very distressing symptom which causes sleep disturbance resulting in morning drowsiness.

MANAGEMENT:

This condition is DOPA responsive and nocturnal dose of levo-DOPA should be tried first as a single dose. If this fails to control the symptoms accurately, carbamazepine may be added in combination. Sleep disturbance is common and addition of clonazepam or zopiclone is both helpful for the symptoms and the sleep. Strong analgesics are sometimes (tramadol) required at night time.

Nocturnal muscle cramp is another common problem that we see every day in our clinical practice. Hypothyroidism should be excluded. Although vitamin E is commonly prescribed, there is no strong evidence that it works. Quinine sulphate (300 mg) at bed time is the drug which is uniformly effective. However, it should be used with caution as long term use in the elderly population can cause subtle hearing loss and thrombocytopenia so appropriate precautionary measures should be taken.

Common medical conditions that should be excluded include:

- Hypothyroidism
- Myopathy
- Neuropathy

Drugs that can cause muscle cramps include:

- Diuretics
- Nifedipine
- β agonists
- Statins

Drugs for restless leg syndrome:

- Steroid
- Mono amino oxidase inhibitors
- Tricyclic antidepressants, SSRIs
- Lithium
- Antipsychotics
- Antihistaminics
- Calcium channel blockers
- Dopamine antagonists

SYMPTOMS:

- Insomnia (10%)
- Fatigue
- Mood disorders like anxiety and depression
- Increased risk of cardiovascular disease

TREATMENT: Is directed towards the underlying causes like iron deficiency should be treated, massaging the legs may be helpful.

Dopaminergic agents: These are mainly taken before sleep. Levodopa, ropinirole (0.25-4 mg) and pramipexole (0.125-0.75 mg) may be used at night time. A long acting drug called rotigotine patch 1-3 mg may be used at night time.

Opioids like codeine, tramadol may be used.

Anticonvulsants:

- Gabapentin and pregabalin may be used in conjunction with dopaminergic drug.
- Benzodiazepine– Clonazepam or Zopiclone may relieve insomnia caused by restless leg syndrome.

So a careful drug history should be taken and acted upon accordingly.

: KEY POINTS :

- Burning feet is a common clinical problem with suboptimal therapeutic response.
- Peripheral neuropathy should be excluded.
- Nocturnal muscle cramp is also common in elder populations and hypothyroidism along with iatrogenic causes should be excluded.
- Restless leg syndrome is uncommon in Indian population.
- Restless leg syndrome is DOPA responsive.

FURTHER REFERENCE:

Marsdew CD *et. al.* (1994) movement – disorders, Oxford Butterworth – Heinemann.

Kumar and Clark – clinical medicine – 5th Ed.

Dr. J M Sheerson – The restless leg syndrome- BJHP April 2011- 72:4-219-223.

Harrison's Principle of Internal Medicine – 17th edition.

Oxford Textbook of Medicine – 5th edition.

25 A PATIENT WITH PARKINSON'S DISEASE

CASE: *A 62 years old patient presented with a gait problem. He has difficulty in getting up from bed and moving about. Of late his activities had slowed down considerably. He could not hold things properly because of shakes in his hand. He was also frequently falling about. He was a non hypertensive and non diabetic. Examination revealed a staring look with mild tremor in the hands. There was significant rigidity in his extremities. Investigation did not reveal any particular abnormality. CT brain scan was normal.*

DIAGNOSIS: Parkinson's disease

DISCUSSION:

Early Parkinson's disease presents with subtle signs and sometimes baffles the clinician. Sometimes it is misdiagnosed as brain stroke, osteoarthritis or age related frailty. Early diagnosis is important as specific treatment is available for this condition and the patients benefit from it.

CLINICAL FEATURES: Three symptoms are classical in this condition-

1) **Akinesia**
2) **Rigidity**
3) **Tremor – often starts unilaterally later on becoming bilateral.**

Later on classical shuffling gait, typical expressionless staring look (Parkinson face), and pill rolling movement of the hands make the diagnosis obvious. Atypical cases present with wide variety of symptoms like prominent axial rigidity (sparing the extremities), frequent falls, features of dementia, and different kinds of gaze palsy. These are known as **Parkinson-plus syndrome**. They do not respond adequately to levodopa therapy and the prognosis is poor. Multiple infarcts in a hypertensive can also cause features of Parkinsonism.

Parkinson Plus:

- **Multisystem atrophy:** With variable degeneration of cerebral and cerebellar.
- **Steel Richardson's syndrome:** Axial rigidity and upward gaze palsy.
- **Shy-Drager Syndrome:** Features of Parkinsonism with significant postural hypotension.

Elderly patients presenting with frequent falls, features of dementia and difficulty in initiating movement. Parkinson plus condition should be thought of.

MANAGEMENT:

Levodopa along with DOPA-decarboxylase inhibitors are the mainstay of therapy (Madopar, syndopa-plus). They should be started early and the dose should be titrated up slowly with increase in frequency depending upon the requirement and response. Although in first few years usually there is no significant problem, with prolonged use drug related side effects like dyskinetic movements and confusional state may become a problem. These are dose related and should be treated with appropriate dose adjustment. These drugs should be used with caution in patients with recent myocardial infarction.

Early use of **dopamine agonists** have also been advocated particularly in relatively young patients without any cognitive problems. The commonly available dopamine agonists are:

- Bromocriptine
- Pergolide (an ergoline-based dopamine receptor agonist)
- Rotigotine, Pramipexole
- Cabergoline
- Ropinirole

They may be started as initial therapy or may be added to levodopa. Cognitive impairment and postural hypotension are the two common side effects.

COMT inhibitors like entacapone may be used as an adjuvant to levodopa. By inhibiting COMT, it prevents peripheral breakdown of levodopa thereby increasing the availability of the drug in the basal ganglion. It has got no role on its own and it has to be prescribed with levodopa. It increases the duration of action of levodopa and its concomitant use may reduce the frequency of levodopa administration. Diarrhoea is a side effect. Tolcapone may cause hepatotoxicity.

Selegiline (Eldepryl) a MAO-B inhibitor was a popular drug in treatment of Parkinson's disease. It is also known to have neuro protective effect. However, in a study published in 1995, concerns were raised, as in that study mortality was high in the selegiline treated group. Since then its use has fallen down significantly. The significance of the study result has been hotly debated and many clinicians would still use it as initial therapy or as combination with levodopa. S/E – insomnia.

In some resistant cases **amantadine** (Amantrel) in the dose of 100 mg thrice daily as an add on therapy may be helpful. Confusional state, leg oedema and livedo reticularis are the common side effects.

In patients with significant rigidity or on and off phenomenon with levodopa, subcutaneous apomorphine may be an option. Domperidone should be co-prescribed to prevent nausea and vomiting caused by apomorphine. This drug is not easily available in India.

Anticholinergic drugs are particularly helpful in tremor. In view of their significant side effects like constipation, confusional state, urinary retention and precipitation of glaucoma, these drugs should be avoided in elderly Parkinsonism for obvious reasons. These are helpful in drug induced Parkinson's disease.

For Parkinson plus syndrome the aforementioned drugs are not effective and the prognosis is uniformly poor.

In addition of specific treatment, general care like physiotherapy, treating underlying depression and constipation should be done accordingly.

In conclusion, patients in relatively younger age group and good biological age dopamine agonists should be the initial drug of choice. Levodopa may be subsequently added to it and with increasing on and off phenomenon, COMT inhibitors may be considered in addition. Whereas in older patients with poor biological age, levodopa is the initial treatment of choice to which COMT inhibitor may be added if needed. In patients are unresponsive to this combination therapy, DOPA agonist should be considered in addition.

CASE: *A 69 years old hypertensive patient presented with history of repeated falls for which he had repeated admissions in the hospital. Frequent change and adjustment of the dose of antihypertensive medicines did not produce any desired results. On examination, he had clinical features of Parkinson's disease with tremor rigidity and classical facial expression. His supine BP was 150/90 mm of Hg which dropped to 106/60 mm of Hg on standing. Routine tests were satisfactory. His cortisol and TSH levels were normal. He was started on Fludrocortisone (0.1 mg) daily along with an advice to use elastic stockings. Anti-Parkinsonism medications were also commenced very cautiously. On follow-up, he was doing well.*

DIAGNOSIS: Parkinson's disease with autonomic failure (Shy-Drager Syndrome) was the working diagnosis.

CASE: *An 81 years old gentleman presented with recurrent falls particularly going down stairs clinically he had features of Parkinson's disease with masked face and rigidity but no significant tremor. Institution of anti Parkinsonian drugs did not produce any appreciable results. However, on careful examination, he was found to have significant defect in downward gaze with some restriction in upward gaze as well.*

DIAGNOSIS: Progressive supra-nuclear palsy (Steel Richardson Syndrome).

This neuro degenerative disorder presents with features of Parkinson's disease, dementia and gaze palsy mainly involving downward or upward gaze. There is no specific treatment. Anti-Parkinsonian medicines are not very effective in this condition.

CASE: *A 74 years old gentleman suffering from chronic vertigo, presented with features of paucity of movement, rigidity and a masked face. Anti-Parkinson drugs were started without a significant improvement. On careful history taking it was revealed that he was also taking stemetil (haloperidol) for last 5 years regularly. The drug was stopped and gradually the patient improved and later on anti-Parkinsonian drugs could be withdrawn.*

DIAGNOSIS: Drug induced Parkinsonism.

Common causes of drug induced Parkinsonism:

- Neuroleptics
- Antipsychotics like haloperidol
- Lithium
- Sodium Valproate
- Fluoxetine (rare)
- Anti-emetics particularly metoclopramide
- Alpha methyldopa
- Chronic exposure to carbon monoxide, manganese

Other secondary causes of Parkinsonism:

- Vascular
- Dementia with lewy bodies
- Post encephalitic
- Repeated Head trauma (Punch-Drunk Syndrome)

- Normal pressure hydrocephalus
- Wilson's disease
- Hypoparathyroidism or pseudo hypoparathyroidism presenting with basal ganglion calcification.

Other treatment options:

In patients not responding to anti Parkinsonian medications and otherwise having a good quality of life, deep brain stimulation (DBS) of the basal ganglion may be tried with good results. The treating clinicians should discuss with the patients regarding this option as it is also available in India now.

Neuro-transplantation of foetal cells and stem cell therapy are the other options although their role in day to day clinical practice has not yet been determined.

: KEY POINTS :

- Early Parkinson's disease is frequently missed in clinical practice.
- Tremor, akinesia and rigidity are the classical symptoms.
- Parkinson plus has a bad prognosis and they do not respond to medical therapy.
- DOPA agonists are the initial drugs of choice in relatively young Parkinson's with good biological age.
- Levodopa is the initial drug of choice in elderly Parkinsonians'.
- COMT inhibitors potentiate the action of levodopa but have no beneficial action on their own.
- Anticholinergics are used in drug induced Parkinsonism but should otherwise be avoided because of their side effect profile.

FURTHER REFERENCES:

- Siderowf A, Stern M – An update on Parkinson's disease. An Internal medicine. 138:651,2003.
- Harrison's Principle of Internal Medicine - 17th edition.
- Oxford Textbook of Medicine – 5th edition.

26 A PATIENT WITH OSTEOPOROSIS

CASE: *A 68 years old lean and thin lady presented with severe back pain for last few years. She finds it difficult to sit straight in the chair. Few months back she had a fracture of the right wrist joint following a trivial injury. Past medical history - total hysterectomy with bilateral oophorectomy at 40 years of age. Investigations showed normal full blood count, normal biochemical parameters, normal glucose and normal renal function. X-ray of L-S spine showed osteoporotic bones with collapse of* L_2 *and* L_3 *vertebrae, Ig Serum Protein (SPE) electrophoresis was normal, calcium level was normal. X-ray chest –NAD, USG whole abdomen NAD, bilateral mammography was normal.*

PROVISIONAL DIAGNOSIS: Senile osteoporosis.

DISCUSSION:

Osteoporosis is a common problem in post menopausal women and usually present with back pain, loss of height because of vertebral collapse, increased incidence of fracture of femur, wrist *etc.*

Common causes are:

- Post menopausal and senile
- Thyrotoxicosis
- Androgen deficiency
- Steroid therapy
- Smoking and alcohol intake

Other risk factors:

- Malabsorption
- Chronic Liver Disease
- Chronic Renal Failure
- Rheumatoid Arthritis
- Cushing Syndrome
- Acromegaly
- Immobility & Immobilization
- COPD
- Osteogenesis imperfecta
- Mastocytosis
- Hyperparathyroidism

- Drugs: Aromatase inhibitor, glucocorticoids, proton pump inhibitors, thiazolidinediones, anticonvulsants, phenytoin, heparin, lithium, steroids, cyclosporine, Selective serotonin re-uptake inhibitors (SSRIs) are also associated with increased fracture risk.

Prolonged use of thyroxin therapy in a euthyroid patient can cause osteoporosis.

CLINICAL FEATURES:

Increased risk of fracture both of vertebral and non-vertebral bones are the main problems of osteoporosis. In addition there are deformities like kyphoscoliosis, shortening of height with buffalo's hump and vertebral pain may also be a common presenting feature.

DIAGNOSIS:

Bone marrow densitometry is the investigation of choice. In osteoporosis the BMD is usually 2.5 standard deviation below the normal value.

Other Diagnostics methods:

- Quantitative CT scan
- Ultrasonography
- X-ray examination like cord fish vertebrae, collapsed vertebrae

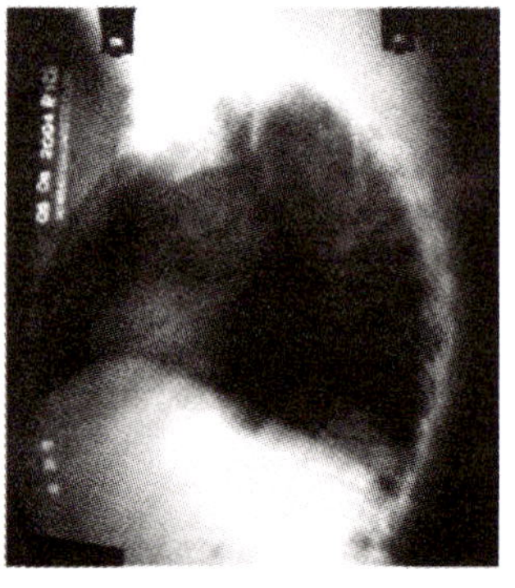

DEXA scan is commonly used and high risk patients like post menopausal woman, premature menopause should undergo evaluation for osteoporosis. Investigations are usually normal. However if there is associated osteomalacia, there will be decreased calcium, phosphate and increased alkaline phosphatase. Osteomalacia is a defect in mineralization of the bone whereas osteoporosis means thinning of bone due to loss of bone matrix.

While dealing with collapsed vertebrae and osteoporotic bones in X-ray spine, following other causes should be borne in mind and excluded with appropriate investigations:

- Multiple myeloma (high calcium, high ESR, M band in electrophoresis).
- Metastatic bone disease breast, lungs, kidneys, prostrate.

In osteoporosis, there is increased excretion of urinary hydroxyproline. However this test is not generally available for routine use. Measurement of bone densitometry is diagnostic. Since the facility of DXA scan is not widely available in all corners of India the treatment of osteoporosis may be started in high risk patients and on strong clinical suspicions after excluding other causes like multiple myeloma or metastatic bone disease.

MANAGEMENT:

It is important to increase dietary calcium and have a healthy diet habit. Smoking should be stopped. Daily calcium supplementation 500 mg to 1 g is helpful even though there is no calcium deficiency. Vitamin D supplementation is needed in the event of concomitant osteomalacia (low Ca, low PO_4, high alkaline phosphatase).

Bisphosphonates are specific treatment for osteoporosis. Cyclical etidronate, alendronate (10 mg) daily and risedronate (5 mg) daily have been shown to reduce the incidence of vertebral fractures in osteoporosis. Alendronate and risedronate should be taken in an empty stomach and the patient should sit upright for some hours in order to prevent oesophagitis. Etidronate is usually given cyclically e.g. 200 mg twice daily for 2 weeks every 3 months. Alendronate and risedronate are available and are superior to etidronate in preventing osteoporotic fractures of bones. Bisphosphonates are the treatment of choice for steroid induced osteoporosis. In patients on long term steroids, they should be concomitantly prescribed to prevent osteoporosis.

Commonly used Bisphosphonates in clinical practice

- Alendronate 70 mg once per week
- Risedronate 35 mg once per week
- Ibandronate 150 mg once per month
- Zolendronate 4 mg IV once per year

Upper GI side effects are common and oral drugs should be given in empty stomach in an upright position. Rarely there may be bony necrosis on prolonged use.

Hormone replacement therapy is the treatment of choice in **post menopausal osteoporosis.** However following the publication of **HERS study,** where it was shown to increase mortality in patients with cardiac problems, this has fallen out of favour. Instead **selective oestrogen receptor modulators (SERM)** are being used more frequently in post menopausal osteoporosis. Unlike oestrogen, it does not have any **adverse effect on breast and uterus.** The dose is raloxifene (60 mg) daily (Evista – BNF).

In severe bone pain, **salmon calcitonin** may be used (Dose 50 mg subcutaneously thrice in a week). Intra nasal calcitonin may also be used.

Other Drugs:

Teriparatide a recombinant form of human parathyroid hormone, in the dose of 20 microgram s/c per day, has been shown to reduce vertebral fracture by 65% and non vertebral fracture by 53% over a median period of 24 months. This drug is very expensive and cannot be used in patients with severe renal failure, hypercalcaemia etc.

Strontium ranelate (Protelos – BNF) in the dose of 2 g sachet per day to be taken at bed time has been recommended for the treatment of postmenopausal osteoporosis. It acts by a dual mechanism of stimulation of osteoblast and inhibition of osteoclastic action.

General Management:

As described before general management of osteoporosis includes ensuring adequate amount of calcium intake, vitamin D intake, regular exercise and cessation of smoking along with excessive alcohol intake. As steroid intake causes osteoporosis, any patient who is on steroid therapy for > 3 months should be assessed properly and preventive therapy should be instituted. In clinical practice, steroids both oral and through inhalation are commonly prescribed. While using oral steroids, osteoporosis prophylaxis is mandatory; its use in patients on long term users of high dose inhaled steroids is not well studied. However clinician should be aware of their association and use his or her judgment while recommending osteoporosis prophylaxis in patients on long term high dose inhaled steroid users. Mechanical maneuvers like using **Taylor's orthopaedic brace** help the pain due to **thoracic vertebral collapse.**

CASE: *A 66 years old lady with past history of hysterectomy and oophorectomy for some benign condition was admitted with a history of back pain. X-ray dorsal spine showed osteoporotic vertebrae with collapsed D_5-D_6 dorsal vertebrae. Her Hb was 7 g%, ESR-120 mm/1st hour, low albumin, very high globulin, high normal Ca level, normal alkaline phosphatase and normal thyroid function tests. In view of anaemia, high ESR and very* *high globulin level, serum immunoglobulin electrophoresis was requested for which showed presence of M-band. Bone marrow examination also showed presence of more than 40% of plasma cells. Bone scan showed presence of multiple hot spots.*

DIAGNOSIS: Multiple myeloma.

DISCUSSION: Routine mammographic screening showed presence of right breast mass and FNAC confirmed the diagnosis of ductal carcinoma. This lady had two malignant conditions. Following oncological consultation, she underwent mastectomy followed by zoledronic acid infusion. She was discharged on dexamethasone and thalidomide. She is under the follow up of an oncologist. In patients with osteoporosis, with high ESR and severe anaemia one should look for other sinister conditions like metastatic bone disease or multiple myeloma.

Duration of Treatment:

Again this is an uncertain area. The general consensus is that a minimum period of 5 years of treatment is required and in some cases it may be even longer.

: KEY POINTS :

- Osteoporosis is common in post menopausal women.
- Fracture femur, wrist and vertebral collapse are the usual manifestations.
- In patients with back pain and collapsed vertebrae, one should consider osteoporosis, multiple myeloma and metastatic bone disease in the differential diagnosis.
- Bisphosphonates decrease the incidence of fracture.

FURTHER REFERENCES:

- Mike Stone- Once weekly treatment of osteoporosis- Hospital medicine - Vol 63 : 4: 2002: 230-232.
- Harrisons Principle of Internal Medicine 17th Edition.
- Oxford Text Book of Medicine 5th Edition.
- Ignac Lgelman- what is new for management of osteoporosis hospital medicine Vol-66 no-5, May 2005. P 284-287.

27 A PATIENT WITH ENCEPHALITIS

CASE: *A 26 years old patient presented with a 2 days history of fever, headache and drowsiness. There was no history of travel in the last few weeks. On examination the patient was having fever of 101 F, unarousable, mild degree of neck stiffness, and no other focal neurological signs. System examination was satisfactory. Half an hour following admission he had an episode of tonic-clonic seizure which was treated with IV diazepam. Routine biochemical and hematological investigations were satisfactory except for mild leukocytosis. Malaria parasite P. falciparum antigen was negative. Urgent CT Scan of brain did not reveal anything specific except for mild generalized edema. Lumbar puncture was carried out which showed mild lymphocytic pleocytosis, mildly elevated protein with normal glucose level, gram stain, AFB stain and India ink stain were negative. HSV antibody, TB PCR and PCR for herpes DNA were awaited.*

PROVISIONAL DIAGNOSIS: Viral encephalitis.

DISCUSSION:

Patients presenting with meningo encephalitis is not uncommon in acute clinical practice and delay in diagnosis and treatment may lead to fatality.

Patients presenting with fever and altered sensorium may be having either:

- **Meningo encephalitis**– *e.g.* viral, bacterial, tubercular and fungal. LP is diagnostic.
- **Toxic encephalopathy**– due to sepsis, enteric fever, malaria and many other systemic infections. LP is usually normal.
- **Acute disseminated encephalitis (ADEM)**– following vaccinations or some viral infections like measles, chicken pox *etc.* Fever is usually absent. History is suggestive. LP may not reveal anything specific. Diagnosis is important as it is treated with IV steroids and IV gamma globulins may have a role in the management.

Investigations:

- Lymphocytosis, > 5 in CSF in viral meningo encephalitis and tubercular meningitis.
- Increased WBC suggests bacterial meningitis and occasionally in ADEM.
- Protein is raised in viral encephalitis. However it is usually less than 80 mg%. Higher protein content with lymphocytosis usually suggests tuberculosis.

- Glucose content is either normal or slightly reduced in viral disease whereas very low glucose with high lymphocyte and protein usually indicates tuberculosis.
- Bacterial, fungal and carcinomatosis meningitis also cause very low glucose.
- Although Gram staining is sometimes helpful, AFB stain has a uniformly low positivity.
- A rising titer of CSF herpes antibody is helpful in diagnosis. However it takes 5-7 days for the titer to rise.
- PCR for TB and HSV DNA are the useful new addition to the list of investigation.
- RBC > 500 cells in the absence of traumatic tap can occur in severe HSV encephalitis.

Radio imaging:

- Ideally an MRI brain scan should be done. If not available CT brain scan is an alternative.
- In MRI scan unilateral and bilateral hyper-intensity in temporal lobes are characteristic of herpes simplex encephalitis.
- Contrast enhanced CT scan can sometimes help to differentiate between viral and tubercular meningitis (basal enhancement in tubercular meningitis). In Japanese encephalitis, there may be bilateral thalamic hemorrhage.

EEG: Although difficult to organize in acute setting, it can give useful clues in differential diagnosis. A focal abnormality in temporal region may indicate HSV encephalitis whereas characteristic diffuse changes may be observed in hepatic encephalopathy.

Viral encephalitis is the most common cause of acute onset of fever, headache, altered sensorium and lymphocytic pleocytosis in CSF (In India TB can also present in this fashion – however onset is usually subacute). Many of the viral infections are self-limiting like EBV, mumps, measles, whereas some of them are quite serious (HSV, CMV) and some are nearly always fatal (Japanese encephalitis, rabies).

Herpes Simplex is the most common cause of isolated sporadic viral encephalitis. So in patients presenting with features of encephalitis and characteristic LP findings, empirical antiviral treatment should be started immediately. Acyclovir is the drug of choice. It is specific for herpes simplex and herpes zoster and does not work in other conditions. The dose is 10 mg/kg 8 hourly. The duration of treatment is 10-14 days. Less than 10 days of treatment can cause relapse of the disease (5% incidence).

Treatment should be started immediately (within 4 days) otherwise the mortality increases. The mortality of untreated cases may be as high as 70% whereas if treated within 4 days of onset the mortality may come down to 20-30%. Renal function should be monitored during therapy.

CMV encephalitis usually does not occur in immunocompetent patients. However, in patients with AIDS or immunocompromised patients like transplant recipients on immunosuppressive therapy, it should be considered in patients presenting with sudden onset of fever with drowsiness and confusional state. Ganciclovir is the drug of choice.

While treating patients with suspected encephalitis, one should also consider ADEM in the differential diagnosis. The history is characteristic. There is usually no fever and history of recent vaccination or viral exanthem is usually present. LP may show leukocytosis.

Treatment is with steroids and IV gammaglobulin may sometimes be indicated.

CASE: *A 26 years old man with history of depression presented to his psychiatrist with increasing abnormal behavior and headache. He also gave history of intermittent fever for last few days. The psychiatrist referred him to us to exclude any organic cause. Examination revealed neck stiffness, unequal pupils, brisk reflexes and bilaterally up going plantars. Urgent CT brain scan with contrast showed mildly dilated ventricles with basal enhancement. LP revealed cell count 86/field mostly lymphocytes, protein 220 mg%, glucose 36 mg%, blood glucose 142 mg%.*

DIAGNOSIS: Tubercular meningitis.

He was urgently treated with IV dexamethasone, 4-drugs TB regime and ofloxacin. Although he had a turbulent course in the hospital but 3 months at follow up he was doing well.

CASE: *A 69 years old HTN, DM lady presented with dysarthria, drowsiness and mild facial weakness on right side. She was diagnosed to have CVA and was admitted in the HDU. In the hospital her sensorium was fluctuating and she was having intermittent fever which was initially thought to be due to urinary catheter related infection. On the 5th day, in view of deteriorating sensorium (not consistent with the CT brain scan findings which showed small infarcts bilaterally) she underwent LP which showed cells 580/field, 80% poly, protein 18 mg%, glucose 46 mg%, blood glucose 246 mg%, Gram stain negative.*

DIAGNOSIS: Partially treated pyogenic meningitis.

In spite of treating her with vancomycin and ceftriaxone she remained vegetative for next 6 months till her death.

The index patient was treated with acyclovir intravenously for 10 days. MRI brain scan showed characteristic features of herpes simplex encephalitis. The patient made a complete recovery.

Acute *Herpes simplex* Encephalitis is a potentially catastrophic condition with high morbidity and mortality if it is not treated early. In addition to routine CSF examinations, PCR has high degree of specificity and sensitivity and may be positive as early as 24 hours of development of symptoms. Apart from characteristic EEG and MRI findings, brain biopsy gives the confirmatory clue. Treatment may be continued for 14 to 21 days and adjuvant steroid therapy may have a beneficial role.

DIFFERENTIAL DIAGNOSIS of Meningo encephalomyelitis:

Infectious causes:

➤ Viral:

- Enterovirus
- Herpes virus
- West Nile virus
- E-B virus
- Japanese B virus

➤ Other infections:

- *Mycoplasma pneumoniae*
- *Bartonella* sp.
- Tuberculosis
- HIV

Non-infectious causes:

- Small vessel vasculitis
- Disseminated encephalomyelitis (presence of leptomeningeal enhancement argues against this disorder)
- Neuromyelitis optica

CASE: *A 41 years old patient was admitted with a history of fever of 2 weeks duration along with headache. The reason of his admission was increasing drowsiness along with vomiting. Clinically there was no focal neurological sign. Hb- 14 g%, WBC- 19000, MRI scan of brain revealed a plain abscess of left parietal lobe with marked localized oedema. He was treated with vancomycin, ceftriaxone and IV steroid, and finally transferred to an advanced neurological centre where he underwent stereotactic brain abscess drainage. The antibiotics were continued and culture report later on grew polymicrobial flora.*

DIAGNOSIS: Intracerebral brain abscess.

DISCUSSION:

Underlying causes

- Trauma
- Sinusitis
- Infective endocarditis
- Dental infection
- Congenital heart disease
- Arteriovenous fistula

Common organisms

- *Streptococcus*
- *Staphylococcus*
- Polymicrobial
- Anaerobic
- *Toxoplasma* in HIV positive patients
- Fungal: *Nocardia* – in immunocompromised patients
- Tuberculosis

DIAGNOSIS:

CT scan with contrast enhancement provides a rapid diagnosis. MRI scan with diffusion weighted imaging may help in differentiating between brain abscess, cysts and necrotic tumours.

TREATMENT:

Stereotactic aspiration for decompression and diagnostic purposes is the treatment of choice and any abscess >1 cm diameter is amenable to such procedure. Antibiotics covering Gram positive and Gram negative organisms should be given for 6-8 weeks duration.

In immunocompromised patients additional cover with trimethoprim-sulphamethoxazole or sulphadiazine (for *Nocardia*), voriconazole (for *Aspergillus*), pyrimethamine plus sulphadiazine (for *Toxoplasma*) should be prescribed depending on the clinical situation. In India, tuberculosis must be considered in the differential diagnosis of brain abscess.

Anticonvulsants are not routinely indicated in brain abscess.

: KEY POINTS :

- Fever with altered sensorium should prompt the physician to do an early LP.
- If viral encephalitis is suspected on the basis of LP empirical acyclovir should be started immediately.
- In India tubercular meningitis is common and should be suspected in patients with headache, fever and altered sensorium of subacute onset.
- In toxic encephalopathy LP will be normal and metabolic and infective causes should be excluded.
- In ADEM there is usually no fever, LP is usually non-diagnostic and steroids should be used for treatment.

FURTHER REFERENCES:

- Harrison's Principle of Internal Medicine 17th edition.
- Oxford Text Book of Medicine- 5th edition.
- M.C. Brouwer *et al.* - NEJM 2014:371:447-456.

28

A PATIENT WITH POLYCYSTIC OVARIAN SYNDROME

CASE: *A 22 years old girl attended the clinic because of increasing weight, and menstrual irregularities. Of late, she has been very much worried about increasing hair growth around her face. Her periods were scanty and she occasionally missed it. Examination revealed an obese girl, with features of early hirsutism. Investigations: normal FSH, high LH, normal prolactin, slightly raised testosterone, normal thyroid function test. She was a non diabetic and her routine haematological and biochemical parameters were normal. Ultrasound examination of pelvis revealed bilateral cystic ovaries.*

DIAGNOSIS: Polycystic ovarian syndrome (PCOS).

PCOS is a rather common presentation in the primary care setting and the patients usually visit their primary care doctor initially before consulting a gynaecologist. The initial work up and diagnosis can certainly be carried out by the physician before referring to a gynaecologist.

USUAL PRESENTING FEATURES ARE:

- Obesity
- Oligomenorrhoea
- Hirsuitism

The diagnosis is important as besides the gynaecological problems they are more liable to develop obesity and infertility. Apart from the above PCOS is also associated with other medical conditions like:

- Insulin resistance and high incidence of gestational diabetes mellitus and type II diabetes mellitus (11% of obese PCOS patients have abnormal glucose tolerance).
- Dyslipidaemia with increased risk of cardiovascular disease.
- Increased incidence of endometrial carcinoma

Examination usually does not reveal anything specific but increased skin pigmentation may be present (acanthosis nigricans).

INVESTIGATIONS:

- LH is characteristically raised.
- FSH is normal.
- Testosterone level is slightly raised.
- T_3, T_4, TSH, prolactin - normal.
- Ultrasound examination reveals polycystic ovaries.

DIFFERENTIAL DIAGNOSIS:

- Ovarian and androgen secreting adrenal tumours (very high level of testosterone).
- Cushing syndrome
- Congenital adrenal hyperplasia.

The last two conditions have characteristic clinical and biochemical features.

MANAGEMENT:

Management is mainly directed as reduction of obesity, treatment of hirsutism with antiandrogen therapy as well as treatment of oligomenorrhoea with attendant infertility and correction of other hormonal and biochemical parameters. It has been shown that even 10% reduction of weight would improve ovarian function with better result from ovarian stimulation therapy; it also reduces the risk of development of diabetes mellitus.

Medical treatment of hirsuitism and acne:

Hirsuitism is due to hyperandrogenism which could be treated with-

- **Oestrogen**
- **Cyproterone acetate** (antiandrogen)- The two preparations can be used in combined shows good result, Dianette (ethinyl estradiol + cyproterone acetate) [BNF].
- **Spironolactone** and **finasteride-** these two may be used as antiandrogens alternatively. Finasteride can theoretically cause feminization of a male fetus so appropriate contraceptive precautions should be taken.
- **Isotretinoin,** topical medications and antibiotics may be used for acne.
- Cosmetic treatment with depilatory creams or electrolysis may be helpful.

Treatment of infertility:

This will fall in the domain of the gynaecologist. Following methods are available-

- **Drugs:** Cyclic use of clomiphene has been used for this purpose with an approximately 50% success rate. Multiple pregnancies and ovarian hyper-stimulation syndrome are the complications (characterized by cystic ovarian enlargement, extravascular fluid accumulation and intravascular volume depletion. This is a life threatening condition needing critical care input).

- **Ovarian surgery:** Traditionally wedge resection of ovaries was the treatment of choice. Newer methods of laparoscopic drilling of ovaries by diathermy are being evaluated.

Newer drugs in PCOS:

Since insulin resistance is the key to many of the metabolic and hormonal problems in PCOS, metformin (500-1500 mg) is increasingly being used in PCOS even in non-diabetic patients. This will help in decrease in weight, correction of metabolic and hormonal imbalance and even help in ovulation. Studies are ongoing to find out its exact role in PCOS.

Causes of Hirsutism:

- **Ovarian**- PCOS, Hyperthecosis, Ovarian tumours
- **Adrenal**- Congenital adrenal hyperplasia, Adrenal tumours, Cushing syndrome
- **Idiopathic**- With elevated testosterone, With normal testosterone

: KEY POINTS :

- PCOS is a common presentation in primary care.
- Hyperandrogenism and infertility are the main features.
- High LH with a normal FSH is characteristic.
- Initial work up and management of hyper-androgenism can be done by primary care physician.
- Metformin is increasingly being used in PCOS because of associated insulin resistance in its pathogenesis.

FURTHER REFERENCES:

- Oxford Textbook of Medicine 5th edition.
- Harrison's Principle of Internal Medicine 17th edition.

29 A PATIENT WITH GROWTH FAILURE

CASE: *A 14 years old boy was brought by his parents because of growth failure. He was otherwise intelligent and active. His parents were of average Indian height. The boy's height was within 2 standard deviations from the mean for his age and gender. Routine haematological and bio-chemical tests including thyroid function test were normal. X-ray of the hands showed normal bone age. Hormonal assessment showed normal FSH, LH, prolactin, testosterone levels. Growth hormone assay following exercise was reported to be normal.*

DIAGNOSIS: Idiopathic short stature.

DISCUSSION: Although patients with growth failure are usually assessed and treated by the pediatricians and endocrinologists, with the availability of synthetic growth hormone injection, primary care physicians are confronting increasing number of adolescent patients with a request from their parents to explore the feasibility of using growth hormone preparation in their children. A working knowledge in this field will be essential for a primary care physician in order to offer a well informed advice. The linear growth of a child depends on parental status and the vast majority of the patients seen in clinical practice are due to idiopathic short stature. However, other causes of short stature also need exclusion by appropriate tests.

Causes of short stature:

- Hormonal causes – hypothyroidism, Growth hormone deficiency.
- Chronic medical conditions like renal failure.
- Genetic disorder like Turner's syndrome.
- Bone disorders - like achondroplasia.

The usual work up should include hormonal assays - FSH, LH, prolactin, cortisol function tests, testosterone, growth hormone assay following stimulation with insulin or arginine in a fasting state.

Clinical examination and chromosomal studies will help to diagnose **Turner's syndrome.** A thorough work up would need expert input from an endocrinologist or a pediatrician.

When to recommend growth hormone therapy?

- Growth hormone deficiency in children.
- Turner's syndrome
- Chronic renal insufficiency in children
- Prader-Willi syndrome

Use of growth hormone in these situations will help to attain their normal height (90% in growth hormone deficient children but not so much in other conditions).

While using growth hormone therapy, one should be careful about its side effects like fluid retention with peripheral oedema, carpal tunnel syndrome, and increase in blood glucose in diabetic subjects. It can also cause headache due to development of benign intracranial hypertension.

Use of growth hormone in other situations like idiopathic short stature does not increase height to an appreciable extent nor does it improve academic activities and should not be recommended.

Use of growth hormone therapy in adults:

Growth hormone deficiency can also develop on adulthood (*e.g.* pituitary tumours and cranial radiation therapy or post partum pituitary deficiency as in Sheehan's syndrome). Deficiency of growth hormone in adults is associated with adverse cardiovascular risk profile, increased LDL, reduced muscle strength and exercise capacity etc. There is a role of growth hormone therapy in adults with proven growth hormone deficiency following a provocative test using insulin. This is a very expensive therapy and the option can be discussed with the patient interested in such therapy before referring him to the endocrinologist.

INVESTIGATIONS:

Measurement of random growth hormone level may not be helpful as its secretion is partial in nature. Subnormal IGF-1 and IGFBP-3 are confirmatory of diagnosis, provocation tests with insulin, glucagon, arginine, and levodopa in a fasting state with a growth hormone level of < 10 μg/litre supports the diagnosis of growth hormone deficiency.

FSH, LH, Testosterone levels along with chromosomal studies (47XXY) in Klinefelter's syndrome may be helpful. Growth hormone suppression test with glucose along with MRI brain scan may help in diagnosing pituitary gigantism.

: KEY POINTS :

- Short stature is a common presentation in clinical practice.
- Idiopathic short stature is the most common variety.
- Growth hormone therapy helps in attainment of final normal height in growth hormone deficient patients and to some extent with patients with Turner's syndrome and chronic renal insufficiency.
- Its use in idiopathic short stature is not very successful.
- There are some indications of its use in adults with growth hormone deficiency.
- The patients should be investigated, treated and monitored by an endocrinologist or a pediatrician with experience in growth disorders.

CASE: *A 32 years old man was referred from a gynaecologist for investigation of infertility. His sperm count in the semen was abnormally low. Examination revealed tall stature, secondary sexual characteristics were abnormal. He had small testis. Investigation revealed: FSH, LH and a low testosterone level. A clinical diagnosis of Klinefelter's syndrome was made and re-referred to the gynaecologist for the consideration of in vitro fertilization. The scope of androgen replacement therapy with testosterone was also discussed with the patient. It was stressed that although testosterone replacement will deal with the problem of osteoporosis, maintenance of muscle mass and ameliorate the symptoms of androgen deficiency like tiredness, weakness and lethargy, it will not increase fertility and gynaecomastia may paradoxically be worsened.*

DIAGNOSIS: Klinefelter's syndrome.

Tall Stature Causes:

- Beckwith-Wiedemann Syndrome
- Soto's syndrome
- Marfan syndrome
- Klinefelter's syndrome
- Pituitary Gigantism

Like short stature, tall stature may be familial. Some of the genetic disorder manifests from the very childhood and other deformities manifests during puberty, adolescence. Specialist endocrinological opinion is needed.

FURTHER REFERENCES:

- Vance ML *et al.* (1999), *Drug therapy— growth hormone therapy in adults and* Children, NEJM 341, 1206 -1216. Ho KKY (2000), Diagnosis of adult growth hormone deficiency, Lancet 356, 1725-1126.
- Kumar and Clark— Clinical medicine - 5th edition.
- Harrison's Principle of Medicine 17th edition
- Oxford Textbook of Medicine 5th edition.

30

CHOOSING THE RIGHT ANTIBIOTIC EMPIRICALLY

CASE: *A 44 years old lady was admitted with 3 days history of fever with chills, headache, and cough with expectoration of yellow sputum along with right sided pleuritic chest pain. Her WBC count was 22,000. X-ray chest showed right middle lobe consolidation. Sputum culture grew Streptococcus pneumonia.*

DIAGNOSIS: Community acquired lobar pneumonia.

DISCUSSION:

Upper respiratory infection, exacerbation of COPD and pneumonia are very common presentations in primary care practice. Mostly they are treated as outpatients but may need admission in case of toxic patients with haemodynamic instability. Choice of antibiotics is empirical as culture sensitivity reports are not available in first 48-72 hours. Initial choice of right antibiotic is very important as it shortens the duration of illness and in serious cases even improves survival.

The three most common organisms that are isolated in chest infection are *Streptococcus pneumonia, H. Influenza & Moraxella catarrhalis. Mycoplasma pneumoniae, Chlamydia pneumoniae, Legionella* group of organisms are the other causative agents. The evidence of penicillin resistant Pneumococcus is on the rise. In addition, 15% of *H. Influenza* strains and virtually all strains of *M. catarrhalis* produce β-lactamase showing in-vitro resistance to amoxicillin. Atypical organisms are usually resistant to penicillin or cephalosporin group of antibiotics. With this background knowledge one should select the antibiotic in a patient with chest infection.

In mild case:

- Amoxicillin may be used in the community.

In severe case:

- A beta-lactamase stable penicillin or cephalosporin should be used e.g. cefaclor, cefuroxime.
- Antibiotic in combination with β-lactamase inhibitor e.g. co-amoxiclav.

Drugs active against atypical organisms: If there is clinical suspicion of atypical infection, addition of another agent will be helpful.

- **Quinolones** - particularly new generation drugs like levofloxacin and they can be given as monotherapy as well. The 2nd generation quinolones like ciprofloxacin or ofloxacin should be avoided as they are not active against S. pneumoniae.
- **Macrolides**

Features suggestive of *Mycoplasma* infection:

- Dry cough.
- Prominent ear symptoms.
- Interstitial changes in X-ray chest.
- Occasional tingling and numbness due to peripheral neuropathy.
- Presence of clumped RBCs in peripheral blood film due to occasional presence of cold agglutinin.

Features suggestive of *Legionella* infection:

- Prominent diarrhoea
- Confusional state
- Hyponatraemia and abnormal LFT
- Interstitial changes in X-ray chest

Whenever suspected on clinical grounds, cover for atypical organisms should be provided.

CASE: *A 72 years old lady was admitted in the ITU with CVA. She was diabetic and hypertensive. She had a GCS score of 7 and was totally nursing dependent. On the sixth day of her admission, she developed fever and respiratory distress. X-ray chest showed right basal patchy pneumonitis.*

DIAGNOSIS: Nosocomial pneumonia probably due to aspiration.

DISCUSSION:

This is a completely different situation compared to the first case in that the patient was seriously ill to start with and the chest infection was nosocomial. In the nosocomial setting, the organisms in contrast to the community acquired organisms are mainly gram negative bacilli. This is due to colonization of oropharyngeal mucosa with gram negative gastrointestinal pathogens which finally find their way to the lungs. Moreover, the chances of aspirating anaerobic flora from the oral cavity are also high. The correct empirical choice of antibiotics in this situation will be –

- The 3rd or the 4th generation cephalosporins in combination with amino-glycosides or quinolones.
- In severe cases, higher group of antibiotics may be chosen, like-

- Carbapenems: imipenem, meropenem
- Ureidopenicillin: ticarcillin + Clavulanate, co-amoxiclav, piperacillin + tazobactam.

  - The incidence of MRSA strain is high in hospital setting particularly those who are ventilated for long and one should consider addition of antibiotics effective against MRSA (e.g. vancomycin, teicoplanin).
  - Although many of the antibiotics like carbapenems, ureidopenicillins are effective against anaerobes, it will be judicious to provide additional anaerobic cover (like metronidazole, clindamycin) in selected cases.

CASE: *A 54 years old gentleman was admitted with history of fever for last 4 weeks. Investigations revealed WBC– 19000 (poly- 90%), ESR– 110, CRP– high, Urine RBC 6-10 per field, ANCA negative, ANF normal. He gave a history of rheumatic fever in childhood. There was an insignificant systolic murmur in the precordium. Echocardiogram showed thickened mitral valve cusps and there was mobile vegetation over the anterior cusp. Blood culture on several occasions were negative (He was on different empirical antibiotics for last 4 weeks).*

DIAGNOSIS: Infective endocarditis.

DISCUSSION:

Infective endocarditis is one of the important causes of fever of unknown origin. Blood cultures are frequently negative because of prolonged antibiotic therapy (before sending blood culture, the microbiologist should be informed, so that special culture medium can be used in patients already on antibiotics).

If the blood culture is positive, it is not difficult to choose the right antibiotics. In culture negative patients, the choice of antibiotics depend upon the most probable causative organisms in that particular case. Majority of infective endocarditis in the native valve are caused by *Streptococcus viridans*. In case of endocarditis in IV drug abusers or infective endocarditis of prosthetic valve, *Staphylococcus aureus* or *Staphylococcus epidermidis* are the causative agents. If there is prosthetic valve of more than one year duration, *Streptococcus, Staphylococcus epidermidis* or fungus are the common causative agents. In elderly patients with genitourinary manipulation or gastro intestinal problems, *Enterococcus* is the suspected organism. In 5% cases, the blood culture may be truly negative because of unusual organisms like *Coxiella burnetii* or HACEK group of organisms. *Streptococcus bovis* is implicated in patients with colon cancer. Colonoscopy should be performed.

Antibiotics:

- **In Streptococcal infection:** Penicillin (for 4 weeks) + Gentamicin (for 1st two weeks)
- **In Staphylococcal infection**
  - **MRSA positive cases:** Vancomycin (IV for 4-6 weeks) or Teicoplanin (IV for 4-6 weeks) + Gentamicin + Rifampicin (orally)
  - **MRSA negative:** Flucloxacillin (IV) + Gentamicin
- **In Enterococcus infection:** Ampicillin (IV) + Gentamicin or Vancomycin (IV) + Gentamicin (for 4-6 weeks)
- **In true culture negative infection:** (due to HACEK group of organism): Ampicillin (IV 1- 2 g) + Gentamicin (for 4-6 weeks)
- **In fungal infection:** Lipid amphotericin (IV for 4-6 weeks)

This patient was treated with IV penicillin, 40 million units in 6 divided doses for four weeks along with 1 g IV amikacin daily for the first two weeks. He made a good recovery but needed mitral valve replacement later on because of development of significant mitral regurgitation.

CASE: *A 64 years old diabetic lady was admitted with fever of 2 weeks. Examination revealed tender swollen left knee joint. Aspiration confirmed septic arthritis with growth of Staphylococcus aureus.*

DIAGNOSIS: Septic arthritis.

DISCUSSION: Septic arthritis is common in diabetic, immunocompromised patients and patients having primary joint disorders like osteoarthritis or rheumatoid arthritis. In India, tubercular arthritis needs to be excluded.

Common organisms:

In children, *Haemophilus* group of organisms may be the responsible agents and the treatment should include cefotaxime to cover the organism.

In adults, the common organisms are *Staphylococcus* followed by *Streptococcus*. In MRSA infection, treatment should be done by vancomycin or teicoplanin. Linezolid may also be used. In MSSA infection flucloxacillin is the drug of choice.

The total duration of treatment is for 6 weeks of which first two weeks should be through IV route.

CASE: *A 55 years old insulin requiring diabetic lady with renal impairment presented with right foot ulcer. The ulcer was painless. There was foul smelling discharge from the ulcer with surrounding necrotic skin tissue around the ulcer. Clinically there was evidence of peripheral neuropathy. Her sugar was not well controlled, urea and creatinine were raised and X-Ray of the foot did not reveal any bony involvement. The culture sensitivity report from the pus was pending. Surgical team was involved and suggested regular dressing followed by wound debridement.*

DIAGNOSIS: Diabetic foot ulcer.

DISCUSSION:

Diabetic foot ulcer and other soft tissue infection is a very common problem in clinical practice and improper treatment may finally lead to life threatening gangrene and amputation. While general wound management strategy is the cornerstone of the treatment, it is equally important to choose the right antibiotic to control the infection.

Common organisms in diabetic foot and other soft tissue infections:

- *Staphylococcus aureus*
- β-haemolytic *Streptococcus*
- Gram negative organisms
- Anaerobes

For mild infection oral clindamycin or second generation cephalosporins may be used for 7-10 days. In more severe infection, intravenous antibiotics in combination should be used.

Common combination used:

- Flucloxacillin + Ceftazidime + Metronidazole
- Cefuroxime + Amikacin + Metronidazole
- Ciprofloxacin + Clindamycin

Many times there is involvement of bones with osteomyelitis and antibiotics with good bone penetration should be chosen, e.g. clindamycin, ciprofloxacin or sodium fusidate. Oral clindamycin along with ciprofloxacin is successful in healing of ulcers with osteomyelitis in 80% of cases. However, surgical debridement will be needed in many cases.

The newer generation of quinolones like moxifloxacin may prove to be a very useful drug in soft tissue infection because of its unique properties of covering gram positive, gram negative and anaerobic organisms. Moreover, it is orally active. While treating diabetic foot, infection specific to diabetes mellitus like necrotizing fasciitis should be considered particularly if there is formation of gas in the tissue planes.

This patient's pus grew MRSA and she was initially treated with cefuroxime, clindamycin and calculated dose of amikacin. She underwent local debridement of the soft tissue. There was no bony involvement. Later on she received 4 weeks of oral ciprofloxacin and clindamycin with good recovery.

Other Skin and Soft Tissue Infection:

Severe skin and soft tissue infection are quite common in diabetic patients, the recently published guidance of IDSA (2014) for the treatment of SSTI is mentioned below.

Recurrent Skin Abscess:

- To exclude local conditions like pilonidal sinus, hidradenitis suppurativa *etc.*
- 5-10 days course of antibiotic according to the culture report.
- 5 days decolonization regime with twice daily intranasal mupirocin, daily chlorhexidine wash.
- Daily decontamination of personal items.
- Neutrophil disorder should be evaluated (like chronic granulomatous disease).

Treatment of or erysipelas and cellulitis:

- For severe infection, MRSA and gram negative cover should be provided *e.g.* vancomycin + meropenem or imipenem.
- In mild cases coverage for streptococcus should be provided (orally). Duration is usually 5 days but may be extended if clinically indicated.
- Anti-inflammatory drugs like steroid may be added in non-diabetic patient.
- In recurrent cellulitis prophylactic oral penicillin or erythromycin or IM benzathine penicillin (monthly) may be considered for 4-5 weeks. Local causes like eczema, venous ulcer, obesity should be treated.

Surgical site infection:

- **Gastrointestinal and genitourinary tract single drug regime**:

  Meropenem (1 g 8 hourly)

  Imipenem + Cilastatin (500 mg 6 hourly)

  Piperacillin + Tazobactam (4.5 g 8 hourly)

- **Combination agent:**

  Ceftriaxone (1 g twice daily) + Metronidazole (500 mg thrice daily)

  Ciprofloxacin + Metronidazole (500 mg IV twice daily)

  Levofloxacin (750 mg IV once daily) + Metronidazole (500 mg IV thrice daily)

  Ampicillin + Sulbactam (3 g 6 hourly) + Gentamicin (5 mg/ kg/ day)

- **Surgical site- extremities:** Following drugs may be used:

  Oxacillin

  Nafcillin

  Cefazolin

  Vancomycin

- **Surgical site infection in axilla and perineum:**

  Ciprofloxacin

  Levofloxacin or

  Ceftriaxone in combination with metronidazole

- **For Necrotizing Fascitis:**

  Linezolid or vancomycin + piperacillin-tazobactam or meropenem or imipenem + cilastatin plus ceftriaxone and metronidazole may be used.

  Penicillin + clindamycin may be used in documented streptococcus infection.

- **Management of Pyomyositis:**

  Vancomycin + an antibiotic covering gram negative enteric organism should be used.

  Local dressing is essential.

- **Treatment of Clostridial gas gangrene or myonecrosis:**

  Debridement of local tissue

  Empirical treatment with vancomycin + piperacillin-tazobactam, ampicillin-sulbactam or carbapenem.

  Definitive treatment – penicillin and clindamycin

  Hyperbaric oxygen therapy is not recommended.

CASE: *A 42 years old patient was admitted in ITU with acute renal failure due to falciparum malaria. He was treated successfully with antimalarials along with daily haemodialysis. He had a central line in-situ for CVP monitoring, TPN and fluid therapy. In spite of clearance of MP, his fever recurred on the 6th day. A diligent search failed to detect any underlying cause on the 10th day, blood culture grew Staphylococcus aureus. The central line was withdrawn and calculated dose of vancomycin was commenced. The tip of the central line also grew Staphylococcus aureus.*

DIAGNOSIS: Catheter related infection.

DISCUSSION: Line related infection is a very common as hospital acquired infection.

Common organisms isolated:

- Coagulase negative *Staphylococcus* : 32-41%
- *Staphylococcus aureus* : 18-31%
- Enteric gram negative bacilli : 10-18%
- *Candida* : 9-11%
- *Pseudomonas* : 4-6%
- *Enterococci* and *Streptococci* : 3-14%
- Other : 8-9%

Although there are guidelines of diagnosing catheter related blood stream infection, the diagnosis is usually made on strong clinical suspicion in a febrile patient with central line. A positive blood culture from a peripheral vein and isolation of the same organism from the removed catheter tip will aid in an accurate diagnosis.

Once the diagnosis is suspected, the line should be removed and sent for culture. Since *staphylococcus* is the most common organism (with increasing MRSA strains), glycopeptides like vancomycin or teicoplanin should be the first choice. If MRSA is isolated, flucloxacillin, the 2nd generation cephalosporin (cefuroxime) or the 4th generation cephalosporin (cefpirome) may also be selected. The duration should be at least for a period of 10-14 days. If fever continues, septic complication like infective endocarditis should be suspected and the duration of antibiotic therapy becomes prolonged.

In ITUs, the incidence of Candida septicaemia is on the rise and if proven, IV lipid amphotericin B or fluconazole (400 mg daily in adults) should be prescribed for 2 weeks. One should remember that the resistance to voriconazole is on the rise and if suspected it should be replaced either by amphotericin or fluconazole.

This patient's fever settled down with the withdrawal of the central line and 10 days treatment of vancomycin. However, he was dialysis dependent for next one month through a separate femoral line.

CASE: *A 58 years old diabetic lady presented with a 4 days history of fever, headache and confusional state. She was presented in an unarousable state, glucose- 310 mg% but no ketoacidosis, Na- 124, malaria negative. Urgent CT brain scan did not reveal any obvious abnormality. Lumbar puncture showed cell count 480/ field, 80% neutrophil; the colour was opalescent, protein- 180 mg%, glucose- 46 mg%, chloride- 106 mg%, Gram stain – Gram positive organisms, culture-awaited.*

DIAGNOSIS: Pyogenic meningitis.

DISCUSSION:

Fever, headache with deteriorating consciousness level is a rather common presentation in hospital practice and meningo-encephalitis or toxic encephalopathy due to systemic infection or metabolic encephalopathy is the common cause. Because of atypical presentation, the lumbar puncture is often delayed and the classical features of pyogenic meningitis are masked or altered because of previous antibiotic therapy. Once the diagnosis of pyogenic meningitis is made (with classical cell count, raised protein and low glucose levels) prompt empirical antibiotic therapy should be instituted.

While treating bacterial meningitis in adults, the common infecting organisms should be borne in mind.

Three most common causes are:

- *Neisseria meningitides*
- *Haemophilus influenzae*
- *Streptococcus pneumoniae*

Other causes:

- *Listeria monocytogenes*
- *Staphylococcus aureus*

In India, tuberculous meningitis should also be considered in the differential diagnosis.

Clinical features suggestive of specific infection:

- Petechial skin rash – *Meningococcus*
- Ear disease, skull fracture – Pneumococcus
- Complement deficiency – *Meningococcus*
- Head injury – *Staphylococcus*
- Elderly, debilitated – *Listeria*
- In immunocompromised – *Cryptococcus*

Common antibiotics for empirical use:

- Intravenous cefotaxime or ceftriaxone.
- Addition of vancomycin with or without rifampicin where serious infection due to penicillin resistant *Pneumococci* is suspected.
- Ampicillin should be added to the regime if Listeria is suspected to be the causative organism.
- Dexamethasone (10 mg) every six hours for first 4 days and the 1st dose should be given prior to the administration of the 1st dose of antibiotic. Use of steroid in bacterial meningitis has shown to reduce the mortality in bacterial meningitis.

The treatment should be continued for a period of 10-14 days.

CASE: *A 48 years old diabetic gentleman was admitted for abdominal pain, distension and vomiting. He was very toxic looking with pulse rate of 140/m, BP 100/60 mmHg. There was prominent abdominal muscle guarding. USG showed distended gall bladder with free fluid in peritoneum. He underwent urgent laparotomy and a perforated and gangrenous gall bladder was removed. He underwent peritoneal toileting. His post operative course was unstable with persistent high fever.*

DIAGNOSIS: Perforated gall bladder with secondary biliary peritonitis.

DISCUSSION:

Intra abdominal infections are common in hospital setting and infections are usually polymicrobial. Common organisms are:

- *Enterobacter, Pseudomonas, Serratia, Citrobacter and Anaerobes.*

The usual antibiotic cover includes:

- β lactam / β lactamase inhibitors, like-
  - Amoxicillin-clavulanic acid
  - Ticarcillin-clavulanic acid
  - Piperacillin-tazobactam [with or without aminoglycoside]
- Carbapenems – Imipenem, Meropenem
- 3rd or 4th generation cephalosporins
  - Ceftazidime or cefepime [if pseudomonas is suspected]
  - Cefotaxime, ceftriaxone.
- Metronidazole cover is sometimes provided in addition, although most of the antibiotics mentioned above have anaerobic cover.

CASE: *A 49 years old lady was admitted with severe upper abdominal pain and vomiting. Investigations revealed Amylase- 2400 (very high),WBC- 20,000, Bilirubin– 2.1 mg%, AST- 104, Alkaline phosphatase- 510, Random glucose- 260 mg%, CRP- 124, LDH- 912, calcium- 6.9 mg% (low), USG- gall stone present, bulky head of pancreas consistent with acute pancreatitis.*

DIAGNOSIS: Acute pancreatitis.

DISCUSSION:

In acute pancreatitis, 80% of the patient recovers without any major problem. However 20% develop severe complications including pancreatic necrosis leading to sepsis and multiorgan failure. A Ranson score of more than 3, APACHE II scoring of more than 8 and CRP more than 120 at the end of the 1st week usually indicate stormy course. Initial management includes supportive therapy with enteral nutrition, antibiotics and drainage of the obstructed biliary tract. In clinical trials imipenem, cefuroxime and combination of ceftazidime, amikacin and metronidazole have been tried. All of them were found to reduce the incidence of sepsis without affecting the overall mortality. The most convincing evidence of efficiency was found with imipenem. Antibiotics with good tissue penetration in the pancreas should be chosen (imipenem, ofloxacin and ciprofloxacin). In severe case, imipenem should be the drug of choice. In infected pancreatic necrosis, antibiotics should be used for 4-6 weeks.

This patient was put on meropenem and later on the culture report from CT guided aspiration fluid showed growth of ESBL producing *E. coli* sensitive to meropenem. He made a full recovery.

CASE: *A 71 years old patient was transferred from another medical facility in an intubated state. He was initially admitted with a CVA which needed intubation. From the 4th day of admission he developed breathlessness and high grade fever which was not remolding. The patient was transferred to the tertiary care for better management. The patient was quite toxic looking and was mechanically ventilated. He was commenced on piperacillin tazobactam and teicoplanin for the fever. 48 hours after admission, his endotracheal tube secretion grew Acinetobacter species. His blood culture also grew the same organism which was resistant to all antibiotics except for colistin. X-ray chest showed pneumatic patch over the right mid-zone.*

DIAGNOSIS: Tube associated pneumonia due to PAN resistant Acinetobacter organism.

DISCUSSION:

Infections due to drug resistant organism in the hospitals are increasing and are becoming a concern throughout the world.

Common causes:

- MRSA (Methicillin resistant *Staphylococcus aureus*)
- Multi drug resistant gram negative organism e.g. *E. coli*, *Klebsiella*, *Pseudomonas*, *Acinetobacter*.

Mechanism of resistance:

- Increased β-lactamase activity
- Porin loss
- Alteration of PBP's
- Efflux mechanism

Classification of β-lactamase:

Group-A	Group-C	Group-D	Group-B
ESBLS, CTX-M TEM, SHV	AMP-C	OX A	NDM, IMP, VIM

ESBL producing gram negative bacteria are a real threat in the Indian scenario and Indian registries suggest that in certain institutions, the rate is as high as 80%. Recently in addition to hospital acquired strains, ESBL producing organisms are also being found in community settings. In addition, co-production of ESBL and AMP C along with ESBL and OX A, are also becoming common which increases the resistance pattern by many folds. These enzymes along with recently described New Delhi Metallo βeta-lactamase producing organisms are even conferring resistance to almost all the commonly used antibiotics including carbapenems leaving only the old drug colistin to be used in a new garb.

: ACTIVITY OF BLI :

BLI	Activity against OXA
Clavulanic acid	**No**
Sulbactam	**No**
Tazobactam	**No**

ACTIVITY OF 3RD GENERATION CEPHALOSPORIN

	ESBL	AMP C	OXA
Ceftazidime	×	×	±
Cefotaxime	×	×	±
Cefepime	×	✓	✓
Cefpirome	×	✓	✓

Combination of Cefepime or Cefpirome with BLI may be effective in treating infection by co-producer of ESBL along with Amp C or OX A.

CLINICAL RELEVANCE OF Β-LACTAMASE PRODUCING ORGANISMS

Mechanism	Producing organism	Affected	Not affected
Common plasmid TEM 1, TEM 2, SEV 1	Gram negative organisms	Amoxicillin Carbapenems	$2^{nd}/3^{rd}$ cephalosporins BL + BLI Monobactam Carbapenem
ESBL producers	*Klebsiella, E. coli*	Above + 2nd + 3rd gen Cephalosporins Monobactams	Cephamycin Carbapenem Tigecycline PBL + BCI
AMP C producers	Enterobacter, Acinetobacter Pseudomonas	Above + BL + BLI Cephalosporin	Cefepime Carbapenem Tigecycline
Metallo β-lactamase	Acinetobacter Pseudomonas	Above + Carbapenem	SM x/TM Aztreonam Colistin

How to prevent emergence of drug resistance:

Since there is no any new antibiotic in the pipeline, judicious and rational use of antibiotics through a well structured antibiotic store and ship programme is the way forward to prevent emergence of drug resistance bugs. Following are the steps that may be adapted towards that effect.

Prevention of infection along with prevention of transmission of infection:

- To avoid unnecessary catheterization
- To renounce central tube, IV as soon as possible.
- Hand washing with alcohol based solution between examinations of each patient. This is a simple yet most important means of prevention of spread of infection..
- Early diagnosis with appropriate specimen culture.

HIT HARD (AS QUICKLY AS POSSIBLE)

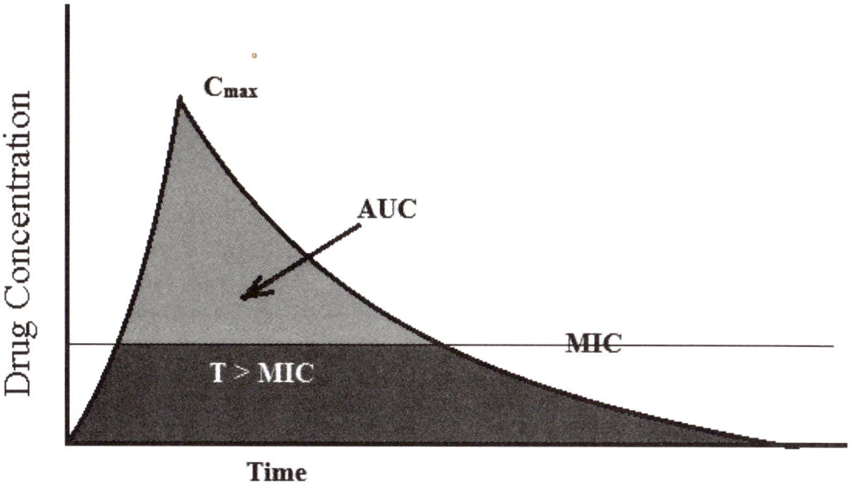

Rational use of antibiotic: 4D

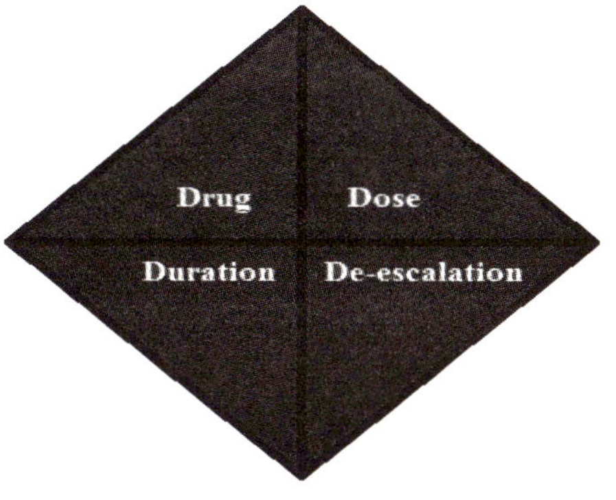

Drug ⇒ initially empirically with broad spectrum, later on as per culture sensitivity report.

Dose ⇒ PK/PD (Pharmacokinetic/Pharmacodynamic) of the drug should be considered, some drugs work by time dependant killing method namely β-lactamase, Carbapenem, Piperacillin, Clindamycin, Macrolides. They should be given by continuous infusion as the drug level should be above MIC about 60% of time in 24 hour.

Some drugs like Aminoglycosides, Quinolones, Vancomycin, Linezolid etc. work by the method of concentration dependent killing where the maximum peak concentration is important for their activity whereas the trough level is related to the side effects of these drugs. These drugs should be given bolus either as once daily or twice dosage.

CHOOSING DRUGS EMPIRICALLY IN HOSPITAL SETTING

No previous hospitalization No risk factors No recent intervention	Low Risk of ESBL PAN resistant Drugs MRSA	Antibiotic β-lactam Co-amoxiclav 2nd gen cephalosporins
H/O Recent Hospitalization H/O Catheterization H/O Antibiotic therapy	Risk of ESBL moderate Risk of pan resistant organism low	Piperacillin-tazobactam BL + BLI Cefepime-tazobactam
Immuno compromised DM, Concur Recurrent Hospital admission Recent interruption	RISK OF ESBL PAN drug resistant organism MRSA high	Carbapenem Colistin Vancomycin Teicoplanin

Right duration ⇒ in majority of infection the duration is for 7-8 days except for infection due to *Pseudomonas* and *Acinetobacter* where they should be given for 14 days.

De escalation ⇒ to discontinue if culture negative, if clinically stable.

Clinical Judgement necessary	To diminish the number of antibiotic. To shorten the duration. To narrow the spectrum.

- Use of MIC based PK/PD doses is important in prevention of drug resistance. The dosing of drugs must be formed above the MIC and not merely above MIC as this may encourage the growth of mutation forming organism thereby giving credence to the concept of mutation preventing concentration which is above the MIC.

- Combination of drugs is something necessary particularly in case of Colistin. Otherwise there is a chance of development of hetero resistance. Common combination with colistin is carbapenem and rifampicin.
- Parenteral to oral switch of antibiotic whenever it is feasible.
- To scrutinise the drug chart daily so that increasing antibiotics dose are stopped as soon as possible.

Different studies have already shown that by observing antibiotic stewardship meticulously, the prevalence of ESBL producing organism, MRSA and PAN resistant gram negative organisms can be reduced

Treatment option for MRSA:

Although MRSA is not a real thought in the Indian scenario, its incidence is rising and the clinician needs to be aware of its occurrence in special situations.

Common condition where it needs to be considered:

- Hospital acquired pneumonia
- Tube related pneumonia
- Skin and soft tissue infection
- IV line related bacteraemia which may be complicated with infective endocarditis
- Complicated intra-abdominal infection

Drugs for MRSA:

- Vancomycin – renotoxic, Redman syndrome if infused quickly
- Teicoplanin – renotoxicity less
- Linezolid – thrombocytopenia
- Daptomycin – does not work in pulmonary infection, may cause myopathy
- Tigecycline – bacteriostatic drug, should not be used in blood stream infection
- Telavancin – found to be equipotent to Tigecycline in VAP (Ventilator associated pneumonia)

Recently Vancomycin resistant strain and Vancomycin intermediate strains with high MIC values have also been described.

Other newer options in the pipeline:

- Ceftobiprole
- Dalbavancin
- Iclaprim
- Oritavancin
- Ceftaroline

Recently community associated MRSA has also been described.

The risk factors are:

- Sports participants
- Children in day care
- Military recruits
- Homosexuals

Drugs used:

- Clindamycin
- Trimethoprim/ Sulfamethoxazole
- Tetracycline
- Rifampicin
- Linezolid

: KEY POINTS :

- Infection is common presentation both in hospital and primary care practice.
- Working knowledge of the probable causative organism should be known to the physician.
- Initial choice of antibiotic should be empirical based on well informed guess.
- Right initial choice of empirical antibiotics will reduce the duration of illness with cost savings and in critical care setting will reduce mortality.
- Local guidelines, prevalence of infection and susceptibility patterns should be the final arbiter in proper antibiotic selection.

FURTHER REFERENCES:

- Gerald L. Mandell (Editor-in-chief), Selected papers from current Infectious disease reports– Current infectious disease reports. Vol. 2: 2003 and Vol. 3, 2003.
- The choice of antibacterial drugs: Med Drugs and Therapeutics Bulletin (DTB), vol. 43: 69, 2001.
- Harrison's Principle of Internal Medicine – 17th edition.
- Oxford Book of Medicine 5th edition.

31 A PATIENT WITH ADDISON'S DISEASE

CASE: *A 68 years old lady was admitted for investigation of weakness of more than 6 months duration. She was on insulin requiring type II diabetic with OA lumbar spine and chronic amoebic colitis. She was on thyroxin replacement. Examination did not reveal anything specific. A thorough search for her weakness and tiredness failed to elicit any cause. She also received 3 months course of antidepressant SSRI (Selective serotonin reuptake inhibitor) without any effect. CT abdomen was normal. Because of her past experience with colonoscopy, she refused to undergo another one. Her tumour markers were normal along with a normal CRP and negative occult blood in the stool. Although normal in the past, her recent biochemistry showed Na^+- 124, K^+- 5.2, Cl^-- 108, urea- 45 mg%. A random cortisol was checked which was low (4 mcg/ml). Blood for ACTH was requested and a short synacthen test was performed which showed suboptimal rise of cortisol at one hour after injection. ACTH report came back as high.*

DIAGNOSIS: Addison's disease.

DISCUSSION:

Addison's disease is not commonly diagnosed in the primary care because of non-specific nature of symptoms in the initial stage and absence of characteristic signs in many patients. A high index of suspicion is needed to detect Addison's disease in the primary care.

The two most important causes of Addison's disease are **autoimmune** (mainly in the western countries) and **tuberculosis** (more prevalent in countries where tuberculosis is common). Other causes are malignant involvement of adrenal gland, haemochromatosis and chronic fungal infection like histoplasmosis. Antifungal drugs like ketoconazole can also give rise to adrenal insufficiency on prolonged use.

Acute adrenal insufficiency occurs due to bilateral adrenal haemorrhage which is a characteristic manifestation of meningococcal septicaemia, (Waterhouse–Friderichsen syndrome (WFS) with purpuric skin rash, hypotension and fever. It can also occur as complication of anticoagulant therapy.

Functional adrenal insufficiency is increasingly being detected in septicaemic patients. However, it is a laboratory diagnosis made by adrenal function test and its importance is to detect the subgroup of septicaemic patients who will benefit from physiological doses of steroid therapy, (hydrocortisone 50 mg IV three times daily × 7 days along with fludrocortisone 0.1 mg orally). However recent trials have suggested against such physiological replacement therapy.

CLINICAL FEATURES:

Weight loss, weakness, tiredness, dizziness due to postural hypotension, abdominal pain is the common presenting features. Sometimes there may be craving for salt, pigmentation (both cutaneous and buccal) are very characteristic, although skin pigmentation may be difficult to detect in dark coloured skin. Pigmentation in the palmer crease marks and occasionally diarrhea may be present.

Biochemical features:

- High urea due to dehydration
- Low Na, high K
- Mild hypoglycaemia
- Mild eosinophilia
- High calcium
- Low random cortisol

Short synacthen test:

Procedure: To check random cortisol at 9 a.m. followed by injection of 250 microgram of synacthen (synthetic ACTH) IM or IV, cortisol estimation after 1 hour of the injection.

Addison's disease is suggested by -

- Low basal cortisol level (less than 6 microgram /100 ml).
- Failure to raise 1 hour post injection cortisol level by more than 7 mcg/100 ml.

1 hr post injection cortisol level of > 21 microgram/100 ml will exclude Addison's disease.

Synacthen is frequently not available in India. In that event the random cortisol level along with other characteristic clinical and biochemical findings should be used to make a provisional diagnosis. High ACTH level is characteristic because of negative feedback mechanism on pituitary gland. In case of secondary adrenal failure, ACTH level will be low. This happens in pituitary tumours. Other features of secondary adrenal failure are:

- absence of skin pigmentation
- absence of postural hypotension
- absence of hyperkalemia
- Intact aldosterone system because it is under renin-angiotensin feedback mechanism rather than pituitary ACTH feedback mechanism.

WHEN TO THINK OF ADDISON'S DISEASE:

- In patients with history of tuberculosis or chronic fungal infections with features of extreme weakness, hypotension or skin pigmentation and weight loss.
- In patients with Type I diabetes mellitus and other autoimmune disorders like hypothyroidism, thyrotoxicosis, pernicious anaemia, premature ovarian failure, presenting with weakness, dizziness and skin pigmentation.
- In patients with malignancy with characteristic features of Addison's disease.
- In patients with characteristic biochemical features like low Na, high K, high calcium and high eosinophil count.
- In patients with abnormal buccal or cutaneous pigmentation.

Many times the non-specific symptoms are passed on as depression, malingering or nutritional. With careful scrutiny of these patients with other characteristic features described above will enable the clinician to detect occasional patients with Addison's disease.

Replacement therapy:

Once diagnosed the patient should be started on immediate replacement therapy with steroids. Steroids dramatically improve the symptoms within 2-3 days time and such therapeutic challenge sometimes confirms the diagnosis.

Usual doses:

MEDICINES	DOSES
Hydrocortisone (Cortisol)	10 mg in the morning (if required). 10 mg in the evening (if required).
Prednisolone	5 mg in the morning additional 2.5 mg may be needed.
Dexamethasone (0.5 mg)	In the morning (usually not used).
Fludrocortisone (0.1 mg)	If mineralocorticoid, replacement is required.

Equivalent doses of steroids:

Hydrocortisone 20 mg ≡ Prednisolone 5 mg ≡ Dexamethasone (0.5 mg)

Dexamethasone has fluid retaining properties and should be avoided in the long term. Patients on IV hydrocortisone may sometimes need to undergo cortisol function test. In that event, hydrocortisone may be replaced with dexamethasone which does not interfere with the estimation of cortisol.

During any stressful event the dose of steroid should be increased temporarily and during operative procedures it should be replaced with parenteral hydrocortisone 100 mg thrice daily in stressed patients or 50 mg thrice daily in otherwise normal patients but unable to take orally. Fludrocortisone 0.1 mg daily may be frequently needed along with steroid in the treatment of Addison's disease.

CASE: *A patient with FUO and adrenal histoplasmosis (The case has been described in the chapter of Fever in clinical practice).*

CASE: *A 56 years old gentleman presented with low grade fever of unknown origin, his BP was low along with low sodium, he had pigmentation of the buccal mucosa, his Hb was low, there was leukopenia and thrombocytopenia, albumin globulin ratio altered, CT scan showed hepatosplenomegaly and bilateral adrenal hyperplasia. His cortisol level was low normal along with elevated ACTH. FNAC from the adrenal gland confirmed the diagnosis of histoplasmosis. He was immediately treated with IV Amphotericin for two weeks followed by oral Itraconazole (200 mg twice daily) for next two years; he was also treated with oral steroids supplementation. At present he is on low dose oral steroid 5 mg daily and itraconazole 200 mg daily, he has gained 8 kg of weight and systemic symptoms have disappeared.*

DIAGNOSIS: Disseminated histoplasmosis with adrenal insufficiency. In West Bengal disseminated histoplasmosis is occasionally encountered and adrenal insufficiency may be a presenting feature in such cases. I have encountered seven such cases including one with histoplasmosis of tongue and majority of them had features of adrenal insufficiency.

CASE: *A 66 years old patient suffering from dilated cardiomyopathy presented with features of slaty discoloration of his skin. His BP was 106/70 mmHg with a Na^+ level of 125 mg% and K^+- 5.1 mg%, he had history of weakness and his ejection fraction on echocardiogram was 25%. Screening for adrenal insufficiency was ruled out by a normal cortisol and ACTH level. His medications included frusemide, spironolactone, β-blocker, amiodarone, aspirin and ACE inhibitor. It is thought that amiodarone was responsible for his skin pigmentation and was withdrawn. At six months his skin pigmentation improved considerably.*

DIAGNOSIS: Amiodarone induced skin pigmentation.

In patient with skin and buccal mucosal pigmentation, Addison's disease should be considered in the differential diagnosis.

Common causes of generalised skin pigmentation:

- Adrenal insufficiency
- Chronic liver disease
- Thyroid disorder
- Haemochromatosis (high ferritin level)
- Drugs- amiodarone, hydroxychloroquine

Classification of adrenaline insufficiency:

- **Primary Adrenaline Failure**
    - Autoimmune infections – tuberculosis, histoplasmosis, metastasis
    - Surgical removal
    - Congenital adrenal hyperplasia
    - Drugs – ketoconazole, metyrapone
- **Secondary**
    - Hypopituitarism due to any cause
    - Steroid therapy

Acute Adrenal Crisis - This is a condition occasionally encountered in clinical practice in the background of severe septic shock and fulminant meningococcal septicaemia (Waterhouse–Friderichsen syndrome). Rarely adrenal haemorrhage due to anticoagulant therapy may be a causative feature. The clinician should suspect this condition if there is profound hypotension in spite of adequate fluid replacement and start high dose hydrocortisone (100 mg IV four times daily) as soon as possible.

Patients with long term steroid may also present with acute adrenal insufficiency during an intercurrent illness like myocardial infarction, acute infection and clinician should double the dose of steroid during any period of stress.

Similarly patients receiving concomitant enzyme inducing drugs like rifampicin, phenytoin should also have their dose of steroids increased lest there will be a possibility of precipitating adrenal crisis, in spite of being on additional dose of steroid.

In patients with hypopituitarism steroid replacement should be commenced first prior to thyroxin replacement as there is a possibility of precipitating adrenal crisis provoked by increased metabolism caused by thyroxin in the absence of adequate steroid.

INVESTIGATIONS:

Classical Symptoms

⇓

Synacthen test (250 microgram cosyntropin IM/IV)

⇓

Subnormal cortisol and aldosterone response

⇓	⇓
High ACTH	Low ACTH
subnormal aldosterone increment	normal aldosterone increment
⇓	⇓
Primary adrenal failure	Secondary Adrenal failure

: KEY POINTS:

- ☞ Addison's disease is an uncommon presentation in clinical practice.
- ☞ Tuberculosis and autoimmune are the two most important causes.
- ☞ Symptoms are non specific in nature.
- ☞ Biochemical changes are characteristic.
- ☞ A good detective work will be needed to diagnose Addison's disease in at risk patient population with suggestive clinical and biochemical features.

FURTHER REFERENCES:

- Oelkers W (1996), Current concepts, Adrenal insufficiency, NEJM 335, 1206-1212.
- Harrisons Principle of Internal Medicine 17th edition.
- Oxford Book of Medicine 5th edition.

32 A PATIENT WITH CARDIAC FAILURE

CASE: *A 60 years old diabetic gentleman presented with acute breathlessness in ITU clinically he was in LVF with wide spread crepts and rhonchi, gallop rhythm and cold extremities. His pulse rate was 140/m sinus and BP- 150/90 mmHg. ECG showed old anteroseptal MI. X-ray chest consistent with LVF. Troponin-T was negative on two occasions. He was treated with mechanical ventilation with addition of PEEP, vasodilators and inotropes like nitroglycerine and dobutamine infusion, frusemide, morphine, IV insulin via continuous infusion pump and low molecular weight heparin. His condition settled over next 48 hours time and eventually transferred to HDU. Echo done in the ward showed dilated LV with global hypokinesia with EF of 36%. He was discharged on medication like ACE-inhibitor, diuretic, beta-blocker, nitrates, aspirin and statins with an advice for a coronary angiogram at a later date.*

DIAGNOSIS: Dilated cardiomyopathy presenting with acute LVF.

DISCUSSION:

Cardiac dysfunction presenting with shortness of breath is a common presentation in hospital and primary care practice. Common causes are IHD, hypertension, dilated cardiomyopathy and valvular heart disease. Atrial fibrillation is a common association. Upto 20-40% of cases have normal systolic function indicating diastolic dysfunction is the cause of cardiac failure in such cases. Diastolic failure should be particularly considered in elderly hypertensive patients and patients with chronic renal failure. The cause of failure is defect in relaxation of cardiac muscles due to stiffness.

Medical therapy of heart failure:

1. Diuretics
2. Vasodilators
3. Digoxin
4. ACE Inhibitors

1. Diuretics:

Diuretics are useful for symptomatic improvement and fluid overload states. Loop diuretics like frusemide, are the commonly used drug and in recalcitrant cases of fluid overload, it can be combined with thiazide diuretics. Combination can cause severe electrolyte imbalance which should be monitored regularly.

2. Vasodilators:

Combination of hydralazine and isosorbide dinitrate was shown to reduce the mortality in clinical studies conducted in mid eighties. However, their uses have been superseded by the use of other drugs. They can still be used in patients who are intolerant to ACE inhibitors.

3. Digoxin:

Its use is particularly useful in patients with A.F. In patients without A.F, it can still cause some symptomatic improvement. Studies have shown that addition of digoxin in patients with cardiac failure reduces the rate of hospitalisation.

4. ACE Inhibitors:

This group of drugs are the cornerstone of treatment in cardiac failure. Since mid-eighties almost all the studies conducted with ACE inhibitors showed both symptomatic improvement and morality benefits. However, proper dose titration is needed and the highest tolerable dose of that particular drug should be used [enalapril 20 mg, ramipril 10 mg, lisinopril 20 mg]. Renal function should be monitored carefully. The 1st dose hypotension is common in patients who have heightened renin-angiotensin activity due to high dose of diuretic therapy. In patients with severe cardiac failure on diuretics, the drug should be commenced in the hospital setting to avoid the 1st dose hypotension. It is contraindicated in pregnancy and should be used with caution in patients with renal bruit as its use in bilateral renal artery stenosis can cause acute renal shut down. In mild renal impairment it can be used (it is a renoprotective drug) but if the creatinine is more than 3.5 mg% it should be avoided. In mild renal impairment, fosinopril may be a safer drug because of its preferential hepatic excretion. 10% of the patients (mainly females) develop dry cough which improves on withdrawal of the drug.

Example: To use low dose in hospital setting – to check urea, creatinine, and electrolytes after 1 week – if satisfactory to titrate the dose upwards.

5. Angiotensin II Blockers (AT2 Antagonists):

These relatively new group of compounds are also effective in treatment of cardiac failure (losartan, valsartan, candesartan, irbesartan). Comparative studies with ACE inhibitors have shown them to be equipotent with perhaps a better side effect profile. Addition of AT2 receptor blocker to ACE inhibitor and β-blocker did not show any additional beneficial effect [vide *Val-HeFT* trial where valsartan was added to ACE inhibitor and β-blocker]. In cardiac failure ACE inhibitors are still the 1st drug of choice and AT2 receptors should be used if the patients cannot tolerate ACE inhibitors).

The beneficial effect of ACE inhibitors and AT2 receptor blockers are due to the role of renin-angiotensin and aldosterone in the remodelling of cardiac muscles.

6. β Blockers:

Many of the adverse effects of cardiac failure are due to activation of catecholamine systems as a compensatory mechanism and beta-blocker if appropriately used have shown to counteract this adverse effect.

Metoprolol (cardio-selective), bisoprolol (cardio-selective) and carvedilol (non cardio-selective with additional vasodilating properties due to α-1 receptor blockade) have been shown to reduce symptoms and improve survival, carvedilol improves mortality in class I as asymptomatic heart failure in patients with recent MI, nebivolol (selective β blocker with nitric oxide donating properties) is also being increasingly used. They are contraindicated in decompensated cardiac failure, heart block, asthma and hypotension. They should be started at a very low dose and gradually titrated upwards. One should remember, it takes few months for them to work and one should not be necessarily worried in the face of minor adverse symptoms. Studies are on comparing selective *vs* non selective β blockers (metoprolol vs. carvedilol) in the treatment of cardiac failure.

7. Spironolactone:

Because of the role of aldosterone in cardiac remodelling, aldosterone antagonist spironolactone has been tried in cardiac failure and in RALES study; it has been shown to reduce the mortality. Addition of spironolactone in the dose of 25 mg per day will be a worthwhile venture in symptomatic patients but practical problems encountered are raising *urea and* K^+ level should be monitored closely. Eplerenone 25 mg a relatively specific mineralocorticoid aldosterone receptor blocker has been shown to reduce mortality in post MI patients with EF of less than 40%. Hyperkalemia is a risk factor. [EPHESUS study]

8. Calcium Channel Blockers:

They do not cause any symptomatic improvement or survival benefit. However felodipine or amlodipine may be used concomitantly for other purposes like control of hypertension. Cilnidipine, a fourth generation of calcium channel blocker, is 50 times more selective than N-type channel blocker.

9. Cardiac Resynchronization Therapy:

In spite of the maximum medical treatment, many patients remain symptomatic. In such patients, other mode of therapy like biventricular pacing should be considered in selected group of patients. In patients with cardiac failure, ventricular asynchrony is commonly present which can adversely affect the left ventricular output. Presence of QRS duration of >140 milliseconds will detect such patients. Biventricular pacing will help resynchronization between the ventricles with improvement of cardiac output along with symptomatic benefit. Careful selection will be essential (sinus rhythm, ECG showing QRS duration of > 140 m sec in precordial leads). This is an expensive treatment and 25-30% of patients will not respond in spite of proper selection. CRT may be combined with internal cardiac defibrillator (COMBO) for the treatment of VF.

Re synchronization therapy with biventricular pacing in patients with cardiac failure not only improves symptoms but also improves survival.

Combination of resynchronization therapy along with ICD (Internal Cardiac defibrillator) device may improve the outcome further. Coronary angiography should be performed as patients with coronary artery disease may benefit from revascularization surgery.

Cardiac transplantation is not a viable option for the vast majority of the patients in India.

10. Management of arrhythmia:

Majority of the death in cardiac failure are due to ventricular arrhythmia or pump failure. Patients, with evidence of ventricular arrhythmias in ECG or 24 hour Holter monitoring, should be referred to the cardiologist for consideration of ICD which has shown to improve survival in such patients. In the absence of such facilities or due to financial constraint, amiodarone should be used as an antiarrhythmic.

11. Other medications:

1. Oral anticoagulants in AF or LV mural thrombus.
2. Drugs for secondary prophylaxis like aspirin, statin should also be used concomitantly.

In spite of the best efforts, the prognosis of cardiac failure is poor with a 1st year mortality rate of 10% following the diagnosis followed by yearly mortality rate of 5% thereafter. This should be explained to the relatives because sudden arrhythmic deaths are common and the relatives may not be mentally prepared for it.

12. Ivabradine:

Recently ivabradine has been shown to improve mortality in patients with EF of less than 35% with high heart rate in spite of β-blocker therapy.

Role of BNP:

Serum B type Natriuretic Peptide (BNP) may help to exclude congestive cardiac failure. This simple and rapid test may be used as screening test for cardiac failure. It has a very good negative predictive value. If negative, cardiac failure may be excluded. A positive test result has to be interpreted in the light of the clinical situation as it may also be positive in other medical conditions.

: Causes of elevated BNP :	: Causes where BNP may be less than expected :
• LV dysfunction • Advanced age • Renal failure • Acute coronary syndrome • Pulmonary disease (ARDS) • Pulmonary embolism	• Obesity • Heart failure where thc causc is upstrcam from LV [e.g. mitral stenosis] • Cardiac tamponade • Constrictive pericarditis

Recently galectin-3 has been proposed as a marker for cardiac failure. However confirmed data are not available as yet.

: KEY POINTS :

- Cardiac failure is common problem in clinical practice.
- EF may be normal in diastolic failure.
- Evidence based treatment protocols are available for cardiac failure.
- Prognosis is poor with high incidence of sudden arrhythmic death.

FURTHER REFERENCES:

- Hunt SA *et al.*- ACC/AHA practice guidelines for the Evaluation and Management of Chronic heart failure of adults – J Am Coll Cardio 38: 2001, 2002.
- Braunwald's Heart disease – A text book on Cardio vascular medicine – 6th edition.
- Update in cardiology – Manuals of Internal Medicine-3rd Feb-Vol-140-N-3[2004].
- Indian Heart Journal-Vol-66. Supp 1. Jan-Feb-2014.
- Harrison's Principle of Internal Medicine- 17th edition.
- Oxford Textbook of Medicine- 5th edition.

33 A PATIENT WITH VASCULITIS

CASE: *A 65-years-old lady presented with a 2 months history of generalized unwell being, joint and muscle ache, weakness, shortness of breath and intermittent fever. She was a known asthmatic stable on inhaler therapy. Her urea & creatinine, checked by her primary care physician, were slightly raised and her liver function test was also deranged for last 2 months.*

Examination revealed an exhausted patient with anaemia, occasional rhonchi in the chest, generalized weakness and tenderness of the muscles and joints but no definite joint deformity. Her BP was 170/100 mmHg. Investigation reveals Hb- 8 g%, WBC 14,000, Eosinophil- normal, ESR 116, CRP 24 (high), creatinine 2.6 mg%, urea 84 mg%, and albumin-globulin ratio was slightly raised. ALT, AST and alkaline phosphatase, uric acid normal, rheumatoid factor, ANF, ASO titre were negative, CPK, calcium, protein electrophoresis were normal, X-ray chest mild left sided pleural effusion. ***Mantoux test was negative. Urine for R/E showed RBC- 12-14/field, protein +. CT lumbosacral spine-OA changes, Sural nerve biopsy- normal***

Her Hb was falling with increasing urea and creatinine and persistent microscopic haematuria. Blood test for ANCA which was sent initially reported to be +ve for pANCA.

She was treated with blood transfusion, IV methyl prednisolone and IV pulsed cyclophosphamide. Because of falling urinary output, she was also receiving intermittent dialysis. Renal biopsy although scheduled, could not be done because of her poor general condition and development of acute perirenal haematoma following dialysis therapy. She was discharged home with an advice of twice weekly haemodialysis and monthly pulsed cyclophosphamide therapy along with high dose of oral steroid. At six months she was readmitted with acute left ventricular failure and could not be resuscitated.

DIAGNOSIS: pANCA positive vasculitis possibly microscopic polyangiitis.

DISCUSSION:

Vasculitis is an uncommon presentation in primary care practice although it is being increasingly detected following the availability of ANCA. These disorders usually present with multisystem involvement, fever and non-specific symptoms and a high index of suspicion is needed to make a diagnosis.

When to think of vasculitis?

> In patients with fever of unknown origin (usual presentation).

> In patients with raised urea, creatinine and urinary abnormality - many times the patients are referred to the nephrologists, who make the final diagnosis.

> In patients with skin rash, purpura necrotic skin lesions along with joint and muscle pain.

> In patients with cavitating or nodular lung lesions along with nose bleeding - they usually present to the chest physicians.

> In young patients with brain stroke or in any patients with undiagnosed peripheral neuropathy or mononeuritis multiplex.

With these backgrounds, request for an ANCA test might sometimes give +ve result.

There are two major staining patterns of ANCA – cytoplasmic (cANCA) directed mainly against proteinase 3 which is mainly found in Wegener's granulomatosis (with 97% specificity and 80% sensitivity) and perinuclear (pANCA) directed against myeloperoxidase, found mainly in microscopic polyangiitis. Unlike c-ANCA, pANCA may be found in other nonvasculitic disorders like autoimmune rheumatic diseases and inflammatory bowel disorders.

Broadly vasculitis is classified according to the size of vessels involved-	
Large arteries	Giant cell arteritis, Takayasu's disease.
Medium arteries	Polyarteritis nodosa.
Medium & small Vessels	Wegener's, granulomatosis. Churg-Strauss syndrome Microscopic polyangiitis.
Small vessels	Henoch - Schonlein purpura Essential mixed cryoglobulinaemia

In addition to the primary vasculitic disorders, there may be many secondary causes of vasculitis like infection, malignancy, drugs, autoimmune disorders etc. Vasculitis may be ANCA positive or ANCA negative.

c-ANCA +ve vasculitis: Wegener's granulomatosis. It may be positive in 25% cases of microscopic polyangiitis and 15% cases of Churg-Strauss syndrome and rarely in polyarteritis nodosa (2%).

p-ANCA +ve vasculitis: Microscopic polyangiitis, Churg-Strauss syndrome and other primary non vasculitic conditions like rheumatoid arthritis, inflammatory bowel disorders.

Large vessel vasculitis:

Giant cell arteritis- In patients presenting with headache, scalp tenderness, ESR should be checked and although uncommon in India, giant cell arteritis should be considered.

- Uncommon in India.
- Elderly patients with headache, scalp tenderness, visual symptoms may be present which may lead to blindness.
- Palpable tender superficial temporal artery.
- Temporal artery biopsy is diagnostic but may be normal because of patchy involvement.
- May be associated with polymyalgia rheumatica, proximal muscle pain and stiffness.
- Jaw claudication pain may be present.
- Treated with steroids

In patients without visual symptoms 30 mg of prednisolone should be used but with visual symptoms 60-80 mg prednisolone should be used, while in polymyalgia, 15 mg of prednisolone is the usual dose. The duration of therapy is usually 2 yrs. with lowest possible maintenance dose.

Takayasu's arteritis:

Common in South East Asian countries as well as in India. Usually presents with pulse-less disease, hypertension, claudication pain in the legs and bruits in the carotids, abdominal and femoral at a younger age with female predominance. In India, tuberculosis has been implicated as a causative factor. It is treated with high dose of steroid with or without immunosuppressives like cyclophosphamide. If there is renal artery stenosis, renal angioplasty may be needed to treat hypertension.

CASE: *A 21-years-old female was referred to us with headache, chest pain and absent pulse over right radial artery, bilateral carotid and femoral bruit. Her BP was 190/110 mmHg in left hand and 130/80 mmHg in right hand. She was treated with ACE inhibitor in a peripheral health centre. We found her BP was low and she complained of fall of urine output for last couple of days. She was immediately admitted and her urea and creatinine were found to be very high. She was also found to have abdominal bruit. Her renal function improved with peritoneal dialysis and aortogram done later on revealed bilateral renal artery stenosis. She was treated with renal angioplasty and calcium channel blocker was substituted for ACE inhibitor as an alternative antihypertensive. She also received steroid and oral anticoagulant. 1 year at follow up, her BP remains well under control.*

DISCUSSION:

This patient had Takayasu's disease with bilateral renal artery stenosis and ACE inhibitor used as antihypertensive caused acute renal shut down. **In any hypertensive patient abdomen should be auscultated and if there is any suspicion of renal artery stenosis, ACE inhibitors should be used with caution and they can cause acute renal shut down in patients with bilateral renal artery stenosis.**

Young patients with unequal or absent pulse, hypertension, chest pain, headache and claudication pain, Takayasu's disease should be considered in the differential diagnosis.

Medium and small vessel vasculitis:

Wegener's granulomatosis: The features are-

1. Necrotising vasculitis of medium and small vessels.
2. Classically causes upper respiratory, pulmonary and renal involvement with nasal discharge, cavitating or nodular pulmonary lesion presenting with haemoptysis and renal failure.
3. Additional features of fever, arthralgia, oral and cutaneous involvement may be present.
4. c-ANCA is characteristically positive.
5. Treated with high dose steroid along with cyclophosphamide (2-4 mg/kg/day) depending upon the severity of the disease activity.

Polyarteritis Nodosa:

1. Has a male preponderance
2. Frequently associated with hepatitis B positivity.
3. Fever, arthralgia, myalgia, abdominal pain are the usual presenting features.
4. Renal involvement may be present in 50% of case.
5. Cardiac involvement may give rise to M.I.
6. Cutaneous involvement in the form of nodule may be present.
7. ANCA is characteristically -ve but may be present in small number of patients.
8. ESR & CRP are high.
9. Renal angiogram may demonstrate aneurysm at the bifurcation of renal arterioles.
10. Treated with steroid and cyclophosphamide.

Churg-Strauss syndrome:

1. History of asthma and eosinophilia is characteristically present.
2. Pulmonary renal involvement is present in 50% of case.
3. Peripheral neuropathy is characteristic sural nerve biopsy (as done in the index case) may be indicated to confirm neuropathy.
4. pANCA is characteristically positive.
5. Treated with steroid and cyclophosphamide.

Small vessel vasculitis:

Some of the small vessel vasculitis present with leukocytoclasis (infiltration of vessels with neutrophils which are fragmented). Examples of leukocytoclastic vasculitis are-

- Allergic hypersensitivity angiitis - due to drugs
- Henoch Schonlein purpura
- Urticarial vasculitis
- Cryoglobulinaemia

Allergic hypersensitivity vasculitis:

- Presents with skin lesions like palpable purpura, bullae and ulcers mainly in the lower extremities. There may be necrosis of the skin.
- There may be fever, arthralgia, pulmonary involvement and renal involvement with microscopic haematuria.
- pANCA may be positive.

Treated with withdrawal of offending drug. Steroids and immunosuppressives may be required.

CASE: *A 61 years lady with h/o RA was admitted in ITU with a probable diagnosis of acute severe asthma. She recently had a chest infection and was treated with cephalosporin. Unfortunately her respiratory syndromes suddenly got worse which led to her admission. She also complained of joint pain on admission. Her pulse rate was 150/m, BP 160/90 with rhonchi and crepts in chest, purpuric and echymotic rash over the lower extremities with suggestion of digital gangrene. ESR and CRP were very high, RA & ANF was negative, urea 106 mg%, creatinine 3.2 mg%, urine RBC++, protein++, X-ray chest showed bilateral round opacities with cavitation.*

Although initially she was diagnosed to have acute severe asthma with flare up of her arthritis, pANCA later on came as strongly positive. She was treated with IV methyl prednisolone followed by oral steroids and pulsed IV cyclophosphamide at monthly interval. Her condition remains stable at 6 months follow up.

DIAGNOSIS: Allergic hypersensitive vasculitis.
Flare up of rheumatoid arthritis with ANCA positive vasculitis.

Henoch-Schonlein Purpura:

- Usually present in children but can affect adults.
- Classically presents with non- thrombocytopenic purpura mainly in the lower extremities, arthritis, abdominal pain and microscopic haematuria due to glomerulonephritis.
- ANCA is negative, IgA may be elevated.
- Treated with NSAIDs and steroids. A small proportion of patients can develop chronic renal impairment.

Urticarial vasculitis:

- Usually present in female.
- The skin lesions last longer than ordinary urticaria. The lesions are usually more painful burning compared to ordinary urticaria.
- Antihistaminics are usually ineffective and steroids are generally required.

Cryoglobulinaemia:

- This is a small vessel of vasculitis commonly occurs in patients with the RA, lymphoproliferative disorders, hepatitis-B & C infections.
- Common presenting features are- arthralgia, vasculitic skin lesions, renal impairment (50%) and hepatic impairment. Raynaud's phenomenon may be a presenting feature.
- High dose of steroids, chemotherapy & plasmapheresis are the therapeutic options.
- Prognosis is guarded.

: KEY POINTS :

- Systemic vasculitis is uncommon presentations in primary care.
- The diagnosis should be considered in patients with prolonged fever, arthralgia, renal and pulmonary impairment along with skin lesions.
- ANCA helps in the diagnosis of vasculitis.
- Steroids and immunosuppressives are the therapeutic options with variable results.

FURTHER REFERENCES:

- Harrison's Principle of Internal Medicine – 17th edition.
- Oxford Text Book of Medicine – 5th edition.

34

A PATIENT ERYTHEMA NODOSUM

CASE: *A 60 years old lady was referred with painful, red erythematous nodules over her legs for the last 2 months. She also had joint pain and low grade fever. Investigations revealed Hb-9 g%, ESR – 96, CRP raised, rheumatoid factor, ANF, ASO titre negative, X-ray chest prominent hilum on both sides. CT scan of thorax revealed multiple hilar and mediastinal glands to exclude the possibility of lymphoma. Her calcium level was normal and Mantoux test was negative.*

DIAGNOSIS: Erythema nodosum – due to acute sarcoidosis (Lofgren's syndrome).

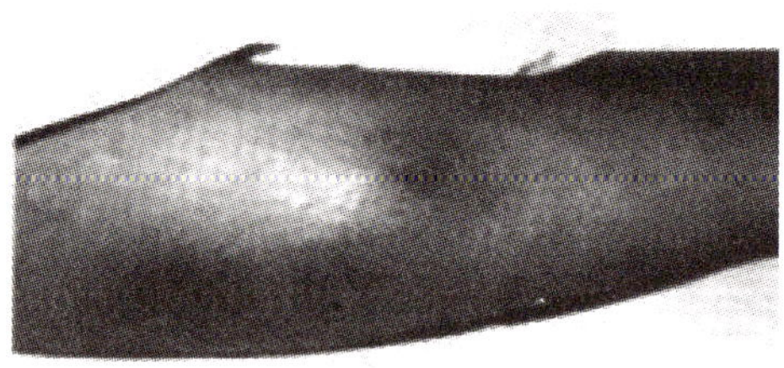

DISCUSSION:

Erythema nodosum is occasionally encountered during outpatient's consultation. They present with painful red erythematous nodules mainly in legs over the skin. Occasionally they can be observed over the upper extremities. Initially they are red but later on they change colour to mauve before fading away. Recurrent fresh crops may appear. Erythema nodosum may be chronic without any underlying cause mainly in females. This variety is known as nodular vasculitis.

Differential diagnosis:

- Nodular vasculitis
- Superficial thrombophlebitis
- Cellulitis
- Septic emboli
- Weber–Christian disease
- Lupus panniculitis
- Cutaneous T-cell lymphoma
- Erythema nodosum leprosum
- Vasculitis

CAUSES:

- Streptococcal infection
- Tuberculosis
- Sarcoidosis
- Leprosy
- Fungal infection like coccidioidomycosis
- Inflammatory bowel disease
- Drugs like oral contraceptives, sulphonamides, penicillin
- Hodgkin's disease

The case described above is a classical example of acute sarcoidosis (Lofgren's Syndrome) which presents with fever, arthralgia, high ESR, erythema nodosum and bilateral hilar lymphadenopathy. This condition has a good prognosis and usually recovers completely with NSAIDS and oral steroid. This lady was treated with steroid and NSAIDS with a very good response in 4 weeks time.

Active tuberculosis can sometimes present with erythema nodosum but much more common presentation is erythema nodosum with strongly positive Mantoux test but no evidence of active tuberculosis. Usually there is a strong family history or a past history of tuberculosis. They respond well to combination of antitubercular drug along with steroids. Most of the patients that I have dealt with fell into this category.

Hodgkin's disease can present with erythema nodosum and one of my patients with treated Hodgkin's disease developed recurrent erythema nodosum which needed long term steroid therapy.

Inflammatory bowel disease, leprosy, fungal infection and drugs can also cause erythema nodosum. Relevant history will help in proper diagnosis.

Pathologically it is a kind of vasculitis involving the deep dermal and subcutaneous vessels and fat (panniculitis).

The patients presenting with erythema nodosum should undergo baseline tests to find out the underlying cause. These are-

- Full blood count ESR, CRP
- ASO titre
- Rheumatoid factor, ANF

- X-Ray chest
- Serum ACE level
- calcium
- Mantoux test
- In difficult cases, biopsy may be helpful.

TREATMENT:

Other medication that may be used:

- Potassium iodide
- Calcium
- Thalidomide
- Cyclosporine
- Hydroxychloroquine

: KEY POINTS :

- Erythema nodosum is an occasional presentation in primary care practice.
- Tuberculosis, sarcoidosis and drugs are the common causes.
- Erythema nodosum along with fever arthralgia and bilateral hilar lymphadenopathy are the classical presentations of acute sarcoidosis which has a good prognosis.
- Erythema nodosum responds well to NSAID, steroid along with the treatment of underlying cause.

FURTHER REFERENCES:

- Bolognia JL *et al.,* Dermatology, Philadelphia, Mosby 2003.
- Callen J.P. *et al.,* Dermatological signs of internal disease, 3rd edition, Philadelphia Saunders 2003.
- Frank J. Dondn, The 5-minute clinical consult, 2012- 20th edition.
- Harrison's Principle of Internal Medicine – 17th edition.
- Oxford Text Book of Medicine – 5th edition.

35 A PATIENT PRESENTING WITH TACHYCARDIA

CASE: *A 34 years old male presented with a history of palpitation of 2 hours duration. He had similar episode in the past which settled on its own within half an hour. Repeat ECGs were normal. Echo, T_3, T_4 and TSH and 24 hours Holter monitoring were normal in the past. Examination revealed a pulse rate of 180/min, no discernable p waves and the QRS complexes were normal.*

He was treated with IV adenosine through a central vein and with a total cumulative dose of 12 mg he was converted to sinus rhythm and repeat ECG showed normal P and QRS configuration.

DIAGNOSIS: Paroxysmal nodal tachycardia.

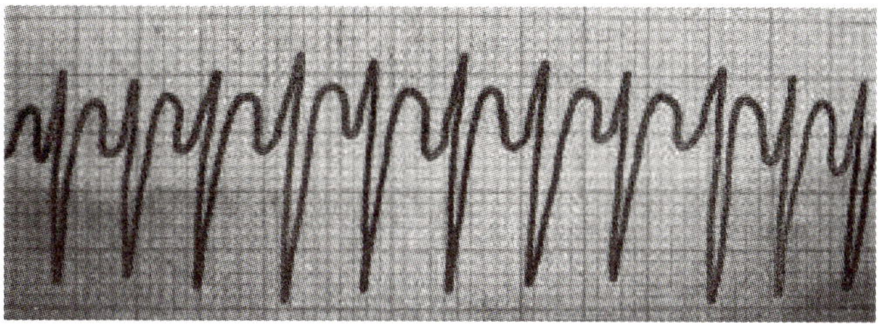

DISCUSSION:

Tachyarrhythmias are very common presentation in hospital practice and most of the times they are being dealt by the physicians rather than the cardiologist.

While dealing with tachyarrhythmias, one should first notice whether it is a broad complex (QRS > 140 ms) or narrow complex. The next thing is to notice whether the rate is regular or irregular?

Narrow complex tachycardia with regular rhythm:

- Sinus tachycardia
- Atrial tachycardia
- Multifocal atrial tachycardia
- Multifocal atrial tachycardia with block
- Atrial flutter with 2:1 or 3:1 block
- Nodal tachycardia

Sinus tachycardia:

Sinus tachycardia is very commonly found in the hospital setting due to fever, infection, dehydration, drugs or thyrotoxicosis. The rate varies from 120-150/min but may be as high as 180/min. ECG shows normal P wave configurations with normal relation to QRS complex.

Atrial tachycardia:

This arises from the ectopic activity in the atrium and the P wave will be different from the normal sinus P wave. The P-R interval will also be shorter.

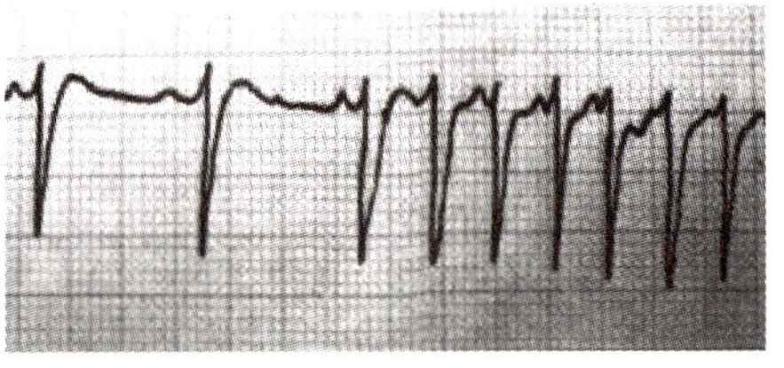

Multifocal atrial tachycardia:

This is due to increased atrial ectopic activity. The rate may vary from 120-180/min. The P waves are of different configurations. This is commonly found in patients admitted with COPD with hypoxia.

Atrial tachycardia with block:

If the atrial rate is very high not all the impulses will be conducted to the ventricles giving rise to variable ventricular rates. If the atrial rate is 300/min, there may be 2:1 conduction to the ventricles with a ventricular rate of 150/min. This arrhythmia typically occurs in digoxin toxicity.

Atrial flutter:

Atrial flutter has a typical atrial rate of 300/min and commonly the ventricular conduction occurs at 2:1 ratio giving rise to a ventricular rate of 150/min. The typical saw-tooth appearance of the flutter waves may not be visible. However, if the conduction is at a slower ratio (3:1 or 4:1) the characteristic flutter waves may be seen. (This can be done by carotid sinus massage or by using vagomimetic drugs).

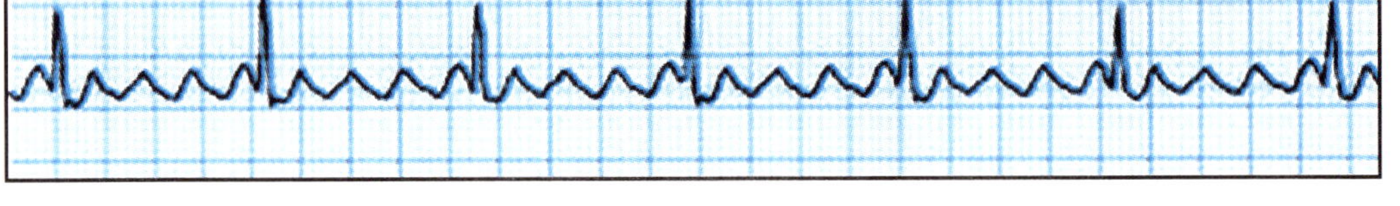

Common causes of heart rate of 150/min:

- Sinus tachycardia
- Supraventricular tachycardia (atrial or nodal)
- Atrial flutter with 2:1 block

Nodal tachycardia:

- **Atrioventricular nodal re-entrant tachycardia**: It is the commonest variety of supraventricular tachycardia. (The case described above). The mechanism is due to the presence of dual conduction pathway inside AV node. They respond to carotid sinus stimulation of drugs like adenosine, verapamil *etc.* The characteristic features are:
    i) Rate of 150-180/min
    ii) P wave usually buried in the QRS complex or seen following QRS complex.

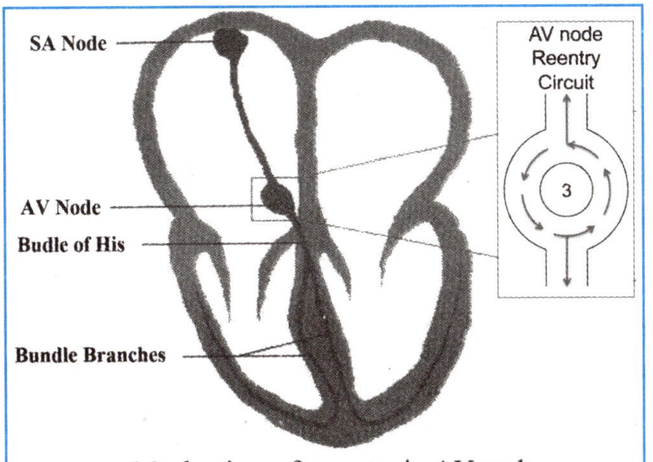

Mechanism of re-entry in AV node

- **Atrioventricular re-entrant tachycardia:** The mechanism is the presence of accessory pathway between the atrium and the ventricle.

The commonest cause of accessory pathway is WPW Syndrome. If tachycardia is due to retrograde conduction, the ECG will be similar to nodal re-entrant tachycardia. However if there is antegrade conduction, broad complex tachycardia will be noticed. Once the patient is converted to sinus rhythm typical features WPW syndrome will be evident in the ECG.

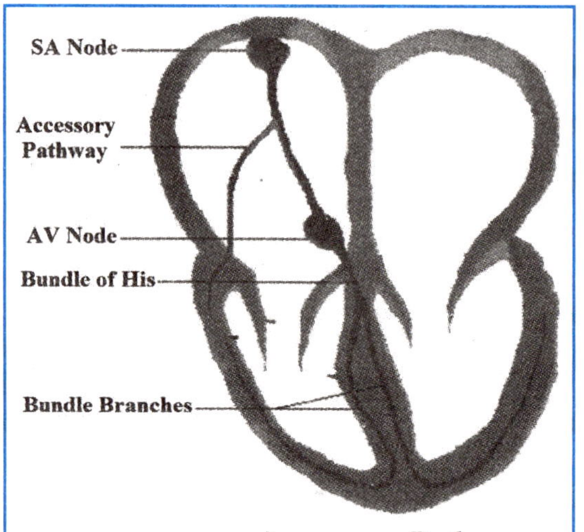

Accessory Pathway

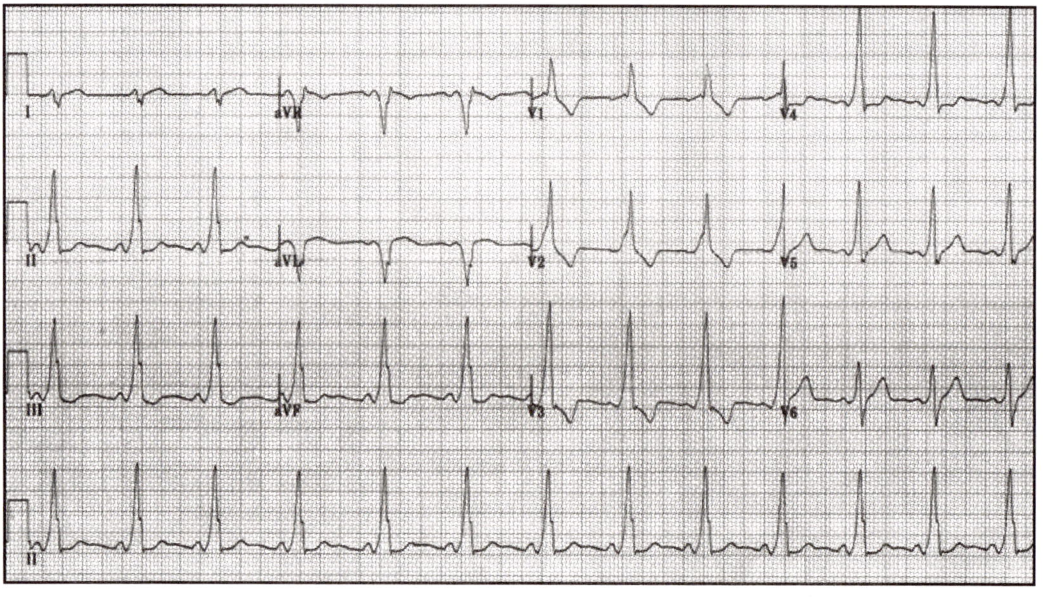

Type A WPW syndrome	Type B WPW syndrome
• Short P-R interval • Delta Wave • Tall R wave in V1	• Short P-R interval • Delta Wave • Negative QRS complex in V1

Other causes of tall R wave in V1:

- True posterior wall infarction
- RBBB
- Right ventricular hypertrophy

Narrow complex tachycardia with irregular rhythm:

Atrial fibrillation is the commonest cause. There may be presence of fibrillary wave. However, in many instances no P waves are visible at all. The rhythm will be irregular.

Common causes of atrial fibrillation and its treatment has to be discussed elsewhere.

Broad complex tachycardia with regular rhythm:

1. Supraventricular tachycardia with aberrant conduction (like RBBB or LBBB)

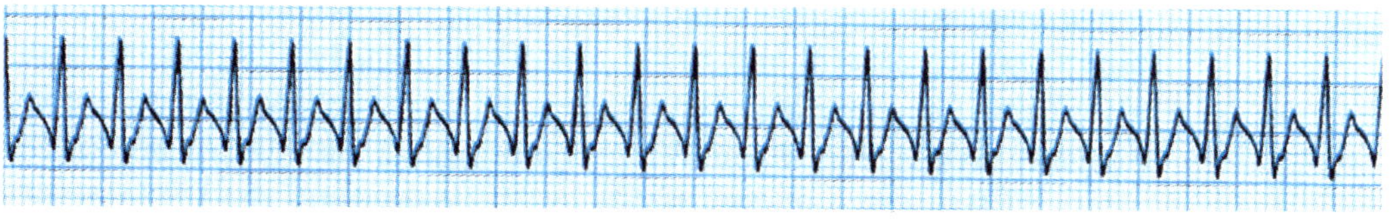

2. Ventricular tachycardia

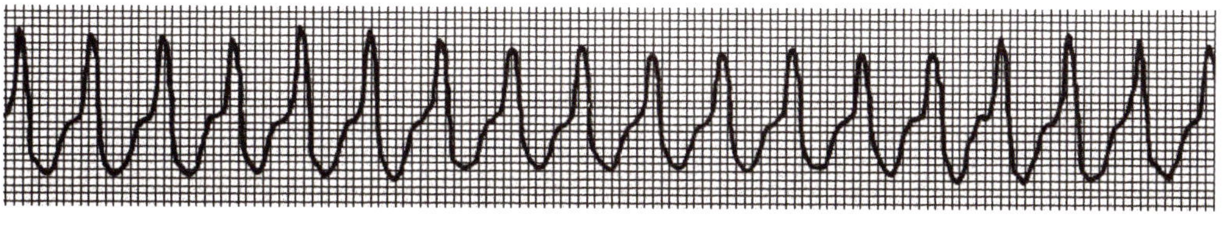

3. Atrial tachycardia with pre-excitation

The rate of ventricular tachycardia varies between 120-300/m and at times it is very difficult to differentiate between VT and SVT with aberrant conduction unless a previous ECG during normal sinus rhythm is in hand.

Common points favouring VT rather than SVT:

1. QRS complex is wider > 160 m sec.
2. Presence of escape beat – that is occasional capture of narrow complex atrial impulse in the rhythm strip.

3. Presence of fusion beat – the ventricle may be captured by both the atrial and ventricular impulse giving rise to a fusion beat which looks different from other QRS complexes in rhythm strip [presence of 2 and 3 are the surest signs of VT].
4. In precordial leads either positive or negative deflection in all the leads (V1–V6). This is known as concordance.
5. If there is one P wave for each QRS complex, the rhythm is SVT rather than VT.
6. If there is RBBB configuration; in VT the initial R wave is taller than the R_1 wave (R R_1) whereas in SVT, the R_1 wave is taller than R wave (R R_1).

In acute situation, if there is any confusion, it is always wiser to treat broad complex tachycardia as VT, as this condition may be life threatening.

There are other special varieties of VT like fascicular tachycardia or right ventricular outflow tract VT.

Broad complex tachycardia with irregular rhythm:

i) Polymorphic VT
ii) Torsades de pointes tachycardia
iii) Atrial fibrillation with RBBB or LBBB
iv) Atrial fibrillation due to pre-excitation

Torsades de pointes tachycardia:

It is commonly seen in acute care setting. Here the cardiac axis rotates over a sequence of 5-10 beats, changing from one direction to another and back again. QRS amplitude also varies similarly, such that the complexes appear to twist around the base-line. The importance of this arrhythmia is that if the underlying cause is not corrected, it can degenerate into ventricular fibrillation. The base line ECG in sinus rhythm shows prolonged Q-T interval.

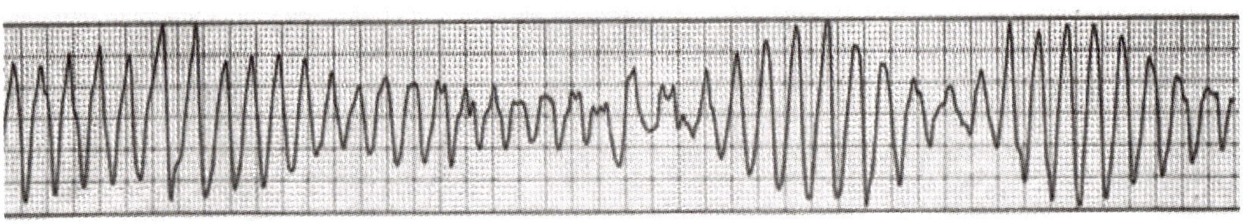

Causes of prolonged Q-T interval:

1. Anti arrhythmic drug – disopyramide, quinine, sotalol,

2. Other drugs – antihistaminics, chloroquine, cisapride.
3. Antibiotics – erythromycin
4. Electrolyte imbalance – low K^+, low Mg^{++}
5. In addition there are rare congenital causes of prolonged Q - T syndrome where patients in their childhood present with repeated syncopal attacks.

CASE: *A 73 years old lady was admitted with a confused and drowsy state. She was diagnosed to have malaria and commenced on chloroquine in the community. She was unarousable peripheral pulse was not palpable. Her K^+ and Mg^{++} levels were low. ECG showed classical torsades de pointes tachycardia.*

This was probably due to multiple factors (Low K^+, low Mg^{++} and recent chloroquine therapy). Chloroquine was stopped, her K^+ and Mg^{++} were corrected and she was finally converted to sinus rhythm.

DIAGNOSIS: Torsades de pointes tachycardia.

Atrial fibrillation with pre excitation:

In patients with WPW syndrome, with atrial fibrillation, there may be broad complex irregular tachycardia if there is antidromic conduction of impulse to the ventricles. The rate may be very high and this is a particularly dangerous situation because it can degenerate into ventricular fibrillation.

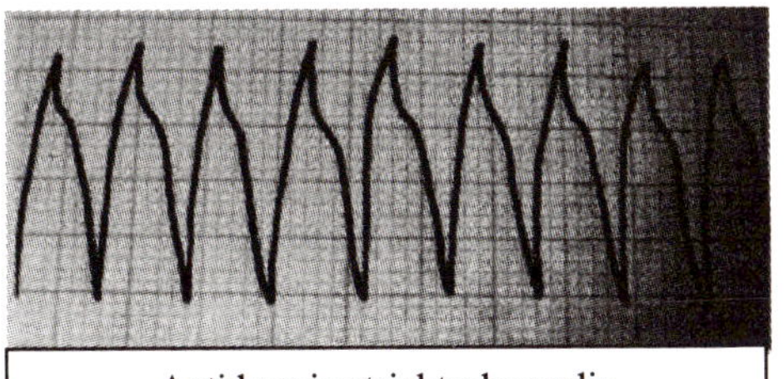

Antidromic atrial tachycardia

This should be borne in mind in patients with WPW syndrome presenting with broad complex tachycardia.

- **Idiopathic VT syndromes**

  Although VT usually occurs in the setting of coronary artery disease, a significant number of patients may occur in other circumstances as well.

- **Idiopathic outflow tract VT (80% RV outflow – 20% LV outflow)**

  It is usually precipitated by exercise stress, and premenstrual period. RV outflow tract VT has a LBBB configuration in ECG while LV outflow tract VT has a RBBB configuration.

- **Idiopathic LV septal/ Fascicular VT**

  It originates in the Purkinje system of left ventricle and has a narrow RBBB configuration in ECG. It is unique in that if responds to verapamil in addition to beta-blocker.

- **VT associated with dilated cardiomyopathy**

  It usually arises from the mitral and aortic valvular regions and less amenable to ablation therapy approached through the endocardium as it usually originals from the epicardium which needs to be accessed through percutaneous route. Drug therapy is usually ineffective although a trial of sotalol or an amiodarone may be given.

- **Bundle Branch Re-entrant VT**

  It originates in the bundle and typically has a configuration of LBBB with a superior axis. It is easily amenable to ablation therapy.

- **VT associated with HOCM**

  Presents with recurrent syncope. Usually there is evidence of non-sustained VT in 24 hrs Holter monitoring and the thickness of septum is usually more than 30 mm. Amiodarone, sotalol and β blockers may be tried. Ablation therapy and preferably ICD implantation is the treatment of choice.

- **Arrhythmogenic right ventricular dysplasia**

  It is genetically determined or may be as a sequence of viral myocarditis ECG shows LBBB pattern in V1 with poor R wave progression from V1 to V6. There may be terminal notching of QRS complex which if prominent may appear separated from the QRS complex and called as epsilon wave.

- **Fascicular tachycardia caused by digoxin toxicity**

  The signature VT caused by digoxin is bidirectional VT. Usually there is narrow complex RBBB pattern in ECG with beat to beat alteration of right to left frontal axis.

- **Long QT syndrome (Congenital and acquired)** – already discussed.

- **Short QT syndrome** – may predispose to VT
- **Brugada syndrome**

  VT originates from RV outflow tract. There is ST segment elevation in V1& V3 in sinus rhythm.
- **Catecholaminergic polymorphic VT**

  There may be bidirectional VT, polymorphic VT or recurrent VT.

: KEY POINTS :

- Tachyarrhythmias are common in hospitalised patients.
- A schematic approach will help to make a definite diagnosis.
- Broad complex tachycardia should be treated as VT until proved otherwise.
- Atrial fibrillation in WPW syndrome can cause very fast wide complex tachycardia which can degenerate into ventricular fibrillation.

FURTHER REFERENCES:

- Braunwald's Heart disease – A Text Book of Cardiovascular Medicine - 6th edition.
- Oxford Book of Medicine – 5th edition.
- Harrison's Principal of Internal Medicine – 17th edition.

CASE: *A 27 years old gentleman was admitted with a history of fever for 10 days. The fever started with low grade mainly in the evening and during admission it was touching 102°F. The fever was associated with headache, vague abdominal pain and dry cough. Examination found normal except for a coated tongue. Investigations showed Hb- 10 g%, WBC- 2800, normal platelet, mildly raised AST and ALT, malaria parasite negative on two occasions, P. falciparum antigen negative. Widal test done on the 7th day was negative. X-ray chest- normal, urine examination normal. He was commenced on IV ceftriaxone and ofloxacin. Blood for malaria parasite was repeated on couple of occasions with negative results. On the 3rd day of admission, BACTEC blood culture report was positive for Salmonella typhi sensitive to ofloxacin and ceftriaxone. Ceftriaxone was continued for 7 days and ofloxacin was changed to oral preparation which he received for total period of 14 days. He was discharged in a stable state.*

DIAGNOSIS: Blood culture positive enteric fever.

DISCUSSION:

Fever is one of the most common presentations in primary care practice and is sometimes the most perplexing of the medical problems encountered in practice. Many times the diagnosis remains unresolved with occasional fatal outcome. The common infections that present with fever to a clinician are usually viral, protozoal or bacterial. While dealing with febrile illness it is important to take history of travel, drug intake and occupation as they may have a bearing in making the diagnosis.

- Travel to certain parts of India: Falciparum malaria.
- Occupation: It is important in certain diseases like leptospirosis.
- Drugs: Ampicillin induced rash in infectious mononucleosis.
- Localizing symptoms: Headache, cough, arthralgia and abdominal pain might pinpoint the diagnosis.
- Pattern of fever: Hectic in abscess, classical malarial fever with chills and rigor may be absent in the initial days.
- Skin rash: Characteristic skin rash may be present in viral infections like measles, rubella, chicken pox, dengue (petechial), rickettsial infections, bacterial infections like meningococcal septicaemia, typhoid fever (uncommonly seen in Indian population).
- Lymphadenopathy may be present in rubella, cat scratch disease, bacterial infections.

- Hepatosplenomegaly: It is common in many acute illnesses but may not be evident in the 1st week.
- Jaundice: in viral hepatitis, leptospirosis and malaria.
- Arthralgia and arthritis: very common in viral fever, fleeting in rheumatic fever.
- Oral cavity: Coated tongue in enteric fever, vesicular lesion in enterovirus infection.

INVESTIGATIONS:

- Leucopenia and thrombocytopenia: viral fever, typhoid and malaria
- Leukocytosis: in bacterial infection
- Atypical monocytes: in infectious mononucleosis
- Eosinophilia – in certain parasitic infections
- Altered LFT: in viral fever, enteric, malaria and leptospirosis.
- Altered urine colour: mustard colour urine and presence of bile salt and pigment in an icteric phase of viral hepatitis when the only symptom will be fever.

In our experience most common cause of acute fever needing hospital admission in Kolkata are viral, enteric and malaria. However, there will be regional variation of disease prevalence in different parts of India.

Our experience with 73 blood culture positive enteric fever over last 5 years (Data in press)

- Organisms isolated: *S. typhi*- 76%, *S. paratyphi*- 24%.
- Symptoms and signs: Fever, headache, abdominal pain, dry cough, dry coated tongue, atypical presentation like cerebellar signs, gastro intestinal bleeding.
- Investigation: Moderate anaemia, leucopenia (24%), lymphocytosis (28%) AST and ALT mildly raised, Widal test in first 10 days 65% positive.
- In vitro culture sensitivity: Amoxicillin– 67%, amoxiclav– 82%, 2nd generation cephalosporins– 95%, 3rd generation cephalosporins 100%, Chloramphenicol– 72%, ofloxacin– 100%, ciprofloxacin– 100%, azithromycin – 100%, co-trimoxazole – 62%.

Our experience of 634 cases of acute severe malaria presenting in ITU/HDU from 1994-2003 (interim report presented in National Critical Care Congress in Bangalore 2000).

Pattern of infection: Almost all of them had *P. falciparum* infection except for 5 patients with *vivax* infection that had drug related side effects due to chloroquine.

Symptoms: Classical fever was present only in 30% of cases. Atypical presentations were common like– gastroenteritis, bronchospasm, acute renal shutdown, respiratory failure due to ARDS, jaundice, unconsciousness.

Investigations: Anaemia, thrombocytopenia, mild hyperbilirubinaemia, variable white cell count.

Management: Quinine was uniformly effective. Most common side effects were tinnitus, nausea and vomiting. Hypoglycaemia was observed more frequently in children and pregnant women. There were two arrhythmic deaths in 1994, where the drug was used in cardiac patients in the absence of suitable alternative during that time. During the later part of the study, **artemisinin** group of compounds were used more frequently. These were more user-friendly and caused fewer side effects. They did not cause any cardiac side effects.

Mortality: Overall mortality was 15%. Mortality was related to organ involvement particularly when more than 3 organs were involved. Combination of ARDS, cerebral malaria and renal failure had the worst outcome (70% mortality).

As it will be noticed that, it may be sometimes very difficult from clinical and initial haematological and biochemical tests alone to pinpoint the diagnosis at least in the initial stages and finally specialized tests will be required. Repeated blood culture and malaria microscopy can yield the final diagnosis.

If the fever persists beyond 3 weeks in spite of thorough search for a cause, it is known as fever of unknown origin (although the definition of FUO has been changed later on- vide next) and it can be a physician's nightmare. Although viral infection sometimes persists beyond 3 weeks the main causes of FUO can be classified under the headings e.g.

- Infection
- Malignancies
- Auto immune disorders
- Factitious and vasculitis, habitual hyperthermia
- Unknown

The percentage of different etiologies varies between countries and in Indian subcontinent 50% of them are due to infection, 22% miscellaneous, 9% connective tissue disorders and 5% undiagnosed. (FUO has been discussed in details later on, in this chapter).

Common causes that need to be excluded by appropriate tests are:

- **Tuberculosis** of different organs is a very common cause of FUO and tuberculosis, like malaria, can be a great mimicker.
- **Amoebic liver abscess:** Commonly missed if there is no localizing symptom like abdominal pain. Hectic rise of temperature, leukocytosis, elevated alkaline phosphatase are the common findings. Early ultrasound examination of abdomen will make an early diagnosis.
- **Infective endocarditis:** Although structural heart disease due to rheumatic heart disease is common in India, the diagnosis of infective endocarditis is often delayed or missed. Heart murmurs, history of valve surgery, IV drug abuse with leukocytosis and very high CRP should indicate for an early ECHO. However, ECHO may be normal and if facilities are available, transesophageal ECHO should be requested for. Repeated blood culture is mandatory.
- Other infections like **brucellosis, kala-azar**, HIV infection etc. should also be borne in mind.
- **Lymphomas** and other solid tumours may present with FUO. CT scan of abdomen or thorax may help in an early diagnosis. In selected cases tumour markers may be requested for as screening test. Bone marrow examination can sometimes detect leukemia otherwise unsuspected. High LDH level may be a pointer towards lymphoma.
- **Connective tissue disorders**: SLE is a frequent diagnosis in FUO and with the availability of ANCA, vasculitis are diagnosed more frequently.
- **Drug fever** can be sometimes confusing and withdrawal of the offending drug may cause miraculous results.
- In addition, other causes like sarcoidosis, granulomatous hepatitis and bacterial prostatitis in elderly may present with FUO.

Special investigation that may be required:

- Urine for AFB and AFB culture.

- Autoimmune screening, ANCA, PSA, other tumour markers.
- CT abdomen
- Bone marrow examination.
- Liver biopsy, skin biopsy, lymph node biopsy.
- Radio-labelled gallium scan or WBC scan. (Not routinely available in most of the centers in India) However, they may be non-specific.

FUO in specialized situations:

In nosocomial setting: FUO in hospitalized patients are common and the special causes that should be considered are:

- Line infections
- Candida septicaemia particularly who are on multiple antibiotics, with central line etc.
- *C. difficile*– diarrhea
- Drugs
- Maxillary sinusitis– due to naso-tracheal intubation.
- Undiagnosed DVT.

Neutropenic fever:

Fever is common, especially those who are on chemotherapy for malignancy. However, they tend to be of much shorter duration compared to classical FUO. Bacteremia, pneumonias, line infection, soft tissue infections are common. Broad spectrum antibiotic cover with or without antifungal should be given if the cause cannot be clearly pinpointed.

HIV associated FUO:

There is a big list of infective causes of fever depending upon the CD-4 count. However, tuberculosis remains the most common one. A specialist opinion will be needed for a proper work up in such patients.

Common infections in HIV:

CD count > 200	Tuberculosis, Candida, Herpes Zoster
CD count 50-200	Toxoplasmosis, Cryptosporidiosis, Pneumocystis carinii
CD count <50	Atypical mycobacterium, Cytomegalovirus

CASE: *A 48 years old man presented with history of fever, cough and possible haemoptysis. X-ray chest showed patchy pneumonitic right base with some elevation of the right dome of diaphragm. Bilirubin- 1.8 mg%, alkaline phosphatase- 612 (high), AST & ALT slightly raised. Hb- 9 g%, WBC- 21,000 (poly 90%). Initially he was treated for chest infection. His condition deteriorated sharply and on closer examination the haemoptysis was found to have anchovy sauce like colour. An urgent USG abdomen revealed big amoebic liver abscess impinging on the right dome of diaphragm. Urgent aspiration along with metronidazole saved him from a life threatening rupture.*

DIAGNOSIS: Amoebic liver abscess with rupture into the right lung.

CASE: *A 19 years old college student was admitted with a history of jaundice and mild confusional state. He was having fever for last 12 days. His blood test for malaria was negative outside. He recently visited Simlipal forest, Orissa with his friends. Blood test in our hospital confirmed falciparum malaria. He was treated with artemether and after a turbulent course he finally made a complete recovery.*

DIAGNOSIS: Acute severe falciparum malaria with multiorgan failure

CASE: *A 62 years old gentleman was admitted with history of fever for more than 3 weeks. Clinical examination did not reveal any specific clue. His WBC was 16,000, ESR-110, CRP high, urine persistent microscopic haematuria (he had prostatomegaly) urea- 62 mg% creatinine- 2.1 mg% (he had chronic hypertension). X-ray chest found normal. He received several courses of antibiotics for suspected UTI. USG of abdomen was normal. Cystoscopic examination failed to reveal any cause for microscopic haematuria. He was commenced on empirical and tubercular therapy for a possibility of genitourinary tuberculosis. At this point his pANCA came back as positive and a renal biopsy showed evidence of vasculitis with presence of glomerulonephritis. He was treated with steroids, pulsed cyclophosphamide and at present he is on remission.*

DIAGNOSIS: pANCA positive vasculitis presenting with FUO.

CASE: *A 60 years old ENT consultant visiting another city of India where malaria was not prevalent. He developed acute febrile illness with severe diarrhea. He was treated locally with IV fluids and antibiotics (with a possible diagnosis of acute infective colitis). After stabilization, he was sent back to Kolkata where he developed further bouts of fever and this time falciparum malaria was confirmed by microscopy and P. falciparum antigen test.*

DIAGNOSIS: Acute severe malaria presenting with acute gastroenteritis.

In endemic areas any febrile illness with confusional state, respiratory distress, jaundice, renal failure, gastroenteritis or anaemia, malaria must be excluded by repeated blood tests. Any travel history to the forest areas should also be taken into account.

CASE: *A 58 years old gentleman was admitted with history of haemoptysis, nose bleeding and fever. Urine examination showed RBC- 6-8/field (he had prostatomegaly) Nasal biopsy: non-specific changes. X-ray chest bilateral cavitating lesions. Urea and creatinine was high normal. Initially we suspected vasculitis like Wegener's granulomatosis and were planning to give him steroid. However, his ANCA was negative and sputum was positive for AFB. He responded to antitubercular therapy.*

DIAGNOSIS: Pulmonary tuberculosis with nasal ulcers– mimicking vasculitis.

Tuberculosis, like malaria, is also a great mimicker and in India it should be considered in each and every case of FUO.

CASE: *A 55 years old engineer from Bangladesh presented with history of FUO of more than 4 months. It was associated with weight loss. Hb- 8 g%, WBC- 2800, Platelet- 94,000, low albumin and high globulin, ESR- 120, CRP- high, X-ray chest NAD, CT abdomen-hepatosplenomegaly and bilateral adrenal mass. Bone marrow changes consistent with chronic infection. Initial treatment with antitubercular drugs was unhelpful. CT guided biopsy from right adrenal revealed Histoplasma capsulatum. He was treated with itraconazole for 9 months and at present he is doing well. His biochemical and haematological parameters had reverted back to normal. Adrenal function test revealed cortisol deficiency and he was also treated with steroid replacement.*

DIAGNOSIS: Chronic histoplasmosis of adrenal gland with adrenal insufficiency, mimicking tuberculosis and presenting with FUO.

CASE: *A 58 years old gentleman presented with repeated fever over a period of last 6 months. Urine showed pus cells and RBC on one occasion and he was treated with antibiotics for a possible UTI. His USG abdomen showed multiple cysts in both kidneys and a suspected haemorrhage in one of the cysts. During his third admission, we decided to do a CT scan which confirmed the USG findings but could not exclude solid mass (shown to be haemorrhage in USG). FNAC confirmed renal cell carcinoma. He underwent nephrectomy and at present is doing well.*

DIAGNOSIS: Renal cell carcinoma presenting as FUO.

CASE: *A 34 years old lady presented with history of irregular fever for > 1 year. Her LFT were deranged. Autoimmune screening was negative, USG abdomen- hepatomegaly. CT abdomen showed multiple nodular lesions in the liver. Liver biopsy revealed granulomatous lesions consistent with granulomatous hepatitis. She is currently on steroids and antitubercular therapy. She is apyrexic now and her LFT has become normal.*

DIAGNOSIS: Granulomatous hepatitis presenting as FUO.

FEVER IN CLINICAL PRACTICE: A PRACTICAL APPROACH WITH RECENT DEVELOPMENTS

Fever of unknown origin: It is one of the most perplexing problems encountered in clinical practice.

Definition: While previously it was defined as any fever of 3 weeks duration with one week's stay in the hospital (Petersdorf *et al.* 1961) but recent criteria for FUO has been changed to any fever which persists in spite of OPD visits on two occasions or three days stay in the hospital for investigation (Durack *et al.* 1991)

It is further classified as –

- Nosocomial FUO: ventilator or tube associated catheter related DVT, Sinusitis, C. difficile diarrhea, CVA pulmonary atelectasis.
- Neutropenic FUO: urine count less than <1000, Perianal abscess, mucositis.
- HIV associated FUO: HIV itself, viral, typhlitis, fungal, neoplasm.

Drug fever: Sometimes drugs mainly in the ITU situation are found to be the main offenders. Common drugs responsible for fever are- allopurinol, isoniazid, heparin, phenytoin, penicillin, hydralazine, quinidine.

Habitual or factitious fever is getting increasingly common as a manifestation of psychosomatic illness. It usually affects young women with a history of low grade fever persisting for months and years, associated with fatigue and myalgia.

Miscellaneous Causes:

- Whipple disease
- Familial Mediterranean fever
- Recurrent Pulmonary Embolism
- Thyroiditis
- Castleman's fever
- Atrial myxoma

Common causes of FUO:

Fungal	Candidiasis, Aspergillosis, Histoplasmosis, Blastomycosis, Mucormycosis, Cryptococcosis
Bacterial	TB, UTI, Infective endocarditis, Hepatobiliary, osteomyelitis, Brucellosis, Salmonellosis, Hidden pus
Viral	Herpes, CMV, EB Virus, HIV
Parasites	Malaria, Toxoplasmosis, Amoebiasis, Leishmaniasis, Trypanosomiasis
Other Infections	Rickettsial, Psittacosis
Vasculitis	Giant cell arteritis, Polyarteritis, Behcet's syndrome
Neoplasm	Hodgkin's lymphoma, NHL, Leukemia, Renal Cell Carcinoma, Metastatic liver disease, Adenocarcinoma of liver, colon etc
Collagen Vascular	**SLE,** Rheumatoid Arthritis, Adult onset Still's disease
Granulomatous disease	Crohn's disease, Sarcoidosis, Granulomatous hepatitis

In Indian background infection, particularly tuberculosis is the most common concern followed closely by collagen vascular disorders and neoplasm.

Apart from history thorough clinical examination also gives useful clues to the diagnosis.

Fever with maculopapular rash – EB Virus, CMV, measles, HIV.

Fever with vesicular rash – *Varicella*, Herpes, Coxsackie virus.

Fever with petechial rash images – Rickettsia, Endocarditis, *Meningococcus.*

Fever with distinctive rash – Lyme disease, Ecthyma gangrenosum.

Fever with Lymphadenopathy – Brucellosis, measles, Rubella, TB, Syphilis.

Fever with hepatosplenomegaly – Malaria etc.

INVESTIGATIONS:

- Full Blood Count
- Hb, WBC, Platelet, Peripheral Smear
- Biochemistry: LFT, uric acid, TSH, protein electrophoresis.
- Inflammatory markers: CRP, ESR, Procalcitonin and other acute phase reactants
- Immunological screening: ANCA, ANF, rheumatoid factor, compliments, gamma Interferon, HIV antibody, Anti-Brucella antibody, PCR.
- Culture Sensitivity: blood, urine, CSF, stool, other body fluid culture.
- Imaging: X-Ray Chest, CT, MRI, Echo cardiogram, PET
- Biopsy, Laparoscopy
- Nuclear medicine: Technetium, Gallium, Indium scan

PET scan is a newer modality in the diagnostic armamentarium. Compared to radio isotope scan, its acquisition time is less. It is particularly helpful in diagnosing vasculitis, malignancy *etc.*

Management:

Frequently no definite cause is forth coming and one needs to embark on empirical therapy particularly when culture negative infective endocarditis, disseminated TB or Giant Cell arteritis are suspected. Steroid and NSAIDs should be considered when auto immune diseases are suspected and infective cancers are excluded. Any low grade fever persisting for more than six months, the clinician should strongly suspect habitual fever.

: KEY POINTS :

- Fever is a very common presentation in clinical practice.
- History of occupation, drug intake and travel can give useful clue in making a diagnosis.
- There is a long list of differential diagnosis in patients with FUO.
- Common causes of FUO are infections particularly TB, autoimmune diseases, vasculitis and malignancies.
- Tuberculosis and malaria are great mimickers.
- Any febrile patient returning following a holiday in the forest area, malaria should be seriously considered in the differential diagnosis.

FURTHER REFERENCE: Harrison's Principle of Internal Medicine, 17th edition.

37 A PATIENT WITH MYOCARDIAL INFARCTION WITH LEFT BUNDLE BRANCH BLOCK

CASE: *A 49 years old patient was admitted with acute central chest pain of 3 hours duration associated with sweating. The pain was radiating towards the left hand. He was a smoker and hypertensive. Examination revealed pulse rate 84/min, BP– 110/70 mmHg, normal heart sounds and chest clear. ECG showed presence of left bundle branch block. Troponin-T was negative on admission. He was treated with IV nitroglycerin and repeat troponin T at 6 hours was positive. He was thrombolysed with streptokinase.*

DIAGNOSIS: Acute myocardial infarction presenting with left bundle branch block.

DISCUSSION:

It is sometimes very difficult to diagnose acute MI in the presence of LBBB. Thrombolysis is indicated in patients with MI presenting with newly developing LBBB or RBBB. While it is relatively straight forward to diagnose MI, presence of pre-existing LBBB, may mask the classical ST changes of MI.

Features suggestive of MI with LBBB:

- If ST segment elevation is more than 5 mm.
- If ST segment elevation shows concavity upward rather than convexity upwards as usually seen in LBBB.
- Normally the ST shifts are seen in the opposite direction from the major QRS complex (discordant) when these changes are concordant; they are specific for acute MI. However in LBBB the major deflection of QRS complex is downwards in V_1, V_2 and V_3 and in acute anteroseptal MI, the ST segment elevation cannot be manifested as concordant ST shift.
- Repeated Troponin T will help diagnose difficult cases during the therapeutic window period of thrombolysis. Troponin is the earliest of the cardiac enzymes to become positive. However, even troponin takes 4-6 hours to become positive. It may remain positive for 10-14 days. So recurrent MI occurring during that window period should be made by serial CPK estimation which normalizes within 72 hours following MI. Troponin may also be elevated in renal failure.

Sometimes ST segment elevation may be due to other causes than MI, *e.g.*

i) **Acute pericarditis**: ST segment elevated in all leads. P-R segment will be depressed.

ii) **Early re-polarization abnormality:** It usually occurs in normal healthy men. Repeated ECGs will not show any evolutionary changes of MI.

iii) **Acute hyperkalemia:** Other features are tall pointed T waves and low amplitude or absent P waves. Clinical picture of background renal failure will be present.

Treatment of ST segment elevation MI:

1. Pain relief
2. Thrombolysis
3. β blocker
4. ACE Inhibitors
5. Statins
6. Primary PTCA

Pain relief:

Morphine and its derivatives are the drugs of choice for pain relief. It is particularly helpful in the presence of LVF. Antiemetics should be coprescribed.

Thrombolysis:

Although the beneficial role of thrombolytic in reducing the mortality has been conclusively shown in clinical trials (ISIS II and GISSI-I) upto one-third of the patient do not get thrombolytic in spite of presenting within the time window. Each and every patient should be thrombolysed if presenting within 12 hours unless contraindicated. Following the publication of ISIS 2 and GISSI studies, streptokinase had been the drug of choice since mid eighties. However fibrin specific agents (recombinant tissue plasminogen activator) like front loaded **alteplase** was shown to be a better drug in terms of maintenance of the patency of the infarct related artery and improved survival. Compared to streptokinase, these agents are more expensive. Recently tenecteplase, a new fibrin specific agent is becoming the thrombolytic of choice in many hospitals in the UK. The main advantage of this agent is that it can given by bolus injection rather than infusion. While treating such patients, time is the most important factor and the door to needle time should be as short as possible.

B-blockers:

In ISIS-1 study immediate use of IV β-blocker 4-6 hours post infarct was shown to reduce mortality by preventing cardiac rupture. Later on, many trials have shown that β blockers when used 7-10 days post MI give long term survival benefits. In clinical practice β blockers are commonly given before discharge as a secondary preventive measure if there is no contraindication.

ACE Inhibitors:

Use of ACE inhibitors in MI with or without LV dysfunction improves survival in the long run and should be commenced as soon as possible.

Statins:

Statins have a definite role in secondary prevention of MI. Its role in acute MI has also been suggested because of its anti inflammatory properties which might help in plaque stabilization.

Primary PTCA:

Primary PTCA in MI is superior to thrombolysis in terms of survival benefit, particularly if it can be done within 90 minutes of presentation (European Society of Cardiology guideline). This facility is usually not available in the majority of the centres in India.

Recent status of Primary PTCA in Indian background: Primary PCI is the treatment of choice in AMI provided the door to balloon time is < 90 minutes. Since this is difficult to arrange in Indian background in majority of patients the strategy could be throbolysed now stent later.

: Different modules of PCI:

- Primary.
- Facilitated ⇒ To thrombolyse and later on to do intervention.
- Rescue ⇒ Thrombolysis now and in the event of ongoing pain, to proceed for PCI within 90-120 minutes
- Pharmacoinvasive ⇒ To thrombolyse now and to transfer to an invasive centre for consideration of PCI when appropriate.

The last option may be considered as a viable option in majority of the patients in Indian background specially having DM.

PCI (Percutaneous Coronary Intervention):

- Percutaneous Coronary Intervention was inferior when compared with CABG in respect to major adverse cardiac and cerebrovascular events (MACCE), MI and death. Repeat revascularization is 2.3 fold higher with PCI.
- Mortality and MI rates were similar with either approach
- Stroke was 3.7 fold higher with CABG
- **Previous trials**
    - BARI (Bypass Angioplasty Revascularization Investigation)

- RAVEL Trial
- CARDIA

➤ Issues in PCI in diabetes

- Coronary arteries tend to be smaller
- Involvement tends to be diffuse
- Atherosclerosis tends to be more progressive, newer lesions
- Lesions tend to be more complex

➤ PCI recommended in diabetics with

- Single vessel disease
- No evidence of involvement of proximal or mid-LAD (i.e. no LIMA)
- Patients with 2 or 3 highly discrete lesions without evidence of diffuse atherosclerosis
- Patients with important contraindications to CABG: previous CABG with patent LIMA and advanced age.

➤ Points for consideration before opting for PCI in diabetics

- Use second generation drug eluting stents
- Use of potent oral anti-platelet agents
- Use a GpIIb/IIIa (or possibly bivalirudin + high dose clopidogrel)
- Cautious about contrast induced nephropathy.

Recent status of management of Acute MI with Thrombolytic:

The goal of successful management of acute MI is early reperfusion with either thrombolytics or catheter based. The ideal timeline for successful thrombolysis would be a door to needle time of 30 minutes or door to balloon time of 90 minutes. Given the paucity of catheter centres, in India (app 500 such centres) and appropriate infrastructure, primary PCI, although a better alternative to maintain reperfusion with an open artery, may not be a viable option. Indian registers suggest that the average time to reach a hospital is approx 300 minutes and the rate of PCI was only 8%. With this background pharmacological intervention is the treatment of choice in majority of patients.

Thrombolytic agents:

1st generation:	Streptokinase Urokinase
2nd generation (more fibrin specific):	Alteplase Anistreplase
3rd generation (Genetic alteration of 2nd generation molecule by Genetic Engineering**)**:	Tenecteplase Reteplase

Indication of Thrombolytic:

- Within first 12 hours of onset of symptoms with ST elevation or newly developed bundle branch block in ECG (Class 1, evidence A).
- Within 12-24 Hrs of onset of symptoms. If the symptoms are ongoing and immediate PCI is not available. (Class II a, evidence C)

Contraindication:

- In ST depression. (Except for true posterior infarction)

Bolus thrombolysis vs prolonged infusion (Reteplase vs Tenecteplase): Advantages of bolus thrombolysis are:

- Pre-hospital thrombolysis possible
- Very early thrombolysis within 1-3 hrs of onset of symptoms may cause reperfusion and patency rate similar to PCI.
- Bolus thrombolysis opens arteries more quickly compared to continuous infusion based thrombolysis (Steady Reteplase vs. Alteplase)

Non-weighted (Reteplase) vs Weighted bolus (Tenecteplase):

- Dose error is less with non-weighted thrombolytics. Dose error increases the side effects of bleeding or decrease the potency (less chance of reperfusion).

Complications of Thrombolytics:

Bleeding is the most serious complication. (Protamine counteracts the effect of Heparin.) Symptomatic treatment and specialist opinion should be taken in the events of life threatening bleeding.

Predictions of bleeding: Advanced age, Height & weight, Female.

DOSAGE:

- Streptokinase- 1.5 million Units IV infusions over 60 minutes.
- Alteplase- 90 min infusion, 15 mg IV bolus ⇒ followed by 0.75 mg/kg (maximum 50 mg) infused over 30 minutes followed by (0.5 mg/kg (maximum 35 g) infused over 60 minutes.
- Tenecteplase- Single bolus dose in 5 second.
  - < 60 kg: 30 mg IV bolus administered over 5 seconds.
  - 60 to 70 kg: 35 mg IV bolus administered over 5 seconds
  - 70 to 80 kg: 40 mg IV bolus administered over 5 seconds
  - 80 to 90 kg: 45 mg IV bolus administered over 5 seconds
  - > 90 kg: 50 mg IV bolus administered over 5 seconds
- Reteplase- 10 units IV bolus over 2 mints ⇒ Repeat 10 units after 30 minutes.

Nitrates:

Nitrates are commonly prescribed for symptomatic relief of angina or for the treatment of LVF. In clinical practice, although it is routinely used in uncomplicated MI, it does not offer any survival benefit.

Concomitant use of anti platelet agents:

The role of Aspirin as an adjuvant was established since ISIS-2 study in mid eighties. Recently clopidogrel added to aspirin was also shown to reduce the rates of cardiovascular events in patients treated with fibrinolytics. (CLARITY – TIMI – 28 trials).

- Aspirin: 162-325 mg loading dose followed by 81-325 mg daily dose.
- Clopidogrel: If < 75 years of age → loading dose of 300 mg followed by 75 mg daily upto 1 year. (In patients of more than 75 years of age → no loading dose is required.)

Although use of heparin along with streptokinase has not been shown to improve the patency rate of the infarct related artery, it is a common practice to use either heparin or low molecular weight heparin in the post thrombolytic period. It can also prevent DVT or formation of mural thrombus in a big anteroseptal MI. Use of IV heparin as an adjunct to TPA has been shown to improve patency rate of the infarct related artery, however. In ASSENT3 study, use of enoxaparin as an adjunct to tenecteplase has shown to improve survival at 30 days post infarct compared to combination of tenecteplase and heparin.

Concomitant Use of Antithrombotic With:

3rd generation Thrombolytic:

- Heparin: 5000 IU IV bolus followed by heparin IV infusion target APTT 50-70 dose or 12000 IU s/c twice daily.
- Low molecule weight heparin Enoxaparin: 30 mg IV bolus then 1 mg/kg s/c twice daily. If patient is more than 75 years old then the dose should be reduced to 0.75 mg/kg s/c twice daily, no bolus is needed. In patients with creatinine clearance of less than 30 ml/min the dose should be once a day.
- Fondaparinux: 2.5 mg IV bolus followed by 2.5 mg s/c once daily.

SUDDEN CARDIAC DEATH

CASE: *A 72 years old patient with known dilated cardiomyopathy with ejection fraction of 23% was recently discharged from the hospital following treatment for increasing breathlessness. In the past he had several admissions with similar symptoms. He was on a protocol wise treatment regime for his cardiac failure except for having an invasive therapy CRT or ICD. Family members were adequately counselled about the progress of his condition. After one week of his discharge he was repeated to have sudden onset of senselessness while going to the bathroom, collapsed and was found to be unresponsive. A doctor from an emergency organization attended him within half an hour and declared him to be dead.*

DIAGNOSIS: Sudden cardiac death in a known patient with dilated cardiomyopathy.

DISCUSSIONS:

Sudden Cardiac Death (SCD) is a major public health challenge throughout the world. It is estimated that worldwide nearly 7 million deaths per year are due to SCD and 50% of all coronary artery disease death are due to sudden cardiac arrest.

- Only 58% thrombolysed
- Only 8% has PCI
- ST Segment Elevation Myocardial Infarction (STEMI) → Mortality 9% at 30 days
- Non ST Segment Elevation Myocardial Infarction (NSTEMI) → Mortality 3.6% at 30 days.

Immediate causes of death:

- Ventricular fibrillation – 25%
- Polymorphic Ventricular tachycardia – 30%
- Torsades de pointes – 10%
- Monomorphic Ventricular tachycardia – 10%
- Pulse less electrical activity – 10%
- Unknown – 5%

Underlying cause: Majority of the causes are due to Ischaemic Heart disease:

a) **Due to Structural heart disease:**
- Ischaemic heart disease
- Hypertensive heart disease
- Valvular heart disease
- Dilated Cardiomyopathy
- Hypertrophic Cardiomyopathy
- Myocarditis
- Congenital heart disease
- Arrhythmogenic Right Ventricular Cardiomyopathy

b) Without any Structural Heart Disease: They constitute 5% -10% of all causes of SCD
- Brugada Syndrome – incomplete right bundle-branch block and ST segment elevation in V_1 and V_2 leads. It is caused by a genetic change in the 'Na' channels which causes action potential changes in the epicardium but not in the endocardium.
- Long Q-T Syndrome – Consists of number of familial disease with genetic variation of different 'Na' and 'K' Channels. The necessary drugs are antipsychotics, antidepressants, antiparkinsonians, chemotherapies etc. In addition hypokalaemia, hypomagnesemia may also cause it.
- Short Q-T prolongation Syndrome – It is recently described and rare.
- Catecholaminergic polymorphic VT – Occurs in childhood days (7-8 yrs of age). It is typically induced by physical stress or emotional stress.

- In addition to VT/VF, supraventricular tachycardia, atrial fibrillation etc. are also common.

The mechanism of arrhythmia is either through increased automacity, triggered activity or by re-entry.

INVESTIGATIONS:

- Sometimes ECG gives clue when fragmented QRS complex in inferior lead, with T wave alternations
- 24 hours Holter monitoring
- ECHO → Ejection fraction of less than 35% is a high risk factor
- CT scan or MRI scan, radio-nucleotide imaging may give further clue.

TREATMENT:

I.C.D (Implantable cardioverter defibrillator) has established itself as a life saving procedure.

Indication: ICD therapy is a Class I indication in patients with structural heart disease and spontaneous sustained V.T

a) Cardiac arrest survivor

b) Structural heart disease with spontaneous VT

c) Post MI > 40 days

- LVEF <30%
- LVEF <40% with nonsustained VT on EPS

d) Non ischaemic cardiomyopathy with LVEF < 35% and NYHA functional class II and III

Other available therapies:

a) Surgical treatment following intraoperative mapping surgery may be an option. However, it has got high morbidity and mortality.

b) Catheter ablation- It is an increasingly adopted therapy. However it needs appropriate mapping. In Indian perspective it may prove to be a valuable option in future given the high acquisition cost of ICD. Moreover, ICD treats VT/VF only, whereas ablation hits at the root cause of its generation.

Pharmacotherapy to reduce arrhythmic mortality:

1. Betablockers: it reduces total as well as arrhythmic mortality (BHAT). Class I drugs like flecainide etc should be avoided as they increase mortality by way of causing pro-arrhythmia.
2. Amiodarone- Reduces arrhythmic death but not total mortality.
3. ACE Inhibitor: In Post MI patients it prevents arrhythmia and reduces overall mortality.
4. Statins: It reduces shocks in patients in ICD.
5. Mineralocorticoid receptor blockage: Eplerenone has been shown to reduce SCD in post MI patients with LVEF < 40% (EPHESUS study)
6. Ranolazine: May have some benefit in reduction of VT/VF although it has not been conclusively proven.

In non-ischaemic Cardiomyopathy:

Beta blockers, ACE inhibitors or ARBs should be prescribed. Amiodarone is of value in secondary prevention of arrhythmic events. Statins and amiodarone reduce the incidence of DC Shock.

In heart failure, a similar line of therapy may be pursued as in non-ischaemic cardiomyopathy. ARB (Angiotensin Receptor Blockers) may not be as good as ACE inhibitors [ELLITE-II Study] and should only be used in case of ACE inhibitor intolerance.

Amiodarone vs ICD:

AVID trial has conclusively proved that ICD has mortality advantage over amiodarone over a 3 years period study. However in subgroup analysis, the advantage was not sustained in patients with EF of more than 35%.

Channelopathies:

➢ <u>Long QT syndrome</u> –

- Betablockers like propranolol in the dose of 2-4 mg/kg/day has been successful in reducing VT/VF.
- Flecainide may be tried if βeta blockers fail.
- Similarly mexiletine which shortens QT segment may be of help.

- Brugada Syndrome – ICD implantation is the treatment of choice Quinidine may be tried.

  Catecholaminergic polymorphic VT/VF- In addition to β blocker therapy sympathetic denervation may be tried.

- Short QT Syndrome – ICD may be the primary therapy.

Cardio Cerebral resuscitation:

- Continuous Chest Compression
- ACLS algorithm
- Aggressive post resuscitation care

Post Cardiac Arrest:

In ED/ICU:

Respiratory Status	Cardiac Status	Neurological Status	Metabolic Status
$SPO_2 > 94\%$ Not necessarily 100% $PaCO_2$ – 40-45 mmHg	SBP > 90 mmHg MAP > 65 mmHg IV fluid Vasopressors	Therapeutic Hypothermia in Comatose EEG, CT Scan	K > 3.5 mol/lit Glucose- 144-180% Mg → supplemental

: KEY POINTS :

- ST segment elevation MI must be thrombolysed if presenting within 12 hours in the absence of any contraindication.
- MI is difficult to diagnose in the presence of LBBB.
- Amongst the cardiac enzymes, troponin is the earliest to become positive.
- 3rd generation bolus thrombolytic have advantages over 1st and 2nd thrombolytics.
- Non-weighted 3rd generation thrombolytics have advantages over weighted 3rd generation thrombolytic.
- In Indian background where primary PTCA is logistically difficult to organize in vast majority of cases, pharmaco-invasive PTCA may be the way forward.

FURTHER REFERENCES:

- Brersmat *et a*l., Acute Myocardial Infarction, Lancet 361: 847, 2003.
- Topol EJ, Acute Myocardial Infarction – Thrombolysis, Heart 83: 122, 2000.
- Jamesd Dalal *et al.*, Role of thrombolytic in reperfusion therapy for management of AMI- Indian Scenario—Indian Heart journal 65 (2013) 566-585.
- Oxford Book of Medicine – 5th edition.
- Harrison's Principal of Internal Medicine – 17th edition.
- Post graduate Medicine: Vol. XXVII, 2013. Coronary artery intervention in diabetes.

38 A PATIENT WITH OBSTRUCTIVE SLEEPAPNOEA SYNDROME (OSAS)

CASE: *A 72 years old doctor presented with history of shortness of breath, lethargy, tiredness and weakness, swelling of legs and sleep disturbance. He had a pacemaker in situ and was treated for cardiac failure and chronic corpulmonale with diuretics, ACE inhibitors and nitrates. Addition of bronchodilators via inhalation and nebulisation did not give him much relief. Examination revealed pulse rate of 72/m, normal heart sounds, bibasilar crepts and pedal oedema. ECG showed paced rhythm, X-ray chest cardiomegaly, Echo- EF 45%. He was admitted for further investigation. In the ward, he was noticed to have pronounced snoring with frequent wake ups. Nocturnal oximetry revealed that he was frequently desatutating throughout the night. A clinical diagnosis of an associated obstructive sleep apnoea was made.*

DIAGNOSIS: Obstructive sleep apnoea syndrome (OSAS).

He was given a trial of nasal CPAP. Although he was uncomfortable in the initial two weeks, he started to improve from the 3rd week and 3 months at follow up, he was a changed man. His BP was better controlled, swelling of legs had gone altogether and he was alert and active as before.

DISCUSSIONS:

Sleep apnoea syndrome (SAS) comprise three main disorders e.g.:

1. OSAS
2. Central sleep apnoea syndrome (CSA)
3. Cheyne-stokes respiration (CSR)

While CSA and CSR occur mainly in patients with CNS disorders, the main risk factor for OSAS is obesity.

Obstructive sleep apnoea is a common clinical condition frequently missed in the primary care practice as it does not always present in its classical form and many times superimposed on other associated medical conditions. Its detection is important however, because it is associated with adverse medical outcome. The incidence of hypertension, neuro-cognitive dysfunction due to recurrent hypoxia, cardiac failure cerebrovascular accident, motor vehicle accidents and occupation hazards increase significantly in patients with OSAS.

The main morbidity and mortality due to OSAS is related to cardiovascular complications like increased prevalence of hypertension, IHD, cardiac failure, arrhythmia and sudden death. In addition, the risk of having CVA is also high. Treatment with nasal CPAP has reduced the incidence of these cardiovascular problems to a large extent.

WHEN TO THINK OF OSAS?

It is common in obese male patients. The main presenting symptoms are unrefreshing sleep with morning headache, drowsiness throughout the day and frequently falling asleep in the workplace. In the elderly the BP goes up and features of cardiac failure are aggravated. A careful history from the spouse often reveals snoring and frequent waking up from the sleep. This condition can also occur in children due to enlarged tonsils and adenoids and may interfere with scholastic performance in the school.

DIAGNOSTIC TOOLS:

- **From clinical history**
- **Nocturnal oximetry:** Oximetry at night time can frequently detect oxygen desaturation due to obstruction. However, it is not a very sensitive test. It can be performed as a baseline test or where polysomnography is not feasible.
- **Polysomnography:** This is the diagnostic test. This usually incorporates EEG, ECG, electrooculogram, Chin-electromyogram, snoring thermistor, pulse oximetry and tibialis anterior electromyogram. If apnoea is documented, a trial of nasal CPAP titration can be undertaken in the second half of the sleep study.

Differential diagnosis:

- Insufficient sleep
- Shift work
- Depression and other psychiatrists illness
- Narcolepsy
- Idiopathic hyper somnolence syndrome

NARCOLEPSY: It usually presents at a younger age characterised by excessive day twice sleepiness along with episodic collapse called cataplexy which may mimic seizure, coma or malingering. The other differential diagnosis is periodic paralysis, myasthenia gravis, TIA etc. Snoring is not a prominent symptom of narcolepsy. Nocturnal polysomnography has got some characteristic features like rapid onset sleep and premature entry into REM sleep.

TREATMENT: Apart from life style changes to ensure proper sleep hygienic, medications like modafinil, dexamphetamine and sodium oxybate may be helpful. For cataplexy, tricyclic antidepressants and SSRI along with venlafaxine may be tried. These drugs are also helpful in sleep paralysis and hallucination.

MANAGEMENT:

The basic mechanism of OSAS is pharyngeal collapse or fall back of tongue and this obstruction can be circumvented by the use of nasal CPAP. Although many patients face problems in the initial period, majority of them eventually overcome them when they find a vast improvement in their quality of life. Nasal stuffiness can be managed with local decongestants, steroids etc.

TREATMENT:

With the advent of nasal CPAP, the treatment of OSAS both symptomatic as well as prevention has been revolutionised. It has been shown that during sleep, if the airway opening pressure is maintained around 5–20 mmHg the problem of OSAS may be circumvented. The modern auto CPAP modules can self adjust the variable measures that may be required during the entire process of sleep for claustrophobic patients newer variants of masks and nasal pillows are also available. However the optimal pressure generation may not be sufficient. The problem of dryness of mouth has been circumvented with an inbuilt-integral heated humidifier in the machine. For morbid obesity, bariatric surgery may be an option.

In patients who cannot tolerate the machine, oral appliances including mandibular advancing and tongue retaining devices may be tried. They act by preventing retroglossal collapse.

Surgical treatment:

The patients with OSAS should undergo ENT assessment for any structural or pharyngeal problems and in appropriate cases uvulo-palato-pharyngo-plasty with the resection of uvula and redundant portion of the soft palate can be done with good effect. In children with OSAS, tonsillectomy with adenoidectomy will cure the condition.

Other treatments:

Control of obesity should be done. In many patients postural care during sleep like sleeping in a lateral decubitus or prone position to prevent tongue fall back, may give partial relief.

OSAS is a condition where proper history taking is very important. The patients are frequently treated with anti-depressants, sedatives, antihypertensive etc. without any relief. A proper history will help to make a correct diagnosis.

: KEY POINTS :

- OSAS is not an uncommon presentation in clinical practice.
- Its detection is important for symptomatic relief as well as prevention of neuro-cognitive and cardiovascular adverse effects.
- One should think of this condition in any obese, male snorer with day time drowsiness.
- Nasal CPAP gives symptomatic relief as well as improves the overall outcome.

FURTHER REFERENCES:

- Mc Nicholas WT, Philupson A – Breathing disorders in Sleep, London, Saunders, 2002.
- TG Quinnell – Narcolepsy and other related conditions, Clinical medicine, Vol. -11, no-3, June 2011.
- J.C. pepperell,- Sleep apnoea syndrome and cardiovascular system, Clinical medicine – Vol. -11, No -3 June -2011.
- Harrison's Principle of Internal Medicine, 17th edition.
- Oxford Textbook of Medicine – 5th edition.

39 A PATIENT WITH CHRONIC HEPATITIS B INFECTION

CASE: *A 29 years old gentleman attended the clinic with non-specific symptoms of abdominal discomfort and weakness. Initial screening test showed altered LFT with bilirubin of 1.8 mg%, AST-141, ALT-123, and USG showed hepatomegaly. Blood test for hepatitis screening profile was sent which showed positive hepatitis B surface antigen, positive hepatitis B e antigen, negative hepatitis B e antibody and high level of hepatitis B DNA. He gave a history of jaundice 15 years back and was not followed up since then.*

DIAGNOSIS: Chronic hepatitis B infection.

DISCUSSION:

More than 400 million people are chronically infected with hepatitis B virus and majority of them are from South East Asia, Indian subcontinent and sub Saharan Africa. A past history of jaundice may not be present in many cases. A history of blood transfusion, previous operation, intravenous drug abuse and history of hepatitis in close contacts should be taken.

Following acute viral infection 90% of the patient will clear hepatitis B surface antigen from their blood within 6 months. Patients with chronic hepatitis B are initially positive for hepatitis B e antigen with high level of hepatitis B DNA in the blood. Eventually hepatitis B e antibody appears in the blood due to antibody response with disappearance of e antigen and hepatitis B DNA. Patients with e antibody, normal liver enzymes and undetectable viraemia are known as normal carriers. They usually do not need any antiviral treatment. In somc of the patients the viral replication continues with persistence of e antigen and high level of HBV DNA. This ongoing infection will eventually lead to liver failure, cirrhosis and hepatocellular carcinoma. Selecting such patients for antiviral treatment is important as it will reduce the complications of chronic infection.

Investigation needed in hepatitis B surface antigen positive patients:

- Liver function test particularly AST and ALT.
- Hepatitis B e antigen.
- Hepatitis B e antibody.
- Hepatitis B DNA (quantitative titre).
- Liver biopsy will be helpful but not essential.

Antiviral treatment should be offered to those with raised AST, ALT (they may be normal in some cases). Positive hepatitis B e antigen and high titre of hepatitis B DNA (the cut off value for treatment varies between the centres).

In precore mutant variety of hepatitis B infection, e-antigen may be negative. However, other features of active viral replication will be present.

ANTIVIRAL MEDICATIONS:

Interferon alpha:

In the dose of 10 million with subcutaneous three times a week or 5 million units subcutaneous daily 3-6 months will induce loss of e antigen in 33% of cases undetectable HBV DNA in 37% of cases and loss of hepatitis B surface antigen in 8% of cases. Even if they are positive for hepatitis B surface antigen the chances of development of cirrhosis or liver cancer drops significantly following seroconversion with loss of e antigen.

Side effects:

- Flu like symptoms
- Alopecia
- Autoimmune disturbance
- Leucopenia

Lamivudine (a nucleoside analogue):

In the dose of 100 mg daily for a period of 1 year will reduce the hepatic inflammatory response significantly and many of the patients will eventually seroconvert. The duration of treatment is controversial. Usually it should be continued for 6-9 months following seroconversion. The main problem with lamivudine monotherapy is the development of drug resistance. This drug can be given even in decompensated liver disease.

Adefovir dipivoxil:

This relatively new nucleoside analogue has been used with success in chronic hepatitis B infection. The dose is 10 mg daily for 48 weeks and the chances of development of drug resistance is low and there are relatively few side effects.

Combination therapy:

Combination of interferon alpha along with lamivudine did not show a significant benefit. Use of this combination for a longer period and combination of two nucleosides are on trial.

Household contacts and close relatives should be checked for hepatitis B surface antigen and vaccinated. There are special protocols for the treatment of babies born of hepatitis B positive mothers which should be followed.

This patient was commenced on lamivudine 100 mg daily 9 months at follow up. He had seroconverted with very low titre of HBV DNA. He remained surface antigen positive however. His liver function had normalized as well. He was advised to continue with lamivudine for another 6 months. He is also under the care of a hepatologist.

Recent treatment recommendation:

Consensus has emerged that no treatment is required for hepatitis B carriers as evidenced by negative Hepatitis B e-antigen, normal ALT and HBV DNA $<10^4$ copies/ml documented serially over time.

Treatment is recommended for patients with Hepatitis B e antigen positive (which may be negative in precore mutant variety), elevated ALT and HBV DNA $>10^5$ copies/ml. Since in compensated cirrhosis treatment with antiviral retards the progress of the disease, it is usually advised to treat the patients irrespective of hepatitis e-antigen status or HBV DNA load although some recommend no treatment if HBV DNA load is $<10^4$ copies/ ml. Similarly in decompensated cirrhosis treatment is recommended in the similar line although defer treatment if HBV DNA load is $<10^5$ copies/ml.

Other drugs that are used in chronic viral infection:

- **PEG interferon** 180 µg/week for 48 weeks.
- **Entecavir** (0.5-1 mg daily) this is more effective than lamivudine as incidence of resistance is low. The treatment should be carried out for indefinite period.
- **Tenofovir** (300µg) daily may be used alternatively as the chances of resistance is low.
- Combination therapy may be used to reduce the incidence of drug resistance.

Common combinations that can be used are:

- Particularly combination of entecavir and tenofovir is a common combination that may be used.
- PEG interferon or interferon with lamivudine.
- Lamivudine with adefovir.
- Lamivudine with either tenofovir or entecavir.
- In HIV co-infection lamivudine should never be used alone.

Response to treatment:

Successful treatment is indicated by very low or undetectable HBV DNA level, loss of e-antigenicity and in 10% of cases hepatitis B e surface antigen negativity. Since there is a controversy regarding duration of treatment, these tests need to be repeated periodically to assess the success of treatment or any relapse.

In pregnancy both standard interferon and lamivudine may be safely used.

Finally for decompensated cirrhosis the patient should be evaluated for liver transplantation.

: KEY POINTS :

- Chronic hepatitis B infection is a common problem in clinical practice.
- Untreated, it can lead to cirrhosis and liver cancer.
- Specific antiviral therapy is available for this condition.
- Entecavir and Tenofovir are the newer option of treatment.

FURTHER REFERENCES:

- Harrison's Principle of Internal Medicine - 17th edition.
- Chronic Hepatitis B infection - The Lancet 2003.
- Oxford Text Book of Medicine - 5th edition.

40 A PATIENT WITH HEPATITIS C INFECTION

CASE: *A 38 years old male hospital staff who recently suffered from amoebic liver abscess, had been complaining of persistent dragging right upper abdominal pain. Investigations revealed persistently raised AST and ALT with evidence of fatty changes in liver in the ultrasound. His hepatitis B surface antigen was negative and HCV antibody was found to be positive. HCV RNA quantitative assay was positive as well.*

DIAGNOSIS: Hepatitis C infection.

DISCUSSION:

Hepatitis C is most commonly transmitted via blood transfusion. However, in a significant proportion of cases, no history of blood transfusion will be available. Transmission through needle prick may also occur. Sexual transmission is much less common compared to hepatitis B infection. The faeco-oral transmission is extremely uncommon.

Hepatitis C infection remains asymptomatic in majority of patients and 15% - 20% of patients get a natural cure. Rest of the patients will develop chronic infection and mildly elevated AST and ALT will be the only marker of the disease activity. Therefore testing for HCV antibody is mandatory in any person with raised liver enzymes.

If positive of HCV antibody, a quantitative assay for HCV RNA will also be required and ideally HCV genotyping should also be done. This is important to predict the response of treatment. Amongst the six genotypes, genotype-I poorly responds to treatment with high relapse rate while genotypes-2 and 3 have a relatively better prognosis in terms of therapeutic response. After confirmation of the diagnosis, liver biopsy is advisable to detect the degree of inflammation and fibrosis as it will be helpful for the post treatment follow up. Moreover, the treatment may even be withheld in HCV positive patients if there is no significant inflammation and fibrosis.

Interferon alpha was the initial treatment available with a suboptimal response rate. Later on its combinations with ribavirin was found to be more effective. Finally it was apparent that weekly injection of interferon was inadequate to maintain sustained blood level to have complete antiviral effect. Recently, **pegylated interferon** in combination of **ribavirin** is the treatment of choice. Pegylated interferon may be effectively given once a week by subcutaneous injection [pegylated interferon 80 mg subcutaneously weekly along with ribavirin 200 mg five times daily]. The treatment is usually offered for 48 weeks and a successful treatment is indicated by HCV RNA negativity after the completion of therapy maintaining at 6 months post-therapy. Serial HCV RNA estimation is not required as they are expensive and the load of HCV RNA does not correlate well with the disease activity.

Pegylated interferon should be avoided in patients with decompensated liver disease and in presence of autoimmune disorders. Because of its propensity to cause autoimmune thyroiditis, a baseline thyroid function test should be checked before commencement of therapy. Ribavirin can cause haemolytic anaemia and during the combination therapy regular monitoring of full blood count and liver function tests should be done.

This patient completed 48 weeks course of combination therapy of pegylated interferon and ribavirin. His latest liver function test was normal and his 6 months post treatment HCV RNA was negative. He is asymptomatic as well.

CASE: *A 46 years old lady attended the clinic for routine preoperative check up for a hernia operation. She had non-specific joint pain along with symptoms of vague weakness but no cardio respiratory risk factors. Investigations revealed Hb- 8.2 g%, bilirubin-2.3 mg%, AST- 84, ALT- 77, alkaline phosphatase- 510 (high), albumin- 2.8 mg% (low), globulin- 4.8 mg% (high), hepatitis B surface antigen negative, HCV antibody-not done as it was not routinely available during that time. ANF-weakly positive, anti-smooth muscle antibody and anti mitochondrial antibody not done because of non-availability, rheumatoid factor was weakly positive. A diagnosis of autoimmune hepatitis was made and the operation was postponed because of abnormal LFT and she was lost to follow up.*

5 years later, she was readmitted with history of haematemesis and melena. During this time her LFT had deteriorated considerably with increase in bilirubin, AST and ALT. Prothrombin time was high, gastroscopy revealed oesophageal varices. There was ascites and other features of portal hypertension. This time HCV antibody was checked from two sources and both were positive.

Classification of autoimmune hepatitis:

Type 1

- ANF is positive- Autoimmune hepatitis.

Type 2a

- ANF negative, anti liver kidney microsomal antibody positive (Anti LKM antibody).

Type 2b

- ANF negative, anti-LKM antibody +ve, HCV antibody positive, HCV RNA +ve.

Type 3

- ANF negative, anti LKM antibody negative, antibody to soluble liver antigen +ve.

FINAL DIAGNOSIS: Autoimmune hepatitis with decompensated liver disease with hepatitis C positivity.

On careful inquiry, she gave history of ruptured ectopic pregnancy 25 years back and she received 2 units of blood transfusion.

This lady might have had Type-1 autoimmune hepatitis with a false positive HCV antibody (because of hypergammaglobulinaemia). The infection could not be confirmed by HCV RNA test because of non-availability of the test during the time of presentation.

This case has been mentioned to stress the importance of chronic hepatitis which can also present with features of autoimmune hepatitis (Type Mb) and in patients presenting with features of autoimmune hepatitis or vasculitis due to cryoglobulinaemia, the clinician should routinely request for HCV antibody test.

Newer treatment for Hepatitis-C:

Alisporivir- It is a cyclophilin inhibitor. It is being researched for potential use in the treatment of hepatitis C. Alisporivir is not immunosuppressive.

Telaprevir and **boceprevir-** these are two protease inhibitors and can be combined the current standard of care, pegylated interferon plus ribavirin. This triple therapy shortens the duration of therapy and may cause prolong virological remission.

: KEY POINTS :

- Hep-C infection can cause chronic liver disease and hepatocellular carcinoma.
- Autoimmune hepatitis and essential cryoglobulinaemia can be associated with hepatitis C.
- HCV antibody should be checked in any patient with altered LFT.
- Hepatitis C has specific treatment.

FURTHER REFERENCES:

- Straden DB; *et al*, Hepatitis C, a brief clinical overview - Review ILARJ 2001: 42: 107-16.
- NICE - guideline on the use of ribavirin and interferon α for Hepatitis C, London: NICE, 2000. www.nice.org.uk <http://www.nice.org.uk>
- Hepatitis C infection, The Lancet Dec, 2003.
- Harrison's Principle of Internal Medicine – 17th edition.
- Oxford Textbook of Medicine – 5th edition.
- British Journal of Hospital Medicine, May 2011, vol.: 72, No. 5.

41 A PATIENT WITH SERONEGATIVE RHEUMATOID ARTHRITIS

CASE: *A 46 years old lady was admitted with 6 months history of pain and swelling of the small joints of the hands including in metacarpophalangeal (MCP) joints. She also had pain and swelling of the knee and ankle joints. She had morning stiffness lasting for at least 1 hour along with a low grade temperature. Her BP was 160/90 mmHg, locomotor system examination revealed swollen MCP joints, effusion of both knee joints with restricted movement of the wrist joints. Investigation revealed Hb- 8.1 g%, WBC- 12,000, platelet- 3.4 lakhs, ESR- 106, rheumatoid factor negative, ANF negative, ASO negative, uric acid normal, ANCA negative, X-ray chest normal, X ray both hands showed soft tissue swelling around MCP joints, periarticular osteoporosis and joint space narrowing. No obvious erosion was found.*

DIAGNOSIS: Seronegative rheumatoid arthritis

DISCUSSION: Pain and swelling of the joints are common clinical presentation and a sizeable number of them would be having rheumatoid arthritis. The diagnosis is important as it has got specific line of management which can prevent the progression of the disease.

The first thing is to identify whether it is an inflammatory arthropathy. Presence of systemic symptoms, anaemia, high ESR, high CRP and high platelet count would indicate inflammatory arthropathy. Presence of morning stiffness, symmetrical involvement of small joints of the hands including MCP joints, presence of characteristic deformities of the hands and positive rheumatoid factor would point towards the diagnosis of rheumatoid arthritis. Rheumatoid nodules or vasculitic skin rash, if present may add to the diagnosis. However rheumatoid factor will be negative in a sizeable number of patients (seronegative rheumatoid arthritis). On the other hand, rheumatoid factor may be false positive in many conditions and clinical assessment is very important in making the final diagnosis.

Clinical features suggestive of Rheumatoid arthritis:

Articular features-

- Usually insidious onset occasionally subacute in nature.
- Clinically symmetrical.
- Classically small joints of the hand, particularly PIP joints but bigger joints are also involved.
- Classical deformities like swan-neck deformity of hand, Z-deformity of thumb, ulnar deviation of hand.
- As far as axial skeletal system is concerned cervical spine is involved but lumbar spine is usually spared

Extra articular features-

- Constitutional symptoms like malaise, low grade fever
- Presence of rheumatoid nodules
- Presence of vasculitis
- Fibrosing alveolitis and bronchiolitis obliterans
- Scleritis, episcleritis
- Pleural and pericardial effusion (exudates with high protein and low glucose)
- Cardiac involvement
- Peripheral neuropathy
- Increased incidence of cancer (lymphoproliferative disorder)
- Felty's syndrome- combination of seropositive rheumatoid arthritis with splenomegaly, leukopenia and leg ulcer.

ASSESSMENT OF DISEASE ACTIVITY:

This is usually measured by duration of morning stiffness, pain and swelling of knee joints. Systemic symptoms in addition to presence of the rheumatoid factor, high ESR, CRP, high ferritin and thrombocytosis may indicate disease activity.

DIFFERENTIAL DIAGNOSIS:

Rheumatoid arthritis should be differentiated from other spondyloarthropathies, reactive arthritis due to IBD, psoriasis and Reiter's syndrome. In these conditions the arthritis is usually asymmetrical and involves other joints, moreover axial skeleton particularly lumbosacral spine is commonly involved. Similarly ankylosing spondylitis with peripheral arthropathy can be differentiated on the same clinical ground. In addition primary vasculitis can also be differentiated by classical clinical pictures and predominant skin involvement and characteristic blood tests (p-ANCA or c-ANCA). SLE usually gives rise to arthralgia smaller than classical rheumatoid arthritis. Osteoarthritis is readily distinguished by classical joint pain in the hip joint, PIP and DIP joint and 1st metacarpophalangeal joints. Moreover, inflammatory signs are usually absent. In septic arthritis, arthritis usually involves a single joint. Reactive arthritis may have similar features.

INVESTIGATIONS:

Apart from rheumatoid factors, anti-citrulline antibody may be positive even if rheumatoid factor is negative. It has sensitivity of 80% with 90% specificity.

Normocytic normochromic anaemia with low calcium and high alkaline phosphatase may indicate disease activity. X-ray of the involved joints is essential to look for any osteoporosis, bony deformity, soft tissue swelling and bony erosions ultrasound examination and CT or MRI scan may be helpful to assess associated synovitis.

Causes of false positive rheumatoid factor:

1. Sjogren's syndrome
2. SLE
3. Tuberculosis
4. Infective endocarditis
5. Kala-azar
6. Malaria
7. Sarcoidosis
8. Hepatitis B
9. Normal persons

This lady's symptoms, clinical and haematological features fitted in well with rheumatoid arthritis although her rheumatoid factor was negative. She was treated with pulsed methyl prednisolone for 3 days. She also received intra-articular steroid injection for the active synovitis of her knee joints and she was commenced on a combination of DMARDs (disease modifying anti-rheumatic drugs). 6 months at follow up, she had been doing well. She was on bi-weekly methotrexate along with hydroxychloroquine and sulphasalazine as DMARDs.

CASE: *A 39 years old lady admitted clinic being referred by her local Physician with a diagnosis of seropositive rheumatoid arthritis. She had had classical symptoms of rheumatoid arthritis for the last three months and her GP made the correct diagnosis on clinical ground supported by a strongly positive rheumatoid factor report. She admitted the clinic mainly for counseling and for discussion regarding different options of treatments.*

PROBLEM: Rheumatoid arthritis → planning for long-term treatment.

DISCUSSIONS:

There has been a recent change in approach in treating rheumatoid arthritis (RA) with aggressively using DMRD either single or in combination. Early in the disease along with NSAID, selective COX2 inhibitors is used and in resistant cases with biological therapy. The aggressive approach has been shown to retard the progression of the disease effectively.

MANAGEMENT:

NSAID: These agents have been useful in controlling the symptoms in RA by way of their anti-inflammatory effect. However with their use, side effects mainly in the form of gastric irritation. Since the gastrointestinal side effects are mediated through COX1 receptors, specific COX2 inhibitory NSAIDs like coxibs have been used successfully in RA. Due to disturbing report of increasing cardiac morbidity with COX2 inhibition, risk-benefit ratio needs to be judged and should be used in appropriate patients with low cardiovascular risk.

DMARDs:

The management of rheumatoid arthritis has changed considerably over the last decade since the availability of newer DMARDs. The old DMARDs like gold, penicillamine, sulphasalazine and hydroxychloroquine has been replaced by methotrexate, cyclosporine, leflunomide and biological therapies like etanercept or infliximab.

In 1996, it was demonstrated that combination of weekly methotrexate along with sulphasalazine and hydroxychloroquine was much more superior to any of the drugs alone in prevention of joint damage without any evidence of increased side effects. Combination therapy may be started as:

- All three drugs starting together
- As step up approach
- As step down approach.

The therapy as stated above may be tailored according to the patient's needs and the doctor's clinical judgment. In difficult cases, combination of bi-weekly methotrexate (10-15 mg) along with daily cyclosporine may be more effective without any added toxicity.

More recently, biological therapy with antibody to tumour necrosis factor (one of the cytokines that perpetrates the joint inflammation in rheumatoid arthritis) has been used with very good effect (both symptomatic and prevention of further joint damage). Two such agents are in clinical use:

- Etanercept 25 mg SC weekly
- Infliximab 3 mg/Kg at 6-8 weeks interval

Both of them cause quick symptomatic improvement. However they are costly and may not be suitable for everyone. Moreover, being immunosuppressives, they may flare up latent tuberculosis. So the patients should be monitored accordingly.

The main facets of treatment are to **reduce pain, maintain the physical function of the joints and prevent deformities**. In this segment the role of physiotherapy, occupational therapy and use of NSAIDs play a very important role. Although they are very helpful for symptomatic relief they do very little to prevent progression of the disease, therefore DMARDs need to be started at early stage of disease.

DMARDs commonly used are:

1) Methotrexate,
2) Sulphasalazine,
3) Hydroxychloroquine,
4) Gold,
5) Azathioprine,
6) Cyclosporine,
7) D-penicillamine,
8) Leflunomide
9) Cyclophosphamide

In addition to these, some biological agent that are used are anti-TNF alpha antibody (adalimumab), Anti-Interleukin-1 (anakinra), B cell blocker (rituximab), blockade of CD 28 pathway & T-cells inactivator (Abatacept- prevents the activation of the T-lymphocytes and blocks the production of T-cells and the tissue destroying chemicals produced by them).

Rheumatologist's opinion needs to be taken before considering the use of these agents as these drugs may cause flare up of some diseases like tuberculosis and some of these may cause delayed cancer as well.

Whether single or combination, and when?

COBRA study has indicated that combination therapy with low dose steroid, methotrexate and sulphasalazine were better compared to sulphasalazine alone. The trial also suggested that, radiological progression starts very early in the disease process and therapeutic intervention should start within a narrow time frame of a window of opportunity.

The recent guidelines suggest that the treatment should be started within 3 months of diagnosis.

Methotrexate: It is the most commonly used drug and has been shown to prevent erosion of bone. The dose is weekly 7.5 mg which can be titrated up to 30 mg/wk. Thrice weekly supplementation with folic acid reduces its gastrointestinal related side effects.

> **Side Effects**
> i) Gastrointestinal disturbance including oral drugs.
> ii) Liver dysfunction.
> iii) Pneumonitis.
> iv) Bone marrow depression.

Therefore 6 weekly screening of liver function and full blood count are mandatory while using methotrexate.

Sulphasalazine: Sulphasalazine is an effective user friendly DMRD to be used in RA. However its efficacy is perhaps less than methotrexate. It can be effectively combined with methotrexate.

> **Side effects**
> i) Agranulocytosis
> ii) Hepatic dysfunction

Dose- 1-3 g/day [to start with 500 g daily]

Hydroxychloroquine: This drug reduces joint inflammation and retard the progression of the disease. It can be used in milder form of the disease and may be combined with other DMRDs.

> **Side effects**
> i) Skin rash
> ii) Retinal toxicity
> iii) Discoloration of skin

Dose- 200-400 mg/day.

Leflunomide: This drug has been found to be as effective as methotrexate and sulphasalazine in randomized trials. This drug can also be used in combination.

> **Side effects**
> i) Leucopenia, thrombocytopenia
> ii) Hepatic dysfunction

Dose- 100 mg daily for three days, then 10-20 mg daily.

Leflunomide can be used alone or in combination with methotrexate. In clinical studies, it was found to be more effective compared to methotrexate. The starting dose is 100 mg daily for 3 days followed by 20 mg daily to continue. When combined with methotrexate a dose of 10 mg may be used. It can cause leucopenia and liver dysfunction and regular Hb, TC, DC, Platelet and LFT monitoring will be mandatory. It is contraindicated in pregnancy. In the event of side effect, cholestyramine may be used to wash it out from the system. I have personally encountered one such patient with severe leucopenia and sepsis. Fortunately this patient responded well to IV antibiotics, granulocyte colony stimulating factor and cholestyramine wash out therapy.

The initial management should be with combination of conventional DMARDs, failing which methotrexate and leflunomide or methotrexate and cyclosporine may be combined. In recalcitrant cases, anti TNF antibody with or without methotrexate should be tried.

Methotrexate should be co-prescribed with folic acid to prevent gastro-intestinal side effect. Periodic liver function test should be done to detect any iatrogenic liver damage.

Parenteral gold and penicillamine have also been found to be useful drugs in retarding diseases progression. However due to side effect profile they are rarely used nowadays. Auranoffin (oral gold) is less effective compared to other DMARDs. More over although it improves inflammation it does not retard radiological disease progression. Minocycline has also some disease modifying activities compatible with that of the antimalarials.

Cyclosporine is effective in the treatment of RA. In view of its side effect profile, it is reserved for the non-responder to first line DMRDs only. On similar grounds azathioprine and cyclophosphamide although effective as DMRDs, are reserved for the patients not responding to the common DMRDs.

Combining DMRDs gives better result than using single drug therapy. However even the risk-benefit ratio of combination therapy should be properly assessed. Currently both 'step-up' or 'step-down' approach are taken depending upon the clinical situations.

Steroids in RA:

Two systemic reviews including 10 randomized controlled trials have shown beneficial effects of steroids both short-term and long-term (more than 3 months). In short-term use, symptomatic improvement is impressive while in long-term use there may be retardation of radiological disease progression. However long-term use is brought with significant side effects and should be selected carefully.

Steroids are commonly given (either pulsed steroid in the form of methyl prednisolone IV for 3 consecutive days or short course of oral steroids for few weeks. It gives quick symptomatic relief before the DMARDs start working which usually take 2-3 months to act.

Biological therapy: Anti cytokine therapy that is active against TNF alpha has been found to be useful drugs in the therapeutic armamentarium. These drugs can be used on their own or in patients already on methotrexate.

Drugs used:

i) Etanercept - 25 mg sc thrice/week.

ii) Infliximab - 3-5 mg/kg IV, repeated at 2 weeks and 8 weeks.

iii) Adalimumab - 40 mg SC alternate weeks.

iv) Anakinra - IL-1 blocker, 100 mg sc once/day.

These drugs are effective drugs in controlling symptoms and modifying disease progression. TNF-α blockers are more effective than IL-1 broker.

Side effects:

i) Flare up of latent tuberculosis.

ii) Formation of dsDNA antibody.

iii) Rarely development of demyelinating disease.

: KEY POINTS :

- Rheumatoid arthritis may be seronegative.
- Clinical diagnosis is important as DMARDs will alter the prognosis.
- Combination therapy is superior to individual therapy.
- Biological therapy is a new addition to the therapeutic armamentarium.

FURTHER REFERENCES:

- W.woh Ck *et al.*, Guidelines for the management of rheumatoid arthritis, 2002 update.
- Arthritis Rheumatic. 46: 328, 2002.
- Harrison's Principle of Internal Medicine- 17th edition.
- Oxford Handbook of Rheumatology.
- Oxford Textbook of Medicine – 5th edition.
- Evidence Based Rheumatology-2004.

PRIMARY PREVENTION OF IHD IN CLINICAL PRACTICE

CASE: *A 50 years old diabetic gentleman attended the clinic for a routine consultation. He was a smoker and hypertensive. He was very worried as his elder brother recently had a massive heart attack and underwent CABG. He was basically enquiring about primary prevention. His BP was 160/90 mmHg, LDL cholesterol- 176 mg%, Triglyceride- 230 mg%, HbA_1C- 7.4%. He did not have any cardio respiratory symptoms.*

DIAGNOSIS: Diabetic, HTN, smoker with a family history of cardiovascular disease.

DISCUSSION: This is a very common cause of consultation in primary care practice and a primary care physician should be able to give appropriate advice regarding the prevention of cardiovascular and cerebrovascular disease.

The drugs commonly used are antioxidants, aspirin, vitamins, anti-lipid preparation along with meticulous control of hypertension and diabetes mellitus. Life style modification also plays a very important role.

Antioxidants:

Of the antioxidants, vitamin E, beta carotene and vitamin C have undergone randomised clinical trials. The most promising data relate to the use of Vitamin E. Although attractive, these data are still inconclusive to warrant its widespread use as a primary preventive strategy.

Vitamins:

Elevated homocysteine level has been associated with increased incidence of cardiovascular events and cerebrovascular events. Experimental and epidemiologic data suggest that supplementation with folic acid, Vitamin B_6 and Vitamin B_{12} is a simple and cheap way of reduction of homocysteine level and this may lead to risk reduction of atherosclerotic disease. However, confirmation from the clinical trials would be needed before recommendation of routine vitamin supplementation. In patients with high homocysteine level, it is definitely an option, however. It appears prudent to ensure adequate dietary intake of folate, Vitamin B_6 and B_{12}.

Aspirin:

In randomised clinical trials, aspirin has been shown to reduce incidence of myocardial infarction and cerebral stroke with a slight increase in gastrointestinal and cerebral haemorrhage. Meta-analysis of 4 clinical trials where aspirin was used as a primary preventive agent also corroborated the same findings. **Therefore one needs to calculate the absolute risk of development of coronary events and if it is more than**

1.5% (calculated from the Framingham risk score) per year; it is perfectly justified to use aspirin in the dose of 75 mg/day. If the absolute risk is less than 1.5% per year, then side effect will nullify the beneficial effects of aspirin. In practical terms, patients with high BP (controlled with medicine) with target organ damage, diabetes mellitus and other risk factors for coronary events, aspirin can be used as a primary preventive measure.

ACE inhibitors:

In the HOPE study, use of ACE inhibitors, ramipril was associated with decreased cerebrovascular and cardiovascular morbidity and mortality in high risk patients. The patients included in the study had evidence of vascular disease or diabetes mellitus plus one cardiovascular risk factor but not overt heart failure or low ejection fraction. In the MICRO-HOPE sub study, diabetic patients were found to have significant vasoprotective and renoprotective effect from the use of ACE inhibitors.

Lipid lowering agents:

Aggressive lipid lowering has been shown to reduce cardiac events in primary prevention trials (WOSCOPS and AFCAPS / TEXCAPS). The value of aggressive lipid lowering as a secondary preventive strategy has been demonstrated well before these trials (4S study).

Based on these data, NCEP guideline for the use of drug therapy is LDL > 160 mg% for those with fewer than 2 risk factors. The target LDL is < 100 mg% in patient with MI, CVA, post CABG and other coronary interventions. In the presence of multiple risk factors with a history of MI, CVA and renal impairment even stringent LDL level of <70% is recommended. Drug therapy may also be indicated if triglyceride level is > 200 mg% in the presence of other cardiovascular risk factors. An American diabetic association consensus recommended meticulous control of diabetes mellitus along with use of lipid lowering agents to maintain the target level of triglyceride < 150 mg%.

Although isolated low HDL level is not the target of therapeutic intervention, it is frequently associated with high triglyceride and LDL levels. This variety of lipid abnormality (HDL, LDL, and triglyceride) is particularly common in Indian population in association with diabetes mellitus (due to insulin resistance). Judicious selection of drugs will enable to increase HDL level along with the reduction of LDL and triglyceride level. This should be borne in mind while treating patients with HDL of less than 35 mg% which is a risk factor for cardiac events.

To note that because of side effect profile, the use of nicotinic acid has been under question in the management of hyperlipidaemia.

Choice of drugs in hyperlipidaemia:

LDL:

- Statins and/or Cholestyramine
- Statin + Cholestyramine + nicotinic acid

Triglyceride:

- Fibrate / Nicotinic acid
- Fibrate and Nicotinic acid

LDL, HDL, Triglyceride:

- Statins: Atorvastatin reduces triglyceride more effectively than simvastatin.
- Nicotinic acid
- Fibrate
- Statin + nicotinic acid

LP (a):

- Fibrate + Nicotinic acid
- Nicotinic acid

HDL:

- Regular exercise
- Nicotinic acid– if associated with high triglyceride level.

Ezetimibe is a new agent that inhibits the intestinal absorption of cholesterol from dietary and biliary sources by impeding the transport of cholesterol across the intestinal wall. Combination of ezetimibe with statin may offer theoretical advantage of incremental lipid lowering from complementary mechanism of action. (Particularly because of frequent non-availability of cholestyramine in Indian market).

Control of hypertension and diabetes mellitus:

These are very important primary preventive strategies and have been discussed elsewhere.

Life style modification:

- Smoking cessation
- Regular exercise
- Weight reduction
- Healthy diet rich in fibre, fruits, vegetables and fish.
- Avoid oily, fried food and reduce the quantity of animal fat intake.

Based on the aforementioned evidence, this patient was judged to be a high risk patient for atherosclerotic disease and he was commenced on aspirin, ACE inhibitor and statin. He was advised to stop smoking, do regular exercise and reduce weight. He was also commenced on oral hypoglycaemic drugs. Unfortunately he was not under any insurance cover or reimbursement scheme and was finding it difficult to cope with the expenses. He was advised to stress on life style modification as much as possible to reduce the necessity of pharmacological intervention. This is a real problem in our country and it is sometimes very difficult to match between what we preach and what we practice. An individualised pragmatic approach is always needed to bridge the gap between the two.

Role of Hormone replacement therapy (HRT):

Although previously HRT was considered to be protective for heart disease, the long term results from HERS and WHI Studies indicate either oestrogen alone or oestrogen + progesterone does not create any special benefit regarding protection of cardiovascular events. On the contrary, there were small but significant hazard of cardiovascular events, stroke and breast cancer on long-term use. Therefore in clinical practice the beneficial role of HRT with regards to post menopausal symptoms and prevention of osteoporosis has to be judged with its long term problem in the light of the patient's clinical condition with the help of input from the gynaecologist.

Markers of coronary risk:

In addition to LDL, LP (A), homocysteine, highly active CRP, high calcium score in CT, Coronary angiogram may be helpful predictors for future coronary events. In addition progress in human genetics hold considerable promise for the risk prediction and individualization of cardiovascular therapy.

Drug interaction:

The chances of having rhabdomyolysis with statins increases with concomitant use of drugs those interfere with its metabolism.

- Erythromycin
- Antifungal
- Immunosuppressive
- Fibrate
- Grape fruits inhibit the metabolism of statins (as it is Cytochrome P450 enzyme inhibitor).
- Co-enzyme Q10 can be given to the patients with statin induced myalgia.

Careful clinical follow up with frequent checking of CPK and LFT should be done.

Side effects of antidyslipidaemic drugs:

Statins	↓↓ LDL ↓ Triglyceride ↑ HDL	Myalgia, arthralgia, elevated liver enzymes, dyspepsia.
Ezetimibe	↓↓ LDL ↑ Triglyceride	Elevated transaminase
Fibrates	↓↓ Triglyceride ↓ LDL ↑ HDL	Dyspepsia, gall stone, myalgia, elevated liver enzymes
Nicotinic acid	↑ HDL ↓ Triglyceride ↓ LDL	Flushing, elevated glucose, varicocele and liver enzymes
Bile acid & sequestrants	↓↓ LDL ↑ Triglyceride	Bloating, constipation, elevated triglyceride
Omega-3 fatty acids (used by some clinicians)	↓ Triglyceride ↑ Bleeding time	Fishy odour

CASE: *A 38 years old male smoker presented to the outpatients clinic with a weight of 96 kg along with a paunch. His BP was 160/94 mmHg, LDL- 164 mg, Triglyceride- 384 mg, HDL- 24 mg, fasting glucose- 115 mg, creatinine- 1.2 mg, TSH- 3.4, uric acid- 7.1 mg, ECG- LVH, ultrasonography showed fatty liver, AST- 67, ALT- 58. He was complaining of joint pain and breathlessness. Family members were warned about short and long term health issues and wanted a medical opinion regarding his present medical issues.*

DIAGNOSIS: Metabolic syndrome with high probability of development of future cardiovascular events and diabetes mellitus.

DISCUSSION:

Metabolic syndrome (syndrome X, insulin resistance syndrome) is a constellation of clinical and biochemical features associated with truncal obesity and is considered as one of the risk factors for development of future cardiovascular events.

Criteria: NCEP ATP III -2001

3 or more of the above
1. Central obesity- waist circumference > 102 cm (M), > 88 cm (F)
2. Hypertriglyceridaemia > 150 mg
3. Low HDL- < 40 mg% (M), < 50 mg% (F)
4. Hypertension
5. Fasting Glucose > 100 mg%

Other associated conditions with metabolic syndrome:

- Non-alcoholic fatty liver disease
- Hyperuricaemia
- Polycystic ovary disease
- Obstructive sleep apnoea

Since metabolic syndrome poses increased risk for cardiovascular events and development of overt diabetes mellitus, vigorous treatment is needed for the risk reduction.

The basic mechanism is increased insulin resistance through truncal obesity. Vigorous exercise should be made to reduce weight through life style modification.

Dyslipidaemia should be treated accordingly. Severely high triglyceride is more commonly prevalent, fibrates may be needed more frequently, statin and nicotinic acid may also be used depending on the LDL and HDL. Blood pressure should be controlled.

Ideally diabetes mellitus should be treated with insulin sensitizer like metformin and thiazolinediones as insulin resistance is at the core of the mechanism for development of metabolic syndrome.

: KEY POINTS :

- Primary prevention forms an integral part of primary care consultation.
- Risk benefit ratio should be assessed before prescribing medication for primary prevention.
- Economic obstacle is a major hindrance in practising evidence based medicine.

FURTHER REFERENCES: Harrison principal of internal medicine – 17th edition.
Oxford text Book of Medicine – 5th edition.

43 A PATIENT WITH HYPONATRAEMIA

CASE: *A 64 years old lady with asthma was admitted with increasing breathlessness. The reason of her admission was increasing drowsiness and confusional state. Examination did not reveal any focal neurological signs. There was no oedema. Na^+ level was 108 mmol/l, K^+- 2.4 mmol/l, urea- 21 mg%, creatinine- 0.8 mg%, Hb- 10.1 g%, PCV- 32, urinary spot Na^+- 41 mmol/l, urinary osmolality- 689 mosmol/kg, plasma osmolality- 230 mosmol/kg. CT brain scan was normal.*

DIAGNOSIS: Hyponatraemic encephalopathy due to SIADH (syndrome of inappropriate antidiuretic hormone) precipitated by chest infection.

DISCUSSION:

Metabolic encephalopathy is a common presentation in clinical practice. Its early recognition is important as inappropriate treatment can lead to increased morbidity and mortality.

Approach to a patient with hyponatraemia:

Hyponatraemia may be due to a measurement artefact due to excess lipids or presence of IgM paraprotein (rarely seen in clinical practice).

Hyperosmolar hyponatraemia:

This is mainly due to severe hyperglycaemia, mannitol infusion and surgical irrigation fluids (post TURP).

Hypoosmolar hyponatraemia (commonly encountered in hospitalised patients):

This may be associated with –

➢ **Hypovolaemia**

- Due to renal loss : Diuretics, cerebral salt wasting syndrome,
  (Urinary Na-high, urinary osmolality-normal)
- Gastrointestinal loss (vomiting)
  (Urinary Na-low, urinary osmolality- high)

➢ **Euvolaemia**

- SIADH: Common in acute care

Causes: Chest infection, CVA, Meningeal infections, Drugs
(Urinary Na concentration-high, urinary osmolality- high)

- Psychogenic polydipsia: (low in psychogenic polydipsia)

➢ **Hypervolaemia-** commonly associated with oedema.

- CCF,

(Urinary Na- low, urinary osmolality- high)

- Liver failure

(In liver failure- urea level will be proportionately low)

- Nephrotic syndrome

(Urate and urea levels will be high – as opposed to SIADH, where they will be low. In liver failure urea level will be proportionately low.)

CLINICAL FEATURES:

Mild hyponatraemia (upto 120 mmol/litre) is asymptomatic. Na^+ level is of less than 120 mmol/litre may cause drowsiness, confusion, convulsion or coma particularly if Na level falls below 110 mmol/litre. Focal neurological sign is not a feature of low Na and its presence should prompt clinician to look for any underlying CNS cause.

DIAGNOSIS: [investigations]

- Electrolytes
- Urea/creatinine
- FBC + PCV
- Plasma osmolality and urinary osmolality
- Urinary spot Na^+

In SIADH:

↓Na, ↓K, ↓Urea, ↓Creatinine, Urinary spot Na (> 20 mmol/litre),

↓Plasma osmolality, ↑Urinary osmolality

Drugs causing SIADH:

- Anti depressants- Tricyclics, SSRI
- Dopamine antagonists-Metoclopramide, Prochlorperazine, Antipsychotics
- Anti-convulsants- Carbamazepine, Phenytoin, Valproate
- Opiates

CAUSES:

- **Pseudohyponatraemia**
  - Hyperglycaemia
  - Mannitol infusion
- **Sodium depletion**
  - **Renal:**
    - Renal loss
    - Diuretics
    - Salt wasting
    - Hypoadrenalism
    - Central Salt wasting
  - **Extra renal:**
    - Gut loss
- **Excess water Intake/ Influx**
  - Inappropriate intravenous fluid
  - Sodium free hypoosmolar irrigation solution
- **Reduced renal free water clearance**
  - **Hypervolaemia:**
    - Drugs
    - Renal failure
    - Hypoalbuminaemia
    - Sepsis with vascular leak
    - Portal hypertension with ascites
  - **Other causes:**
    - Cardiac failure
    - Nephrotic syndrome
    - Hypokalaemia
    - Hypopituitarism
    - SIADH

Exercise induced hyponatraemia

Vigorous exercise can cause ADH release. It may be further compounded if fluid resuscitation is done by intake of free water.

Nephrogenic SIADH is a recently described condition characterised by continuous activation of AVP receptor (V_2R) [as opposed of loss of function as in nephrogenous diabetes insipidus] leading to anti-diuresis with persistent hyponatraemia.

Management of symptomatic hypoosmotic hyponatraemia:

It is very important to know the volume status of the patient as the treatment will differ in different groups.

In hypovolemic patients (like patients with vomiting), normal saline infusion will be needed. In patients with hypovolemic hyponatraemia with oedematous state, fluid restriction along with treatment of the underlying cause will correct it.

Vasopressin receptor blockers are new group of drugs for the treatment of hypovolemic hyponatraemia.

In euvolemic patients (commonly SIADH), fluid restriction is the treatment of choice (1.2 litre/24hr).

Demeclocycline, by causing nephrogenic diabetes insipidus, can theoretically be used but it is not helpful in acute situation because of its slow onset of action.

Severe symptomatic hyponatraemia is a medical emergency as it can cause death. Hypertonic saline (3%) should be used slowly and cautiously along with injection of frusemide (to increase free water clearance). The rate of correction should be less than 12 mmol/litre as more rapid correction may lead to central pontine myelinolysis, a demyelinating disorder of brain stem with high morbidity and mortality. The typical history is that the patient's condition improves for the first few days following hypertonic saline infusion but starts deteriorating later on with features of cerebellar signs, pseudo bulbar palsy and Parkinsonism. MRI scan shows characteristic changes. Therefore routine round-the-clock hypertonic saline infusion must not be given in patients with hyponatraemia.

There are different calculations available for Na^+ replacement. In clinical practice, the requirement is established by checking Na^+ level twice daily following infusion of 100 ml of 3% saline.

Over correction of hyponatraemia must be avoided. The correction should stop as soon as serum Na^+ reaches 125 mmol/litre.

Management with persistent hyponatraemia:

- Fluid restriction-in SIADH
- Demeclocycline- 600 mg – 1.2 g/day
- Lithium
- Vasopressin receptor antagonist

Vasopressin receptor antagonists (Vaptans) work on V_2R receptors [there are 3 subtypes of vasopressin receptors– V_1a, V_1b and V_2]. The vaptans are classified as selective working on V_2R receptors and non-selective (V_2R and V_1a receptors). Both increase renal water clearance without any significant impact on renal electrolyte loss. Both are effective in the treatment of hyponatraemia with normal and increased plasma volume.

We have recently performed a study on the use of tolvaptan in the dose of 15 mg daily in patient put under our care with hyponatraemia due to SIADH, in addition to standard treatment for SIADH. It was found that the target Na^+ of 130 mmol/litre was achieved quicker (48 hrs earlier on average) compared to standard therapy.

Our experience of low Na^+ in ITU:

- Most cases are due to SIADH- due to chest infection, CVA, meningitis.
- Vomiting due to different causes.
- Post operative patients (mainly elderly orthopaedic patients with fracture neck of femur receiving prolonged dextrose infusion), post TURP.

One must remember that in CVA, hyponatraemia may also be caused by a condition known as cerebral salt wasting syndrome (due to liberation of brain natriuretic peptide) rather than dilutional due to SIADH and one should always check the volume status before restricting fluid as it may have detrimental effect in hypovolemic patients with cerebral salt wasting syndrome. These patients may need saline infusion instead of fluid restriction.

CASE: *A 52 years old gentleman was admitted with 4 days history of vomiting. The reason for his admission was increasing drowsiness and one episode of convulsion. His Na^+ was 105 mmol/litre. Liver function was slightly deranged. Urinary Na^+ was 26 mmol/lit, urinary osmolality high, PCV within normal range. CT brain scan was normal. In view of severe symptomatic hyponatraemia, he was very cautiously treated with 3% saline with a target rate of correction of less than 12 mmol per 24 hours. Within 48 hours he improved* *with a Na^+ level of 121 mmol/l. Unfortunately, the improvement was short-lived. On the 4th day his consciousness level deteriorated. His Na^+ level was hovering between 121-126 mmol/l. No other cause could be detected to explain the deterioration. MRI scan of brain was done later on showed evidence of demyelinating lesions in the brain stem. He had a prolonged stay in the hospital developed features of pseudobulbar palsy and remained nursing dependent on discharge.*

This patient possibly had hyponatraemic encephalopathy which was corrected slowly with appropriate precaution. His late deterioration was probably due to central pontine myelinolysis (CPM). The message is that although CPM is rare, the threat is real and it can occur even following restriction of fluid only. With this background knowledge, one should attempt to correct hyponatraemia in his clinical practice.

CASE: *A 21 years old student was brought by his patients because of abdominal swelling. Examination revealed a distended urinary bladder. USG of abdomen showed hugely distended bladder, bilateral hydroureter and hydronephrosis. He underwent detailed urological check up under an urologist and no obvious cause for obstruction was found (IVU, micturating cystourethrogram and cystoscopy). His Na^+ level was persistently in the range of 124-128 mmol/l. Urinary osmolality was low; plasma osmolality low normal, urinary spot Na^+ was non-diagnostic. On careful enquiry he disclosed history of polyuria. He was admitted for water deprivation test.*

[Principles of water deprivation test: 8 hours dehydration with hourly plasma and urinary osmolality measurement. After 8 hours, injection vasopressin given IM followed by hourly measurement of plasma and urinary osmolality continued.

Result: Normal persons will maintain plasma osmolality while concentrating urine > 800 mosmol/kg during dehydration unenhanced by vasopressin. In central diabetes insipidus, urine will fail to concentrate with dehydration while plasma osmolality rises, this will be corrected by vasopressin with a urinary osmolality > 800 mosmol/kg.

[Those with nephrogenic diabetes insipidus behave as central DI initially but do not concentrate urine after vasopressin while those with psychogenic polydipsia generally respond normally.]

On the fourth hour of water deprivation, he became very restless and violent and desperately started craving for water to drink. An abbreviated water deprivation test showed a normal response. However, the diagnosis was quite obvious by then. He admitted drinking huge amount of water surreptitiously for last 3 years which he did not disclose to anyone in the past. A diagnosis of compulsive water drinking with dilutional hyponatraemia with functional hydronephrosis and hydroureter was made. He was referred to a psychiatrist for further management.

DIAGNOSIS: Compulsive water drinking with hyponatraemia.

: KEY POINTS :

- Hyponatraemia is common in hospitalized patients.
- SIADH is frequently caused by chest infection, CVA and meningitis.
- Treatment of hypoosmolar hyponatraemia depends on the volume status of the patient.
- Severe hyponatraemia can cause death.
- Correction of symptomatic hyponatraemia should be cautious as it can cause CPM.

FURTHER REFERENCES:

- Ad rogue H.L. *et al.* (2000) – Hyponatraemia – NEJM 342:1581.
- Harrison's Principle of Internal Medicine, 17th Ed.
- Medicine International.
- S.G. Ball – Hyponatraemia - J.R. Coll physic Edin 2010 Vol-40, issue 3 – 240-245.
- Oxford Textbook of Medicine – 5th edition.

44 A PATIENT WITH ACUTE OLIGURIA

CASE: *A 56 years old lady was transferred from another medical facility with a history of decreased urine output over last 24 hours. She underwent abdominal hysterectomy 3 days back. On the 2nd post operative day, she had a bout of fever with chill. She was on IV fluids, IV aminoglycoside and cephalosporin, intramuscular diclofenac as analgesic. She was a known hypertensive with normal preoperative renal function. Her BP was 120/80 mmHg, pulse rate 120/min, clear chest, no oedema, Hb- 8.9 g%, WBC- 21000 with poly 90%, urea- 131 mg%, creatinine- 3.6 mg%, K^+- 5.2, Na^+- 128, coagulation profile-normal, urinary spot Na^+- 40 mmol/l, urine for routine examination- no active sediment, occasional brown-muddy pigmented granular cast. Urgent USG of abdomen revealed slightly enlarged kidneys with no obstructive change.*

DIAGNOSIS: Acute postoperative renal failure of unknown cause.

DIAGNOSIS:

Acute oliguria is a common problem in hospital practice. It is also commonly encountered in community practice as well. It is a medical emergency with attendant high morbidity and mortality. On many occasions it is potentially preventable.

It is very important to be aware of the basic principles in the diagnosis and initial management of the condition.

The main causes are divided into: Pre-renal, Renal, Post-renal.

1. **Pre renal** – volume depletion due to any cause.

2. **Renal** – acute tubular necrosis or due to intrinsic renal disease. The list is long. Common causes are-

    - Hypotension – Ischemic insult
    - Nephrotoxic drugs
    - Renal parenchymal disease – vasculitis, glomerulonephritis, interstitial nephritis
    - Renal vein thrombosis
    - Hepatorenal syndrome
    - Myeloma, uric acid nephropathy, acute pyelonephritis, atheroembolism, malignant hypertension, rhabdomyolysis

3. **Post renal** – Bladder outlet obstruction

RIFLE CRITERIA- It is a criterion to assess renal function in critical care settings.

In acute oliguria, clinical examination is very important as retention of urine is a very common cause which can be easily treated with catheterization. Similarly in a hospitalized patient with restlessness and oliguria, blocked urinary catheter should be excluded first before embarking on further tests of ARF.

Secondly, one needs to exclude between ARF and CRF. History is important. In ARF, kidney size is usually normal or enlarged whereas in CRF they are usually small and contracted (except in diabetic nephropathy and amyloidosis). Severe anaemia is common in CRF. Evidence of bone disease (renal osteodystrophy) in X-rays goes in favour of CRF. It is well known that CKD predisposes to AKI; vice-versa is also true.

Once ARF is confirmed, urgent USG of abdomen is needed to exclude obstructive causes particularly in post operative renal failure. It may disclose hydronephrosis, hydroureter or distended bladder due to prostate enlargement.

Differentiation between pre-renal and renal cause is equally important, as early pre-renal oliguria can be successfully treated with fluid challenge.

Characteristic urinary indices in pre-renal and renal oliguria:

Parameters	Pre-renal	Renal
Urinary Na^+ (mmol/l.)	< 20	> 40
Fractional excretion of Na^+%	< 1	> 1
Ratio of urinary to plasma urea	> 40	< 20
Ratio to urinary to plasma creatinine	> 1.5	< 1.1

In pre-renal oliguria, due to intact tubular function, there is increased absorption of Na and water by the tubules leading to low urinary Na and increased urinary osmolality. However, these tests may be misleading in patients with diuretic or dopamine infusion.

INVESTIGATIONS:

Urine microscopy:

- Presence of active urinary sediments – glomerulonephritis, vasculitis.
- Presence of eosinophils – acute interstitial nephritis.
- Absence of RBC but blood test positive in patients with trauma – rhabdomyolysis.

Examination of blood:

- Eosinophilia – acute interstitial nephritis.
- High CPK – Rhabdomyolysis
- ANCA – Vasculitis
- Anti-glomerular basement membrane antibody – Goodpasture syndrome
- High urate – Uric acid nephropathy (particularly after chemotherapy for leukaemia or myeloma
- ANF – SLE
- LDH – renal infarction
- Cryoglobulin – cryoglobulinaemia
- Ig electrophoresis – myeloma
- Microangiopathic – HUS (Haemolytic Uremic Syndrome) picture in blood film.

Classification of Acute Kidney Injury (AKI) and Chronic Kidney Disease (CKD):

State of AKI	Serum creatinine	Urea output
1.	1.5-1.9 × baseline or ≥ 0.3 mg/dl above baseline	< 0.5 ml/kg/Hr for 6-8 hrs
2.	2.0-2.9 × baseline	< 0.5 ml/kg/Hr for more than 12 hrs
3.	≥ 3.0 × baseline, ≥ 4.0 mg/dl or initiation of renal replacement therapy	< 0.3 ml/Kg/Hr for≥ 24 hrs or anuria for ≥ 24 hrs

CKD	Definition	GFR (ml/min/ 1.73 m^2)
1	Kidney damage with normal GFR	≥ 90
2	Kidney damage with mild decrease in GFR	60 - 89
3A	Mild to moderate decrease in GFR	45 - 59
3B	Moderate to severe decrease in GFR	30 - 44
4	Severe decrease in GFR	15 - 29
5	End stage renal disease	< 15

Relationship between AKI, CKD and Cardiovascular disease:

Since AKI may lead to CKD in the long term irrespective of the cause of AKI, the survivors of AKI should be followed up closely with regular urinary albumin- creatinine ratio testing, using renoprotective drugs like ACE inhibitors, low sodium diet. This is important for the prevention of cardiovascular morbidity that is associated with CKD as well. Cautious use of diuretics, nephrotoxic contrast agents, NSAIDS and early use of markers to detect kidney injury, is the way forward as a preuretric measure.

MANAGEMENT:

- Once the diagnosis of ARF is established and obstructive causes excluded. Volume status of the patient should be determined by using CVP monitoring. Early aggressive fluid resuscitation in pre-renal failure will help open up the kidneys with restoration of urinary output. Strict intake and output measurement must be done otherwise it can cause fluid overload.

- Following fluid challenge, continuous use of IV frusemide may be tried [100 – 200 mg IV infusion or 10 – 40 mg infusion per hour]. This should be abandoned if there is no result within 4-6 hours. Frusemide must not be given in a volume depleted patient. Frusemide frequently converts oliguric failure to non-oliguric failure. However the benefit of this conversion is still hotly debated.

- **Use of renal dose dopamine:** Renal dose dopamine frequently increases urinary output without improving the prognosis. It has no reno-protective effect except for using as an inotropic agent, its use as a diuretic agent in ARF is debatable and has declined in the western countries although commonly used in India.

- **Choosing the right fluid for resuscitation:** Theoretically colloids are preferable as they remain in the vascular space and improve peripheral circulation. While this may be true for simple hypervolaemia like diarrhoea, in septic patients because of the leaky capillaries they may escape in the tissues and cause accumulation of fluid in tissue spaces including the lung interstitial tissue with adverse consequences. Therefore in sepsis, crystalloids are preferable. Use of albumin as a resuscitation fluid is also controversial since the Cochrane meta-analysis of the use of human albumin in patients with hypovolaemia, hypoalbuminaemia and burn showed 6% increase in mortality compared to the use of crystalloids. One trial showed improved outcome with 20% albumin in patients with cirrhosis, ascites and bacterial peritonitis. In general, crystalloids should be preferred and in selected cases colloids may be used with caution.

In spite of all these measures, if oliguria persists, one should contemplate renal replacement therapy. At this stage, involvement of nephrologists is essential.

Types of renal replacement:

- Continuous haemodiafiltration
- Intermittent haemodialysis
- Peritoneal dialysis

Intermittent haemodialysis causes fluctuation of BP and can increase the tubular damage further. So in haemodynamically unstable patients, continuous haemodiafiltration is the treatment of choice. Peritoneal dialysis can also be used but it may be difficult in patients with abdominal operation and ascites. Moreover fluid removal is sometimes unpredictable. Nevertheless in Indian setting it is frequcntly used because of non-availability of other facilities.

Haemodialysis, using biocompatible membrane is associated with better outcome as cellulose membrane can activate complement with untoward effect on the patient. In patients with sepsis and severe lactic acidosis additional benefit may be gained by using HCO3 buffered replacement solution rather than lactate based solution.

Appropriate choice of RRT is important in the management which should be decided by the nephrologists.

General management:

- Prevention of infection
- Use of appropriate antibiotics
- Stress ulcer prophylaxis
- Maintenance of nutrition

In patients with renal replacement therapy, proper nutrition is essential as protein catabolism is substantial. While main calorie requirement should be derived from carbohydrate and fat, moderate amount of protein supplementation can be safely provided in patients on dialysis. The patient described above had ARF due to multiple factors including sepsis. Early cautious fluid challenge along with frusemide infusion did not help. She needed intermittent haemodialysis in the ITU and started dialysis 10 days following admission. She received adjusted dose of meropenem along with other supportive measures. NSAID and amikacin were withdrawn. She also needed 6 units of blood transfusion. 2 months following discharge her renal function was normal.

In her case possibly, renal failure was due to multiple factors like dehydration, sepsis, use of NSAID and aminoglycoside. One needs to be careful while using NSAID, aminoglycosides, ACE inhibitors, glycopeptides in post-operative dehydrated patients which may lead to acute renal shut down.

: KEY POINTS :

- Aggressive fluid resuscitation will prevent acute tubular necrosis in patients with pre-renal failure.
- Obstructive cause should be excluded in patients with acute oliguria by clinical examination followed by USG examination.
- Renal dose dopamine is now out of fashion in treating acute oliguria due to intrinsic cause.
- In post operative patients certain drugs should be used with caution.
- Blood tests and urine examination will give important clues to the cause of ARF.
- AKI may progress to CDK or may cause CKD later on, so close follow up is needed.

FURTHER REFERENCES:

- Khahr. S *et al.* (1998), acute oliguria, NEJM Vol. 338, 671-676.
- Huges H.D. (1997) – Editorial, Acute renal failure – The promise of new therapy, NEJM – 336, 870-871.
- Harrison's Principle of Internal Medicine – 17th edition.
- Kumar and Clark, Clinical Medicine – 5th edition.
- S. Chawla *et al.*, Acute kidney injury and chronic kidney decease as interconnected syndrome, NEJM – July 3 2014: 371: 58 – 66.

45

ADVERSE DRUG EFFECTS IN CLINICAL PRACTICE

CASE: *A known patient with rheumatoid arthritis was admitted with disease flare up for methyl prednisolone pulses. Her X-Ray chest showed old calcified lesion in both upper lobes. Following 3 days course of methyl prednisolone, her symptoms improved dramatically. On the 6th day, just before discharge, she developed a cough with high rise of temperature. The discharge was deferred and an antibiotic was prescribed. Unfortunately her fever persisted with increasing cough. On the 7th day she was toxic and a repeat X-Ray showed bilateral shadowing in both upper lobes consistent with tuberculosis. On enquiry, she gave a history of TB 20 years back.*

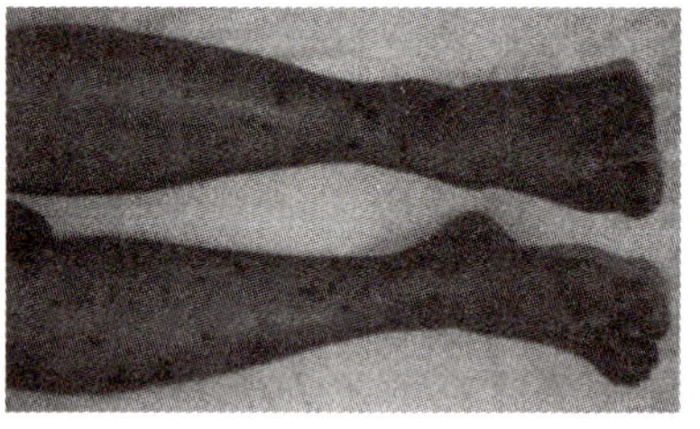

DIAGNOSIS: Reactivation of TB following high dose of steroid.

DISCUSSIONS:

Tuberculosis is a common problem in India which may lie dormant without any overt manifestation. While using high dose steroids or planning for long term steroids, careful enquiry must be made about this disease. X-Ray chest and a mantoux test (for long term steroid use) should be done before commencement of steroid. Appropriate precautionary measures like use of chemoprophylaxis with (isoniazid) INH should be done in suspicious cases. Infliximab (used in rheumatoid arthritis and IBD) is the other drug that can also cause similar effect.

This patient was treated with 4 drugs anti TB regime and responded successfully.

CASE: *A 48 years old Type II diabetic lady was seen with leg oedema. Her kidney function was normal, TSH normal, LFT normal, urine for albumin– trace, Echo normal. Increasing dose of frusemide and spironolactone did not help. She was on losartan, gliclazide and pioglitazone. The oedema subsided following discontinuation of pioglitazone.*

DIAGNOSIS: Drug induced oedema of legs.

DISCUSSIONS:

Pedal oedema is a common problem in clinical practice and the lay persons always associate with some sinister pathology in the kidneys. Before embarking on any specific tests, one should take a thorough drug history. Although the list of drugs causing oedema is long, in my experience, three common drugs associated with oedema are:

- Calcium channel blockers
- Glitazones [thiazolidinediones]
- Steroids

Thorough history taking may obliviate the necessity of detailed investigations.

CASE: *A 54 years old gentleman with a history of dilated cardiomyopathy on treatment attended the clinic with bilateral chest pain. Examination revealed painful gynaecomastia. Before requesting for hormonal assay, a drug history revealed intake of spironolactone.*

The drug was stopped and after one month, his symptoms disappeared and no further sophisticated investigations were asked for.

DIAGNOSIS: Drug induced gynaecomastia.

Common drugs causing gynaecomastia:

- Spironolactone
- Oestrogen therapy for prostatic cancer
- Testosterone blockers for prostatic cancer
- Digitalis
- Isoniazid

CASE: *A 51 years old gentleman presented with aches and pain all over the body. He had history of MI 6 months back. Rheumatological investigations were normal. CPK was high, BP normal, ESR and CRP normal. Drug history revealed intake of atorvastatin. The pain disappeared within 10 days of discontinuation of atorvastatin.*

DIAGNOSIS: Drug induced myalgia.

DISCUSSIONS:

Statins can cause myalgia and occasionally myositis with elevation of CPK. Combination with fibrates increases the chance of myositis. Reduction of dose may sometimes help in reduction of symptoms. At times the drug needs to be replaced by other lipid lowering agents.

Other drugs causing muscle pain:

- Steroids
- Interferon – for the treatment of hepatitis (it usually causes flu likes symptoms)
- Zidovudine
- Diuretics – can precipitate acute gout. While treating symptomatic hyperuricaemia, one needs to avoid diuretic based antihypertensive regime.

CASE: *A 40 years old lady attended the clinic with history of recurrent headache. She was on migraine prophylaxis for last 2 years with flunarizine and β-blocker. CT brain scan was normal. On careful enquiry, it was found that she was taking ergotamine on regular basis (she was advised to take it on as and when basis only). Following discontinuation of regular ergotamine, her daily headache subsided. She was advised to take sumatriptan during acute attack of migraine.*

DIAGNOSIS: Medication overuses head-ache (MOH) due to ergotamine.

One should remember even regular use of triptans can cause similar problems.

Common drugs causing headache:

- Nitrates
- Nicorandil
- MOH due to ergotamine and triptans
- Dipyridamole
- Any vasodilator

CASE: *A 50 years old gentleman attended the clinic with history of cough, sneezing, nose block and frequent itching. He recently underwent CABG 6 months back. On examination NAD. Anti-allergies gave partial relief. He was on ACE inhibitor which has replaced by losartan. The symptoms remained unabated. Finally aspirin was replaced by clopidogrel with eventual relief of his symptoms. On enquiry, he gave history of allergic disorders in his childhood.*

DIAGNOSIS: Aspirin sensitivity in an atopic person.

DISCUSSIONS:

Aspirin hypersensitivity is quite common (upto 30%) in atopic persons. It can manifest as different kind of allergic reaction. The clinician needs to be aware of this as aspirin is a very commonly prescribed drug for primary and secondary prevention of cardiovascular disease.

In my experience ACE induced cough is much more common than described in the western literature, this needs to be explained to the patients before prescribing it.

β blocker both oral and eye drop used in glaucoma can precipitate bronchospasm in a stable asthmatic. The only manifestation may be cough. Change of medication will solve the problem.

CASE: *A 36 years old gentleman was admitted with 10 days history of fever treated with ciprofloxacin. The reason of his admission was increasing confusional state. During hospital admission, he was apyrexic but very much confused. The provisional diagnosis was viral or metabolic encephalopathy. Clinical examination was entirely normal. CT scan of brain and lumbar puncture were normal. His symptoms improved quickly with withdrawal of ciprofloxacin.*

DIAGNOSIS: Drug induced confusional state due to ciprofloxacin.

The list of drugs causing confusion is long. We have come across five cases of ciprofloxacin induced neurotoxicity in last 10 years. Recently cefepime a very effective 4th generation cephalosporin in hospital practice, has also been shown to cause reversible neurotoxicity. Artemisinin group of anti malarial can also cause reversible neurotoxicity (2 cases in our experience).

Other common drugs causing confusional state:

- Sedatives in elderly
- Antiparkinsonian drugs
- Anticholinergic
- Steroids

Proper drug history is very important in dealing with patients with confusional state.

CASE: *A 42 years old hospital staff complained of repeated attacks of hyper pigmented lesions mainly in his body following episodes of cough and cold. On enquiry it was found that his GP used to prescribe him septran (trimethoprim and sulfamethoxazole). The lesions use to occur in the same area of his body.*

DIAGNOSIS: Fixed drug eruption due to trimethoprim, sulfamethoxazole.

He was advised to avoid septran and since then he did not have any recurrence.

Causes of fixed drug eruption:

- Sulphonamides
- Tetracycline
- NSAIDS
- Phenolphthalein

CASE: *A 51 years old lady presented with history of itchy skin rash over last 4 weeks. Examination revealed purpuric rash over the lower extremities. Anti-allergic medication was not helpful. She was receiving treatment for hypertension and hyperuricaemia with amlodipine and allopurinol respectively.*

DIAGNOSIS: Allopurinol induced vasculitic skin rash.

Itchy skin rash is a very common manifestation of drug reaction. Examples are:

- **Urticarial rash** – Penicillin, ACE inhibitors, aspirin
- **Vasculitic rash** – Carbamazepine, phenytoin, allopurinol (usually presents with fever, skin rash, arthralgia, eosinophilia, lymphadenopathy and hepatitis).

CASE: *An 11 years old boy with recently diagnosed epilepsy on phenytoin was admitted with fever, lymphadenopathy, purpuric skin rash and arthralgia. He was diagnosed to have viral fever. He had eosinophilia and later on developed features of hepatitis. Phenytoin was withdrawn and steroid was commenced. His epilepsy was controlled with IV midazolam. After his symptoms were controlled he was cautiously changed to carbamazepine to which he did not develop any untoward effect.*

CASE: *A patient diagnosed to have polymyalgia rheumatica controlled on 10mg of prednisolone developed pulmonary tuberculosis possibly because of reactivation. She was started on standard 4 drugs regimen. From the 3rd week onwards, although her fever subsided the aches and pains of the original disease started to increase. Initially, it was thought to be due to hyperuricaemia caused by pyrazinamide. Her uric acid level was normal. Eventually her symptoms were controlled by doubling the dose of prednisolone which was again brought back to normal following completion of rifampicin therapy.*

DIAGNOSIS: Pharmacokinetic interaction between rifampicin (liver enzyme inducer) and steroid, increasing the metabolism of steroid.

Rifampicin is a strong enzyme inducer and can increase the metabolism of certain drugs with adverse clinical effect. This has to be borne in mind by the physician while co-prescribing rifampicin with other drugs (barbiturates, carbamazepine are the other enzyme inducers).

Common interaction in clinical practice:

- Rifampicin - Steroid
- Rifampicin - oral contraceptive
- Rifampicin - anti retroviral drugs

The dose of the medication may need to be increased in order to maintain their efficacy otherwise flare up of the primary disease or failure of contraception may result.

Significant drug interaction due to enzyme inhibitors

- Cyclosporine toxicity may be precipitated due to enzyme inhibition by ketoconazole, diltiazem and erythromycin.
- Lovastatin may cause myopathy due to enzyme inhibition by erythromycin, cyclosporine.
- Cisapride may cause ventricular tachycardia – due to enzyme inhibition by ketoconazole, erythromycin.

Other clinically significant pharmacokinetic interaction in clinical practice

Amiodarone - increases digoxin level and may precipitate toxicity
Amiodarone - increases anticoagulation affect of warfarin
NSAID - Potentiates the action of warfarin
Quinidine - Potentiates the action of digoxin
Verapamil - Potentiates the action of digoxin

The list of drug interaction is long and any standard text book of pharmacology may be consulted in this regard.

Adverse drug reaction leading to skin rash is a common problem in critical care setting where the patients are on multiple drug therapy and it is sometimes very difficult to find out the endpoint drug causing cutaneous reaction. It is estimated that drug rashes occur with a frequency of 10% in intensive care units. In addition acute dermatological conditions cause acute skin failure like Steven Johnson syndrome and toxic epidermal necrolysis also need ITU admission with high mortality rates.

Common causes of erythematous drug rash: They usually present with symmetrical erythematous, maculopapular rash.

- Penicillin
- Cephalosporin
- Gentamicin
- Erythromycin
- Amphotericin
- Co-trimoxazole
- Phenytoin, Carbamazepine, lamotrigine
- Thiazides, frusemide
- Allopurinol
- Tricyclic antidepressants, SSRI's

Drug reactions with eosinophilia and systemic symptoms (DRESS)

They present with systemic symptoms with pyrexia, lymphadenopathy and eosinophilia mucous membranes are usually spared. There may be hepatitis, thrombocytopenia, nephritis, pericarditis and pneumonitis. Steroids may be helpful in the treatment.

Causes of DRESS syndrome:

- Lamotrigine,
- phenytoin,
- carbamazepine,
- barbiturates
- Sulphonamides
- Allopurinol
- Diltiazem
- NSAIDS
- Atenolol

Drugs causing urticaria:

- Penicillin, Cephalosporins
- Tetracycline, Sulphonamides
- Phenytoin, Carbamazepine, lamotrigine
- Vancomycin
- Aspirin, NSAIDS
- ACE inhibitors

BLISTERING RASHES:

Steven-Johnson syndrome and toxic epidermal necrolysis:

They are almost exclusively caused by drugs. There are typically target lesions and there is also commonly involvement of the mucous membranes of the body. Lesions with less than 10% blisters are classified as S-J syndrome whereas cases with more than 30% lesions are called TEN.

The treatment is generally supportive with regular involvement of ophthalmologists if eyes are involved. Mortality ranges from 5% to 40%. Steroids, immunosuppressive drugs and immune-modulators have been tried without success.

Common causes of S-J syndrome and TEN:

• Lamotrigine	• NSAID
• Phenytoin	• Allopurinol
• Carbamazepine	• Penicillin
• Phenobarbital	• H_2 antagonists
• Sulphonamides	• Nevirapine
• Tetracycline	

Other drugs causing blistering diseases: **(Pemphigus like symptom)**

• Penicillamine	• Captopril	• Rifampicin

Steroids may be helpful for the treatment.

In addition to the drugs, pemphigus (aged 40-60 yrs) and pemphigoid (older persons) may present with blistering conditions of skin.

Pustular rash in ITU, Causes:

- Penicillin, cephalosporin
- Tetracycline
- Carbamazepine
- Calcium channel blockers
- Quinolones
- Macrolides

Purpuric rash in ITU

Drug induced vasculitis usually cause purpuric rash.

Causes:-

- Beta lactamase antibiotics
- Sulphonamides
- Erythromycin
- Carbamazepine
- Frusemide, thiazides

: KEY POINTS :

- Adverse drug reaction is a common problem in clinical practice.
- Delay in its detection can cause unnecessary investigations.
- Thorough drug history should be a part and parcel of medical consultation.

FURTHER REFERENCES:

- Goodman and Gillman - The Pharmacological Principles of Therapeutics - 9th edition, Philadelphia.
- Harrison's Principle of Internal Medicine - 17th Edition.
- Colin Bigham *et al.* - Cutaneous drug reaction in intensive care BJHM, Vol-74, No-6, June-2013, P-340-346.
- Oxford Text Book of Medicine – 5th Edition.

46 FOUR PATIENTS WITH CEREBROVASCULAR ACCIDENT

CASE: *A 71 years old gentleman was admitted to the hospital because he was unarousable in the morning. He was a known diabetic, hypertensive and on medication. Examination revealed right sided flaccid weakness with up going plantar on the same side. He was in sinus rhythm with a BP of 186/100 mmHg and no carotid bruits or cardiac murmur. His FBC, urea, electrolytes, random glucose, cardiac enzymes, were within normal range. ECG showed LVH. Urgent CT brain scan showed large infraction in the left middle cerebral artery territory.*

DIAGNOSIS: Non haemorrhagic infarction in left MCA territory.

CASE: *A 58 years old diabetic and hypertensive patient was admitted with history of vomiting, dizziness and headache. Examination revealed BP 170/96 mmHg, small pupil on the right, positive cerebellar sign like intension tremor on the right, sensation to pin prick was diminished on the left upper and lower extremities and on the right side of the face. He had an abnormal voice, with a sluggish palatal reflex and accumulation of secretion in the oropharynx. Routine investigations were normal. CT brain scan revealed small infract in the right medulla of brain stem.*

DIAGNOSIS: Brain stem infarction due to occlusion of the posterior circulation with right sided lateral medullary syndrome (Wallenberg's syndrome).

(Same sided cerebellar sign, Horner syndrome, vagal nerve involvement with bulbar palsy, loss of pain and temperature on the same side of the face and on the opposite side in the extremities. This is due to infarction of posterior inferior cerebellar artery, infarction involving a wedge shaped area in the lateral part of medulla. The artery is a branch of vertebral artery).

CASE: *A 62 years old diabetic, hypertensive and hyperlipidaemic patient presented with mild weakness along with numbness of his left hand. His speech was slightly dysarthric. Examination revealed mild facial asymmetry with mild weakness of his left hand grip. CT brain scan showed small infarct in right basal ganglion region.*

DIAGNOSIS: Lacunar infarction.

CASE: *A 61 years old lady presented in an unconscious state. She had a preceding history of severe headache which led to collapse. Examination revealed comatose patient with neck stiffness and bilateral upgoing plantars. CT scan revealed evidence of extensive subarachnoid haemorrhage.*

DIAGNOSIS: Subarachnoid haemorrhage.

DISCUSSION:

Cerebrovascular disease is a very common presentation both in hospital and primary care practice. Diagnosis is not difficult if they present in a classical way. However in comatose or semi comatose patient, other causes like **hyponatraemia, hypo or hyperglycaemia, drug overdose, cerebral infections including malaria need to be excluded by appropriate tests.**

Many patients present with transient symptoms lasting for less than 24 hrs. The Transient Ischemic Attacks (TIA) can occur repeatedly and are known to be the warning sign of an impending cerebrovascular accident. In these patients, proper risk factor modification can reduce the incidence of CVA.

T.I.A in carotid artery territory (anterior circulation)

- Transient monocular blindness (amaurosis fugax)
- Dysphasia
- Unilateral weakness
- Facial asymmetry

T.I.A in vertebrobasilar artery territory (posterior circulation)

- Diplopia
- Dizziness, vertigo, tinnitus
- Dysarthria
- Bilateral motor weakness or sensory signs

Patients with such symptoms should be thoroughly investigated with lipids, glucose, ECG, echo, carotid doppler and the risk factors including hypertension should be modified as much as possible. The target BP should be preferably 130/80 mmHg and LDL cholesterol < 100 mg%. Aspirin will reduce the incidence of further attack with addition of dipyridamole having an additional effect.

Though slightly superior to aspirin, the beneficial effect of addition of clopidogrel to aspirin has not yet been conclusively demonstrated in secondary prevention of stroke. However, this combination is justified in selected patients with ischemic heart disease where combination of aspirin with clopidogrel had been found to be beneficial. Clopidogrel is much more expensive compared to aspirin. Patients with symptomatic TIA and stroke with carotid artery occlusion more than 70% (assessed by carotid Doppler, CT angiogram, MR angiogram or cerebral angiogram) may benefit from carotid endarterectomy. Although this is not a commonly done procedure in India, the option should always be discussed with the patients.

Patients, who have atrial fibrillation or demonstrable clot in LV cavity, should be anticoagulated. Aspirin and other antiplatelet agents work better in atherosclerotic plaques of carotid arteries where the clot is platelet rich. While in left ventricular or left atrial clots that are found in atrial fibrillation or ventricular aneurysm are mainly fibrin rich and anticoagulants are clearly superior to antiplatelets in these situations.

The recurrence rate of further brain attack following an episode of TIA or stroke is 5% in the 1st year followed by a yearly rate of 3%. In western countries, use of anticoagulants has reduced the recurrence of stroke in patients with atrial fibrillation. The INR has to be maintained between 2 to 2.5.

Presentation of CVAs in clinical practice:

1. **TIA**
2. **Haemorrhage –**
   - Focal – Primary intracerebral haemorrhage (PICH).
   - Global – Subarachnoid haemorrhage (SAH).
3. **Infraction –**
   - Total anterior circulation infarction (TACI).
   - Partial anterior circulation infarction (PACI).
   - Lacunar artery infarction (LACI).
   - Posterior circulation infarction (POCI)

These patients are frequently seen by the primary care physician in the community and finally referred to the hospital.

MANAGEMENT:

Immediate management plan:

Initial screening tests as mentioned above.

CT scan or MRI brain scan: CT scan is the imaging technique of choice as it detects presence of blood immediately. This is important as in non-haemorrhagic infarction there is a role of thrombolysis with recombinant tissue plasminogen activator (rtPA) if presenting within the first 3 hours. CT scan can exclude haemorrhage before thrombolysis is commenced. Disadvantage of CT scan is that it may fail to detect if the infarction is evolving, it may also fail to detect small lacunar infarcts and after 10-14 days of haemorrhage, the CT picture may be isodense thereby missing the diagnosis of initial cerebral haemorrhage. This will be important in those patients who present late after 10-14 days and the decision regarding anticoagulation needs to be taken (haemorrhagic infarction). MRI scan on the other hand fails to detect blood early but better in detection infarction earlier than CT scan, it can detect small lacunar infarcts better and can demonstrate presence of blood even after few weeks. So MRI scan may probably be needed in subsequent follow up studies in selected group of patients.

Emergency management of cerebral infarct:

Following an ischemic stroke, there is immediate cessation of blood supply in the affected territory. Surrounding the infarct zone, there is an area of ischemic zone (ischemic penumbra zone) which is also susceptible to further occlusion leading to the extension of the infarct territory resulting in poor outcome. The mainstay of treatment is to prevent this to happen as much as possible. As no specific drug has been found to prevent this, one should strive for meticulous general management in the initial few days that will definitely improve the outcome in patients with stroke.

Managing comatose patients:

- Head end should be raised.
- Frequent oral toileting should be done.
- If needed orotracheal intubation needs to be done.
- NG tube should be inserted for gastric aspiration. Enteral feeding should be avoided initially for the risk of aspiration.
- If there is evidence of increasing intracranial pressure, IV mannitol (20%) 100-300 ml should be given. Round the clock mannitol may not be helpful and may even be counterproductive. In selected cases artificial ventilation and therapeutic hyperventilation may be carried out with a target $PaCO_2$ is very low (< 25 mmHg), it can cause cerebral vasoconstriction thereby increasing the ICP instead.
- If CT scan shows cerebellar haematoma or any subcortical haematoma, urgent neurosurgical opinion should be taken.
- In non-haemorrhagic infarction, aspirin (150-300 mg) should be given through the NG tube.
- Pyrexia, hypoxia, infection, hyperglycaemia etc may cause extension of the infarct zone and every attempt should be made to bring down the temperature by

paracetamol or sponging. Hypoxia should be corrected by oxygen therapy. Glucose should be kept within 150 mg%. Dextrose drip should be avoided and frequently insulin via infusion pump will be necessary to keep the blood glucose under control.

- Although control of hypertension prevents stroke in acute stroke patients there may be increase in blood pressure as a part of homeostatic autonomic response. It should not be lowered in the initial 7-10 days as it might cause further extension of stroke.
- Seizures complicate 5-10% of the strokes. It is not yet known whether antiepileptic should be given prophylactically. As seizures commonly occur in sub-cortical infracts, antiepileptic may be prudently used in big subcortical infarcts. Phenytoin, diazepam, carbamazepine, valproate and more recently levetiracetam may be chosen as therapeutic agents.
- Chest infection due to respiratory or urinary tract infection due to catheterization should be treated with appropriate antibiotics. Avoidance of routine catheterization in stroke patients has also reduced the incidence of nosocomial infection rate in our ITU, considerably. Patients with incontinence should have an external drainage while those with retention, catheterization has to be done. Proper positioning of the patients and avoidance of oral feeding in first few days has also reduced the incidence of aspiration pneumonia in our unit.
- DVT prophylaxis: Silent DVT is common in paralysed patients. Heparin or low molecular weight heparin reduce the incidence of DVT but increase the risk of haemorrhagic transformation of the infarct zone significantly. One should use other methods like 'antiembolism' stocking as a preventive strategy.
- Prevention of pressure sores: It is important to prevent pressure sore by using special mattress and by meticulous nursing care.

Once the patient stabilizes, other problems like persistent urinary incontinence should be treated with anticholinergics like oxybutynin, tolterodine or darifenacin. Muscle stiffness may be helped with baclofen. Early physiotherapy of shoulder joints will prevent painful frozen shoulder in the future. Painful hand due to shoulder hand syndrome (reflex sympathetic dystrophy) can be helped with a course of methylprednisolone. Multi disciplinary approach involving physiotherapist, occupational therapists and dieticians will help in early rehabilitation with a much improved outcome. A well organized stroke unit can coordinate the activities of different disciplines in a well-orchestrated manner and deliver the goods to the patients on secondary prophylactic measures (like aspirin, statins, antidiabetics and antihypertensive). In patients with non-haemorrhagic embolic stroke, anticoagulants should be considered after two weeks post infarction to avoid the possibility of haemorrhagic transformation in the initial days. Different aids and appliances might help the patients to lead a reasonably useful life. Stroke units are lacking in majority of places in India and provision of such in the district and teaching hospitals will definitely improve the outcome.

The **management of subarachnoid haemorrhage** is different from usual stroke management. Urgent neurosurgical referral should be done for consideration of cerebral angiogram with a view to do aneurismal clipping. Meanwhile, increased intracranial pressure should be treated accordingly. Antiepileptic cover should be given for first 6 weeks. There are three major complications of SAH:

- **Rebleeding**– Strict blood pressure control will be needed to prevent rebleeding.
- **Cerebral vasospasm**– Vasospasm distal to the bleeding vessel can cause delayed deterioration with complications like drowsiness and hemiparesis. Calcium channel blocker nimodipine 60 mg four times a day can reduce the incidents of vasospasm and should be started early. If the patient with SAH develops deteriorating consciousness level, an urgent repeat CT scan should be performed to exclude rebleeding, cerebral infarction due to vasospasm or obstructive hydrocephalus. If there is evidence of vasospasm, BP should be raised on the upper side of normal and volume depletion, if any should be corrected.
- **Obstructive hydrocephalus**– This complication should be treated with ventriculoperitoneal shunting.
- **SAH**: It needs expert input from neurologist and neurosurgeons.

PROGNOSIS: It varies with different varieties of stroke.

TACI: 60% death, 30% disability, 10% independence.

PACI: 20% death, 30% disability, 50% independence.

LACI: 10% death, 30% disability, 60% independence.

POCI: 20% death, 20% disability, 60% independence.

Role of neurocritical care in managing medical and neurosurgical emergencies:

In India, at the secondary level majority of the critical care units are general and the doctors need to handle neurological emergencies as well. A brief discussion on neurological care will be relevant in this regard.

NEUROLOGICAL AND NEUROSURGICAL CONDITION THAT MAY NEED ADMISSION IN ITU:

- Traumatic Brain Injury
- Traumatic Spinal Injury
- Subarachnoid haemorrhage
- Intracerebral haemorrhage
- Postoperative neurosurgical patient
- Malignant middle cerebral artery stroke
- Posterior fossa stroke
- Cerebral venous thrombosis
- Status epilepticus
- GB Syndrome
- Myasthenia gravis
- Intensive care acquired weakness
- Critical care neuropathy

Traumatic brain injury:

The outcome depends upon the severity of injury, age and secondary infections, hypoxia, hypercapnia, hypotension and intracranial hypertension. It has been shown that management in a dedicated neuro critical care unit reduces the mortality up to two fold compared to management in general critical care unit.

Regular neurosurgical input is needed as in the event of very high intracranial pressure, decompressive craniectomy may be needed.

Traumatic spinal injury:

Although the majority of cases, surgical management will be needed, medical input is also essential in the initial management like respiratory support and hemodynamic support with a target mean arterial pressure of 85-90 mmHg for at least 7 days, nutritional support, and DVT prophylaxis.

Intracerebral Haemorrhage:

The initial management goals of some trials have shown that surgical evacuation in ICH does not alter the overall prognosis (STICH trial). However smaller trials have shown favourable response in cases of superficial haemorrhages.

Subarachnoid Haemorrhage:

Glasgow Coma scale is the greatest predictor for survival. 10-20% of patients need immediate intubation on admission. The chance of rebleeding is 4% in first 24 hrs, 1% thereafter in unsecured aneurysm.

Hydrocephalus develops over days and is treated by ventriculoperitoneal shunt or insertion of external ventricular drain.

For vasospasm triple H therapy (hypertension, haemodilution and hypervolaemia) should be instituted.

Arterial thrombosis or embolism:

Occurs more commonly following coiling and is treated with aspirin, clopidogrel and/or anticonvulsants. Electrolyte imbalance may occur either due to cerebral salt wasting syndrome or SIDAH.

Neurological causes needing ITU care:

Malignant middle cerebral artery strokes is fatal in 80% of cases. In CT scan, hypo density over 50% of the territory in the MCA region, would predict development of malignant MCA stroke. In addition to aggressive medical therapy decompressive hemicraniectomy has been recognised to improve outcome in younger patients with reduced mortality and improve neurologically. 3 trials that have shown such effects are, DESIMAL, DESTINY and HAMLET.

Cerebral venous thrombosis:

This condition can cause life threatening intra cranial hypertension and needs neuro-critical care monitoring. This is the condition where anticoagulation either with heparin or low molecular weight heparin will be needed in spite of evidence of intracranial bleeding which is a secondary consequence of venous outflow obstruction. Repeated lumbar puncture or surgery may be needed for raised ICP.

Status epilepticus:

It is a common condition needing neuro critical care management. It is a continuous seizure activity lasting for > 5 minutes. Encephalitis is the most common condition.

Guillain-barré syndrome:

Neuro critical care management is essential in GB syndrome. Respiratory function should be monitored closely. Vital capacity < 20 ml/kg, maximum inspiratory mouth pressure less than 30 cm of H_2O or maximum expiratory pressure less than 40 cm of H_2O, are indication of close monitoring as they frequently need intubation and ventilation. Cardiac monitoring is also essential as symptomatic bradycardia needs pacing.

Myasthenia Gravis:

Close observation of this condition is required in neuro critical care regarding fatigability, cough swallowing, oxygen saturation, development of any sepsis, and drug monitoring (like verapamil, quinine, timolol, aminoglycoside– which may exacerbate myasthenia gravis). Treatment with steroid, physostigmine, IV immunoglobulin or plasmapheresis should be carried out from neuro critical care unit. In refractory cases 'rituximab' may be necessary.

APPROACH:

On admission	Monitoring	Management goals
Adequate resuscitation	Cardiac monitoring	Sedation, analgesic, propofol and fentanyl
Baseline investigation	Pulse oximetry	If sedation upto 24 hr
	Invasive arterial monitoring	Midazolam and morphine if sedation for > 24 hr
	Urinary catheterization, CVP measurement	Respiratory support
	Intracranial pressure monitoring	• PEEP less than 5cm of H_2O • $FO_2 < 0.5$ • $PaO_2 > 65$mmHg • $PaCO_2 = 30\text{-}32$ mmHg • Intracranial pressure < 25 mmHg • Cerebral perfusion pressure > 60 cm/day • Core temperature– 25-27°C • Tight glucose control • Tight control of seizure • Early enteral feeding • Optimum hemodynamic and volume status

MANAGEMENT:

Step 1:

Lorazepam 4mg IV bolus (can be repeated once)

Step 2:

Phenobarbital IV 10 mg/kg

or

Phenytoin infusion IV 15 mg/kg

or

Fosphenytoin infusion 15 mg/kg

or

Valproate infusion – 25mg/kg

Step 3 (Refractory status 60-90 minutes):

- Propofol IV bolus then infusion @ 5-10 mg/kg
- Thiopental IV bolus 100-250 mg over 20 seconds, with further bolus every 2–3 minutes.

Midazolam IV bolus 0.1–0.3 mg/kg, then infusion.

: KEY POINTS :

- Brain attacks (stroke) are common presenting problems at primary, secondary and tertiary level of care.
- CT scan will differentiate a non haemorrhagic stroke from a haemorrhagic one.
- Ischemic stroke may be due to atherosclerotic or embolic as in atrial fibrillation.
- Ischemic stroke in sinus rhythm should be treated with aspirin while embolic stroke due to atrial fibrillation should be anticoagulated in the long run.
- Thrombolytic therapy can be used in selected group of patients with brain attack.
- Subarachnoid haemorrhage needs input from neurologist and neurosurgeon.
- Patients with stroke need secondary preventive measures which will reduce the incidence of strokes.
- In India, we need more organised stroke units to improve the outcome of such patients.

FURTHER REFERENCES:

- Johnston S.C.: Clinical practice – Transient ischemic attack, NEJM 347: 1687, 2002.
- Adem SHP *et al.* guidelines for the early management of patients with ischemic stroke— A scientific statement from the stroke council of the American, Stroke Association, Stroke 34, 1056, 2003.
- Rothwell pm *et al.* – Analysis of pooled data from the randomized controlled trials of endarterectomy for symptomatic carotid stenosis, Lancet 361: 107, 2003.
- A Sadek *et al.* – The role of neuroscience intensive care in trauma and neurosurgical condition – BJHM-74, oct-2013, 552-556.
- A Sadek *et al.* – The role of neuroscience intensive care in neurosurgical condition – BJHM-74, oct-2013, 558-563.
- Harrison's Principle of Internal Medicine 17th edition.
- Oxford Text Book of Medicine 5th edition.

47 A PATIENT WITH OBESITY

CASE: *A 51 years old gentleman weighing 116 Kg was admitted with gradual drowsiness over a period of last 15 days. During admission he was unarousable. His pulse rate was 96/min, BP 166/90 mmHg, chest showed few basal crepts, distended and obese abdomen, peripheral oedema present. His blood gas showed $PaCO_2$ of 109 mmHg, PaO_2 61 mmHg, HCO_3 38 mmol/lit. ECG and X-ray chest were normal. His TSH and electrolytes were within normal limits.*

DIAGNOSIS: Type II respiratory failure due to hypoventilation as a result of obesity.

He was treated with non invasive ventilation later on requiring endotracheal intubation and ventilation. He was finally weaned off from the ventilator with great difficulty. On discharge he was put on calorie restricted diet, intermittent non invasive ventilation and antiobesity drugs like orlistat and sibutramine. 6 months at follow up, he lost 18 Kg of weight and hardly required any non invasive ventilatory support.

DISCUSSION:

Although it is said that malnutrition is the major problem in our country obesity is also becoming increasingly a common problem in clinical practice, particularly in the urban white color population. It is significantly associated with increased morbidity and mortality.

Problems associated with obesity:

- Osteoarthritis.
- Increased tendency to DM and hypertension with added cardiovascular morbidity.
- Obstructive sleep apnoea.
- Increased incidence of gall stones.
- Fatty liver.

Common causes of obesity:

Most common cause is mismatch between the energy intake and expenditure due to faulty dietary habit or lack of exercise. Hypothyroidism and Cushing's syndrome needs exclusion by appropriate tests. Rare genetic causes like Laurence-Moon-Biedl syndrome, Prader-Willi syndrome and Frolic syndrome can also cause obesity. Certain drugs like steroids, oral contraceptives, lithium and other antipsychotics, antidepressants and certain antiepileptic drugs can also cause obesity. Use of insulin is also associated with weight gain in diabetic patients. While evaluating a patient with obesity one should take a thorough drug history.

How to measure obesity?

- Body Mass Index: This is derived by dividing patient's body weight in kg by square of the patient's height (in meter).

  BMI = Weight in Kg ÷ (Height in meter)^2.

  According to western standards,

  over weight- BMI 25 to 29.9 and
  obesity- BMI more than 30.

  [By India standard, the values may be a bit lower]

- Waist hip ratio.

- Waist circumference- Women whose waist lines are over 31.5 inches and men whose waist lines are over 37 inches should watch their weight as increasing waist line is associated with increased risk of heart disease. In simple terms, abdominal obesity is particularly associated with increased risk of heart disease.

- Anthropometric measures like triceps skin fold thickness and mid arm muscle circumference.

How does obesity predispose to cardiovascular risk?

In obesity, particularly of central type there is increased incidence of insulin resistance which in turn causes hypertension, raised LDL and triglyceride reduced HDL and glucose intolerance. This metabolic syndrome is known as **syndrome-X.** These metabolic changes in turn lead to adverse cardiovascular outcome.

How to tackle obesity?

Life style modification:

- Proper dietary advice with caloric restriction.

- Increase physical activity- with daily aerobic exercise of 45-60 minutes. The treadmill burns the calories most. Frequent exercise in short bursts (10 minutes each) may be helpful for obese patients.

Drugs: Two groups of drugs are used.

- Centrally acting appetite suppressants like **sibutramine 10 mg** daily may cause weight loss. It works on serotonin receptors and may cause dry mouth constipation and insomnia. It should be avoided in patients taking SSRI group of antidepressants.

Locally acting on gut, like **orlistat,** inhibits intestinal lipase thereby causing fat malabsorption. Steatorrhoea is a problem and it may inhibit absorption of other drugs if administered concomitantly. It is of particular help in controlling blood glucose in type II diabetic patients. The dose is 120 mg twice daily immediately after major food intake.

These two drugs can also be combined to have additive effect.

Drug therapy should be used if the BMI is >30. In patients with other associated risk factors, BMI of 27 should be the cut off point for commencement of drug therapy.

In morbid obesity (BMI >35) in view of the greatly increased cardiovascular risks, surgical intervention may be indicated (standard bariatric surgeries).

Examples of such surgeries are:

- **Vertical banded gastroplasty** (this procedure narrows the stomach and allows only small amounts of food to pass through).
- **Roux-en-Y gastric bypass graft**- This involves creating a small stomach pouch that serves as a reservoir and connects directly to the intestine (extensive gastric bypass). This procedure also limits the amount of food that a person can consume. Complication like vomiting, dumping syndrome and nutritional deficiency are common following surgical procedures.
- **Laparoscopic gastric banding** is a new procedure that avoids surgical incision. While treating obesity, the main thrust should be given to the life style modification as drug therapy is expensive. The patients should be motivated with regular counseling. The long term risks should be explained properly in order to motivate the patients.

: KEY POINTS :

- Obesity is increasing in the Indian urban population.
- It increases the risk of development of diabetes mellitus and other cardiovascular problems through the mechanism of insulin resistance.
- Abdominal obesity is a good predictor of long term cardiovascular risks.
- Life style modification is the first approach in treating obesity.
- In high risk patients, anti obesity drugs may be used.

FURTHER REFERENCES:

- Harrison's Principle of Internal Medicine-17th edition.
- Oxford Text Book of Medicine-5th edition

48 NUTRITION THERAPY IN HOSPITALISED PATIENTS

CASE: *A 56 years old alcoholic patient was admitted with features of hepatic encephalopathy following an episode of variceal haemorrhage. He was initially resuscitated with IV fluids, blood transfusion and somatostatin infusion. After stabilization of his condition over next 48 hrs, nutritional therapy was considered. He was treated with intravenous dextrose (with multivitamins), 20% lipid infusion and branched chain amino acids. On recovery, he was started on enteral nutrition containing branched chain amino acids. He was discharged after 3 weeks and on his subsequent outpatient visit he did not have any evidence of encephalopathy. He had evidence of gross malnutrition however. He was cautiously resumed on high protein diet and vitamin supplementation. Branched chain amino acid was discontinued. Further follow up after 2 months did not show any evidence of encephalopathy and his nutritional status had recovered to some extent.*

DIAGNOSIS: Malnutrition associated with chronic liver disease.

DISCUSSION:

Nutritional deficiency is common in hospitalized patients. It is estimated that upto 40% of the hospitalized patient suffer from some degree of malnutrition which in term adversely affects the mortality and morbidity. Provision of proper nutritional support improves the overall outcome in such patients. Since proper advice and assistance from a well trained dietician is not always available in many centres, it is the responsibility of the treating physician to provide the guidance about proper diet therapy.

How to assess nutritional status?

The first step is to find out the nutritional status of the patient. This is done by

- **Anthropometric method**
  - Mid arm skin-fold thickness over the triceps muscle.
  - Arm muscle circumference.
- **Laboratory tests**
  - **Serum albumin**

    Limitation of serum albumin – It has got long half life so it is not suitable in acute illness. In critical care situations there is shift towards formation of acute phase proteins at the expense of albumin synthesis. Therefore low albumin may be an indicator of severity of underlying condition rather than nutritional status. Estimation of CRP in these situations may be helpful. **(Low albumin with low CRP may indicate nutritional status, while low albumin with high CRP**

indicating underlying disease activity). Moreover, administration of intravenous fluids can reduce the albumin level by dilution effect.

- **Pre-albumin**

  It has a shorter half life and is a sensitive indicator of protein energy deficiency. However it may be decreased in liver disease, hyperthyroidism and inflammation.

- **Transferrin**

  It has a shorter half life than albumin. It may be increased in pregnancy, iron deficiency etc.

- **Retinol-binding protein**

  It is a sensitive indicator of short time protein deficiency. It may also be altered in liver disease, renal disease and inflammation.

- **Immunological function**

  Total lymphocyte count, delayed cutaneous hypersensitivity.

- **Blood tests**

  Estimation of K^+, Na^+, Ca^{++}, Vitamin B_{12} and folate levels.

How to assess nutritional requirement?

Onc can use the traditional formula of Harris-Benedict to calculate the basal energy expenditure (BEE) of a patient.

Male : BEE = 66.67 + 13.75W + 5H – 6.76A

Female: BEE = 665.1 + 9.56W +1.85H – 4.68A

H= height in centimetres, W= actual weight in kg, A= age in years.

Energy expenditure (EE) is then calculated by multiplying BEE with factor F (F stands for extra metabolic stress from various conditions). BEE increases by 10% for each degree centigrade rise of temperature from the normal.

- In infection, F = 1.2 – 1.8
- Surgery, F = 1.1 – 1.2
- Trauma, F = 1.3 – 1.6
- Burn injury, F = 1.5 × 2.0 (40% - 100% body surface area burn)

In clinical practice, the approximate requirement of energy is derived from the following chart:

- In healthy men - 22 kcal/kg/day
- In Sepsis - 24–30 kcal/kg/day
- In MODS -30 + 5 kcal/kg/day
- In pancreatitis with sepsis - 30 + 5 kcal/kg/day
- In burn - 40 kcal/kg/day

Example: In an average 60 kg Indian patient with sepsis –

- Calorie requirement: 1800 kcal
- Protein 1-1.5 g/kg
- Fat 30%-50% of energy
- Carbohydrate 30% -70% of energy

Having calculated the amount of calorie requirement one should then proceed for proper nutritional therapy.

Which route?

Although parenteral nutritional therapy was popular in early eighties, for last one decade the pendulum has swung in favour of enteral route. The reason behind it is that gut mucosa works as a physiological barrier and in the event of non utilization of gut; there is mucosal atrophy which in turn leads to easy permeation of bacterial toxins into the portal circulation finally finding their way to the liver. These toxins ultimately lead to cytokine stimulation enhancing the cascade of sepsis with development of MODS. Enteral nutrition maintains the gut mucosal integrity and thus may prevent the inflammatory cascade. Unfortunately there are some conditions where enteral nutrition cannot be persuaded on.

Contra indications of enteral feeding:

- Intractable vomiting
- Severe diarrhoea
- Intestinal obstruction
- Peritonitis
- Severe pancreatitis with malabsorption.

In such cases parenteral nutrition should be persuade. These two routes are not mutually exclusive and they can be effectively combined with the main energy source provided by parental route while gut mucosal function maintained by the enteral route.

In post operative patient, mere absence of bowel sound is not a contraindication of enteral nutrition. One should start slowly and observe the effect. If there is gastric distension, one should reduce the amount of feed and use a prokinetic like metoclopramide etc. If these methods are not effective, one should try post pyloric feeding with naso-duodenal or naso-jejunal feeding. (These special feeding tubes can be negotiated upto the jejunum at the bed side).

In post surgical patients where prolonged nutritional therapy is anticipated, perioperative jejunostomy tube can be inserted prior to closure of the abdominal wound. In patients with brain stroke with swallowing problems or in patients with oesophageal cancer, percutaneous endoscopic gastrostomy (PEG) can be done for long term feeding.

How to proceed enteral feeding?

It can be accomplished by two ways:

- Bolus
- Continuous infusion

Bolus method is commonly used in our country because of its easiness to use. It can cause gastric distension and aspiration. It can cause metabolic instability in diabetic patients. Continuous infusion on the other hand is a more physiological way of delivering the feed. It is better tolerated in diabetic patients. It can theoretically cause proliferation of gastrointestinal flora because of continuous inhibition of gastric acid.

Which kind of enteral food?

There are two kinds of enteral formula

- Polymeric
- Monomeric

In polymeric formula, there is intact protein, fat and carbohydrate as starch. Because of high osmolality, these formulas can cause diarrhoea. The digestive systems need to be active as well. In patients with maldigestion and malabsorption monomeric formulas may be tried instead (elemental diet). These formulas contain pre-digested food like amino acids, oligosaccharides and fatty acids.

Condition where monomeric formulas are used:

- Malabsorption
- Severe pancreatitis
- Crohn's disease

Examples – Peptamen, Novasource peptide etc.

In spite of the best efforts many patients still cannot tolerate enteral nutrition and parenteral nutrition is reserved for them. Like enteral feed, the constituents of TPN are carbohydrate, fat and amino acids (supplied as a source of protein). Vitamins and trace elements are frequently added to them.

Monitoring:

Following parameters need regular monitoring during TPN:

- Glucose– Random glucose should preferably maintain around 110-120 mg%. If needed insulin should be added to the solution.
- Liver function test– prolonged TPN can cause hepatic steatosis.
- Daily electrolytes.
- Random triglyceride– especially if the patient is on lipid infusion. The level should be kept below 400 mg% if possible. In pancreatitis, there is no contraindication of fat infusion provided the lipid level is kept below the target level.

NUTRITION IN SPECIAL CIRCUMSTANCES:

In burn, pressure sore, cancer patient's high caloric enteral feeds with high protein content is needed.
Example– Resource high protein, Ensure plus protein etc.

In patients with renal failure:

Predialysis patients– low protein, low salt, low K^+ containing feed like Nepro, neutrenal.

Patients on renal replacement therapy– High protein, low salt, low K^+ containing diet.

Example – Suplena, nutrenal CRF.

In patients with respiratory failure:

Excessive carbohydrate increases CO_2 production thereby may cause difficulty in weaning from ventilator. Carbohydrate content of the feed should be reduced in such patients (50% energy from carbohydrate, 50% from fat).

In diabetic patients:

Special formulas are available for diabetic patients with low carbohydrate content.

Example- Diabetic resource, Nutrical DM, Glucerna etc.

In hepatic failure:

In patients with cirrhosis with malnutrition– High protein containing diet.

In patients with grade I or II encephalopathy– In hepatic encephalopathy aromatic amino acid can form false neurotransmitters and can exacerbate encephalopathy. Branched chain amino acids (BCAA) can prevent this with improvement of the encephalopathy.

Special preparations containing BCAA are– Resource hepatic, Fresubin heap.

In grade-iv encephalopathy, BCAA can be used as IV infusion.

E.g. Aminoplasmal heap.

In patients with pancreatitis:

In severe cases, TPN needs to be used with monitoring of triglyceride level. However enteral nutrition should be attempted whenever possible. Naso-jejunal feeding is the preferred method as delivery of food beyond the ligament of Tietz does not cause pancreatic stimulation. In addition to maintain gut mucosa, it may also inhibit pancreatic exocrine secretion by negative feedback mechanism called 'iliac break'. If the patient is undergoing pancreatic necrosectomy, the surgeon should be advised to put a feeding jejunostomy for feeding purpose. In severe malabsorption elemental formulas can be used.

Immunonutrition:

Arginine, glutamine, omega-3 fatty acids and nucleotide RNA constitute immunonutrition. They maintain the immunological function of the gut and prevent bacterial translocation from the intestine to the portal circulation. In conditions like burn, trauma, sepsis and post gastrointestinal surgery their use may reduce the hospital stay. Total mortality may not be affected however. Their routine use in aforementioned cases is still hotly debated.

Example– Reconvan.

Example of parenteral preparations (for practising doctors):

- PNA-16: Provides high energy because of presence of 50% dextrose and amino acids.

  (The calorie content may further be increased by adding lipids to it, e.g. Celipid 20% 500 cc).
- Vitrimix & Nutriflex-peri: Provides moderate amount of energy. The advantage is that they can be given via peripheral veins.

  (Any solution containing more than 10% than 10% of dextrose should be given via a central vein to prevent thrombophlebitis).
- Lipofundin (20%) & Intralipid (20%): 500 cc will provide 500 kcal of energy.
- Omegaven: Parenteral immunonutrition
- Dipeptaven: Parenteral immunonutrition (this should be avoided in hepatic encephalopathy).
- Celicel: Provides trace elements.

CASE: *A 30 years old gentleman with ruptured liver abscess and MODS in ITU.*

Weight – 80 kg, Height – 183 cm,

BEE 1950 kcal + Stress factor (1.5)

Calorie requirement = 2410 kcal/kg

EN + TPN→ which one?

In this patient PNA 16 + 20% Celipid was selected (because of high energy requirement). Later on it was supplemented with enteral formula in the form of immunonutrition. Gradually the amount of enteral feeding was increased and TPN was discontinued.

CASE: *A 56 years old patient with variceal bleeding and hepatic encephalopathy.*

Weight – 61.5 kg, Height – 170 cm,

BEE – 1380 kcal/day

TPN + EN → which preparation?

Initially TPN was used with 20% Intralipid, aminoplasmal heap and 10% dextrose with vitamins. With improvement of his condition, he was offered oral nutrition with resource heap. He recovered well and was discharged. On subsequent follow up he was treated with resource high protein.

CASE: *A 55 years old patient with pancreatitis.*

Weight – 55 kg, Height – 170 cm,

BEE – 1150 kcal/day stress factor 1.5;

Metabolic goal – 1650 kcal/day

TPN + EN → which one?

Initially treated with TPN (nutriflex special). Later on peptamen (elemental) was used through surgically placed jejunostomy tube.

In the Indian context, it may not be possible to provide these expensive formulas in a sizeable number of patients. Provision of blended homogeneous food may be used in such patients as an alternative.

CASE: *A 65 years old was admitted with Crohn's disease and leading to severe malnutrition. Clinically he was cachexic with a weight of 51 kg, Hb– 7.9 g, Albumin– 2.1 mg%, Low Calcium, potassium, phosphate and magnesium level. He was treated with blood transfusion and TPN was commenced. Within 72 hrs he started developed breathlessness along with cardiac arrhythmias. Repeat blood tests showed further fall of his potassium, magnesium and phosphate levels. Arrhythmias were corrected following replacement of potassium, magnesium. His confusional state improved by giving thiamine supplementation. At the time of presentation, since IV phosphate preparation was not available in Kolkata (now it is available), phosphate enema was applied hoping that it may replenish the depleted phosphate store to some extent.*

DIAGNOSIS: Refeeding syndrome.

DISCUSSION:

Refeeding syndrome occurs due to institution of either TPN on enteral nutritional therapy in severely malnourished patients which may even cause mortality if the clinician fails to make a proper diagnosis.

Mechanism: In starvation there is a switch from carbohydrate to fat and protein metabolism which leads reduction of lean body mass and depletion of intracellular magnesium, phosphate, potassium and thiamine although the blood levels may remain apparently normal due to extracellular body fluid. During refeeding there is hyperglycaemia and secretion of insulin which further drives phosphate, magnesium and potassium to the intracellular compartment thereby causing sudden depletion of these elements in the extracellular compartment since thiamine is used in glucose metabolism there is depletion of thiamine as well. This depletion leads to the symptoms of cardiac arrhythmia, cardiac failure, severe musculoskeletal weakness, anaemia confusional and delirium state (thiamine deficiency) that constitutes refeeding syndrome.

Treatment:

Clinicians should be aware of this condition and start feeding slowly targeting supply of 50% of energy requirement in the initial period and slowly build the target up. NICE recommends starting nutrition with a target of 10 kcal/kg/day and slowly increase it. Since hypophosphataemia is the main cause of the syndrome, it should be replaced by intravenous infusion. Mg^+, K^+ and Ca^{++} should also be supplemented in order to prevent Wernicke's encephalopathy. Associated nonketotic hyperglycaemia, if present should also be treated.

: KEY POINTS :

- Malnutrition is common in hospital patients.
- Malnutrition adversely affects the overall outcome of the patients.
- Provision of proper nutritional therapy improves mortality.
- Enteral feeding is more physiological route of delivery.
- Choosing the right preparation is important in individual patients.
- Immunonutrition may be helpful in cancer, burn or trauma patient.
- While feeding malnourished patients, refeeding syndrome should be kept in mind.

FURTHER REFERENCES:

- Harrison's Principle of Internal Medicine – 17th edition.
- Oxford Text Book of Medicine – 5th edition.
- Willet WC *et al* (1997) Dietary assessment methods – American journal of clinical nutrition 65 (supplement 4).
- Santa WW (1997) Nutritional support NEJM 336 : 41-48
- Payne James JJ et al (2000) — Artificial nutritional support in clinical practice, 2nd ed. Greenwich medical media Ltd.
- Clare Ormerode *et al.* Refeeding syndrome BJHM. Vol 71, No 12 Dec 2012.

49 PRE-OPERATIVE RISK EVALUATION

CASE: *A 62 years old doctor with diabetic cardiomyopathy was referred by a neurosurgeon to the clinic for pre-operative cardiac risk assessment. He had severe back pain radiating towards the thighs and MRI scan of lumbosacral spine showed degenerative disc disease at multiple levels along with severe lumbar canal stenosis. Since his symptoms were unabated with maximum medical and physical therapy, the patient was desperate to undergo surgical treatment at any cost and hence the referral for preoperative risk assessment. His BP was 120/80 mmHg, presence of 3rd heart sound, basal crepitations present along with mild ankle oedema. He was breathless with slightest exertion.*

ECG– LBBB, Echo– EF 20%, dilated LV with generalized hypokinesia, X-ray chest– hugely dilated heart. Haematological and biochemical parameters were satisfactory. He was on oral nitrates, ACE inhibitors, digoxin, aspirin diuretics and oral hypoglycaemics.

DIAGNOSIS: Dilated cardiomyopathy with lumbar canal stenosis and sciatica for preoperative risk evaluation.

In view of the severely compromised cardiac status, he was considered to be a very high risk case for any surgical procedure under general anaesthesia. He was advised against any surgical intervention under general anaesthesia. He was also advised to explore other possible means of pain relief and referred to a pain clinic for further management.

DISCUSSION:

Although pre-operative check up falls under the domain of anaesthetists, in India very frequently the primary care physicians are involved in the pre-operative management.

It is a very common practice in our country to have the physician present in the theatre during the procedure at the request of the surgeons and the relatives. So it is incumbent upon the physician to be aware of the different predisposing risk factors of any surgical procedures during the intraoperative and immediate perioperative period. The main thrust is of course on the immediate cardio-respiratory problems during intra and post-operative period.

Common cardiac problems encountered in clinical practice:

1. Hypertension
2. IHD
3. Cardiac failure
4. Arrhythmias
5. Valvular heart disease

Common respiratory problems encountered in clinical practice:

1. Asthma
2. COPD

Pre operative evaluation:

The first step is to take a proper history including history of chest discomfort, anginal pain, breathlessness, exercise tolerance, history of smoking etc.

Cardiac risk evaluation:

History of myocardial infarction is an important risk factor of post operative cardiac complications. Elective operation should be deferred for the initial six months following MI. In case of emergency surgery, maximum antianginal protection should be given if the operation is performed within that period.

In patients with stable angina who can perform exercise stress test upto stage II, the risk of any adverse cardiac event during the perioperative period is low. Betablockers have been shown to reduce perioperative cardiac complications and should be routinely included in the regimen if not contraindicated. Preoperative BP should be meticulously controlled. Data from the cardiac surgery registry indicate that in patients with multi-vessel coronary artery disease, revascularization (PTCA or CABG) prior to the non cardiac surgery reduces the mortality. Clearly this is not an option in most of the Indian patients and the emphasis should be given on optimization of the medical therapy, as much as possible before any non cardiac surgical procedure. Patients with valvular heart disease with (class I and II symptoms), tolerate non-cardiac surgical procedures well. However the risk of complications is high in patients with class III and IV symptoms. This is particularly true in patients with critical aortic stenosis and mitral stenosis where post operative pulmonary oedema and even sudden death have been reported. If feasible, surgical correction of the valvular lesion should be done before any non-cardiac procedure. One should also remember to give infective endocarditis prophylaxis in patients with valvular heart disease and patients with prosthetic valves. In case of hypertrophic obstructive cardiomyopathy, intravascular volume should be maintained during the intra operative period to prevent fall in cardiac output due to increase in outflow obstruction as a result of volume depletion. Oral anticoagulants should be discontinued and replaced by low-molecular weight heparin prior to any surgical procedure and they can be resumed after few days following surgery.

Asymptomatic ventricular arrhythmia in the pre-operative ECG does not have any major significance unless it is a manifestation of underlying cardiac failure. Correctable causes like hypokalaemia or hypomagnesaemia should be looked for and treated accordingly.

The patient should be evaluated with an Echo and the presence of LV failure should be meticulously treated prior to operation. Presence of atrial fibrillation does not pose any major intra or perioperative problem provided the rate is reasonably well controlled with medication. Presence of asymptomatic bifascicular block (right bundle branch block with left axis deviation) is a common cause of referral to the physicians. In the absence of any syncopal attack, prophylactic temporary pacemaker implantation is not routinely required although the provision of emergency pacemaker insertion should be kept ready in the OT. In patients with history of syncope or with other indications for permanent pacemaker insertion, prophylactic temporary pacing is mandatory. Clinical judgement will always be required in decision making as in our experience insertion of prophylactic pacemaker even in asymptomatic patients with cardiac dysfunction may be life saving particularly if the patient is undergoing prolonged general anaesthesia for difficult surgical procedures. In patients with permanent pacemaker, preoperative evaluation of the pacemaker function is essential.

Risk Factors:

1. Presence of MI within last 6 months.
2. Presence of 3rd heart sound.
3. Presence of multiple ventricular ectopics in patients with cardiac failure.
4. Class III and IV symptoms in patients with valvular heart disease.

Pulmonary evaluation:

In asymptomatic patients with no prior history of any pulmonary disease, routine X-ray chest is not mandatory in patients <60 yrs old. In patients with chronic pulmonary disease following tests should ideally be done prior to any surgical procedures under general anaesthesia.

- X-ray Chest
- Lung spirometry (FVC, FEV_1, FEV_1 and FVC ratio)
- Blood gas analysis

If FVC is < 1 litre and $PaCO_2$ > 47 mmHg, the incidence of post operative pulmonary complication is high. The patient should be advised to stop smoking prior to the operation and be treated with chest physiotherapy, bronchodilators and antibiotic therapy prior to the surgical procedure. The post operative complications can be reduced upto 50% if aforementioned therapy is given before the surgical procedure. Post operative pulmonary complications are common following upper abdominal surgery and if needed the patient should be observed in ITU as they may need ventilatory assistance. This is particularly true in patients who are undergoing repair of big incisional hernia of abdomen.

Other haematological or biochemical evaluations-

1. **Full blood count:** This is routinely done pre operatively. Polycythemia with Hb of more than 16 g% is associated with increased post operative morbidity and mortality. Polycythemia should be corrected pre operatively.

   Severe anaemia also leads to increased morbidity and mortality. In adults and children older than 3 months, preoperative Hb should be targeted at 9 g%. In younger patients, Hb should be around 10 g%. Coagulation profile should be checked routinely although in asymptomatic individuals without any prior history of any bleeding disorders, these tests can give predictions of intra-operative bleeding. Antiplatelets like aspirin should be discontinued few days prior to the surgery. Haematological opinion should be sought if the platelet count is less than 60,000.

2. **Liver function test:**

   It is a good practice to check base line liver function test, as asymptomatic liver function abnormalities are common. This will help the anaesthetist to select appropriate anaesthetic agents, sedatives and post operative analgesics. Serum albumin level may be predictor of adverse post operative outcome particularly in patients undergoing major abdominal surgery and nutritional therapy should be provided prior to such surgical procedures in patients with lower albumin level.

3. **Hepatitis B and C screening, HIV screening:**

   This should be routinely done pre-operatively. Post operative infective hepatitis (both B and C) are common in our country (both transfusion and non transfusion related). On the other hand, prevalence of asymptomatic hepatitis B carrier state is also common in India. Pre operative check up of hepatitis B and C status is therefore important from medicolegal point of view.

4. **Renal function test:**

   Urea and creatinine should be routinely checked as post operative complications rise in the presence of azotemia. Dehydration should be avoided. Avoidance of certain drugs (like NSAID, aminoglycosides) and appropriate dose adjustment of antibiotics will be needed. Infusion of hypotonic saline (0.45% saline) prior to angiographic procedure might reduce the incidence of radio-contrast induced kidney damage. Nephrological consultation will be needed in such cases.

5. **Blood glucose:**

Blood glucose should be controlled prior to the surgical procedure. Detailed protocols for pre operative management of diabetes are available in standard text books and these should be consulted for proper reference.

Finally many patients are anxious and stressed before any general anesthetic procedure. Encouraging and reassuring words from the primary care physician work as a tremendous psychological booster for the patients going for surgical procedure.

A PRACTICAL APPROACH FOR THE INTERNISTS

During preoperative assessment following questions needs to be addressed, such as:

Whether the surgery is-
a) Elective b) Urgent c) Emergency

Surgical risk factor-
a) High risk b) Intermediate c) Low risk

Preoperative risk scoring

There different scoring systems are being used, like– ASA, Goldman Cardiac Index etc.

ASA:

1. Fit & Healthy
2. Mild or severe or incapacitating system disease.
3. Moribund- not expected to survive
4. Age > 70 yrs.

Other associated medical conditions:

1. Diabetes Mellitus
2. Addison's disease
3. Active Thyroid
4. Pulmonary/Cardiac complication
5. Hepatic complications
6. CNS complications

Goldman's Cardiac Risk Index:

Risk factors	Points	Score	Mortality
Age > 70	5	0 - 5	0.9 %
MI within last 6 months	10	6 - 11	5.6%
S_3 gallop or jugular venous distention	11	12 - 25	3.8%
Aortic stenosis	3	> 26	78%
Non sinus rhythm	7		
>5 premature ventricular contractions/minute	7		
PO_2 < 60 or PCO_2 > 50 mmHg ;K<3 or HCO_3 <20 mEq/L; BUN > 50 or Cr > 3.0 mg%, or CLD or bedridden from noncardiac causes	3		
Intraperitoneal, aortic, thoracic operation	3		
Emergency operation	4		

Clinically exercise tolerance is a simple tool for risk factor assessment. Patients with poor exercise tolerance has increased perioperative morbidity.

PRE-OPERATIVE TREATMENTS:

Cardiac factors in surgery:

- Control of B.P. <150/90 with medication like β blocker Ca Channel blocker.
- IHD– should be treated with β blockers and nitrates.
- Rhythm problem should be treated.
- Heart failure should be treated.

Renal factors in surgery:

In patients with renal impairment, haematocrit should be maintained around 15% to 20%. Preoperative packed cell transfusion should be used with frusemide. Patients may also need preoperative albumin under IV frusemide. NSAID and IV contrast should be avoided. Dialysis may be offered pre-operatively if $K > 5.5$, HCO_3 is < 15 and if there is fluid overload.

Hepatic disorders:

The operative morbidity depends upon the Child Pugh Score in patients with chronic liver disease (based on albumin, bilirubin, prothrombin time, ascites and encephalopathy and classified into A, B and C category). There is another scoring system called MELD which depends upon cause of liver disease, bilirubin, INR and creatinine.

Surgery needs to be avoided in patients with MELD score of more than 8 or Child Pugh Class B and C.

If surgery is at all contemplated in milder form of liver disease, following principles should be adopted e.g.

1) Platelet at least > 50,000
2) Ascites must be minimized
3) Electrolytes must be corrected
4) Nutrition must be optimized
5) Renal function must be stabilized.

Pulmonary risk factors:

1) Age > 80 yrs
2) Obesity: BMI > 27 kg/m^2

3) Poor exercise capacity
4) Smoking
5) Cough and wheezing
6) REV_1-/FVC = <70%
7) $PaCO_2$ >45 mmHg

Pre-operative management-

- Smoking cessation
- Pre-operative antibiotics may be needed
- Physiotherapy
- Inspiratory muscle training
- Steroids in asthma

Other risk factors:

1) Obstructive sleep apnoea
2) Neurological impairment
3) Immunosuppression

Other associated treatments:

1) Pain control
2) Glycaemic control
3) Role of naso gastric decompression
4) TPN – in selected cases
5) Prevention of DVT

: KEY POINTS :

- Protocol driven pre-operative assessment reduces pre-operative and post-operative complications.
- Physicians should be aware of the common cardio-respiratory risk assessment protocols.

50 A PREGNANT LADY WITH SEVERE HYPERTENSION

CASE: *A 25 years old primigravida at 34 weeks of gestation presented with increasing headache and swelling of her legs. The obstetrician got her admitted for observation and the medical team was involved for further management. She did not have any past history of hypertension, diabetes mellitus or any kind of renal disease. Since 24th week of pregnancy, her BP was noticed to be high and she was on methyldopa. Examination revealed BP of 170/110 mmHg, pedal oedema present. Investigations include FBC normal, platelet normal, urea and creatinine normal, uric acid– 8.1 mg% (high), bilirubin normal, AST and ALT slightly elevated, urine examination– protein++, USG normal foetal movement, no local signs in the liver or kidneys.*

DIAGNOSIS: Pre-eclamptic toxaemia (PET) with severe hypertension.

She was treated with increasing dose of methyldopa, since her BP remained uncontrolled, sublingual nifedipine and nitro-glycerine infusion were commenced sequentially with non-invasive BP monitoring. Her liver function test, uric acid and platelet counts and coagulation profile were monitored regularly. On the third day of following admission, she underwent caesarean section and observed in the ITU during the immediate post operative period. The antihypertensive medications were gradually needed to be tapered off and before discharge her BP was maintained at 140/90 mmHg with methyldopa therapy only.

DISCUSSION:

It is not uncommon to have obstetric patients developing acute problems requiring input from the medical team and physicians should be aware of those conditions and conversant with the management plans.

The common problems encountered are:

- Usual range of medical problems
- Acute surgical emergencies and
- Specific obstetric problems.

While treating such patients, one should remember that during pregnancy, the normal range of physiological variables change, so the therapy is guided to different end-points and both mother and foetus are affected by the pathology and subsequent treatment. The mother's welfare takes precedence over the foetal concerns as foetal survival is dependent on optimal maternal management.

Data from Woodlands Hospital ITU/HDU over a period of 5 years (1998-2003):

Obstetric complication	Medical conditions
Number- 48 cases Eclampsia HELLP Syndrome Post-operative pulmonary oedema Post-partum haemorrhage Sepsis with MODS Pregnancy related jaundice Pregnancy related hypertension	Number- 34 cases Asthma Drug Overdose DVT with pulmonary embolism Falciparum malaria with MODS Enteric fever Rheumatic mitral valve disease Anaesthetic complications Myasthenia gravis GB syndrome Pancreatitis

Common physiological changes during pregnancy:

Cardiovascular

Systolic BP	:	-5 mm Hg.
Mean BP	:	-5 mmHg.
Diastolic BP	:	-15 mmHg.
CVP	:	no change
Pulmonary wedge pressure	:	no change
Heart rate	:	+ 15%
Stroke volume	:	+ 30%
Cardiac output	:	+ 45%
SVR	:	- 15%

Respiratory

Tidal volume	:	+ 40%
Respiratory rate	:	+ 10%
Minute volume	:	+ 50%
Oxygen consumption	:	+ 20%

Blood gas

Ph	:	no change
PaCO2	:	- 10 mmHg

Haematological

Blood volume	:	+ 40%
Haematocrit	:	- 0.06
Plasma albumin	:	- 5 g/*l*.

In addition, there is also change in renal blood flow and due to change in blood volume and altered protein binding, drug metabolism also changes during pregnancy.

MONITORING SPECIFIC CONDITIONS:

Severe preeclampsia:

Hypertension, proteinuria and oedema after 20 weeks of gestation constitute preeclampsia. Frequently physicians are involved in the management. This is a potentially serious condition and if inappropriately treated can lead to increased morbidity and mortality.

Monitoring- Frequent BP monitoring, urine output measurement and meticulous monitoring of fluid balance is essential. Because of decrease in oncotic pressure in pregnancy, there is proneness to develop a pulmonary oedema with inadvertent fluid administration. These patients are prone to develop ARF and urine output should be kept under close observation. As urea level falls during pregnancy, creatinine is a better guide for monitoring renal function. One should also monitor the O_2 saturation as they are prone to aspiration. Commonly used antihypertensive drugs are alpha methyldopa and labetalol (α and β blocker). If labetalol is available then prazosin (α blocker) can be used instead. During severe hypertension, nitroglycerine or even sodium nitroprusside may be used as intravenous infusion with proper monitoring of BP. sublingual nifedipine is frequently used in this situation. Although it is user-friendly, it may aggravate post partum haemorrhage due to uterine atony. Moreover it may interact with $MgSO_4$.

Classification of blood pressure-

Class	Diastolic	Systolic
Mild	90-99 mmHg	140-149 mmHg
Moderate	100-109 mmHg	150-159 mmHg
Severe	>110 mmHg	Systolic > 160 mmHg

Classification of proteinuria-

24 hr urine > 300 mg/mmol

Protein: creatinine ratio > 30 mg/mmol

Mechanism- The mechanism is not fully understood. Essentially it is alteration of balance between thromboxane and prostacyclin in the mother which causes hypertension (anti-aldosterone effect of progesterone), vasospasm, increased endothelial permeability, platelet aggregation and thrombophilia. Consequent to these there is inadequate placental blood supply that causes intrauterine growth retardation.

Drug treatment for hypertension:

Labetalol:

- Oral – 200 mg hourly up to maximum 1600 mg.
- IV – 20 mg bolus followed by 40 mg bolus 10 minutes later, then 80 mg bolus every 10 minutes until desired response, maximum of 220 mg.

Hydralazine:

- IV – 5-10 mg every 15-20 minutes.

Nifedipine:

- Oral – 10 mg, maximum 120 mg/day

Other drugs:

- Oral α-methyldopa
- Oral – prazosin
- IV nitro-glycerine
- IV Sodium nitroprusside

Multisystem effects of preeclampsia-

CNS	Eclampsia (seizure) Cerebral Haemorrhage Cortical blindness Retinal blindness
Renal	Renal Cortical necrosis Renal tabular necrosis
Respiratory	Pulmonary oedema
Liver	Jaundice, HELLP syndrome
Coagulation	DIC
Placenta	Placental infarction
Baby	Preterm birth Intrauterine growth restriction

Eclamptic fit is a medical emergency and must be treated in ITU with IV diazepam or phenytoin. $MgSO_4$ infusion is increasingly being used by the obstetricians. Physicians should be cautious as overdose can cause respiratory paralysis. Loss of ankle jerk is a clinical indicator of such event. Calcium gluconate is an antidote for this side effect.

Prevention of Eclampsia-

Following the MAGPIE trial, it is now recommended that all patients with severe preeclampsia or severe hypertension should be treated with intravenous $MgSO_4$ if birth is planned within 24 hrs. Deep tendon reflexes and respiratory effects should be monitored.

Dose: $MgSO_4$- 4 g IV over 5 minutes followed by IV infusion of 1 g/hr for 24 hrs.

During eclamptic fit $MgSO_4$- IV 2-4 g and rate of infusion may be increased upto 1.5 g/hr.

Prevention:

- Aspirin 75 mg daily (except for in acute stages where chances of bleeding is high)
- Calcium supplementation
- The role of statin (pravastatin) is being explored in ongoing trial (antagonist to endoglin– vascular endothelial growth factor)

HELLP syndrome is a complication of severe eclampsia, characterized by thrombocytopenia, haemolysis, elevated liver enzymes and microangiopathic haemolytic anaemia. This condition should be differentiated from septicaemia with DIC or haemolytic uremic syndrome (please vide the chapter of haemolytic uremic syndrome). If this subgroup of eclamptic patients complains of abdominal pain and vomiting, haemorrhage in the liver should be seriously considered. Regular monitoring of coagulation profile, renal function test and liver function test are essential.

Peripartum haemorrhage is an important cause of maternal morbidity and mortality. As blood volume increases during pregnancy, significant drop of BP does not occur until more than 35% of the blood volume is lost. Most of the cases of maternal deaths are due to underestimation of blood loss. As uterine flow is not auto regulated inotropes should be used with caution as they can cause placental ischemia. Ephedrine does not affect the uterine flow significantly and therefore ideally the drug of choice in such situations. However, inotropes and vasopressors like epinephrine, nor-epinephrine, dopamine or dobutamine should not be withheld if clinically indicated.

Acute liver disease of pregnancy is mainly due to acute fatty liver of pregnancy, hepatitis and associated with HELLP syndrome. In our country Hepatitis E infection carries a particularly high risk of mortality. While monitoring liver function in pregnancy one should remember that alkaline phosphatase increases during pregnancy and therefore AST and ALT are better indicators of liver function.

While managing sepsis during pregnancy if the foetus is viable, supra normal maternal haemodynamics should be achieved (higher cardiac index and oxygen delivery). Therapy should be guided by serum lactate level and SVO_2 of more than 70% (mixed venous oxygen saturation) or SaO_2 of more than 95% (arterial oxygen saturation). Rising lactate and falling SVO_2 indicate tissue hypoxia and increased oxygen extraction by the tissue. Emergency caesarean section in such situation will dramatically reduce the oxygen demand of the mother (it will increase SVO_2 by 5%-8%). Clearly the removal of dead foetus by caesarean section in order to save mother's life needs proper consent from the patient and the relatives. Septic abortion is not uncommon in India and should be kept under appropriate antibiotic cover. Although noradrenalin is the ideal vasopressor in vasodilated septic patients, dopamine is a useful alternative in our country as it is much cheaper.

Common respiratory problems during pregnancy (pregnancy specific):

- Amniotic fluid Embolism (rare)
- Tocolytic pulmonary oedema (Rare)
- Preeclampsia complicated by pulmonary oedema
- Pulmonary Oedema due to puerperal cardiomyopathy
- Obstetric sepsis with ARDS

Risk increased in pregnancy:

- Venous thromboembolism
- Asthma
- Pulmonary oedema due to heart disease
- Aspiration

Asthma frequently exacerbates during pregnancy and while treating acute asthma oxygen saturation should be kept above 95%. The patient should be managed in an upright position leaning forward in a table thereby taking uterus off the IVC (which may cause obstruction to the venous return). Steroids, aminophylline and β-stimulants can be used safely in pregnancy. Intravenous Beta stimulants can rarely cause pulmonary oedema and theophylline can cause foetal tachycardia, however.

Post operative DVT is not so uncommon and can sometimes lead to pulmonary embolism. Sudden onset of respiratory distress in a post operative patient should lead one to suspect silent DVT with pulmonary embolism.

Acute febrile illness is common in India and naturally can occur during pregnancy. Malaria should be excluded by repeated blood tests. Quinine and chloroquine in therapeutic doses are quite safe during pregnancy. During quinine therapy, frequent blood glucose monitoring should be done to detect early hypoglycaemia. During febrile illness, blood culture should be done routinely as we have detected few patients with blood culture positive enteric fever responding to appropriate antibiotic therapy.

Rheumatic heart disease is common in India and patients with stable mitral valve disease may decompensate during pregnancy due to increase in blood volume. Moreover, during 3rd stage of labour extra 500 ml of blood is auto transfused which may precipitate acute LVF. In case of aortic stenosis, due to fixed cardiac output, sudden drop in BP can have catastrophic result. This may be particularly true in case of epidural anaesthesia and quick fluid resuscitation is essential. MR and AR are better tolerated. Congenital heart disease with pulmonary hypertension (PA pressure of > 50 mmHg) is poorly tolerated and it is advisable to avoid pregnancy in such situations.

Isolated ASD, VSD or PDA without pulmonary hypertension is generally well tolerated. During caesarean section in patients with mitral valve disease, intra-operative meticulous attention to fluid balance and BP monitoring is essential as in our experience post operative pulmonary oedema is common and needing ITU management.

During the third stage, one should be careful regarding the use of ergometrine as it increases systemic vascular resistance (SVR) thereby increasing regurgitant lesions while bolus syntocinon (oxytocin) can reduce SVR and worsens cardiac output in patients with fixed cardiac output status (aortic stenosis). If indicated from the obstetric point of view, it should be used as infusion.

It is sometimes necessary to treat cardiac arrhythmias as they may cause cardiac decompensation. Lignocaine, digoxin, verapamil and adenosine can safely be used in pregnancy. Amiodarone can be used in resistant cases. It may cause fatal hypothyroidism, however.

Management of cardiac arrest in pregnancy is no different from non-pregnant women. Few points should be noted however.

- Intubation may be difficult.
- Aspiration is common and application of cricoid pressure is necessary before endotracheal intubation.
- The patient should be tilted 30° laterally with application of wedge on the right side. This is to displace the gravid uterus which may cause aortocaval compression and impede venous return.
- Emergency caesarean section should be performed if resuscitation is unsuccessful within 5 minutes.

CASE: *A 26 years old primigravida at 36 weeks of pregnancy had been complaining frequent dizzy spells. While undergoing an ultrasonographic examination, she was fainted and needing hospital admission for 24 hours. Her BP was low and she responded to fluid therapy. No obvious cause was found to account for her dizziness and hypotension. While she was on the operating table, she started sweating and fainted again. Her BP was 60/40 mmHg. The medical team was called. The foot end was elevated and she was put on left lateral position. Intravenous fluid was given. Her BP came back to normal. She underwent caesarean section in a left lateral tilt and finally made an uneventful recovery.*

DIAGNOSIS: Supine hypotension syndrome.

DRUGS – WHICH CAN SAFELY BE USED IN PREGNANCY

	Safe	With caution	Contraindicated
• **Antibiotics:**	Cephalosporin Amoxicillin Erythromycin	Quinolones Metronidazole	Sulphonamides Chloramphenicol Gentamicin
• **Antihypertensives:**	Alphadopa Labetalol Prazosin	Beta blockers Calcium channel blocker.	ACE inhibitors
• **Antimalarials:**	Chloroquine	Quinine	
• **Antiarrhythmics:**	Digoxin Lignocaine Verapamil	Amiodarone	
• **Antitubercular:**	Rifampicin Ethambutol INH		Streptomycin
• **Anticoagulants:**		Heparin LMW heparin	Warfarin (1st and 3rd trimester)
• **Anti inflammatory analgesics**	Aspirin (may prevent eclampsia) (avoid in 3rd trimester)		Indomethacin (particularly in 3rd trimester)
• **Antiepileptic**		Carbamazepine Phenytoin Barbiturate	Valproate

Carbamazepine and phenytoin have also been reported to have teratogenic effect. However, in the absence of any absolutely safe antiepileptic drugs, carbamazepine and phenytoin may be used with caution explaining to the relatives about the probable effect of the drugs on the foetus.

CASE: *A 34 years old lady was admitted with breathlessness of relevant onset. She was also complaining of falling urine output. She was suffering from infertility and was under gynaecologists for assisted reproduction. On examination her BP was 90/60 mmHg, albumin 2.4 g/dl, Hb- 9.4 g%, creatinine-1.2 mg, USG abdomen showed bilateral pleural effusion and ascites.*

DIAGNOSIS: Ovarian hyper stimulation syndrome.

DISCUSSION:

Ovarian hyper stimulation syndrome is an increasingly recognised condition found in clinical practice since assisted reproductive technologies, particularly the gonadal stimulating hormones therapy, are increasingly used in the treatment of infertility. It is characterised by leaky capillaries with hypoalbuminaemia, polyserositis and hypotension and in severe cases may lead to acute lung injury with ARDS. Treatment is supportive with albumin infusion, haemodynamic support, parenthesis and close observation with respiratory function which may need non-invasive or any invasive ventilatory support.

Preconception care for healthy woman- Role of physician

Frequently healthy women suffering from medical condition take option from their primary care physicians before planning for conception. Hence physicians should be adept with the common clinical conditions that are prevalent in the community in order to provide useful suggestions.

General recommendations:

- **Folic acid** supplementation should be recommended prior to conception upto the first trimester of pregnancy. It reduces the incidence of neural tube defects.
  Risk factors for development of neural tube defects-
  - Diabetes mellitus
  - Obesity
  - PHO of delivery of baby with neural tube defect
  - On an antifolate drugs like phenytoin, trimethoprim, azathioprine.
- **Smoking** > 10 cigarettes/days increases the incidence of still birth. If women stop smoking by 15 weeks of gestation the risk of small baby and preterm birth decreases.
- **Alcohol** causes a condition called foetal-alcohol syndrome (growth retardation and neurological disturbance). Appropriate advice should be given in this regard.

- **Body mass index**– Both under weight and over-weight can pose problem during pregnancy and advice of regular physical exercise and healthy diet should be given accordingly.
- **Maternal age**– Mothers older than 35 years, have increased risk of infertility, impaired growth, miscarriage and maternal complications whereas pregnancy at a very young age is also faced with similar problem.

Patients with hypertension planning for pregnancy

Systolic BP should be kept below 160 mmHg. ACE inhibitors or AT_2 receptor blocker should be stopped (teratogenic) and changed to either methyldopa, calcium channel blockers or labetalol. Use of aspirin 75 mg/day will reduce the risk of preeclampsia.

Patients with diabetes mellitus (Type I and Type II)

There is 2-3 fold increased incidence of foetal malformation. A meta-analysis of studies of HbA_1C showed stepwise risk of malformation according to HbA_1C. **35% risks with HbA_1C of 6%, 65% risks with HbA_1C of 9% & 12% risk with HbA_1C of 12%.**

The goal of management will be, to maintain HbA_1C at a near normal level (4.2%-6.2%), to prescribe folic acid, aspirin and to give lifestyle advice.

Drugs that are may be safely used-

In Systemic Lupus Erythematosus:

Planning for pregnancy is essential. Those with pulmonary hypertension should avoid pregnancy. Those who are on mycophenolate should be changed to azathioprine. Anti-inflammatory analgesic should not be used during 1st trimester and 3rd trimester (risk of premature closure of ductus arteriosus). Preparation containing misoprostol should be absolutely avoided. Steroid, azathioprine, hydroxychloroquine and cyclosporine are safe during pregnancy.

In epilepsy:

No antiepileptic drug is absolutely safe in pregnancy. The most teratogenic drugs like valproate should be changed to relatively safe drugs like phenytoin. Ideally, attempts should be made to withdraw antiepileptic drugs 6 months prior to congestion in women who are seizure free for number of years with a normal EEG and CT scan of brain. Neurological input will be needed in this regard. Folic acid supplementation should be routinely given.

- Valproate – Neural tube defects – avoided
- Lamotrigine – Oral cleft, SJ Syndrome – avoided
- Carbamazepine – Neural tube defects – to use with caution
- Phenytoin – Cleft lip, foetal anticonvulsant syndrome

In heart disease:

Women with mechanical heart values must avoid warfarin in 1st trimester of pregnancy (due to teratogenic effect). Low molecular weight heparin may be used instead. Alternately the regard of Low molecular weight heparin (up to 3 months) → warfarin (2nd trimester) → Low molecular weight heparin (3rd trimester) may also be used. Aspirin may be continued clopidogrel although not increased in pregnancy, may be continued in patients with drug eluting stents, statin (till date) should be avoided during pregnancy.

Risks of maternal mortality in congenital heart disease:

<table>
<tr><td colspan="2">Low risk (< 1% mortality)
• Pulmonary stenosis,
• Atrial septal defect (ASD),
• Ventricular septal defect (VSD),
• Patent ductus arteriosus (PDA),
• Successfully repaired septal defect
• Cohabitation tetralogy of Fallot.</td></tr>
<tr><td>Significant risk (1-10% mortality)
• Mechanical valve
• Single right ventricle
• Fontan's surgical procedure
• Marfan syndrome</td><td>High risk (contradicted, mortality >10%)
• Pulmonary hypertension
• LVEF < 30%
• Aortic aneurysm
• Severe intraluminal aortic stenosis</td></tr>
</table>

Four generic risk factors:

- Cyanosis
- NYHA – class>II
- EF < 30%
- Previous adverse cardiovascular event

The final decision regarding conception should be taken after through discussion between the cardiologists, obstetrician and the family members.

Patients with chronic kidney disease:

Chronic kidney disease adversely affects the outcome of pregnancy. Associated hypertension and diabetes mellitus should be controlled meticulously. Drug treatment may be changed like substitution of mycophenolate to azathioprine. Ideally patients with chronic kidney disease should be advised to have pregnancy early in their life before it progresses to stages III/IV of the disease.

There are umpteenth numbers of chronic medical conditions that may prevail during pregnancy which is outside the scope of discussion in this book. Close liaison with the obstetrician is essential to appropriately deal with such condition.

Women with mental illness on medication may conceive. Usually in majority of the cases the benefit of continuation of antipsychotic drugs outweighs the attended risk. However certain precautions may be taken like avoidance of high risk teratogenic drugs like Valproate. Prolactin raising drugs like sulphide, amisulpride and risperidone should be changed. Lithium levels need monitoring more frequently. Blood glucose should be monitored more frequently as these patients on medications are now prone to develop gestational diabetes.

: KEY POINTS :

- Obstetric patients may sometimes pose specific problems needing input from the physician.
- End point of the treatment goals may be different because of changed physiological variables in pregnancy.
- While treating, both maternal and foetal well being should be taken into consideration although in difficult situations, maternal wellbeing takes precedence over the foetal well being.
- Management should be done with joint consultation with the obstetrician.
- The physician should be aware of the list of drugs which can be safely used in pregnancy.
- No drug is absolutely safe during pregnancy. Drugs should only be prescribed if they are absolutely essential.

FURTHER REFERENCES:

- Saunder's Manual of Critical Care Medicine, 2003.
- Shoemaker's Text book of Critical Care Medicine – 4th edition.
- Alina Vais – Preconception care for healthy women and those with medical condition – BJHM – Vol 74, No 6 June 2013.
- Luchinda Green - Preconception care for healthy women with maternal health condition, BJHM – Vol 74, No 6 June 2013.
- Rhidian Jones – Peripartum management of pre-eclamptic patient. BJHM – Vol 74, No 6 June 2013.
- Harrison's Principle of Internal Medicine – 17th edition.
- Oxford Text Book of Medicine – 5th edition.

51 A PATIENT WITH MELAENA

CASE: *A 72 years old gentleman on aspirin was admitted with history of passage of black stool for last 3 days. On examination, he looked pale; his pulse rate was 110/min, BP-110/70 mmHg. Abdomen- soft, epigastric tenderness present with increased bowel sounds. Investigations revealed Hb of 6.9 g%, WBC- 10,800, normal platelet counts, normal coagulation profile, normal liver function test, normal creatinine with raised urea, amylase was normal. USG examination of abdomen did not reveal anything specific. After transfusing him with 3 units of blood, gastroscopy was performed which showed a large posterior duodenal ulcer.*

DIAGNOSIS: Duodenal ulcer presenting with melaena.

DISCUSSION: Acute upper gastrointestinal haemorrhage is not uncommon presentation in day to day hospital practice. Common causes encountered are:

- Peptic ulcer
- Variceal bleeding
- Mallory Weiss tear
- Oesophagitis, gastritis and duodenitis
- Vascular
- Tumours

There is often history of steroid and NSAID ingestion. Any bleeding beyond the attachment of ligament of treitz usually causes melaena rather than haematemesis. However massive small intestinal bleeding can also cause haematemesis. While dealing with such patients haematemesis should be differentiated from haemoptysis as it may sometimes confuse the clinical picture. Haemoptysis is usually of bright red in colour.

Bleeding from Mallory Weiss tear may be bright red colour. Haematemesis is acidic where as haemoptysis is alkaline in nature.

Relevant history taking usually solves the issue. In peptic ulcer disease there may be history of aspirin, NSAID and steroid intake. In patients with chronic liver disease, variceal bleeding is the cause although in 25% of case peptic ulcer disease may co-exist. Sudden haematemesis (with bright red colour) following vomiting or retching points towards the diagnosis of Mallory Weiss tear.

Recent history of aortic-graft insertion would suggest aorto-duodenal fistula. Presence of telangiectatic lesion in the mouth may indicate hereditary haemorrhagic telangiectasia. Presence of Virchow's nodes in the neck may point towards an underlying gastric malignancy. Other causes like gastric antral vascular ectasia, Dieulafoy's lesion, gastric lymphoma etc needs endoscopic examination for proper diagnosis.

In critically ill patients, upper gastrointestinal bleeding is a common problem and it is usually multifactorial like severe thrombocytopenia due to DIC, in septicaemic patients, stress ulceration and use of anticoagulants like heparin *etc.*

INVESTIGATIONS:

- Full blood count
- Coagulation screening
- Liver function test
- Urea, creatinine, electrolytes
- Gastroscopy

MANAGEMENT: While the diagnostic work up is on, full resuscitative measures should be taken. Haemodynamically unstable patient should be preferably managed in High Dependency Unit with CVP monitoring. Fluids in the form of crystalloids (Normal saline) should be given with appropriate CVP monitoring.

Blood transfusion should be targeted at an Hb level of approximately 10 g%. Endoscopy should only be done after appropriate fluid resuscitation otherwise it can cause morbidity particularly in elderly population.

Majority of the patients presenting with upper Gl bleeding settle with conservative treatment. However, occasional patients need endoscopic therapy. The situations are:

- Bleeding oesophageal varices.
- Peptic ulcer with stigmata of recent haemorrhage.
- Vascular malformations.

TREATMENT FOR BLEEDING PEPTIC ULCER:

Injection of adrenaline (1:10,000)- This is very effective in controlling bleeding. Addition of sclerosant like polidocanol, ethanolamine does not give any additional benefit. On the contrary they can cause necrosis of the injected area.

Heat probe - Application of heat probe over the bleeding area is an equally effective way of securing haemostasis. Application of Argon Plasma Coagulator (APC) via an endoscopically placed catheter is one of such ways of securing haemostasis.

However, combination of injection of adrenaline and application of heat probe does not add on to the efficacy of each other.

Indication of endoscopic therapy: Not all patients will need endoscopic therapy. There are certain endoscopic stigmata of impending re-bleeding with attendant high mortality. The stigmata are:

- Active spurting haemorrhage.
- Non bleeding visible vessel
- Adherent blood clot over the arterial defect.

The aforementioned findings are associated with high chance of re-bleeding which may prove catastrophic.

MEDICATION:

- Gastric pH should be kept above 6.8 as acid environment destabilizes the clot. Injecting omeprazole (bolus 80 mg followed by 72 hours infusion in a dose of 8 mg/hr) has been shown to reduce the incidence of re-bleeding. H_2 blocker although widely used do not decrease the risk of re-bleeding from duodenal ulcers.
- Continuous infusion of somatostatin has been shown to reduce the incidence of re-bleeding. The mechanism of action is by reduction of mesenteric blood flow and suppression of acid secretion.
- Tranexamic acid, by way of its antifibrinolytic activity with stabilization of the blood clot, can reduce the chance of re-bleeding.

SURGICAL THERAPY:

Now-a-days, it is rarely needed. However in occasional elderly patients, medical therapy along with endoscopic therapy may fail. In such situations emergency surgery is the way forward. In duodenal ulcer, under running of the ulcer with pyloroplasty and in gastric ulcer, partial gastrectomy is all that is required. Vagotomy is not done nowadays because of acid suppressing effects of proton pump inhibitors.

In critically ill patients stress ulcer bleeding is common and the risk factors are mechanical ventilation, renal failure and coagulopathy. The best treatment is prophylactic use of H_2 blockers, sucralfate and antacids.

After successful treatments, the patients should receive *H. pylori* eradication therapy. PPI should be prescribed with NSAID in patients needing long term NSAID.

The index patient underwent gastroscopy which showed a moderately large posterior duodenal ulcer and the endoscopist thought it to be prudent to be treated with local adrenaline injection therapy. He received blood transfusion and fluid resuscitation and fortunately there was no recurrence of the GI bleeding. He was given a course of *H pylori* eradication therapy and was discharged with 6 months course of omeprazole therapy.

CASE: *A 66 years old gentleman was admitted in a shock state with massive haematemesis and melaena. Clinically there was evidence of jaundice and ascites. After resuscitation with fluids and blood transfusion, he underwent gastroscopy which showed evidence of grade III oesophageal varices. His liver function test was deranged with raised bilirubin, raised AST and ALT and low albumin. His prothrombin time was raised. He was found to be positive for hepatitis B surface antigen and the alpha fetoprotein was markedly raised. Ultrasound examination of abdomen showed evidence of chronic liver disease with ascites. Additional information from CT scan was suggestive of a hypodense lesion of liver consistent with hepatoma.*

DIAGNOSIS: Variceal bleeding in a patient with hepatitis B positive. Chronic liver disease with hepatoma of liver.

He was treated with somatostatin infusion, variceal band ligation along with general supportive measures. FNAC from the hypodense lesion from liver confirmed hepatoma. Following discharge, he underwent repeat band ligation after 8 weeks. Although he was stable, the poor prognosis was explained to the relatives. He remained under regular follow up by an oncologist.

DISCUSSION: Variceal bleeding accounts for 10-30% of upper GI bleeding. The mortality rate varies from 40% to 70% prognosis depends upon the underlying hepatic function status which can be determined by CHILDS CRITERIA.

Child-Turcotte-Pugh Scoring System to assess severity of liver disease

Clinical and Laboratory measurements	Points scored for increasing abnormality		
	1	2	3
1. Encephalopathy (grade)	None	1-2	3-4
2. Ascites	None	Mild or controlled by diuretics	At least moderate despite diuretic treatment
3. Prothrombin time (sec. prolonged)	< 4	4-6	> 6
4. Albumin (g/dl)	> 3.5	2.8-3.5	< 2.8
5. Bilirubin (mg/dl)	< 2	2-3	> 3

Total Score: 5-6 (Grade-A), 7-9 (Grade-B), 10-15 (Grade-C)

Factors associated with high risk of first variceal haemorrhage:

- Red sign, red wale mark on varices.
- Childs class.
- Varices size.

MANAGEMENT:

Endoscopic therapeutic approach (sclerotherapy or ligation of varices) for acute control of bleeding is effective in about 90% of cases.

Infusion of **octreotide** (100 microgram bolus followed by 50 microgram/hour for 48 hours, followed by 100 microgram subcutaneously every 8 hours for total 72 hours) is also effective particularly when it is combined with sclerotherapy or band ligation. Alternatively intravenous **terlipressin** (a synthetic vasopressin analogue) may also be used instead of octreotide. It is superior to vasopressin and does not need nitroglycerine along with it. Somatostatin infusion is another option.

In severe bleeding, as a temporary measure, **balloon tamponade** may be used to control bleeding pending definitive therapy with band ligation. ***Sengstaken Blakemore Tube*** is the device traditionally used for this condition. However, the four-lumen ***Minnesota tube insertion*** is the safest of the available devices because it allows continuous aspiration of secretions that tend to collect proximal to the oesophageal balloon. Patients should be endotracheal intubated to protect the respiratory tract and the position of the partially inflated gastric balloon should be confirmed radiographically before full inflation. One should remember that it is a temporary measure and the tube should be removed as soon as possible.

Transjugular intrahepatic portosystemic shunt (TIPS), a non surgical means used in severe cases An expert hands can cause hepatic decompression in 90% of cases with control of severe variceal bleeding.

For **prevention of re-bleeding,** beta blocker (propranolol - will reduce the re-bleeding by about 40%) along with nitrate is used. Repeat variceal ligation may be done.

CASE: *A 91 years old otherwise fit patient presented with episodic melaena and haematochezia. He had history of diabetes mellitus, asthma and old CVA for which he was on clopidogrel. Initial gastroscopy showed small vascular ectasia, a very unlikely source of bleeding. Colonoscopy revealed multiple colonic diverticulitis, again an unlikely source of bleeding as the blood was seen to be coming from above the ileocecal valve. 10 years prior to admission, he was investigated for malabsorption and was found to have multiple jejunal diverticulitis. Mesenteric angiography was avoided in view of past history of acute renal failure following aminoglycoside therapy for a chest infection. He underwent enteroscopy from the upper end. The scope could be negotiated up to mid ileum and the test confirmed the source of bleeding from the jejunal diverticulitis.*

DIAGNOSIS: Small intestinal bleeding due to jejunal diverticula.

Capsule endoscopy and push enteroscopy are the two recently developed tests that will be very helpful for investigation of small intestinal bleeding. In this particular case, capsule endoscopy was avoided because it is relatively contra indicated in the presence of jejunal diverticulitis for fear of obstruction.

CASE: *A 51 years old gentleman presented with haematochezia with a history of central abdominal and right iliac fossa pain for last 6 months. Clinical examination was satisfactory. Hb was 8.1 g%, normal WBC and platelet count, high ESR and CRP, liver function test showed low albumin and mildly raised AST and ALT. Urea was high but creatinine normal. USG abdomen NAD. Colonoscopy could be negotiated in the terminal part of ileum which showed discrete ulcers. Biopsy report was consistent with Crohn's disease. He was treated with blood transfusion, mesalazine and other supportive therapies and finally discharged home in a stable condition. Within the next six months he was admitted twice with haematochezia. A repeat colonoscopy yielded identical findings. Small bowel enema did not add anything specific. After detailed counseling he was persuaded to have Capsule Endoscopy to make sure no other associated organic lesions have been missed. Detailed discussion was needed because of prohibitive cost of Capsule Endoscopy by Indian standards. Capsule Endoscopy confirmed extensive ulceration in the terminal part of small intestine. By this time AFB culture report from the biopsy specimen came back positive for Mycobacterium tuberculosis. 4 drugs ATD regime was commenced and found better in 6 months follow up.*

DIAGNOSIS: Tubercular enteritis presenting as recurrent haematochezia.

DISCUSSION: The source of small intestinal bleeding is sometimes difficult to detect as it is out of reach of the routine investigative tools. It sometimes become challenging in clinical practice to find out the source of bleeding once gastroscopy and colonoscopy yield negative results.

CASE: *A 71 years old patient presented with dizziness followed by collapse which was found to be due to sudden massive melaena. In gastroscopy and colonoscopy NAD. The patient continue to have melaena and haematochezia, RBC tagged scan was not helpful in locating the bleeding sites. He was considered to have mesenteric angiogram, capsule endoscopy or push enteroscopy. Finally it was decided to subject him to push enteroscopy for its therapeutic potential. He was referred to a gastroenterologist in another city experienced in this procedure. He was found to have ileal ulcer which was treated with local adrenaline injection therapy with ultimate cessation of bleeding.*

DIAGNOSIS: Bleeding ileal ulcer diagnosed by enteroscopy.

Causes of small intestinal bleeding:

- Vascular lesions as described above
- Neoplasm (commonly benign)- leiomyomas, leiomyosarcoma are most common
- Lymphoma
- Polyps (associated with Peutz-Jeghers syndrome)
- Carcinoid
- Metastatic -melanoma
- Breast cancer
- Ovarian cancer etc

Infection and inflammatory lesion:

- Crohn's disease
- Tuberculosis
- Cytomegalovirus

Others:

- Meckel's diverticulum
- Vasculitis
- Ischaemic ulcers
- NSAID related ulcers
- Small bowel diverticulum
- Haemobilia
- Small intestinal varices due to liver cirrhosis, portal vein thrombosis.

How to investigate: Ulcers, strictures and tumours can be detected by conventional studies like- small bowel enema and CT scan. However, flat lesions (like vascular lesions) will be difficult to detect by these methods (Diagnostic yield 5-10%). Angiography has a 50% success rate, provided there is active bleeding at a rate of 0.5 ml/minute and in 25% of cases where there is no bleeding. Technetium-99m is successful in approximately 75% of cases in diagnosing Meckel's diverticulum. 60-70% of the small intestinal lesions are within the reach of standard endoscopy. Push enteroscopy with specially designed enteroscope allows examination of the entire jejunum. Intra-operative enteroscopy can increase the diagnostic yield to 75-80%.

Wireless video-endoscopy is a new technique for visualization of small intestine, providing diagnosis in 50-60% of cases. The patient swallows a capsule which has got a light source, lens digital receiver and transmitter. It transmits 50,000 digital images over 8 hour's period to a sensor and data recorder worn by the patient. The data is finally downloaded and interpreted by the computer finally to be viewed through a video recorder by the physician within one hour.

In spite of meticulous attempts no cause of bleeding may be found in a small number of patients.

CASE: *A 51 one years old patient was admitted with intermittent epigastric pain, acidity, flatulence and recent history of black stool. His Hb was 8.1 g%, liver function test was normal. Gastroscopy demonstrated severe gastric erosion at the pyloric end and rapid urease test was positive for H. pylori infection.*

DIAGNOSIS: *H. pylori* related gastric erosion presenting with melaena.

DISCUSSION:

H. pylori related upper gastro intestinal diseases are a common problem encountered in clinical practice. Common conditions associated with *H. pylori* infections are-

1. Gastric ulcer, erosion
2. Duodenal ulcer
3. Gastric carcinoma
4. Mucosa Associated Lymphoid tissue (MALT), lymphoma

Possible associations are:

1. Gastro esophageal reflux diseases
2. Esophageal carcinoma
3. Non ulcer dyspepsia
4. autoimmune gastritis with pernicious anemia
5. Iron deficiency anemia
6. Controversial associations are IHD and cerebrovascular accidents.

In any patient with upper gastro-intestinal symptoms, gastroscopy should be done early if the symptoms are not remitting easily with symptomatic treatment or relapsing following cessation of H_2 blocker or proton pump inhibitor therapy. The diagnosis is done with rapid urease test done at gastroscopy and treatment should be done immediately. The regime includes triple or quadruple therapy.

Common regime used:

Proton pump inhibitor twice per day + amoxicillin 1g twice perday + clarithromycin 500 mg twice per day or metronidazole 500 mg twice per day (if allergic to penicillin).

If all the four drugs are used for 10 days → eradication 81.3%.

PPI + Bismuth citrate (420 μg) + Metronidazole + Tetracycline for 10-14 days (De Noltab)

Rate of eradication → 84 %

Since many patients can't tolerate all the four drugs at a time, sequential therapy has also been suggested which includes

PPI- twice daily + Amoxicillin twice daily × 5 days. Followed by-

PPI- twice daily + Metronidazole + Tinidazole twice daily + Clarithromycin 500 mg twice daily × 5 days.

The eradication rate is 84.3 %

H. pylori eradication therapy not only prevents relapse of the disease and symptoms but also helps in the prevention of malignancy.

: KEY POINTS :

- Gastrointestinal bleeding is a common presentation in clinical practice.
- Most of the bleeding sources are detected by gastroscopy or colonoscopy.
- Gastric, duodenal or variceal bleeding has definite protocol treatment.
- Small intestinal bleeding source is difficult to detect.
- Video assisted capsule endoscopy and enteroscopy are two recently developed techniques to detect small intestinal bleeding source.

FURTHER REFERENCES:

- Management of haematemesis and melaena- K Palmar, PG. Med. J, 2004, 80 : 399-404.
- Modern management of oesophageal varix - P J Gow, R.W. Chapman, PG Medical journal 2001, 7 7 : 75-81.
- Harrison's Principles of Internal Medicine
- Quarterly review of French Medical and Pharmaceutical News vol.62 no.3 Aug 2014.

52 A PATIENT WITH SUBCLINICAL HYPERTHYROIDISM

CASE: *A 36 years old obese lady attended the clinic because of palpitation. She also complained of vague musculoskeletal pain. Examination revealed pulse rate of 106/min, BP 120/80 mmHg, no thyroid goiter. Biochemical and haematological parameter were normal. TSH 0.01 mIU/L or μIU/ml (↓), T_3 and T_4 in the high normal range. ECG showed sinus tachycardia. USG thyroid gland NAD, on further questioning she admitted that she was taking thyroxin tablet (100 microgram) for weight reduction.*

DIAGNOSIS: Subclinical hyperthyroidism (factitious).

DISCUSSION:

Suppressed TSH (< 0.1 mIU/L or μIU/ml) in the face of normal T_3 and T_4 is a common biochemical abnormality encountered in clinical practice. Clinicians are often in a dilemma particularly if the patient is clinically euthyroid as well. Proper history taking, drug therapy and enquiry about other associated co-morbid conditions should be done meticulously in order to treat this condition.

Causes of suppressed TSH (< 0.1 mIU/L with normal T3 and T4 levels):

- Thyroxin therapy.
- Multinodular goitre.
- Suppressive thyroid hormone therapy in patients with thyroid cancer.
- Subclinical hyperthyroidism.
- Sick euthyroid syndrome.

Sometimes TSH level is not related to thyroid problem altogether. TSH may be suppressed in severe illness unrelated to thyroid, with high doses of steroid and dopamine (which can suppress TSH). TSH may also below in hypothalamic or pituitary dysfunction. In 20% of healthy young females in the 1st trimester of pregnancy TSH may also be low.

Problems with persistently ↓TSH with normal T_3 & T_4 (subclinical hyperthyroidism):

Persistently low TSH is associated with increased cardiovascular and musculoskeletal morbidities. Moreover in the long term it can even cause cognitive impairment. The incidences of atrial fibrillation and cardiac failure are high in the long run. The incidence of osteoporotic fractures is also common.

How to tackle the situation?

Whenever treating patients with thyroxin, the target TSH should be kept between 0.3 to 3.0 micro IU/ml and the dose of thyroxin should be adjusted accordingly. However when the patient is getting thyroxin as suppressive therapy for thyroid cancer, the TSH should be kept below 0.1 microIU/ml. In case of multinodular goitre, there is a point in favour of suppressive therapy although the risk benefit ratio of such therapy should be assessed periodically. Other non-thyroid causes of suppressed TSH should be ruled out.

In patients with endogenous subclinical hyperthyroidism where other causes have been ruled out, there is as yet no consensus of opinion regarding the treatment. Expert opinions suggest that in the event of atrial fibrillation or decreasing bone mass due to osteoporosis or unexplained weight loss, there is a point in favour of treatment either with oral anti-thyroid medication or radio-iodine. The problem is recurrence of symptoms following its discontinuation and so the treatment has to be for an indefinite period. In such cases, thyroid function test has to be monitored every 6 months.

CASE: *A 67 year old lady presented with history of fever and throat pain along with difficulty in deglutition. A course of antibiotic for a presumed diagnosis of pharyngitis did not yield a favorable result and her fever and throat pain continued. Examination revealed tachycardia along with tenderness over the anterior aspect of the neck. Her WBC count was normal and ENT consultation didn't reveal anything specific to account for her symptoms. Her T_3 and T_4 were found to be mildly raised along with a high ESR & CRP. Ultrasonography of the neck was apparently normal. Radio isotope scan of thyroid gland showed diminished uptake by the thyroid gland. She received a course of NSAID, β blocker and tapering dose of steroid over two weeks with relief of her symptoms. Six weeks following the event her thyroid function became normal.*

DIAGNOSIS: Sub acute thyroiditis (de Quervain's thyroiditis).

This condition is occasionally encountered in clinical practice and sometimes missed if the clinician is not aware of it. Classical features are throat pain with local tenderness over the thyroid gland, fever and features of mild thyrotoxicosis the ESR is high and there is diminished uptake of the thyroid gland in radio isotope scanning. Treatment is with NSAID a short course of steroid and β-blockers may be needed. Periodic thyroid function test needs to be done as a portion of patient may develop hypothyroidism.

Other causes of thyroiditis:

- Acute – Bacterial infection, Radiation
- Sub acute – Postpartum, Mycobacterial
- Chronic – Hashimoto's thyroiditis, Riedel's thyroiditis

Drugs causing thyroiditis:

- Amiodarone
- TNF-alfa
- Interferon

In clinical practice occasionally abnormalities of thyroid function like raised T_3 and T_4 level with normal TSH are encountered. In patients without any evident of thyrotoxicosis, this is due to changes of thyroxin binding protein due to different conditions. Measurement of free thyroxin level usually settles the issue.

Common causes of euthyroid hyperthyroxinemia:

- Pregnancy
- Oestrogen
- Cirrhosis of lever
- Hepatitis

SUBCLINICAL HYPOTHYROIDISM: More commonly mildly elevated TSH level with normal T_3 and T_4 level, is encountered in clinical practice. The patients are either asymptomatic or very mildly symptomatic. The clinician needs to decide regarding thyroxin replacement therapy in such patients. If the patient has definite symptoms of hypothyroidism, the decision is easy. In asymptomatic patients, one needs to take into consideration of the following things.

- Presence of anti-thyroid antibody.
- Elevated levels of lipids particularly cholesterol.
- Whether the patient is pregnant or not.
- History of infertility.

In patients with anti-thyroid antibody, presence of raised lipids levels and in patients with pregnancy or infertility mildly elevated TSH (5-10) should be treated. In ischemic heart disease, the introductory dose should be 125 mcg daily. TSH level should periodically monitored as suppressed TSH level, as described before will have adverse consequences. Thyroid function should be routinely monitored in men more than 65 years old, women more than 35 years of age and during pregnancy.

: KEY POINTS :

- Subclinical hyperthyroidism and hypothyroidism are common clinical dilemmas in clinical practice.
- Sick euthyroid syndrome should be considered in the differential diagnosis in appropriate cases.
- Sub clinical hyperthyroidism should be treated in selected cases mainly in patients with osteoporosis and atrial fibrillation.
- Subclinical hypothyroidism should be treated in presence of anti-thyroid antibody, increased cholesterol, pregnancy and infertility.
- Thyroid function test should be routinely checked in middle aged women, elderly men and in pregnancy.

FURTHER REFERENCES:

- Hyperthyroidism - David S Cooper, Lancet 2003, 362; 459 - 68.
- Subclinical hyperthyroidism - *to treat or not to treat*, E.H. Hoogerndorn *et al*., Post grad med: 394 - 398 Journal 2004: 80.
- Subclinical hyperthyroidism - A.D. Tott NEJ M – Vol. 345, N - 7, August 16 -200, P-512-517.
- Subclinical hypothyroidism - David S Cooper, NEJM Vol. 345, No 4 July 26, 2001.
- Harrison's Principle of Internal Medicine – 17th edition.
- Oxford Textbook of Medicine – 5th edition.

53 A PATIENT WITH SEDATIVE OVER DOSE

CASE: *A 71 years old diabetic and hypertensive gentleman was admitted in a comatose state. Examination revealed unconscious patient with Glasgow Coma Scale of 6, pupil non-reacting to light, deep reflexes absent, plantars unresponsive, no neck stiffness. Initial investigations– high blood glucose (280 mg%), electrolytes normal, blood gas analysis normal, normal liver function test, urea and creatinine raised, urine ketone negative, ECG– hypertensive changes, cardiac enzymes normal. CT brain scan was normal. He was given IV naloxone without any response. Next he was given IV flumazenil (total 2 mg over 10 minutes) to which he opened his eyes. Over the next few days he was treated with supportive therapy and he became conscious after 72 hours. His stay in the ITU was complicated with aspiration pneumonia, renal failure needing haemodialysis and nosocomial sepsis. Fortunately he could be sent home in a stable condition. He admitted to have taken 46 diazepam tablets.*

DIAGNOSIS: Diazepam overdose.

DISCUSSION:

Accidental and deliberate self poisoning for attempted suicide is a common problem encountered in hospital practice and the internists should be able to deal with the initial management of such case before requesting for specialist opinion. While it will be impossible to deal with all kinds of poisoning encountered in a hospital setting in this book, general initial management scheme for any patient presenting with poisoning has been described.

Many of these patients present in an unconscious or semiconscious state and reversible medical conditions like hypoglycemia, hyperglycemia, electrolyte imbalance, myocardial infarction or cerebrovascular accident should be excluded.

EPIDERMIOLOGY:

In 2005, in India 113 914 estimated cases of poisoning with insecticides were reported although overdose may occur with any medicines or substances; pesticide poisoning is still the commonest in the Indian scenario, due to easy availability of them.

Poisoning may occur by way of inhalation (toxic fumes), ingestion, absorption and infection and it can be either due to homicidal, suicidal, accidental or occupational. While dealing with a patient of unknown poisoning a clinician should try to identify generic symptoms (toxidromes) in order to find out the brand group of those substances. Common toxidromes are –

Cholinergic toxidromes effects- Diarrhoea, urination, miosis, bradycardia, bronchospasm, emesis, lacrimation, sweating salivation.

Common elements:

- Organophosphates irreversibly binds to cholinesterases
- Carbamates – Reversibly binds to cholinesterases
- Pesticides

Anticholinergic toxidromes effects- Dry mouth, mental status changes, mydriasis, fever, tachycardia, hypertension, urinary retention, seizures.

Common drugs: atropine, antispasmodics, antihistaminics, antipsychotics, tricyclic antidepressants.

Sympathomimetic drugs effects: Hypertension, tachycardia, hyperpyrexia, mydriasis, delirium

Common chemicals responsible: substances of abuse like cocaine, amphetamine.

CNS depressants result: Respiratory depression, miosis.

Common chemicals responsible: opioids, sedatives.

(It should be noted that while symptoms of anticholinergics and sympathomimatics are similar. However while dryness of skin is common in the former group, sweating is a common feature of the later group.)

Glasgow coma scale (GCS) should be used to assess the level of consciousness. General examination may be give some clues like –

Constricted pupil:

- Morphine and its analogues
- Organophosphorus and Carbamates

Dilated pupil:

- Tricyclic antidepressants
- Anticholinergics
- Antihistaminics

Cerebellar signs with nystagmus:

- Alcohol
- Antiepileptics

Convulsions:

- Tricyclic antidepressants
- Theophylline
- Antihistaminics

Hyperventilation:

- Aspirin
- Amphetamine
- Cocaine

Increased Salivation:

- Organophosphorus poisoning

Bradycardia:

- Digoxin
- Beta blockers
- Calcium Channel blockers
- Organophosphorus

Tachycardia:

- Tricyclic antidepressants
- Hypoglycemic agents
- Amphetamines
- Cocaine

Extrapyramidal syndromes:

- Phenothiazines
- Metoclopramide
- Haloperidol

Hyperthermia:

- Amphetamine
- Cocaine
- Neuroleptic malignant syndrome
- Serotonin syndrome

Clinical examination also gives useful clues:

	Sign	Toxin Poison
Colour	Pink	Cyanide
	Red	Rifampicin
	Blue	Aniline, methemoglobinemia
	Yellow (Jaundice)	Paracetamol, $CuSO_4$, hepatotoxic drugs
Odour	Garlic	Arsenic
	Sweet	Ethanol
	Bitter	Cyanide, Carbon monoxide
Urine Colour	Brown	Myoglobin
	Black	Phenol
	Red	Rifampicin
	Green/Blue	Copper Sulphate, Methylene blue

LABORATORY TEST: Routine laboratory tests also give useful clues *e.g.*

- **Respiratory acidosis**: indicates intake of respiratory depressants like sedatives and hypnotics.
- **Metabolic acidosis (high anion gap)**: occurs in ethylene glycol, methanol and salicylates.

Increased osmolar gap: High osmolar gap is found in ethanol, ethylene glycol and methanol poisoning. Osmolar gap is the difference between the calculated osmolality and measured osmolality. The value is usually < 10.

Calculated osmolality = 2(Na + K) + Glucose (in mmol) + urea (in mmol).

In addition, blood should also be sent for analysis of common toxicological substances prevalent in that area.

ECG and X-ray chest should be done routinely. ECG may show MI, heart block or specific arrhythmias while X-ray chest may show aspiration pneumonia which is commonly associated with sedative overdose.

MANAGEMENT:

- Decontamination of skin
- Decontamination of eyes
- Gastric decontamination

Initial management:

- **Airway should be protected** and the patient should be intubated if necessary and ventilated if there is respiratory depression.
- **Circulation should be maintained** with IV fluid along with inotropes and vasopressors to maintain the BP.
- In an unconscious patient with unknown poisoning IV **naloxone** (opioids antagonist) and IV **flumazenil** (benzodiazepine antagonist) should be used and in appropriate case their use may sometimes pay rich dividends. In cases of diazepam poisoning, IV flumazenil (0.2 mg) can cause transient arousal, thereby confirm the diagnosis. It is mainly used as a diagnostic purpose and should be avoided in patients with history of epilepsy.
- **Gastric lavage** should be collected if the patient arrives within 1-2 hours of overdose. It is contraindicated in poisoning due to corrosive and caustic agents.

- **Activated charcoal** (0.5-1 g/kg of body weight) directly and reversibly absorbs most substances except iron, lithium and pesticides. It also interrupts enterohepatic circulation of many toxic substances. It may create concentration gradient that allows diffusible substances already absorbed into the bloodstream to return to the intestinal lumen for elimination (intestinal dialysis).
- **Multiple dose charcoal** may be indicated (50g 4 hourly) in life threatening overdose with carbamazepine, theophylline, quinine and phenobarbitone.

Activated Charcoal	
Effective	**Not so effective**
Carbamazepine	Lithium
Diazepam	Iron
Digoxin	Alcohol
Salicylate	Lead
Theophylline	Hydrocarbons
Tricyclics	Caustics

- **Whole bowel irrigation** (using non-absorbable ethylene polyglycol) is indicated in certain overdoses like lithium, iron ingestion of large dose of enteric coated drugs like theophylline.

Methods to increase drug excretion:

- **Urinary alkalinization**: 1 litre of sodium bicarbonate (1.26%) is given over 3 hours; 20-40 mmol of potassium is added as it is difficult to produce alkaline urine in the face of hypokalaemia. The target urinary pH is 7.5 or more. Drugs that are eliminated by this method are – Phenobarbitone, Salicylates.
- **Haemodialysis** may be indicated in phenobarbitone, salicylates, lithium and ethylene glycol overdose. It is less effective when the toxin has large volume of distribution, large molecular weight or high protein binding.
- **Charcoal haemoperfusion**: may be helpful in overdose of theophylline and carbamazepine.
- **Peritoneal dialysis**: Alcohol, long acting salicylates, lithium.

- **Exchange transfusion** – may be considered in fatal irreversible toxicity when the patient is deteriorating in spite of best supportive therapy e.g. in arsenic or sodium chlorate poisoning.

Specific Antidotes:

Morphine and related substance	Naloxone
Benzodiazepines	Flumazenil (for diagnostic purpose)
Organophosphorus	Atropine and pralidoxime chloride
Carbamates	Atropine
Acetaminophen	N-acetylcysteine
Beta blockers	Glucagon, adrenaline
Calcium channel blockers	Calcium

- **Chelation** for elimination of heavy metal poison.

BAL – Arsenic Leak, Copper Mercury

EDTA – Cobalt, Iron, Cadmium

Desferrioxamine mesylate – Iron

DMSA – Lead, Mercury

- **Supportive Care**

Management of Cardiac problems:

Cardiac toxicity is common in many overdoses e.g. TCAs, anti histamines, pesticides, cardiac medicine. ECG gives useful clues regarding rate, rhythm, QRS Complexes, QT Intervals.

For tachycardia (commonly due to tricyclics)-

- Patient should be maintained at 7.40-7.45 pH with sodium bicarbonate
- Lignocaine may be used for ventricular tachycardia
- Isoprenaline may be used for torsades
- Defibrillation for ventricular fibrillation

For bradycardia:

- Patient should be maintained at 7.40-7.45 pH
- Temporary pacing may be needed
- Resuscitation should be continued for at least 1 hour

Procedures not done now-a-days:

- Forced diuresis – Can cause fluid overload
- Acid diuresis – previously done for amphetamine and phencyclidine. May produce myoglobinuria and renal failure.

Our experience of poisoning over 4 years Period in an urban private hospital catering to the needs of middle class population:

Total number of cases	**54 cases**
Mortality	2
Sedative	33
Tricyclic antidepressant	9
Phenobarbitone	2
Organophosphorus compounds	5
Muriatic acid	3
Phenol	1

Total mortality was two. One patient died of multiorgan failure due to severe diazepam overdose. The second patient died of cardiovascular collapse due to multiple overdoses of sedatives and tricyclics. Rest of the patients responded to supportive therapy. Two patients with muriatic acid poisoning needed surgical intervention later on. Sedative overdose was particularly common in young females.

Patients recovering from self poisoning must have psychiatric assessment prior to discharge to evaluate the mental health status and risk of further suicidal attempts at a later date.

CASE: *A 63 years old gentleman was admitted from the railway station where he was found to be lying unconscious in the railway compartment. He was returning from a holiday trip. A fellow passenger mentioned that he was absolutely normal in the train, had his breakfast and enjoyed a cup of tea from an outside vendor couple of hours before the final arrival. Examination revealed deeply unconscious patient, deep reflexes lost, pupil sluggishly reacting to light, no neck stiffness. Finger prick glucose was normal, normal blood gas analysis, normal ECG, electrolytes normal, CT brain scan normal. A lumbar puncture was planned. However, before the LP, diagnostic injection of flumazenil made transient arousal of the patient, thereby confirming diazepam poisoning. With supportive therapy, the patient made a complete recovery in next 72 hours and was discharged home. He reported to have lost his purse with money and valuables.*

DIAGNOSIS: Diazepam poisoning.

: KEY POINTS:

- Drug overdose is a common problem in hospital practice.
- It should be considered in any patient presenting with unconscious state.
- Empirical antidote in suspected cases may help to clinch an exact diagnosis.
- Protocolized treatment schedules are available for the treatment of individual poisoning.
- Psychiatric counseling is needed before discharge to assess risks for future suicidal attempts.

FURTHER REFERENCES:

- Churchills Pocket Book of Toxicology - Alison Jones, Paul Dargan
- Critical Care Medicine – Saunderis *et al.*

54 AN ELDERLY MAN WITH CONFUSIONAL STATE

CASE: *An 82 years old patient with past history of MI was admitted with confusional state. He had a brief spell of diarrhoea which responded to norfloxacin-tinidazole therapy. While in the toilet during his diarrhoeal episode he had a brief fall without any apparent injury. On examination, no definite abnormality was found. His Na^+ was 122 mmol/lit, K^+ was 3.2 mmol/lit, Troponin T- negative, ECG- old anteroseptal MI with no fresh changes. In spite of correcting his hyponatraemia, he remained mildly confused and after 48 hours of hospital admission he underwent a CT brain scan which revealed acute subdural haematoma. He was referred to the neurosurgeon for necessary action.*

DIAGNOSIS: Acute confusional state due to metabolic encephalopathy along with subdural haematoma.

The relatives were not keen on any surgical intervention because of his age and frailty and they discharged him home against medical advice. In elderly population subdural haematoma may occur even without any history of apparent head injury and clinician should request for a brain imaging in an elderly patient with confusional state.

DISCUSSION: With increasing number of elderly population in the community, the primary care physician or an internist will be confronting with geriatric problems more frequently into their day to day clinical practice. Department of geriatric is still in its nascent stage in India, the young and freshly graduated clinicians are not always adapted to tackle the problems arising in this population. Few salient points in the management of the care for the elderly have been discussed over here. While dealing with the medical problems in the elderly, one should remember body reserves decreases with aging–

Function	% less than normal
Basal metabolic rate	16%
Cerebral blood flow	25%
Cardiac output	30%
Muscle strength	15-30%
GFR	31%
Vital capacity	44%

The physiological functions of most of the organs decline with age. The functional reserve of the organ systems of the body decreases. While this can cope with restful activities in the day to day life, during stress or diseased state it may become compromised. Example: mild post operative dehydration may precipitate acute renal failure in elderly patients with apparently normal preoperative renal function.

With aging there is also disordered physiological homeostatic control mechanism. Example: loss of postural adjustment of BP leads to frequent falls in the elderly.

There is decreased barrier function of the body. This makes an elderly person more susceptible to infectious agents and injury.

Immune function is also compromised which leads to altered body response to infection. Frequently in elderly population a serious infection is not associated with any leukocyte response. Ability to maintain the core temperature of the body is frequently compromised and many times these patients do not mount a temperature in the event of an infection in the body.

Due to cerebral aging with cell loss in important higher brain centers and deceased cerebral oxidative metabolism, acute confusion is very common presentation in elderly population, suffering from an unassociated illness. If the clinician is unaware of it, the underlying precipitating cause may be missed.

CAUSES OF ACUTE CONFUSION:

- Any metabolic derangement like hypoxia, electrolyte imbalance, hypoglycemia or hyperglycemia etc.
- Pneumonia or any chest infection.
- Urinary tract infection.
- Myocardial infarction, cardiac failure.
- Drugs– anticholinergics, sedatives, anti-parkinsonian drugs (levodopa), tricyclic antidepressants, digoxin, diuretics, beta blockers, NSAIDs.
- Subdural haematoma or any kind of cerebral trauma.
- Cerebrovascular accident.

Chronic subdural haematoma: Characteristically occurs in elderly population. There may not be a proper history of head injury. There is accumulation of blood in the subdural space following an insignificant injury, which may enlarge and can give pressure effect.

CASE: *An 83 years old gentleman was admitted with history of fall and dizziness. On admission, he was also mildly confused. Investigations did not reveal any abnormality. CT brain scan showed age related atrophic changes. X-ray cervical spine showed cervical spondylosis. A provisional diagnosis of TIA with cervical spondylosis was made. Before discharge, a routine ECG, which was originally missed during initial admission, showed evidence of acute inferior MI. Troponin-T was requested and was found to be strongly positive.*

DIAGNOSIS: MI presenting with fall and confusional state.

One should remember that in elderly population because of autonomic neuropathy pain may be absent in MI. ECG and cardiac enzyme is mandatory in any elderly patients with fall, postural drop of BP and confusional state.

CASE: *A 78 years old lady with osteoarthritis and chronic ill health was admitted to the hospital. She was noticed to be acutely confused. Examination did not reveal any focal neurological signs; she was apyrexic with normal WBC count. Her Na^+ was 126 mmol/lit. CT Brain scan was normal. Routine X-ray chest showed right lower lobe pneumonia.*

DIAGNOSIS: Pneumonia presenting as an acute confusional state.

Another common cause of confusional state in the elderly is disturbance of fluid and electrolyte balance and frequent inappropriate ADH secretion (SIADH) leading to hyponatraemia. It is well known that SIADH leading to hyponatraemia is quite common in older population particularly after pneumonia, surgery, trauma and sometimes spontaneous. Disease manifestations may be different in the elderly population. Thyrotoxicosis in elderly may not present in the classical way. Atrial fibrillation of cardiac failure may be the only manifestation. Thyroid function may also be deranged in euthyroid patients (sick euthyroid syndrome) who are seen more frequently in the elderly population.

Another common problem in elderly female population is osteoporosis and tendency to have fracture at the slightest provocation. There may be definite history of fall in fracture neck of femur and clinician should be aware of it and prescribe appropriate prophylactic treatment. Because of altered pharmacokinetics and pharmacodynamics, the drug delivery differs in the elder population with altered hepatic metabolism and renal excretion. This along with diminished functional reserve of the organ systems, drug related side effects are common. These patients are usually on multiple drugs and drug related interaction is frequently observed in this population.

Examples: Acute renal failure is quite common with NSAID, ACE inhibitors, aminoglycosides in patients with apparently normal renal function and mild dehydration or post operative state. Radio contrast related renal failure is also occasionally encountered in clinical practice following routine coronary angiogram and the clinicians should be careful about it.

Example of drug interaction with OHA in elderly diabetics:

Decreased renal excretion of glibenclamide causes increased hypoglycemic event. Plasma bound drugs transiently increase free sulphonylurea increasing risk of hypoglycemia are-

- NSAID's
- Salicylates
- Fluconazole
- Fibrates
- Allopurinol

Drugs whose renal elimination is impaired with aging:

- Digoxin
- ACE inhibitors
- Aminoglycoside
- Vancomycin
- Lithium
- Frusemide

Drugs whose hepatic metabolism is impaired with advanced age:

- Amlodipine
- Nifedipine
- Diazepam
- Morphine
- Phenytoin
- Propranolol
- Theophylline

Drugs whose sensitivity is altered in advanced age:

Decreased	Increased
β blockers	H_1 antihistamines
β agonist	Benzodiazepines
Frusemide	Warfarin
Vaccines	Neuroleptics

Elderly patients in critical care units have higher mortality rates than the average. This is due to coexisting medical conditions like dementia, diabetes, cardiac failure and cancer. There is increased incidence of sepsis, aspiration pneumonia, ventilator associated pneumonia, gastrointestinal bleeding and pressure sores.

Degenerative brain disease, cognitive impairment from isolation and loneliness, atherosclerotic brain disease like stroke are common accompaniment of the elderly population and the physician dealing with the elderly patients should be caring and sympathetic and should not cast aside the patient with neglect and indifference.

CLINICAL ASSESSMENT OF AN ELDERLY PATIENT:

Clinicians should be well adept in dealing with elderly patients as the number of elder patients is increasing day by day due to the increasing life expectancy of the population. During assessment of such patients a quick overview will help to access the functional status of the patients –

Assessment of functional status:

- Ability to stand up from the chair and walk
- Activities of daily living like bathing, dressing, feeding, housekeeping, shopping *etc.*
- Assessment of the mental function by mental test scoring.
- Assessment of hearing and vision.
- Assessment of nutrition.
- Assessment of bladder and bowel function.
- Assessment of integrity of the skin, presence of pressure sores.

Frailty– Frailty is progressive decline in physiological resource and functional ability with increasing vulnerability to disease and death. While assessing an elderly patient, assessment of frailty is a very important fact in the diagnosis, overall prognosis and counseling the relatives regarding the possible adverse outcome of the disease.

The Canadian Society of Health and Aging (CSHA) Clinical Frailty scale:

1. Very fit
2. Well without any active disease
3. Well with treated co morbid condition
4. Appreciably vulnerable but not frankly dependant.
5. Mildly frail with limited dependence on others in daily living activities.
6. Moderately frail with instrumental and non-instrumental help is needed for daily living activities.
7. Severely frail with completely dependent on others.

FRAILTY SYNDROME

- Falls
- Delirium and dementia
- Poly-pharmacy
- Incontinence
- Immobility
- End-of-life-care

Frequent fall is a common problem in elderly patients' due to–

- Poor vision
- Postural hypotension
- Balance and gait problems– cervical spondylosis, lumbar spondylosis, peripheral neuropathy, old CVA, muscle atrophy
- Medication – sedation
- Cardiovascular – arrhythmia
- Neurological – epileptic attacks.

Frequently encountered problems in elderly patients:

- **MEDICAL:** Falls, immobility, osteoporosis, Osteoarthritis, incontinence, increased incidence of MI, diabetes, CVA, pressure sore, Cancer, nutritional deficiencies.
- **PSYCHOLOGICAL:** Dementia, depression, delirium.
- **SOCIAL:** Social isolation, End of life decisions.

Urinary Incontinence: It is a common problem in elderly population. Before going for detailed investigation, one needs to exclude reversible causes of incontinence like –

- Urinary infection
- Atrophic vaginitis
- Faecal impaction
- Delirium
- Polyuria due to diabetes mellitus
- Drugs – diuretics

Types of urinary incontinence:

- Stress incontinence
- Urge incontinence
- Mixed incontinence (combination of both stress and urge incontinence)
- Overflow incontinence

Stress incontinence is usually due to weak detrusor muscles of the pelvic floor or as an aftermath of gynaecological operation. Incontinence is produced by coughing, straining etc. It is treated with pelvic floor exercise, anti-cholinergic drugs like oxybutynin, tolterodine, darifenacin groups of drugs. However one must be aware of the fact that these drugs may cause retention of urine. Surgical intervention in gynaecological patients may sometimes be helpful.

Urge incontinence is due to detrusor muscle hyper activity. It is manifested by sudden irresistible urge to void with resultant incontinence. Bladder retraining programme with asking the patient to void every 2-3 hours may be helpful. Anticholinergics may have additional beneficial effect.

Overflow incontinence– This may be either due to obstructive uropathy like BPH or urethral stenosis. It can also be due to detrusor muscle weaknesses due to neurological causes like diabetic mellitus, alcoholism, Vitamin B_{12} deficiency, multiple sclerosis etc. Before embarking on therapy urodynamic study is warranted as the treatment will vary. In overflow incontinence due to prostate enlargement TURP or urethral dilatation in case of urethral stenosis will be helpful. Whereas, in neurological causes of overflow incontinence, these procedures will lead to permanent incontinence with severe impairment of quality of life. In these instances, spinal nerve stimulation, cholinergic drugs like carbachol or bethanechol, which stimulate the detrusor muscles, may be partially helpful. Intermittent self catheterization failing which permanent catheterization will be the last resort.

Pressure Ulcers are common in elderly bedridden patients and it is frequently a cause of medical litigation in cases of hospitalized patients. It is mandatory that during admission pressure areas should be noticed for any preexisting pressure sores and should be documented in the bed head ticket with signature from the relatives. Common predisposing factors are frailty, CVA with bed ridden conditions, malnutrition, fracture pelvis, urinary incontinence and oedema. Staging of ulcer is important for the treatment purpose.

Stage I – mild erythema

Stage II – partial thickness dermo-epidermial

Stage III – full thickness

Stage IV – Deep, involvement of subcutaneous tissues, muscles with necrosis.

Treatment will vary from local meticulous dressing with frequent change of postures to wound debridement and necrosectomy depending on the depth of involvement and presence of infection. Preventive measures must be ensured in all bedridden elderly patients with the use of ripple mattress and should be well documented in the bed head ticket for medicolegal purposes.

Nutritional assessment is important in elderly patient and nutritional supplements should be used on nutritionally deficient patients. Particular care should be taken with regard to osteoporosis, Vitamin D deficiency and Vitamin B_{12} deficiency. Assessment of osteoporosis is particularly important in elderly women where the risk of osteoporotic fracture is very high.

Other associated issues in elderly patients:

- Immunization- mainly for pneumonia, influenza.
- Cancer Screening- checking of PSA, PAP smear, mammography.
- Assessment of psychological problems- like depression loneliness should also be assessed which are frequently present in these patients due to various reasons.
- Assessment of social problems- a very important in view of the emerging concept of nuclear family in this subcontinent over the last 3 decades. The elderly patients are frequently left alone creating a huge problem like the western countries which faced this problem 6 decades ago. Although it is the societal responsibility to tackle this problem, a clinician should also look at their problems sympathetically and try to provide his or her best input while dealing with the individual patient.
- 'End of life decision' issues: This must be discussed in mentally and intellectually competent patients with regard to the patients' last wishes regarding 'organ donation', 'do not resuscitate', 'do not ventilate' issues.

While dealing with elderly patients, it is imperative for every clinician to take utmost care, sympathy and empathy and provide adequate time for consultation and for hearing to their problems.

: KEY POINTS :

- In clinical practice, increasing number of elderly patients is being encountered in modern times.
- Clinical manifestation may be different in the elderly population.
- Drug therapy should be cautious in view of increased incidence of side effects.
- Confusional state, depression and degenerative brain disease are common presentation in the elderly.
- Elderly patients should be dealt with care, sympathy and empathy.

FURTHER REFERENCES:

- Acute Medical Illness in Old Age- edited by Alan J. Sinclair, K. W. Woodhouse, 1995.
- Geriatric Medicine – Problems and Practice – M.S. John Pathy, Paul Finucane, 1989.
- Brockle Hurst's Text Book of Geriatric Medicine and Gerontology – 6th Ed.
- Laura M Pal *et al.* – Clinical Medicine, Vol. 14 – Nov 13, June 14 2014
- Harrison's Principle of Clinical Medicine, 17th edition

55 A PATIENT WITH MEDIASTINAL MASS

CASE: *A 46 years old doctor presented with history of persistent cough for last 6 weeks. He was also complaining of occasional chest pain for last three weeks. He was a non-smoker. Initial investigations showed normal Hb, urea, electrolytes, uric acid but LDH were high, ECG normal. X-ray chest showed widening of the mediastinum. A contrast enhanced CT thorax confirmed presence of anterior mediastinal mass suggestive of lymph nodes, without any other focal lesion in the lungs. CT guided FNAC from the mass confirmed Non-Hodgkin's Lymphoma. He was immediately referred to the oncologist. After undergoing staging with abdominal CT scan, he was commenced on chemotherapy. 6 months at follow up, he was doing well; X-ray chest and CT Thorax have shown regression of the mediastinal mass with disappearance of cough.*

DIAGNOSIS: Non Hodgkin's Lymphoma presenting with mediastinal mass.

DISCUSSION:

Mediastinal mass or hilar lymphadenopathy is a common radiological finding in X-ray chest encountered in the day to day clinical practice. Approximately 50% of them are malignant and they usually present with symptoms of cough, chest pain, dyspnoea or superior venacaval syndrome, rest are benign and they are usually detected on routine X-ray chest examination.

While dealing with such cases, the exact location of the mass is important so as to know the cause of the lesion.

Anterior mediastinum:

- Lymph nodes
- Retrosternal thyroid
- Thymus
- Teratoma

Middle mediastinum:

- Aortic aneurysm
- Cysts

Posterior mediastinum:

- Neurofibroma
- Para vertebral abscess

Associated symptoms are also important e.g. presence of myasthenia gravis might indicate thymus. Joint pain, erythema nodosum may indicate acute sarcoidosis.

The next step would be to do a contrast enhanced CT scan of thorax, which would immediately differentiate between a tumour and an aneurysm.

It can also be helpful in diagnosing teratoma. However, it may not be able to reliably differentiate between a solid and a cystic lesion. In myasthenia it will not be able to differentiate between thymic hyperplasia and tumour. MRI scan has got no special advantage except for in cases where intravenous contrast cannot be given and in posterior mediastinal neurogenic tumour where it has definitely got an edge over CT scan.

Tissue diagnosis would be the next step and CT guided FNAC has got a sensitivity of approximately 80% and specificity of nearly 100%. There is a small chance of having pneumothorax as a complication of the procedure. If CT guided FNAC is not possible or does not yield any diagnostic results, there are other options such as—

- Scalene (supraclavicular) lymph node biopsy even if there is no palpable gland is present. The sensitivity in diagnosing lymphoma or sarcoidosis is nearly 70-90%.
- Mediastinoscopy– This is particularly helpful in staging lung cancer. It has got a moderately low sensitivity and a negative test does not rule out malignancy.
- Surgical biopsy through thoracotomy is the gold standard for the final diagnosis. The attendant morbidity can be reduced by the application of newer technique such as video-assisted thoracotomy. Needless to say that the sensitivity and specificity of surgical biopsy is 100%.

The index patient was referred to the oncologist and on the basis of the FNAC report he was started on chemotherapy after staging the disease with appropriate tests. Six months at follow up, he was doing well with regression of the mediastinal mass on X-ray chest and CT thorax. Subsequently he was symptom free.

DISCUSSION:

Non Hodgkin Lymphoma (NHL): NHL includes several lymphoproliferative malignant disorders with different clinical and histological appearances.

Histological classification:

- Lymphoplasmacytic lymphoma.
- Follicular lymphoma.
- Mantle cell lymphoma / MALT lymphoma.
- Diffuse large β cell lymphoma.
- Burkitt's lymphoma.
- Anaplastic large T-cell lymphoma.

Clinical presentation: The patient can present with lump anywhere in the body. The most common site is lump in the neck (25%). There may be extra nodal involvement as well like gastrointestinal tract, head, neck, skin and involvement of the Waldeyer's ring. The patient may also present with B symptoms (night sweat, weight loss > 10% and fever).

Histological classification:

- Tumour type and disease bulk
- Increasing age
- Poor performance status
- High LDH level
- Bone marrow involvement

MANAGEMENT:

Follicular lymphomas- Only few patients with follicular lymphomas present early to be treated with radiotherapy. Most of the patients usually present with disseminated disease and they are being treated with different chemotherapeutic regimes which include combination of Cyclophosphamide, Vincristine, Prednisolone (CVP); fludarabine or anthracycline containing regimes. Rituximab (Chimeric human- murine IgG, monoclonal antibody that binds specifically to B-cell surface antigen CD 20) is combined with the usual chemotherapeutic regimes (Rituximab + CHOP-showed 95% response rate in one trial).

Diffuse large B-cell lymphoma: For stage I and II disease, two strategies are undertaken-

- Doxorubicin containing chemotherapeutic regime e.g. CHOP followed by involved field radiotherapy *e.g.* 3 cycles of CHOP + Radiotherapy.
- 8 cycles of CHOP without radiotherapy.

Both the strategies have equivalent results.

For advanced disease, the most effective treatment is CHOP and addition of rituximab has shown to improve in survival in one trial.

Gastric lymphoma of MALT type:

Eradication of H pylori infection causes regression of lymphoma in majority of the patient. However, close surveillance needs to be taken as they can transform into large B cell lymphoma.

Discussion on Hodgkin's Lymphoma:

Clinical presentation:

- Bimodal age of onset.
- Presence of asymptomatic lump anywhere in the body.
- Mediastinal mass of X-ray chest.
- May present with B symptoms like night sweating, fever and weight loss etc.

WHO classification of Hodgkin's disease:

- Nodular lymphocyte predominant.
- Classical Hodgkin lymphoma– Nodular sclerosis, mixed cellularity, lymphocyte rich or lymphocyte depleted.

Stages of Hodgkin Lymphoma:

- Stage I – Involvement of lymph node region or lymphoid structure.
- Stage II – Two or more lymph node region on the same side of the diaphragm.
- Stage III – Lymph nodes on both sides of diaphragm.
- Stage IV – Involvement of extra nodal sites.

  A – No symptoms. B – Fever, night sweats and weight loss.

Poor prognostic markers:

- Increasing age
- Low albumin level
- Raised WBC count (>15,000) or lymphopenia
- Low haemoglobin
- Stage 4 disease

TREATMENT:

In stage I and II disease, the treatment of choice is radiotherapy. However, although initial response is good, there is high incidence of relapse rate. Relapse rate can be reduced by using combination of chemotherapy and radiotherapy.

In advanced disease, the treatment of choice is combination chemotherapy. Different regimes used are –

- MOPP – the oldest regime (1960)
- ABVD – Adriamycin, bleomycin, vincristine, dacarbazine (started in 1970)
- BEACOPP – (Bleomycin, etoposide, doxorubicin, cyclophosphamide, vincristine, procarbazine and prednisolone). This regime has been found to be superior to the

other regimes. However the side effect profile is also higher. This regime should be reserved for the high risk patients. Consolidation radiotherapy can also be given to patients with advanced disease with good results.

While treating lymphomas one should keep in mind the complication of treatment with cytotoxic drugs which include secondary malignancies, cardiac diseases, endocrinological diseases and infertility.

Comparison between ABVD and BEACOPP:

For ABVD / Against BEACOPP	Against ABVD / For BEACOPP
Relatively non-toxic	Significant higher relapse rate
Low risk of infertility	Significantly lower initial response
Less neutropenia	More need for salvage therapy and an
Lesser risk of mid day myelodysplasia	autologous stem cell transplantation

Important side effects of ABVD treatment:

- Adriamycin – Dose dependent Cardio toxicity
- Bleomycin – Pulmonary toxicity
- Vinblastine – Peripheral neuropathy
- Dacarbazine – Arm pain after infusion

Relapse:

In younger patients with relapse; platinum based chemotherapy with an autologous stem cell transplant may be an option.

Two randomised trials have shown that BEAM (carmustine, etoposide, cytarabine, melphalan) autologous stem cell transplantation has a superior 3 yrs disease free survival compared to dexamine (BEAM and non-BEAM). In carefully selected cases BEAM autologous stem cell transplantation can be an excellent salvage therapy.

Treatment in older patients with co-morbidities:

In older patients non-bleomycin regimes like ChlVPP (Chlorambucil, Vinblastine, Procarbazine and Prednisolone) may be tried. There is also evidence that bleomycin omitted regime (AVD) with granulocyte stimulating factors may produce reasonable outcome. Other options in elder patients include VEPEMB (vinblastine, cyclophosphamide, pregnenolone, procarbazine, etoposide, mitoxantrone and bleomycin) may be an alternative option which has been recently evaluated.

PET adapted approach:

It is an excellent staging modality in Hodgkin's disease and may help in modifying treatment regularly. RAPID trial suggests that patients with I-II A stages, if PET negative after 3 cycles of ABVD, may stop further treatment and avoid involved field radiotherapy. RATHL trial is assuring whether bleomycin can be omitted from ABVD regime in stage II-B-IV discuss who are negative for PET scan after two cycles of ABVD.

Brentuximab vedotin:

It is exciting antibody drug conjugate which links a monoclonal antibody to CD30 to microtubule toxin. As a single agent it has got excellent overall response rate of 75% with complete response in relapsed, refractory Hodgkin's lymphoma, post autologous stem cell transplantation. It is currently used as a bridge therapy to autologous stem cell transplantation. Studies are afoot to compare ABVD require versus AVD plus brentuximab. Peripheral neuropathy and neutropenia are its main side effects.

: KEY POINTS :

- Mediastinal lymphadenopathy is common radiological findings in clinical practice.
- Tuberculosis, sarcoidosis, lymphoma and some benign conditions should be considered in the differential diagnosis.
- Early diagnosis is important as with modern chemotherapeutic regime the prognosis of lymphoma has improved considerably.

FURTHER REFERENCES:

- Edgar R Black *et al.* - Diagnostic strategies for common medical problems, 2nd Ed.
- B. Linda S Evan S, Barry W. Hancock, C. Lancet, Non-Hodgkin Lymphoma 2003, 362: 139 - 46.
- Lynn Yung, David Linch, Lancet– Hodgkin's Lymphoma 2003.
- V.T. Devila Jr., NEJM – Hodgkin's disease – clinical trials and travails Vol. 348, No. 24, 2375 - 2376.
- Toby A Epe *et al.* Classical Hodgkin's Lymphoma: past, present and future perspectives. BJHM-74, oct-2013, 558-563.
- Harrison's Principle of Internal Medicine – 17th edition.
- Oxford Text book of Medicine – 5th edition.

56 A PATIENT WITH EPILEPSY

CASE: *A 9 years old boy was referred from a district where he was found to be unconscious with right sided weakness, developed suddenly. His BP was found to be 160/90 mmHg and initially a diagnosis of CVA was made and urgently referred to this hospital. There was no history of head injury, history of epilepsy or family history of epilepsy. He did not suffer from any significant illness and very agile and active when he arrived at the hospital approximately 3 hours following the incidence, he was fully conscious and there was no focal neurological sign, no neck stiffness. His BP was 110/70 mmHg. Investigations showed normal biochemical and haematological parameters. CT scan of brain was normal, EEG showed focal sharp-wave activities consistent with simple partial epilepsy. He was started on carbamazepine and discharged home with an advice to attend the clinic in 8 weeks time with an MRI brain scan.*

DIAGNOSIS: Simple partial seizure (Idiopathic).

DISCUSSION:

Epileptic seizure is a common clinical problem and very frequently internists and primary care physicians are involved in the management with periodic consultation from the neurologist. Status epilepticus is usually dealt with internists, intensivists or neurologists involved with critical care.

While dealing with epilepsy, one should first differentiate seizure from syncope (discussed previously). Correctable metabolic causes like hypoglycemia electrolyte imbalance, hypoxia, metabolic, acidosis, alcohol intoxication or withdrawal, drug withdrawal should also be borne in mind. Head injury, subdural haematoma, cerebrovascular accident should also be considered in appropriate settings. In young patients and children, congenital structural abnormality of the brain needs to be considered.

- Tuberous sclerosis
- Sturge-Weber syndrome.
- West's syndrome.
- Lennox-Gaustaut syndrome

A thorough family history of epilepsy is worth taking. A history from the eye witness gives useful clues to the diagnosis.

INVESTIGATIONS:

FBC, urea, electrolytes, glucose, liver function test and serum drug levels (for drug overdose like tricyclic antidepressants, or antiepileptic drugs if the patient is already on anti epileptic drugs should be done.

EEG is the most useful investigation tool for exact diagnosis. It should be done 48 hrs after the attack otherwise it can give inappropriate results. EEG may need to be repeated or done with maneuvers like photic stimulation, hyperventilation, sleep deprivation etc. and with special electrodes like (temporal and sphenoidal). In spite of specialized EEG techniques, EEG may be normal in 10% of cases.

Structural **imaging of the brain** by CT or MRI scans is another diagnostic tool. In acute situations, CT is handier and excludes any gross underlying structural problems like stroke, bleed or tumour. However it may miss subtle abnormalities and there may be necessity of doing an MRI later on to find out abnormalities like mesial sclerosis, demyelination, a small brain tumour, a small tuberculoma or cysticercosis (both are common causes of seizure disorder in India) which may be missed by the CT scan.

CLASSIFICATION: Epilepsy is broadly classified as: Partial and Generalized.

A) **Partial:** Partial or focal epilepsy may be of two types –

- Simple- where there is focal motor or sensory deficient.
- Complex- there may be psychic component and abnormal behavior with loss of consciousness (the patient cannot recollected the incidents later on).

Both these types can be complicated with generalized tonic clonic seizure, known as simple or complex partial seizure with secondary generalization.

B) **Generalized:** It may be of two types –

- Absence seizures - It is associated with brief period of unresponsiveness with rapid recovery. Seizure may be precipitated by hyperventilation. This type of seizure is often complicated with generalized tonic-colic seizure.
- Primary generalized - There is generalized tonic clonic seizure to start with as opposed to partial seizures with secondary generalization.

Different causes of convulsion:

- Idiopathic
- Trauma
- Tumor
- Cerebrovascular disease
- Dementia
- Multiple Sclerosis
- Alcohol
- Metabolic: hyponatraemia, hypernatraemia, hypocalcemia, hypoglycemia.

Epilepsy meds to be differentiated from different varieties of syncope (discussed in the chapter of syncope), pseudo seizure, migraine and transient ischaemic attack.

MANAGEMENT:

Should we start treatment following the first seizure?

There are certain conditions where it needs to be started sooner *e.g.*

- Structural brain lesion
- Family history of seizure
- Partial seizure
- EEG abnormality.

In other situation watchful waiting can be done.

Which medication?

For partial seizures following medication may be tried:

- Phenytoin
- Carbamazepine
- Sodium valproate
- Oxcarbazepine (has less toxicity)

For generalized seizure (absence attacks) -

- Ethosuximide
- Sodium valproate (This is preferable as it is also effective against generalized tonic-clonic seizure which is a common accompaniment of absence attacks)
- Primidone

Dosage of Commonly Used Antiepileptics:

- Clobazam : 30-60 mg / day
- Valproate : 150-300 mg / day
- Carbamazepine : 600-1600 mg /day
- Phenytoin : 150-300 mg/ day
- Phenobarbital : 60-180 mg/ day
- Levetiracetam : 1000-3000 mg/day
- Oxcarbazepine : 600-2400 mg /day

What to do if the seizure is not adequately controlled?

The dose of the drug should be increased to the maximum therapeutic level and if there is no control, another drug should be added and the dose slowly built up. Once the full dose is achieved the initial drug may be slowly taken off. However if the risk of further epileptic attack is high and not acceptable, the combination of two drugs may be continued. Clinical judgement will be needed to make the final decision and a neurologist must be involved. Rarely addition of third drug may be necessary.

Drug level monitoring:

This is needed for phenytoin, carbamazepine, phenobarbital and ethosuximide, with a view to ascertain compliance and dose adjustment in patients with poor control of epilepsy on multiple drug therapy. The therapeutic level should be interpreted with caution as many patients have well controlled seizure in spite of having sub-therapeutic levels while some will tolerate the drug in spite of having drug levels above therapeutic level.

When to stop therapy?

Again this is sometimes a difficult decision and clinical judgement will be needed. Usually the patient should be fit free for at least 2 years before baking decision regarding withdrawal. Factors those might have to decide in favor of withdrawal are-

- Idiopathic epilepsy and starting in childhood.
- Normal EEG
- No structure lesion in brain scan
- Seizure controlled with one medication

The chance of recurrence India in these group a patient is approximately 25% (80% of this recurrence will occur in the 1st year of following discontinuation). The decision should be individualized were and should be taken by a neurologist.

How to withdraw the medication?

The doses should be that tapered off slowly. For phenytoin, carbamazepine, lamotrigine, valproate and vigabatrin the dose should be reduced by about 10% every 2-4 weeks. Barbiturates, diazepam and ethosuximide should be tapered by 10% every 4 to 8 weeks. When the patient is taking combination medication there should be a gap of at least one month before the second drug should be started to be tapered off, following the withdrawal of the first drug. During pregnancy the pro and con of continuing antiepileptic medication is well controlled epileptic should be discussed with the patient and in patient willing to conceive, folic acid supplementations should be commenced prior to planning for conception.

Pregnancy & antiepileptic drugs:

No Drug is absolutely safe as all of them will have some teratogenic effect. Of particular importance is that of valproate which is associated with neural tube defect and partial agenesis of corpus callosum. Carbamazepine is associated with spina bifida. Phenytoin and phenobarbital are associated with cleft lip and cleft palate.

In clinical practice phenytoin and carbamazepine are the most commonly prescribed drugs. However the possible side effects should be explained to the patients. And folic acid supplementation should be routinely given in order to prevent neural tube effects.

The medication used as adjunctive in partial seizure:

- Sodium valproate
- Gabapentin
- Lamotrigine
- Levetiracetam
- Tiagabine

Common side effects of commonly used antiepileptics:

Phenytoin- ataxia, cerebellar signs, gum hyperplasia, folate deficiency, osteomalacia, pseudo-lymphoma, drug rash, enzyme inducer à may cause drug interaction.

Carbamazepine- sedation, drug rash, hepatic problems, hyponatraemia, enzyme inducer à may cause drug interaction.

Valproate- liver dysfunction, tremor, alopecia, contraindicated in pregnancy.

Drug rash may be serious with carbamazepine and phenytoin and leads to Steven Jenson syndrome. In that event of drug rash alternate medication like Gabapentin, valproate on levetiracetam may be tried as an alternative.

CASE: *A 73 years old hypertensive lady was admitted with history of sudden onset of unconsciousness following a brief episode of headache. Immediately after admission to ITU she started to have convulsion. She was given bolus dose of phenytoin which failed to control the seizure. She was intubated and ventilated; her convulsion was finally controlled with continuous midazolam infusion. CT scan of brain showed evidence of a big* *subcortical haematoma over the right parietal region. She was treated with hyperventilation. Her BP was controlled with IV nitroglycerine and she was finally extubated. After a prolonged hospital stay, she was discharged home with comprehensive domiciliary nursing support. She was on phenytoin along with other medications on discharge. Repeat CT brain scan showed partial resolution of the cerebral haematoma.*

DIAGNOSIS: Post cerebral bleed epileptic attack.

Etiology of epilepsy in elderly population:

- Cerebrovascular accident.
- Brain tumours (primary and secondary).
- Subdural haematoma due to subtle head injury.
- Secondary causes like hypoxia, low Na and other metabolic causes.
- Degenerative brain disease

MANAGEMENT: Long term treatment for 1st symptomatic seizure is more controversial in elderly patients. Since recurrent seizure may cause serious injury and more prolonged post-ictal state, it is perhaps justifiable to treat such event. Fortunately, remote symptomatic seizure due to old CVA (the most common cause) is usually well controlled with single antiepileptic drug.

The 1st line medication:

- **Phenytoin** - It is user friendly. However is has got most of side effects. Furthermore it has got non-curvilinear dose-response relationship whereby small dose adjustment may increase the serum drug level out of proportion resulting risks of side effects.
- **Carbamazepine** - It is an effective drug. However it can cause drowsiness and the dose should be build up slowly.
- **Sodium valproate** - It is an effective drug in the elderly population. Unlike phenytoin and carbamazepine it is not an enzyme inducer, so drug interaction are less common.
- **Lamotrigine** - It is also a useful drug in elderly population. It is not an enzyme inducer. It can cause idiosyncratic skin reactions and insomnia.

Other second line alternatives in elderly:

- **Gabapentin**
- **Levetiracetam**
- **Topiramate**

Other Antiepileptic Drugs:

- Tiagabine- add on for refractory epilepsy
- Pregabalin- add on in partial seizures
- Zonisamide - add on in partial seizures, may causes Stevens-Johnson syndrome.
- Felbamate- as a last line drug, may causes aplastic anaemia, liver failure.

CASE: *A 47 year patient with history of chronic alcoholism, recently on abstinence therapy was admitted with convulsion, confusion, fever and tachycardia. Other causes of epileptic fit were excluded my appropriate tests. CT scan of brain was normal. He was treated with IV diazepam and infusion, IV fluids with vitamin $B_1B_6B_{12}$ injection and other supportive therapies to control of his symptoms. He was discharged with tapering doze of chlordiazepoxide to prevent further epileptic attacks.*

DIAGNOSIS: Delirium tremens in a patient with alcohol withdrawal state.

Other CNS effect of alcohol:

- Wernicke's encephalopathy- confusional state, opthalmoplegia, diplopia.
- Korsakoff's psychosis- features of amnesia
- Dementia
- Cerebellar degeneration
- Marchiafava Bignami syndrome
- Peripheral neuropathy
- Myopathy
- Susceptibility towards subdural haematoma

Alcohol withdrawal is the only treatment available. However majority of conditions are not fully reversible. In cases of Wernicke's encephalopathy and Korsakoff's psychosis thiamine supplementation is essential. Glucose infusion without thiamine must be avoided as it may complicate the symptoms further. In spite of treatment, while Wernicke's encephalopathy is reversible, Korsakoff's psychosis is not fully reversible.

CASE: *A 61 years old lady was admitted with history of vomiting followed by confusional state. She was noted to have one episode of convulsion at home which was the main reason of her admission. Examination did not reveal any focal neurological sign. CT brain scan was normal. Her Na^+ level was 106 mmol/litre. Rests of the test reports were satisfactory. She was treated with IV fluids and sodium replacement with complete recovery in next 72 hours. Before discharge her Na^+ level was within normal limits and she was not discharged on any antiepileptic medication.*

DIAGNOSIS: Convulsion due to hyponatraemia.

CASE: *A 58 years old lady was referred to the ITU with history of repeated convulsive episodes. She had a history of headache of recent onset, drowsiness for last few days. Examination revealed bilateral extensor planters, unequal pupil size with evidence of right sided 6th nerve palsy. Biochemical and haematological parameters were normal. CT brain scan showed bilateral small ring enhancing lesions in the parietal and frontal lobes. MRI scan showed multiple ring enhancing lesions in both the cerebral cortex and brain stem. Consideration of tuberculoma was high in the differential diagnosis. Mantoux test was positive in moderately high dilution. Anti-cysticercal antibody was negative. She was treated with IV mannitol, IV dexamethasone and 4 drug anti-tubercular regime and phenytoin (IV initially followed by oral). Following 2 weeks of hospital treatment, she was discharged home. 3 months at follow up she was doing well with good resolution of ring enhancing lesions in repeat MRI Scan.*

DIAGNOSIS: Multiple tuberculoma presenting with status epilepticus.

CASE: *A 21 years old man was admitted in the middle of the night with status epilepticus. He was intubated and ventilated. This convulsion was controlled with IV midazolam infusion and IV phenytoin. Subsequent MRI scans revealed characteristics of cysticercosis (initial CT scan showed evidence of localized edema only). He made good recovery except for having aspiration pneumonia. He was treated with albendazole 400 mg twice daily for 4 weeks. At present he is doing well.*

DIAGNOSIS: Status epilepticus due to cerebral cysticercosis.

Management of status epilepticus: This needs to be managed in critical care unit with consultation with an intensivist or a neurologist. For details of management, one should consult a neurological or critical care test book. Drugs commonly used have been mentioned here-

IV Diazepam

IV Midazolam

IV Lorazepam

IV Phenytoin

IV Fosphenytoin

IV Phenobarbitone

In uncontrolled cases, IV thiopentone may be used with appropriate monitoring; similarly IV propofol may also be used. These patients should be intubated and ventilated before commencing such medications.

Role of surgery:

There is a role of Epilepsy Surgery in drug refractory cases if the focus can be exactly located with the help of investigation like FDG PET Scan or SPECT scan. The most common cause of refractory epilepsy is due to mesial temporal lobe epilepsy secondary to hippocampal sclerosis. Specialist opinion is needed for this purpose.

FURTHER REFERENCES:

- Diagnostic Strategies for Common Medical Problems, 2nd ed., Edgar R Black et al.
- Lecture Notes in Endocrinology, 5th edition, William Jeffcoate, Male sexual function, P 193 - 201.
- Harrison's Principle of Internal Medicine, 17th edition.
- Oxford Textbook of Medicine, 5th edition.

57

A PATIENT WITH IMPOTENCE

CASE: *A 32 years old businessman attended the clinic with history of recent onset of loss of libido and impotence mainly during sexual intercourse. He did not suffer from any significant past medical history. He was non diabetic, non hypertensive and was not on any medication. Recently he had major problem in his business and was quite depressed and anxious. Examination did not reveal anything specific. He had normal secondary sexual characteristics. Biochemical and haematological parameters were normal. Serum testosterone and prolactin levels were within normal limits.*

DIAGNOSIS: Psychogenic impotence, due to situational depression and anxiety.

He was reassured and counselled and treated with a course of anti-anxiety medication with the suggestion of using sildenafil if things did not improve within next few weeks.

DISCUSSION:

Erectile impotence is a common cause of consultation in clinical practice. Psychogenic cause is the most frequent cause although the clinician needs to exclude organic causes as well.

Common causes of impotence are:

- Psychogenic
- Depression
- Organic
- Peripheral vascular disease
- Diabetes Mellitus
- Peripheral neuropathy
- Spinal cord injury
- Multiple sclerosis
- Endocrinal causes with low testosterone levels
- Prolactinoma
- Prostatic surgery
- Drugs – Spironolactone, cimetidine, β-blockers, thiazides, digoxin etc.
- Alcoholism

Thorough history and clinical investigations will help to find out the cause. Initial investigations that might be helpful are:

- Routine FBC, LFT, urea, creatinine, blood glucose.
- Testosterone, prolactin, FSH, LH levels
- Measurement of testicular size.

In vast majority of cases, treatment may be carried out with the aforementioned test reports. However, in occasional cases further investigation may be needed and specialist opinion should be sought for.

Common investigations of impotence are:

- Penile pressure
- Penile Doppler ultrasonography
- Cystometry
- Nocturnal penile tumescence (NPT)

In NPT one looks for spontaneous erection during REM sleep. Presence of erection during REM sleep rules out organic impotence and points towards a psychogenic cause. Another important clue favouring psychogenic impotence is ability to have a normal erection during masturbation while failure during intercourse. Premature ejaculation is usually psychogenic.

Management of impotence:

Majority of patients will improve with anti-anxiety treatment and counselling only and detailed investigation and drug therapy will not be needed at least in the initial period. If symptoms persist, one needs to investigate these patients and embark on drug therapy.

Drug therapy for erectile impotence:

- Diabetes mellitus
- Parkinson's disease, multiple sclerosis, pelvic injury, spinal cord injury, post prostatectomy
- Renal failure

Treatment options available are:

- Intracavernosal injection of alprostadil (Prostaglandin E)
- Intra urethral administration of alprostadil
- Intracavernosal injection of papaverine
- Oral and sublingual drug therapy

These oral drugs are available:

- Sildenafil 25 mg, 50 mg
- Vardenafil 5 mg, 10 mg, 20 mg
- Tadalafil 10 mg, 20 mg

These drugs are phosphodiesterase-5-inhibitors and act by increasing intracavernosal guanosine monophosphate activity.

These drugs have comparable efficacy. Sildenafil should be used as a first line failing which the other two drugs should be used. These drugs should be avoided in patients with unstable coronary artery disease or recent MI. These drugs are contraindicated in patients on nitrate as the combination can lead to severe hypotension. Headache and dizziness are the common side effects. These drugs should be taken 30 minutes before the act.

Sublingually effective drug: Apomorphine 2 mg, 3 mg.

This drug acts centrally stimulating CNS dopamine receptors thereby increasing peripheral parasympathetic flow with the resultant relaxation of corpus cavernosus smooth muscle, corporal engorgement and erection. It should be taken 10 minutes before the act. Although less effective than the oral drugs, it may be a useful alternate in patients on nitrate therapy. Combination therapy of oral and sublingual therapy is not indicated. It can cause dizziness and headache and should be avoided in patients with recent MI or in patients on centrally acting dopamine agonists.

Most patients presenting with impotence have normal libido and their testosterone level would be normal. Administration of testosterone in such patients will be not only ineffective but also illogical, as it will heighten the desire without enhancing the performance.

CASE: *A 46 years old post MI patient presented with enlargement of his breasts of recent onset. Examination revealed bilateral gynaecomastia. Investigation revealed normal FSH, LH, prolactin, testosterone and TSH levels along with normal creatinine and liver function test. As his medications contained* spironolactone *for cardiac failure, it was stopped. His gynaecomastia resolved within next 2 months of time.*

DIAGNOSIS: Drug induced gynaecomastia (Spironolactone).

Common causes of gynaecomastia are:

- Obesity– local fat accumulation may cause gynaecomastia
- Lipoma
- Neurofibroma
- Male breast carcinoma

Investigations:

Blood FSH, LH, Prolactin, Testosterone, LFT, Urea, Creatinine, T_3, T_4, TSH, PSA.

Other causes of gynaecomastia are:

- **Physiological**
  Puberty
  Old age
- **Medical**
  Testicular failure (Klinefelter's syndrome)
  Pituitary failure/tumour (Prolactinoma)
  Thyroid problem
  Hepatic failure (chronic liver disease)
  Adrenal tumour
  Prostate cancer
  Hermaphroditism
- **Drugs:**
  Cimetidine, Ranitidine
  Isoniazid
  Spironolactone
  Statins
  Calcium channel blockers
  ACE Inhibitors
  Digoxin
  Androgen/ Oestrogen
  Anabolic steroids
  Ethanol

TREATMENT:

In case of accumulation of adipose tissue reassurance should be given to the patient. In true gynaecomastia, suspected offending drug should be withdrawn.

Drugs:

- **Danazol** 10 mg twice daily initially followed by 200 mg twice daily for 2-6 weeks.
- **Tamoxifen** 20-40 mg for 2-6 weeks may also be tried in puberty gynaecomastia.
- **Mastectomy** for suspected carcinoma.
- **Cosmetic surgery** for increased adiposity.

CASE: *A 56 years old postmenopausal lady presented with galactorrhoea. Investigations revealed high prolactin level and MRI scan showed small pituitary adenoma. There was no visual field defect. She was referred to a neuro surgeon for follow up.*

DIAGNOSIS: Pituitary adenoma presented with prolactinoma with galactorrhoea.

Causes of galactorrhoea:

- **Physiological**
  Post pregnancy, Nipple stimulation
- **Pituitary tumours**
  Micro and macro prolactinoma and hypothalamic

Medications:

Dopamine antagonists
Metoclopramide,
Domperidone
Phenothiazine
Atypical antipsychotics
SSRI
Calcium channel blockers
α-methyldopa
Isoniazid
Ranitidine
Oestrogen

Diseases:

Hypothyroidism
Cushing syndrome
Chronic liver disease
Renal failure
Ectopic prolactin secretion
Other cause of non-milky discharge from the nipple should be excluded (like mastitis, intraductal papilloma or carcinoma)

Investigations:

- Hormonal assay– TSH, FSH, Prolactin, LFT, Creatinine, Cortisol
- Visual field testing
- MRI scan of Brain

Treatment:

Offending drugs should be withdrawn. Dopamine agonists may be tried in pituitary micro adenoma *e.g.*

- Bromocriptine – 1.25 mg daily to stent with upto 2.5-5 mg daily

- Cabergoline – to start with 0.5 mg weekly followed by biweekly (Continuous high dose of cabergoline may cause valvular heart defect)

Surgery:

For pituitary macro adenoma trans-sphenoidal surgery is the treatment of choice. Alternately radiotherapy may be tried with 20-30% success rate.

: KEY POINTS :

- Impotence is a common clinical problem.
- Majority of cases are due to psychogenic causes.
- Phosphodiesterase inhibitors are useful in treating impotence.
- These drugs should be avoided in patient taking oral nitrates.

FURTHER REFERENCES:

- Franck J Dominea 5 minutes clinical consultation -2012, 20th edition.
- Harrison's Principle of Internal Medicine - 17th edition.
- Oxford Text Book of Medicine – 5th edition.

58

A PATIENT WITH POLYCYTHAEMIA

CASE: *A 48 yrs old police officer presented in the clinic with headache, dimness of vision and numbness in the hands of few months duration. His relatives had noticed him to be flushed in his face. He was hypertensive, smoker and used to drink on regular basis. Examination revealed pulse rate of 72/ minutes, BP 170/100 mmHg, normal heart sounds, looked flushed, no organomegaly, no lymphadenopathy. Investigation revealed Hb of 18.6 g%, PCV- 0.58, WBC normal, platelet normal, Urea, Creatinine, LFT all are within normal range, Blood gas analysis was normal, neutrophil alkaline phosphatase was normal, bone marrow examination was normal. X-ray chest normal, USG abdomen normal.*

DIAGNOSIS: Polycythaemia in a smoker and hypertensive ?Gaisbock's syndrome.

His BP was controlled with appropriate medication. He was advised to stop smoking and in view of his symptoms he underwent periodic venesection to maintain his PCV below 49%. He is asymptomatic at present.

DISCUSSION: Polycythaemia is occasionally encountered in clinical practice. PCV is a better indicator of erythrocytosis than Hb level and a PCV of more than 0.52 in men and 0.49 in women will be considered as significant erythrocytosis. The symptoms are mainly due to high plasma viscosity like headache, visual symptoms and poor circulation in the extremities. Very high PCV can be a predisposing factor of brain stroke.

CAUSES:

It can be with increase in red cell mass:

- **Primary** - Polycythaemia rubra vera (PRV).
- **Secondary** - Due to increased erythropoietin levels –

Relative: Dehydration due to fluid loss.

Absolute:

1. Hypoxia due to any cause - high altitude, COPD (pulmonary cause), excessive smoking, congenital cyanotic heart disease, right to left shunt.

2. Due to erythropoietin secreting lesion e.g. renal cell carcinoma, uterine fibromyoma, Cerebellar hemangioblastoma.

3. Drugs - Erythropoietin injection

It can be with normal red cell mass: Due to plasma volume contraction e.g. dehydration, diuretic overdose, Gaisbock's syndrome (association with hypertension, smoking, alcoholism).

INVESTIGATIONS: In addition to the routine biochemical and haematological tests and chest x-ray, one should also do –

- Blood gas analysis
- Erythropoietin levels (low in PRV, in secondary causes).
- Red cell mass - normal in Gaisbock's syndrome.
- USG abdomen.
- CT brain if cerebellar haemangioma is suspected.
- Blood for neutrophil alkaline phosphatase (NAP) activity and vitamin B_{12} binding protein - (high in PRV)
- Bone marrow examination.

Diagnostic work up:

In patients with polycythaemia ideally one need to measure RBC mass by radioactive labeling study using Cr 51 labelled autologous red blood cells. In case of relative polycythaemia it will be normal, if RBC mass is high, the next step would be to measure erythropoietin level. If it is high then the secondary causes as mentioned earlier should be excluded by appropriate test [X-ray, echo, blood gas analysis, CT scan of brain and abdomen etc]. In polycythaemia rubra vera, erythropoietin will be suppressed, bone marrow examination will settle the issue.

Points favouring PRV:

- Increased red cell mass (may not be routinely available in all centres).
- Low erythropoietin level
- Splenomegaly
- Increased platelets
- Bone marrow - increased megakaryocytes.
- Increased neutrophil alkaline phosphatase.
- Increased vitamin B_{12} binding protein.

General management of polycythaemia:

- Avoidance of smoking.
- Avoidance of diuretic as antihypertensive.
- Regular venesection to keep PCV below 0.49.
- Management of the underlying cause like hypoxia.

Management of PRV: This needs to be treated by haematologist. Drugs used are –

- Hydroxyurea
- Busulfan
- Radioactive phosphorus (P^{32})

(In very elderly population only as it can cause acute leukaemia)

CASE: *A 19 yrs old girl with inoperable VSD with balanced shunt used to attend the clinic for routine medical checkup. Although her cardiac symptoms were stable, she had been complaining of increasing headache, usual problems and joint pains. Her Hb is 19.3 g%, PCV- 0.55 and Uric acid- 7.4 mg% (due to increased red cell mass). She underwent venesection and started on allopurinol with symptomatic improvement.*

DIAGNOSIS: Secondary polycythaemia due to hypoxia in congenital cyanotic heart disease.

CASE: *A 49 yrs old smoker and hypertensive attended the clinic with increasing shortness of breath and headache. Clinically he looked flushed with a BP of 170/110 mmHg. Chest was with scattered rhonchi bilaterally. His O_2 saturation was 88%, Hb 18.6 g%, PCV 0.56. His X-ray chest and CT thorax showed evidence of multicystic pulmonary disease. He has treated with bronchodilator inhaler and nebulisation theophylline, antihypertensive, with an advice to stop smoking. He also received periodic venesection. A surgical consultation ruled out any surgical intervention because of extensive bilateral involvement with cysts.*

DIAGNOSIS: Secondary polycythaemia due to multicystic lung disease.

CASE: *A 67 years old patients was admitted with a history of TIA. His platelet count was found to be very high. Bone marrow examination was consistent with essential thrombocythaemia. He was positive for JAK2 V617F mutation.*

DIAGNOSIS: Essential thrombocythaemia.

He was treated both with aspirin (to prevent thrombosis), hydroxyurea, followed by anagrelide and subsequently by hydroxyurea. At present he is under hematologists' follow up and doing well.

Clinical features of essential thrombocythaemia:

- Female preponderance.
- Features of both thrombosis like TIA, and haemorrhage.
- Erythromelalgia due to microvascular occlusion
- Mild Splenomegaly: huge splenomegaly usually indicates another myeloproliferative disorder.
- 50% of patients express JAK2 V1617F Mutation.

Thrombocytosis:

Occasionally thrombocytosis is encountered in clinical practice. Common causes of thrombocytosis are-

- As an inflammatory marker in patient with rheumatoid arthritis, Crohn's disease.
- In cases of active bleeding.
- Post splenectomy and hyposplenism
- Essential thrombocythaemia.

: KEY POINTS :

- Polycythaemia is relatively uncommon in clinical practice.
- PRV should be differentiated from secondary causes.
- Urgent venesection may improve morbidity in patients with polycythaemia with high haematocrit.

FURTHER REFERENCES:

- Spivak SL Polycythaemia vera : myths, mechanism's and management. Blood 100 : 4272, 2002.
- Harrison's principles of internal medicine -15th edition - Anaemia and Polycythaemia.

59

A PATIENT WITH MYASTHENIA GRAVIS

CASE: *A 51 yrs. old gentleman presented with 6 months history of generalized muscle weakness aggravated with increasing activities. He was finding it difficult to keep his head straight with a tendency to drop forward. In the evening time he was finding it difficult to keep his eye lids open. He was also having double vision on lateral gaze. Examination revealed bilateral ptosis, bilateral weakness of lateral gaze and weakness of neck muscles. Prolonged conversation caused nasal intonation of his speech. Motor and sensory examinations of the extremities were normal. Investigations revealed normal haematological and biochemical parameters. CPK- normal, X-ray chest- normal. CT scan of thorax was suggestive of enlarged thymus. EMG was consistent with myasthenia gravis. Acetylcholine antibody report came back as strongly positive.*

DIAGNOSIS: Myasthenia gravis with bulbar involvement.

DISCUSSION:

Myasthenia gravis, an autoimmune disease, resulting in muscle weakness is an uncommon presentation in clinical practice although generalized asthenia and weakness is very commonly encountered in clinical practice. On careful history taking a minority of them may be found out to be suffering from organic disorders like myopathy on myasthenia gravis.

PATHOGENESIS:

There is decreased number of acetylcholine receptors (AchRs) at the synaptic junctions which lead to a characteristic weakness. In 85% of cases, the AchR loss is AchR antibody mediated and in 15% cases AchR antibody is apparently absent (although there is transfer of disease from seronegative myasthenic mothers to their babies and improvement of such patients with plasma exchange). Recently IgG antibodies to muscle specific Kinases (Musk) have been detected in those who are AchR antibody negative. These antibodies may be responsible for the inhibition of AchR clustering, consistent with the pathogenic action of MG.

Symptoms and signs:

- Weakness in different group of muscles
- Exercise induced fatigue
- Dysphagia
- Weakness of neck muscles
- Difficulty in breathing and features of hypoventilation
- Low breath count

Differential diagnosis:

- Myopathy (high CPK)
- Motor neuron disease (EMG)
- Neuropathy (NCV study, Lumbar puncture).
- Thyroid dysfunction (T_3, T_4, TSH)

Diagnostic tests:

- EMG – single fiber EMG is positive in more than 90% of cases.
- AchR antibody – positive in 85% of cases.
- CT scan may show thymoma.
- Edrophonium test – injection of edrophonium (IV) improves muscle function.

Ocular Myasthenia: Occasionally myasthenia involves only the eye muscles. AchR is negative in 50% of cases. Diagnosis will be dependent on edrophonium test if single fibre EMG is not available.

MANAGEMENT:

Pharmacological treatment: Oral long acting acetyl cholinesterase inhibitors are the drug of choice (Pyridostigmine 30-60 mg 4 hourly). Excessive dosage can cause cholinergic crisis. Abdominal pain and diarrhea may be troublesome symptom.

Role of thymectomy: It is ideally indicated in patients with thymic hyperplasia or thymoma who are also +ve for AchR antibody. It may also be indicated in AchR antibody negative patients whose symptoms are inadequately controlled by pharmacological therapy.

Immunosuppressive therapy: Indicated in suboptimal result following surgery or patients declining surgery.

Medication:

- **Corticosteroids** – It should be started with a small dose and the dose should be built up slowly to avoid myasthenic crisis.
- **Azathioprine** – It is a slow acting drug and has steroid sparing effect.
- **Cyclosporine** – may be used if azathioprine is ineffective.
- Cyclic IV **cyclophosphamide** (monthly)
- **Mycophenolate mofetil** has been recently used with success.

Plasma exchange and IV gammaglobulin infusion: These two methods have been found to be equally effective in randomized controlled trials. These methods may be helpful in myasthenic crisis or before preparing the patients with high AchR antibody titre before thymectomy.

The index patient was seen by neurologist, who suggested preoperative plasmapheresis in view of high AchR antibody titre. The patient underwent plasmapheresis for 5 days followed by thymectomy. He made reasonably good recovery and he was discharged on pyridostigmine, low does prednisolone and azathioprine. 6 months at follow up, he made almost 80% recoveries and immunosuppressive therapy was discontinued.

CASE: *A 66 yrs. old lady was transferred from another medical centre with severe episodic hypoventilation. She had all the relevant tests with negative results (EMG, NCV, CT thorax, T_3, T_4, TSH, CPK). In the ITU, she was found to be hypoventilating with drowsiness and raised P_aCO_2 level and needed intubation. Injection of neostigmine IV was found to increase the respiratory rate. Repeat EMG (single fibre EMG was not available). MRI brain, NCV were all normal. In view of the therapeutic response to neostigmine, she received IV methylprednisolone and plasmapheresis without any positive result. Meanwhile AchR antibody titre came back as negative. She remained on artificial ventilation. In this desperate situation, she was given 5 days course of IV immunoglobulin and surprisingly following this therapy she started responding and was off ventilator in the next 5 days.*

However, there was a further twist to the story with her complaining of severe pelvic girdle pain for 2 days followed by flaccid paraparesis, a feature suggestive of transverse myelitis. She was again given IV methyl prednisolone. After two months of hospital stay, she left hospital in a wheelchair bound state with a final diagnosis of myasthenia gravis followed by acute transverse myelitis. Multiple senior level consultations at different stages could not offer any satisfactory explanation of such atypical presentation of myasthenia gravis and above all even if the initial diagnosis was correct, what was the correlation between her myasthenia gravis and subsequent development of acute transverse myelitis.

PROBABLE DIAGNOSIS: Myasthenia gravis followed by acute transverse myelitis.

Other causes stimulating myasthenia:

1. **Congenital myasthenia syndrome** – Ach receptor deficiencies, slow channel and low affinity fast channel related problems.
2. **Hypo and hyperthyroidism**

3. **Lambert Eaton syndrome** – which is a presynaptic disorder with predominant involvement of proximal group of muscles of lower extremities. Eyes are involved in 70% of cases. Autoimmune involvement with dry mouth or impotence may also be present. Deep reflexes are absent. Repetitive Nerve stimulation test shows-incremental rather than decremental nerve stimulation response. This syndrome is caused by autoantibodies against P/O type calcium channels at the motor nerve terminals. It is commonly associated with small cell carcinoma lungs. The treatment is by plasmapheresis or 3, 4 diaminopyridine and pyridostigmine.

4. **Botulism** – may have similar features.

5. **Neuro asthenia** – which is a non organic disorder may simulate myasthenia.

Associated conditions:

MG may be commonly associated with thymoma, thymic hyperplasia, Hashimoto's thyroiditis, Graves disease, rheumatoid arthritis, SLE. Clinicians should do appropriate tests in order to exclude these conditions.

Drugs that flare up myasthenic symptoms and should be avoided:

- Aminoglycosides
- Non depolarizing muscle relaxants like Atracurium, Vecuronium
- Betablockers
- Penicillamine
- Quinine
- Botulinum toxin
- Local anesthetics like xylocaine.

CASE: *A 41 years old lady presented with fever and breathlessness. Her chest X-ray showed a mediastinal mass along with right lower lobe pneumonitic changes. Antibiotics were started but she developed Type II respiratory failure needing ventilatory support. She was successfully extubated by developed repeated respiratory failure needing reintubation and ventilation in spite of clearance of her chest infection. CT guided FNAC from the mass suggested either lymphoma or more probably thymoma. Since her Ach receptor antibody which was sent later on, was strongly positive, she underwent 5 sessions of plasmapheresis followed by removal of her mediastinal mass which was proved to be thymoma following thoracotomy. Post operative period was surprisingly uneventful and she was put on incremental dose of steroid and pyridostigmine. 4 weeks during post discharge follow up she was doing well.*

DIAGNOSIS: Thymoma with myasthenia gravis presenting with respiratory failure without presence of any other classical features of myasthenia.

CASE: *A 60 years old lady presented with history of transient weakness of left leg along with tingling sensation which was persisting, MRI brain and L.S. Spine did not reveal any gross abnormality and she had a provisional diagnosis of T.I.A. In the ward, she developed repeated type II respiratory failure needing ventilatory support. It was initially thought that it was probably a manifestation of obstructive sleep apnea which she had had in the past. However, with a view to exclude any neuro muscular abnormality she underwent bedside EMG and NCV studies and to our surprise she was found to have features consistent with AIDP (Acute Inflammatory demyelinating polyneuropathy). She was offered I.V. Immunoglobulin for 5 days and finally she could be weaned off from ventilation.*

DIAGNOSIS: AIDP presenting atypically with acute respiratory failure.

CASE: A 36 years old lady presented with respiratory distress and generalized muscle ache for some duration. Her CPK level was very high and subsequent EMG report was consistent with polymyositis. She was treated with steroid and azathioprine with good improvement.

DIAGNOSIS: Polymyositis with week intercostal muscles leading to respiratory failure.

CASE: *A 65 yrs. old gentleman presented with respiratory failure needed BiPAP therapy. Neurological evaluation showed presence of wasting of small muscles of hands. EMG later on proved it to be a case of motor neurone disease.*

DIAGNOSIS: Respiratory failure due to motor neurone disease.

In any patients presenting with muscle weakness and respiratory failure, myasthenia gravis, polymyositis, motor neurone disease and poly neuropathy (both AIDP and CIDP) should be considered in the differential diagnosis.

Myasthenic crisis:

This may be precipitated by some intercurrent infection. It can also be due to over medication with pyridostigmine (known as cholinergic crisis). The patients should be treated in ITU, anticholinesterase medications stopped and should be provided with respiratory support if needed. Plasmapheresis or IVIg may help to hasten the recovery.

: KEY POINTS :

- Myasthenia gravis is uncommon in clinical practice.
- Associated thymic pathology should be looked for.
- Thymectomy is useful in Ach receptor positive patients with thymic hyperplasia.

FURTHER REFERENCES:

- Harrison's Principle of Internal Medicine – 17th Ed.
- Oxford Text Book of Medicine.

60 ACUTE PHASE PROTEINS IN CLINICAL PRACTICE

Acute phase response: Acute phase response is a generalized term used to describe a series of diverse local and systemic events those accompany with inflammation and tissue damage. These changes also include synthesis of specific liver derived acute phase proteins and these proteins are measured in clinical practice to assess the severity of inflammation. The synthesis of these acute phase proteins are stimulated by cytokines like interleukins and tumour necrosis factor predominantly derived from the macrophages at the site of injury. There are approximately 30 such acute phase proteins, although only few of them are in clinical use. During inflammation there are a group of proteins whose levels decrease as a result of decreased synthesis. They are called negative acute phase proteins. Albumin, pre-albumin, retinol binding protein and transferrin fall in this category.

Common acute phase proteins that increase during inflammation:

- C-reactive protein
- Complement
- Fibrinogen
- Serum amyloid A protein
- Alfa-1-antitrypsin
- Ferritin

Clinical use of acute phase response:

- They are mainly used to diagnose various inflammation and infective condition.
- They are helpful to differentiate organic from functional disease (normal in irritable bowel syndrome, soft tissue rheumatism etc).
- They are helpful in monitoring the therapy.

Laboratory measurement of acute phase response:

ESR and plasma viscosity: ESR is the laboratory measurement of the rate of sedimentation of RBC which is dependent on aggregating of RBC by different acute phase response proteins like fibrinogen, α-2 macroglobulin and immunoglobulin. It is a very common parameter used in clinical practice. However it has got limitation like -

- It is influenced by several parameters like presence of abnormal immunoglobulins as in myeloma.
- It can be influenced by drugs, sex and lipids in the diet resulting in circadian rhythm.
- It mainly reflects the change in fibrinogen level which as an acute phase response protein is slow to rise with persistence for a long time. As a result, in acute

inflammation ESR is slow to rise and may persist for long. It may give erroneous result, where fibrinogen is consumed as in DIC. It is useful in chronic inflammation or infective diseases.

Causes of very high ESR:

- Myeloma
- Tuberculosis
- Giant cell arteritis
- Malignancy
- Infection like infective endocarditis, inflammatory arthritis and gout ESR is high, where as in osteoarthritis it is usually not elevated. ESR may be moderately high in anaemia.

CRP is **only slightly raised in:**

- SLE
- Ulcerative colitis
- Leukaemia
- Dermatomyositis
- Graft versus Host Disease

Plasma viscosity: It is also heavily dependent on fibrinogen and other group of proteins. However it is not affected by red cells and independent of sex and much easier to standardize.

C-reactive protein (CRP): It rises very quickly following inflammation and comes down quickly following treatment thereby making it suitable acute phase response protein for diagnosis and monitoring the therapy. In infective endocarditis, falling CRP titre is helpful in monitoring therapy. In a similar fashion it is also helpful in prognostication of acute pancreatitis.

In SLE, CRP is usually not raised and rise of CRP in SLE would indicate intercurrent infection.

CRP may also be helpful in prognostication in patients with unstable angina where its level is usually raised.

Role of CRP in clinical practice:

- To differentiate organs from functional Disorders like IBD & IBS
- To diagnose infection, inflammation and malignancy
- To follow up: the effect of treatment

Very high CRP is found in:

Inflammatory	
	Rheumatoid arthritis
	Polymyalgia rheumatica
	Crohn's disease
Necrosis	
	Myocardial infraction
	Acute Pancreatitis
Trauma	
	Surgery
	Burns
	Fracture
Malignancy	
	Multiple myeloma
Infection	
	Many bacteria e.g. infective endocarditis, tuberculosis.

Newer molecules as markers of inflammation: Recently interest has generated about the role of newer molecules as a marker of inflammation like procalcitonin, interleukin-6 etc and they have been shown to be of promise in detecting sepsis, systemic inflammation as well as prognostication in sepsis and various other medical conditions.

Causes of increase in procalcitonin (Pro CT):

- Sepsis, systemic inflammatory response syndrome (SIRS), burn, pancreatitis.
- Medullary carcinoma of thyroid.
- Aspiration pneumonia and ARDS.
- Small cell carcinoma of lung.

In sepsis Pro CT, it is not only helpful in diagnosis, persistently raised Pro CT may indicate severity of the disease thereby indicating a poor prognostic marker (may be helpful in acute severe pancreatitis, hospital acquired pneumonia etc). The value of Pro CT as an inflammatory marker has been compared with CRP, IL-6, lactate and pentraxin-3 and has been found to be superior to all of them in terms of sensitivity, specificity, positive and negative predictive value (sensitivity 89%, specificity 94%, negative predictive value 90% and positive predictive value 94%).

Different Acute Phase Proteins	
Increased	**Decreased**
α_1 antitrypsin	Albumin
Fibrinogen	Pre-albumin
Prothrombin	HDL
Complements c_3 c_4 c_5	LDL
Haptoglobin	
Ceruloplasmin	
C-reactive proteins	
Ferritin	

: KEY POINTS :

- Acute phase response proteins are important tests for diagnosis, prognostication and follow up of many clinical conditions.
- In clinical practice, CRP has better discriminating value than ESR.
- Procalcitonin and IL-6 are useful new markers which may prove superior to CRP.

FURTHER REFERENCES:

- Acute phase response- Rosamonde Banks et al, Oxford Text Book of Rheumatology, Vol. 1 (4.1 - P 361 -367).
- Procalcitonin and calcification gene family of peptides in inflammation infection and sepsis, K L Becker *et al*, Journal of Clinical Endocrinology and Metabolism, 89(4); 1512 - 1525, 2004.

61 A PATIENT WITH URTICARIA

CASE: *A 30 years old Bangladeshi patient attended the clinic with a history of severe itching of the body, rash and facial swelling along with a burning sensation. During the attack, his skin became red, itchy and on scratching there were formation of visible marks. He identified that eating certain food stuffs caused these attacks. Examination was satisfactory, skin showed urticarial rash in upper extremities and presence of dermatographism on scratching the skin. Investigations revealed normal FBC with eosinophil count of 16%. T_3, T_4, TSH, ANF, and other baseline biochemical parameters were normal. On detailed enquiry, he was found to have specific food allergy and he was treated with corticosteroids and anti-histaminics with good symptomatic relief.*

DIAGNOSIS: Severe chronic urticaria with dermatographism.

DISCUSSION:

Urticaria is a common presentation in clinical practice. It is characterized by, itchy red swelling of various size and shape and it is usually transient in nature. It is caused by mast cell degranulation as a result of immunological stimulation. It can also be immune complex mediated, in which symptoms usually occurs 4-7 days following exposure.

CLINICAL PICTURE:

Sudden onset of itchy swelling is the hall mark. The lesions are smooth, raised and non-scaly wheals may occur anywhere in the body. Urticaria may occur alone or with angioedema, with classical swelling of the face. Laryngeal oedema may be life threatening. While urticaria occurs in superficial dermis, angioedema refers specially to localised deep tissue swelling.

Although the cause of urticaria is mainly due to release of histamine which is IgE mediated, it can also be triggered by neurogenic causes or by direct stimulation by opiates or strawberries. Angioedema, on the other hand, is due to release of bradykinin. Infection, trauma and ACE inhibitors (by way of preventing the breakdown of bradykinin) are the significant causes of angioedema. It must be remembered that there is a general misconception that urticaria in particular is rarely due to allergy.

DIFFERENT VARIETIES:

➢ **ACUTE URTICARIAS:** Causes are-

- **Drugs:** Penicillin, cephalosporins, aspirin, toxoid, insulin, quinine, morphine, codeine.

- **Food:** Fish, nuts, chocolates, sea fish, tomato, strawberries, milk, cheese, spices, yeast, dyes and food additives like tartrazine (a synthetic lemon yellow azo dye).
- **Infection:** Viral, protozoal, UTI.
- **General:** SLE, lymphoma, polycythaemia.
- **Congenital / Hereditary:** Hereditary C_1 esterase inhibitor deficiency.

➢ **PHYSICAL URTICARIAS:**

- **Dermatographism:** simple pressure on the skin produces urticaria (photo reference).
- **Solar, cold, heat urticaria:** urticaria develops in response to sweating, exercise, emotions – difficult to treat.

➢ **CHRONIC NON-ALLERGIC URTICARIA (more than six week's duration):** Very frustrating to treat. These patients are otherwise healthy. Elimination of diet/ drug should be tried.

Causes non-allergic urticaria and angioedema:

Urticaria with angioedema	Angioedema alone
• Stress (50%-70%). • Infections like *H. pylori*. • Physical pressure • Drug induced e.g. NSAID, opioids. • Vitamin B_{12} deficiency • Iron deficiency • Thyroid disorders • Liver disease • Mastocytosis • Hypocomplemententemic vasculitis. • Cholinergic, Idiopathic	• Stress. • Infection. • Hereditary due to C_1 esterase inhibitor deficiency. • Drugs: ACE inhibitors, Statins, Proton pump inhibitors, NSAIDS. • Acquired angioedema: myeloma, lymphoma.

INVESTIGATIONS:

- FBC,
- Eosinophil,
- ANF,
- T_3 T_4 & TSH,
- LFT,
- Autoantibody,
- C1 esterase inhibitor,
- Stool for R/E,
- X-ray chest.

MANAGEMENT:

Urticaria without angioedema:

- Non sedating long-acting antihistamines *e.g.* cetrizine.

If still symptomatic

↓

- Add on sedative anti-histaminic *e.g.* hydroxyzine, chlorpheniramine

If still symptomatic in stressed persons

↓

- Add on doxepin, mirtazapine

If still symptomatic

↓

- Add on H_2-receptor blockers
- Add on montelukast.
- Add on calcium channel blockers
- amitriptyline

If still symptomatic in stressed persons

↓

- Add on cyclosporine, tacrolimus

If still symptomatic in stressed persons

↓

- Add on IV immunoglobulin or omalizumab.

Urticaria with angioedema:

The initial management would be the same. In recalcitrant cases, one needs to consider tranexamic acid up to 1 g four times/day or androgen in place of tranexamic acid.

Role of steroids:

It should be used only in emergency. Adrenaline should be reserved for emergency.

Role of Immunosuppressive Therapy:

Cyclosporine is of value. Alternatively tacrolimus may be appropriate.
Other agents that may be used in arterial vasculitis are:

- Chloroquine
- Hydroxychloroquine
- Dapsone
- Methotrexate
- Omalizumab

Topical therapies like doxepin cream with potent H_1 and H_2 antagonist property or menthol in aqueous lotion may also be used.

In hereditary angioedema, treatment is carried out in similar fashion. Prophylaxis with tranexamic acid with monitoring of liver function may be tried. Danazol and stanozolol are potential alternatives.

If attacks are frequent intravenous weekly C_1 esterase inhibitor is appropriate. Acute attacks may also be treated with C_1 esterase inhibitor or with icatibant, a bradykinin antagonist which is administered subcutaneously.

Patients with cold urticaria should avoid swimming and participating in winter sports.

: KEY POINTS :

- Urticaria is a common problem in clinical practice.
- Food allergy, drug allergies are the common causes.
- Chronic recurrent urticaria is frustrating to treat.
- Elimination in diet and avoidance of the offending drugs are the mainstay of treatment.
- Acute angioneurotic oedema is a medical emergency and should be treated with IV steroid and in some cases with adrenaline.

FURTHER REFERENCES:

- Dermatology in practice: Anthony Villeor.
- Clinical dermatology: Rona M Mackie– 4th edition.
- G Spickeft–urticaria and angioedema—The Journal of Royal College of Physician [Vol.-44 1 March 2014]
- Harrison's Principle of Internal Medicine: 17th edition.
- Oxford Book of Medicine: 5th edition.

62 A PATIENT WITH HYPOPITUITARISM

CASE: *A 65 years old diabetic lady was admitted with unwellbeing, swelling of legs and recurrent vomiting with drowsiness. She had been deteriorating over the last few months with increasing headache and history of loss of consciousness on one occasion. Initial CT brain scan was reported to be normal. On admission, she looked puffy, pale, oedematous and systemic examination did not reveal anything specific. Her BP was 160/90 mmHg. Investigations: Hb- 8.6 g%, Na- 122 mmol/lit (low), K- 3.8 mmol/lit, LFT, amylase, urea, creatinine all are normal, urine- glucose+++, trace of albumin and ketones, TSH- 0.03 (low), T_3 and T_4 (low normal), in X-ray chest and USG abdomen NAD.*

She was treated with IV insulin via syringe pump and normal saline infusion, within the next 6 hours she developed severe symptomatic hypoglycemia with increasing drowsiness which was corrected along with correction of hyponatraemia with partial improvement of her symptoms. A repeat CT scan of brain was suggestive of enlargement of pituitary gland. MRI brain scan confirmed the presence of a pituitary space occupying lesion with evidence of recent haemorrhage in it. At this point, baseline hormonal assessment was done which showed- FSH 3.8 IU/l (normal post menopausal level more than 30 IU/l), low LH level, prolactin 68 IU/litre (normal - less than 20 IU/l), 9 am cortisol level 3.6 IU/l (low), ACTH level (low). Plasma growth hormone level, ADH level and hormonal stimulation test was not done in this patient.

DIAGNOSIS: Pituitary adenoma with features of hypopituitarism.

DISCUSSION:

This lady was initially thought to be suffering from diabetic nephropathy along with diabetic gastroparesis with recurrent vomiting leading to hyponatraemia with metabolic encephalopathy. However investigation revealed that this lady was suffering from hypopituitarism with multiple hormonal deficiencies. With hind sight her recent spell of unconsciousness was probably related to pituitary haemorrhage as evident in the MRI brain scan. Her severe hypoglycemic episode due to low dose insulin was probably a reflection of insulin hypersensitivity in the face of cortisol deficiency.

Upon diagnosis she was commenced on prednisolone (10 mg) followed by thyroxin 25 microgram (initial dose). Within 72 hours she had symptomatic improvement. She became more alert and conscious. Her mobility improved and she was referred to the neurosurgical team for consideration of trans-sphenoidal surgery of the pituitary tumour.

Hypopituitarism is an uncommon presentation in clinical practice. Before discussing about pituitary dysfunction, we should first recapitulate the normal physiology of pituitary-hypothalamic system which would help to clarify the pathological conditions.

Pituitary hormones secreted from the anterior pituitary gland:

- Growth hormone
- FSH
- LH
- ACTH
- Prolactin

Hormone secreted from posterior pituitary gland (actually secreted from the hypothalamus and stored in pituitary stock):

- Antidiuretic hormone
- Oxytocin

Hypothalamic control of pituitary gland:

Stimulating effect	Inhibiting effect
• Cortisol releasing hormone • Thyrotropin releasing hormone • Gonadotropin releasing hormone • Growth hormone releasing hormone	• Prolactin release inhibiting hormone • Growth hormone release inhibiting hormone.

Lesions of Pituitary gland:

- Growth hormone secreting adenoma.
- Prolactin secreting adenoma (micro-prolactinoma and macro-prolactinoma). Sometimes there is secretion of both prolactin and growth hormone from the adenoma.
- ACTH Secreting lesion.
- Cushing's disease (ACTH secreting micro-adenoma).
- Nelson's syndrome - In patients with past history of bilateral adrenalectomy, there may be hypertrophy of ACTH secreting glands due to negative feedback mechanism.
- Rarely FSH, LH or TSH secreting tumour.
- Chromophobe adenoma- sometimes pituitary adenomas are non-secreting and non-functioning and the features are due to hormone deficiencies (as in this case). There may be involvement of pituitary stalk with resultant ADH deficiency (diabetes insipidus). Due to the presence of simultaneous cortisol deficiency, the full manifestation of diabetes insipidus will not manifest (cortisol is needed for excretion of water load from the kidneys). It is only after cortisol supplementation the patient will develop classical features of diabetes insipidus. In non functioning adenomas, one may find prolactin level to be high. This is because of hypothalamic extension of

the lesion and as prolactin is under inhibitory control from the hypothalamus (via dopaminergic neurone), the prolactin level will be increased. However the increment will not be as high as in case of prolactinoma where the level may increase several hundred folds. (The index patient has slightly elevated prolactin level indicating pituitary stalk lesion rather than prolactinoma).

Other causes of raised prolactin level:

- Physiological- pregnancy
- Drugs- dopamine antagonist and dopamine receptor blocking drugs metoclopramide, haloperidol, domperidone.

CLINICAL EXAMINATION:

- Visual perimetry may reveal bitemporal field defect. X-ray skull- enlargement of sella turcica. MRI and CT Brain scan (MRI is better).
- Hormonal assay- ACTH, FSH, CH, Prolactin, GH, ADH, Cortisol, T_3, T_4, TSH.
- Na, K, Urinary and plasma osmolality.
- In case of suspected deficiency, hormonal stimulation test *e.g.* assay of growth hormone, ACTH following insulin induced hypoglycemia.
- In case of hormonal excess, hormonal suppression test *e.g.* estimation of growth hormone following glucose load or arginine infusion. In case of diabetes insipidus, water deprivation test may be done (discussed in the chapter of hyponatraemia).

Causes of pituitary hypothalamic dysfunction:

- Hypothalamic dysfunction
- Kallmann syndrome - due to deficiency of LHRH (anosmia, hypogonadism).
- Hypothalamic tumour.

Craniopharyngioma:

Tumour of the remnants of Rathke's pouch (mainly presents in childhood with headache and variable combination of pituitary hormonal deficiency).

Pituitary adenoma:

- Functioning - gigantism, acromegaly, prolactinoma, Cushing's disease.
- Non- functioning - chromophobe adenoma.

Post-partum pituitary necrosis: (Sheehan's syndrome)

Still common in rural India, where obstetric facilities are poor. This condition occur following post-partum haemorrhage which leads to pituitary necrosis with features of pituitary failure. This condition should be considered in a post partum patient with non-specific symptoms of weakness, alopecia, persistent amenorrhea, anaemia *etc.* Granulomatous disorders like sarcoidosis, eosinophilic granuloma of pituitary gland can cause features of pituitary failure (classically diabetes insipidus). Head injury can cause diabetes insipidus. Secondary deposits can rarely cause pituitary deficiency.

CASE: *A 36 years old patient was admitted in the ITU with head injury following a road traffic accident. CT Brain showed no obvious intracranial lesion. Over the next few days he developed polyuria. His plasma Na was 155 mmol/l, plasma osmolality 287 mmol/kg and urinary osmolality 301 mmol/kg. He was diagnosed to have trauma induced diabetes insipidus and responded well to SC vasopressin therapy.*

DIAGNOSIS: Diabetes insipidus caused by head injury.

CASE: *A 27 years old lady was admitted from a rural set up where she was initially admitted with history of drowsiness, weakness and anaemia. She delivered a baby 7 months back and the delivery was complicated with severe post-partum haemorrhage, which was managed conservatively. She had amenorrhea since her last child birth. Examination revealed pale and puffy lady and was drowsy. Investigations revealed Hb- 7.8 g%, Na- 123 mmol/l, TSH- 0.01, T_4- low, T_3- low, cortisol low normal, FSH and LH low. She was diagnosed to have Sheehan's syndrome and started on prednisolone (10 mg) followed by thyroxin and cyclical oestrogen and progesterone (with the consultation of gynaecologist). She also received 3 units of blood transfusion. She made a good recovery and was discharged home in a stable condition.*

DIAGNOSIS: Sheehan's syndrome.

Clinical features of Pituitary tumours:

- Due to hormone excess *e.g.* Acromegaly, Gigantism.
- Due to hormone deficiency *e.g.* Diabetes insipidus.
- Due to local pressure effect *e.g.* Visual field defect, multiple cranial nerve palsy, if cavernous sinus is involved cause headache, hypothalamic involvement may cause weight gain and drowsiness and diabetes insipidus by way of pituitary stalk involvement.

CASE: *A 57 years old post menopausal lady attended the clinician with history of galactorrhoea. Her prolactin level was found to be high. She was found to be on PAN-D (pantoprazole + domperidone) for long. The drug was stopped with subsidence of galactorrhoea.*

DIAGNOSIS: Drug induced high prolactin level causing galactorrhoea

CASE: *A 55 years old post menopausal lady presented with history of galactorrhoea. Her prolactin level was high, MRI brain scan revealed micro-prolactinoma. Her visual perimetry was normal. Neurosurgical assessment suggested conservative management with cabergoline. She was advised as yearly follow up with visual perimetry and MRI brain scan along with regular measurement of prolactin level. She is on twice weekly cabergoline (0.5 mg) with normalization of prolactin level and subsidence of galactorrhoea.*

DIAGNOSIS: Micro-prolactinoma resulting galactorrhoea.

MANAGEMENT:

Although hormone replacement is needed in individual hormone deficiency syndrome, mainstay of the treatment is localization of the pituitary tumour and its surgical removal. Nowadays trans-sphenoidal resection is the preferred route although in large tumours trans-frontal route may have to be chosen. Sometimes surgery may be supplemented with external beam radiation. Implantation of radioactive Yttrium, (Y90) via trans-sphenoidal route is another alternative way of treatment. Surgery must be followed by replacement therapy with steroid, thyroxin and in some cases cyclical estrogen/progesterone therapy. In micro-prolactinoma, bromocriptine is the drug of choice. Although it causes resolution of infertility, galactorrhoea and amenorrhea, in cases of macro-prolactinoma, trans-sphenoidal surgery would still be needed to counter the local pressure effect. In acromegaly, although somatostatin analogues may biochemically reduce the growth hormone level, surgery is needed for symptomatic improvement.

Individual diseases:

- **Acromegaly** - Classical case is easy to diagnosis and the real challenge is to diagnose it early before the typical features appear. Headache, jaw pain, heel pain, arthritis, visual field defects are the manifestations. CT/MRI brain scan would detect a pituitary tumour, while growth hormone level following glucose load or arginine infusion will confirm the diagnosis.

- **Prolactinoma** - Usually presents with headache, impotence in males and amenorrhea with infertility in females. Prolactin level is very high. Microadenoma may be treated with bromocriptine while macroadenoma needs surgical intervention like trans-sphenoidal surgery.

: KEY POINTS :

- Pituitary tumours are rare in clinical practice.
- Good amount of detective work including good history taking, brain imaging and hormonal assay studies will be needed for its early detection.
- Abnormal biochemical tests can give some initial clues for its detection.
- MRI brain scan has an edge over the CT brain scan in detecting pituitary tumours.

FURTHER REFERENCES:

- Lamberts *SWJ, et al.* (1998) - Pituitary insufficiency, Lancet 352: 127 - 134.
- Kumar and Clarke— clinical medicine— 5th edition.
- Harrison's Principle of Internal Medicine – 17th edition.
- Oxford Textbook of Medicine – 5th edition.

63 A PATIENT WITH ULCERATIVE COLITIS

CASE: *A 56 years old patient presented with intermittent bloody diarrhoea for last few years which was treated with oral metronidazole and quinolone with relief of symptoms during such episodes by his local practitioner. During one such episode he attended the clinic because of associated painful swelling of his knee and ankle joints along with ulcers over his shin bone. Examination revealed swollen hot right knee joint and left ankle joint. Abdomen was slightly tender. He looked pale. Investigations revealed Hb- 7.1 g%, WBC-16,000, Poly 90%, ESR & CRP was high, albumin– low, urea, creatinine and uric acid was normal, potassium 2.4 mmol/l, rheumatoid fact negative, ASO titre negative, normal, X-ray chest– old treated Koch's lesion (he had a past history of tuberculosis). Aspiration of fluid from the knee joint– cell counts raised, no pus cells, gram stain– negative.*

DIAGNOSIS: Reactive arthritis due to inflammatory bowel disease.

He underwent blood transfusion, IV ofloxacin, IV metronidazole, IV hydrocortisone and TPN therapy. His knee joints were injected with steroid. After stabilization of his medical condition, he underwent colonoscopy which revealed pan-colitis and the biopsy showed classical picture of ulcerative colitis. He was started on oral mesalazine. IV steroid was switched over the oral therapy and finally tapered off over next one month. Dermatologist thought that the cutaneous lesions over the skin was due to pyoderma gangrenosum and advised us to continue with the same therapy. Azathioprine was also added but withdrawn due to side effects. Over the next 2 years he had several admissions with exacerbation of ulcerative colitis each time responding to conservative measures.

At one point infliximab (Anti TNF antibody) was considered but rejected because of past history of tuberculosis (even during steroid therapy he received INH prophylaxis). During his last admission, he was quite toxic needing ITU care and during that time, cyclosporine was added to the regime. Of late he has been doing well. He is on yearly colonoscopic surveillance. The family members have been apprised of the risk of colon cancer in the future. The option of total colectomy with ileoanal anastomosis as the only preventive measure for the cancer had been discussed in details but the patient's relatives and the patient were not keen to have it.

Brief discussion of ulcerative colitis:

Ulcerative disease is characterized by continuous diffuse mucosal inflammation of the colon. It usually affects people of 20 to 40 yrs age group. It has got a prominent psychosomatic background with flare up of the disease during mental stress, smoking etc. Clinical features of UC is bloody diarrhoea not responding to usual anti-infective medicines and the severity score is judged by number of stools per day (>6 is characteristic of severe disease), fever, resting tachycardia (>100/min, indicates severe attack) and high increase of ESR (>30 mm/h). The disease process involves whole colon including rectum.

Crohn's disease by contrast, is a discontinuous disease with patchy transmural involvement of whole of intestine. Genetic factor may be involved in its causation (mutation of chromosome 16, 5 and 10). Smoking increases the risk of Crohn's disease. It is manifested by fever of unknown origin, abdominal pain, diarrhoea, mouth ulcer, intestinal obstruction, perianal pain and fistula (inflammatory, fistulating and fibrostenosing). Biopsy shows sarcoid like granuloma.

Features suggestive of Ulcerative Colitis:

- Bloody diarrhoea
- Fever, anaemia, tachycardia – in severe cases
- Nutritional deficiencies
- Colonoscopy – Collar-button ulcers, loss of haustration, pseudo-polyp formations

Features suggestive of Crohn's disease:

- Features of ileo-colitis with right iliac fossa pain, palpable mass.
- Fever, leukocytosis along with features of intestinal obstruction due to stricture.
- Fistula formation with adjacent organs or urinary bladder.
- Jejuno-ileitis with features of intestinal malabsorption.
- Perianal disease with anal fissure, perianal abscess.
- Gastro-duodenal disease with features of anorexia, nausea, vomiting.
- Colonoscopy reveals aphthous ulcers, cobble stoning and stricture formation.

Extra intestinal manifestation of inflammatory bowel disease:

- Erythema nodosum
- Pyoderma gangrenosum
- Reactive arthritis
- Ankylosing spondylosis
- Uveitis, episcleritis
- Cholelithiasis
- Sclerosing cholangitis, biliary cirrhosis
- Urolithiasis
- Metabolic bone disease
- Increased incidence of deep vein thrombosis.

INVESTIGATIONS:

Serological markers: pANCA and ASCA antibodies are frequently found to be positive in IBD. P-ANCA is more often found to be in pancolitis.

MANAGEMENT:

Sulphasalazine and 5-aminosalicylic acid (5-ASA) preparations are the mainstay of treatment (mesalazine, olsalazine and balsalazide). 5 ASA preparations are equal in terms of efficacy. 5 ASA rectal preparations are also available and rectal suppositories are used in distal colitis with efficacy greater than steroid enema. Side effects like headache, nausea, Steven Johnson's syndrome, rarely agranulocytosis may occur with these groups of drug. Renal function needs monitoring.

TREATMENT:

Antibiotics: Occasionally in disease flare up, metronidazole and ciprofloxacin may be helpful. Metronidazole is particularly helpful in fistulous and perianal diseases.

Steroids: It is very useful for acute attack. Intravenous hydrocortisone followed by oral prednisolone (40 mg starting dose) is the usual agent. However, oral budesonide, in view of its extensive hepatic first pass metabolism may be preferred because of its low systemic toxicity.

Immunosuppressive drugs:

- **Azathioprine:** 2-3 mg/kg has a steroid sparing effect. It is slow to act. It can cause leucopoenia. Periodic monitoring of full blood count, liver function test will be necessary.
- **Methotrexate:** In the dose of 25 mg/week is a suitable alternative in patients intolerant to azathioprine. Regular monitoring of full blood count and liver function test is mandatory.
- **Cyclosporine:** It is the most effective of the immunosuppressives. Its onset of action is quick and can be given either intravenously or orally. The low dose regime (2-3 mg/kg) has lesser toxicity compared to the standard 4 mg/kg dose schedule. Kidney function should be monitored regularly.

Biological therapy: **IV Infliximab** (anti TNF-alpha antibody) may be used in recalcitrant cases, where surgical treatment is not feasible. It can cause reactivation of TB and should be avoided in patients with past history of tuberculosis. The cost is prohibitive by Indian standards. They may have a role in UC.

Probiotics: Crohn's disease is treated in the similar line except for the role of 5-ASA is doubtful. Prolonged use of metronidazole and ciprofloxacin may be helpful in healing of perianal fistulating lesions specific nutritional therapy (with elemental formulas) may have a therapeutic effect on Crohn's disease.

Newer immune suppressive therapies:

- Dapsone
- Adalimumab
- Certolizumab pegol inj.

Drugs that may be used in pregnancy:

- Sulphasalazine with folic acid supplementation
- Steroids
- Azathioprine if indicated.

Surgery:

In ulcerative colitis it may be indicated in acute flare up of UC with toxic mega colon. It is a medical emergency which might need urgent colectomy. It is a serious condition and while treating patients with UC the clinicians should be aware of it (X-ray abdomen shows distended colon with diameter more than 6 cm). Panproctocolectomy is curative and abolishes the risk of colon cancer in the future. Patients unwilling to undergo such procedure should undergo regular colonoscopic surveillance to detect early cancer. In Crohn's disease surgery is not curative hence conservative approach should be taken. Small intestinal resection with anastomosis is a frequently needed procedure.

CASE: *A 42 years old male presented with bloody diarrhoea, fever and abdominal pain. Recently he was on a holiday trip to sea side and was taking outside food regularly. Examination revealed abdominal tenderness with increased bowel sounds. Investigation revealed high WBC count, stool examination reveal pus cells, RBC and trophozoites and cyst of Entamoeba histolytica. He was treated with IV fluids, IV metronidazole and IV ofloxacin with symptomatic relief within 48 hours.*

DIAGNOSIS: Amoebic colitis.

DISCUSSION: Acute diarrhoeal illness is very common in clinical practice and clinician should be aware of the approach in such patients as some of them can lead to chronic illness and sometimes life threatening condition.

Diarrhoea may be of small intestinal and large intestinal origin. **In small intestinal diarrhoea, the volume may be large and in large intestinal diarrhoea the stool amount is small and frequent along with tenesmus.** Again diarrhoea may be toxin mediated where there may not be any fever or abdominal pain or it may be due to invasion of the mucosa which usually gives rise to pain, fever and bloody diarrhoea.

Example of small intestinal diarrhoea (infective): Giardiasis, viral, cholera *etc.*

Example of large intestinal diarrhoea (infective): Amoebiasis, *Shigellosis*, *Salmonellosis*, *Campylobacter* (both small intestinal and large intestinal) *etc.*

Example of toxin mediated diarrhoea: Cholera, staphylococcal diarrhoea, *E. coli* exotoxin induced diarrhoea, *Clostridium difficile* toxin induced diarrhoea (in severe cases it can cause bloody diarrhoea, intestinal obstruction etc.). In any patient on prolonged antibiotic therapy (mainly cephalosporin, clindamycin and quinolones) one should be aware of this condition and treat them promptly with oral vancomycin or metronidazole. *C. difficile* toxin estimation is not routinely done in many centres in India.

Example of diarrhoea due to mucosal invasion: Amoebiasis, *Salmonella*, *Shigella*, verotoxin producing strain of *E. coli* (due to 015747 strain). (One should also remember that enteroinvasive strain of *E. coli* can produce toxin which can produce Haemolytic Uraemic Syndrome (HUS) with haemolysis and renal impairment and the clinician should be aware of this condition in patients with acute diarrhoea followed by renal failure).

Sometimes acute diarrhoea may lead to a chronic phase occasionally seen in giardiasis. Tropical sprue is one such condition affecting visitors of the Western World to tropical countries. Non-tropical sprue is a somewhat similar condition affecting local residents of the tropical countries. In both the conditions definite causative organisms may not be found and they respond to long term tetracycline and folic acid therapy. Cryptosporidiosis is self limiting diarrhoea in an immunocompetent host. However in patients with AIDS, it may lead to chronic voluminous diarrhoea with weight loss. One should therefore always check for HIV antibody status in patients with chronic diarrhoea with weight loss.

CASE: *A 65 years old lady from North Bengal was admitted with chronic diarrhoea and generalized oedematous state with swelling of her face, legs, hands and abdomen. She was having breathlessness. She had an Echo in the past showing pericardial effusion which was drained. Investigations at that time did not reveal anything specific. Examination revealed generalized anasarca. Her Hb was 6.2 g%, urea, creatinine was normal, serum albumin– 2.0 g% (very low), rest of the liver function test was normal, 24 hour urinary* *albumin not raised, ANF and ANCA– negative. Ig Electrophoresis for M band was negative, Echo– presence of a big pericardial effusion, X-ray chest– bilateral pleural effusion, ECG– normal, Stool– undigested food materials++, Fat globules++, no organism, HIV status– negative, CT scan of pancreas– normal, amylase, lipase– normal.*

DIAGNOSIS: Protein losing enteropathy with gross hypoalbuminaemia, probable underlying cause- non tropical sprue.

She was treated with blood transfusion, vitamin and calcium supplementation, high protein containing enteral nutrition. She also underwent pericardiocentesis with continuous drainage for 48 hrs with relief of her breathlessness. She was put on short course of metronidazole (which she received many times in the past) and long term tetracycline and folic acid. She was reviewed after 3 months with no evidence of recurrence of her old problems. Her Hb was 9.6 g%, Albumin 3.2 g%, mild residual pericardial effusion and above all no oedema or diarrhoea. By retrospective thinking in terms of improvement following therapeutic challenge, we thought it to be a case of non-tropical sprue.

CASE: *A 46 years old recently diagnosed diabetes mellitus attended the clinic with chronic abdominal pain, weight loss and diarrhoea over the last few months. He drank alcohol only socially. Investigations revealed, random blood glucose of 215 mg%, slightly raised amylase, lipase and liver enzymes. Stool– globules++ (a feature of malabsorption). The stool was frothy, greasy and offensive. X-ray Abdomen showed abdominal calcification. CT abdomen confirmed pancreatic calcification with presence of calculi. ERCP showed dilated tortuous pancreatic duct with stricture. It was opined by the gastroenterologist that endoscopic therapy would not be successful in this case and he was referred to the surgeon for pancreatico-duodenal anastomosis. Following surgery he was pain free and with pancreatic enzyme supplementation, his diarrheal symptoms improved and he has gained weight.*

DIAGNOSIS: Chronic diarrhoea due to chronic calcific pancreatitis with diabetes mellitus.

DISCUSSION: While dealing with chronic diarrhoea *maldigestion (due to pancreatic insufficiency) should be differentiated from malabsorption.*

Causes of maldigestion: Due to pancreatic insufficiency due to various causes.

Causes of malabsorption: (The list is very long and only the common clinically encountered conditions have been mentioned here).

1. **Small intestinal–**
   Giardiasis,
   Jejunal diverticulosis,
   Blind loop syndrome,
   Coeliac disease,
   Small intestinal tuberculosis and Crohn's disease,
   Small intestinal resection,
   Small intestinal lymphoma,
   Tropical and non-tropical sprue

2. **Large intestinal–**
   Chronic amoebiasis
   Ulcerative colitis

Small and large intestinal ischemia, caecal neoplasm (left sided colonic neoplasm usually causes constipation).

There are rare endocrine causes of chronic diarrhoea such as VIP secreting tumours of intestine (VIPOMAS), serotonin secreting tumours of intestine (Carcinoid syndrome – intermittent diarrhoea, flushing of skin and skin rash) and should be considered in the appropriate setting. Lactose intolerance, food allergy and laxative abuse should also be considered in the differential diagnosis.

INVESTIGATIONS:

- Simple blood tests may indicate malabsorption *e.g.* FBC, calcium, ferritin, Vit-B_{12}, folate levels (folate levels may be high in jejunal diverticulosis because of increased production by the bacteria), stool examination for fat globulin, microscopy and 72 hr faecal fat excretion study (cumbersome and not generally done in routine clinical practice).
- Other less frequently performed tests – (14)C-D-xylose breath test. Xylose absorption test.
- Gastrointestinal series *e.g.* gastroscopy, colonoscopy, duodenal or jejunal biopsy, small bowel enema, enteroscopy.
- Pancreatic function test (not a frequently performed test).
- Pancreatic imaging with ultrasound, CT and endoscopic procedures (*e.g.* ERCP).

Once diagnosis is made, treatment is directed accordingly and detailed discussion is outside the scope of this book.

CASE: *A 45 years old woman from Bangladesh presented with anorexia, weight loss, mouth ulcer and generalized swelling of her body. She was complaining of diffuse abdominal pain. Examination revealed presence of pallor, mouth ulcer with angular cheilosis, oedema of legs and mild ascites. Investigations revealed Hb- 7.4%, albumin- 2.4 g%, urea and creatinine were normal, TSH and LFT were normal except for low albumin, calcium- low, ferritin- low, serum folate and vitamin* B_{12} *is low. CT scan abdomen revealed thickened mesentery and thickened terminal ileum. Barium follow through was consistent with Koch's or Crohn's or lymphoma of the terminal ileum. After discussing about the possible likelihood with the relatives, she was started on empirical anti-TB medication and started along with intensive nutritional replacement therapy. After a brief period of improvement she was discharged only to come back in 4 weeks time with features of intestinal obstruction. She underwent laparotomy where extensive involvement of the mesentery and terminal ileum was detected. The surgeon did a small intestinal resection, anastomosis along with omentectomy as much as possible and detected a very poor prognosis. After undergoing a turbulent post-operative course she finally recovered. Before discharge, the histological report came back as gastrointestinal stromal tumour (GIST) of small intestine and mesentery. Oncologist was involved and she was commenced imatinib.*

DIAGNOSIS: Gastrointestinal stromal tumour presenting with small intestinal obstruction.

DISCUSSION: GIST although uncommon in the clinical practice, may present to the clinicians with various gastrointestinal symptoms. GISTs are the most common mesenchymal tumor and are highly resistant to conventional chemotherapy or radiotherapy.

CLINICAL FEATURES: This condition usually affects patients over 50 years of age with no particular sex predilection. The commonly affected sites are-

1) Stomach- 50%.
2) Small bowel – 25%.
3) Colon and rectum- 10%.
4) Mesentery and omentum- 10%.

The patient may present with anemia, bloating and symptoms of obstruction and malabsorption as in the index case. Aggressive GIST may metastasize in liver and rarely to lungs and bones.

DIAGNOSIS: Routine radiological investigation with CT scan may pick it up. It may also be diagnosed incidentally during gastroscopy.

MANAGEMENT:

Surgical- Once diagnosed surgical resection is the treatment of choice. Since these lesions rarely metastasize to the lymph nodes, routine lymph node biopsy is not required.

Medical- Imatinib, a tyrosine kinase inhibitor, is the drug of choice in the dose of 400 mg twice daily. Imatinib achieves disease control in 70-80% of cases of advanced GIST with a survival rate in the range of two years to three years.

Imatinib resistant cases are difficult to treat. Alternative kinase inhibitors like sunitinib may also be tried. Newer inhibitors like dasatinib, nilotinib are on the horizon.

: KEY POINTS :

- Diarrhoeal illness is very common in clinical practice.
- Acute diarrhoea may be toxin medicated or due to mucosal invasion.
- Increasing use of colonoscopy has enabled us to diagnose inflammatory bowel disease at an earlier stage.
- In chronic diarrhoea, malabsorption due to various causes, maldigestion due to chronic pancreatitis, food intolerance, lactose intolerance and irritable bowel syndrome should be excluded.
- In chronic diarrhoea with marked weight loss, AIDS should be excluded in appropriate background.

FURTHER REFERENCES:

- Navarro F, Hanaver SB –Treatment of inflammatory bowel disease, safety and tolerability issues – Am Journal Gastroenterology - 98 (Supp 12) – 518, 2003.
- Harrison's Principle of Internal Medicine – 17th edition.
- Oxfords Text Book of Medicine- 5th edition.
- Brian P. Rubin *et al*: Gastrointestinal Stromal Tumor, Lancet 369-1731-41.
- Jason Blindsery *et al*.- Atrial Septal Defect in adults, The Lancet vol. 369-9569-Amt14. 1244-1246.

A PATIENT WITH JAUNDICE

CASE: *A 43 years old gentleman was admitted with history of fever followed by jaundice. Before his illness he was working in a remote place in Assam (North Eastern region of India) and drank water from a suspected contaminated well (A history which the patient gathered later on from the local residents). The reason for his transfer to our hospital was rising bilirubin (45 mg%) along with a creatinine of 3.2 mg% and a WBC count of 30,000. Examination revealed a toxic looking patient, deeply jaundiced with palpable liver. USG abdomen showed hepatomegaly. Urine examination revealed occasional RBC, pus cells and trace of protein. Virological markers (Hepatitis B, Hepatitis C, Hepatitis A, Hepatitis E and HIV antibody) were negative. Liver function test showed bilirubin of 64 mg% (highest ever I have come across). AST and ALT markedly raised, alkaline phosphatase raised, prothrombin time raised, amylase and lipase- normal, ANF, anti-smooth muscle antibody and anti-mitochondrial antibody were negative. He never gave any history of alcohol or illicit drug intake. Initially biliary sepsis was considered but repeated blood culture was negative and repeat ultrasound failed to demonstrate any biliary or hepatic obstruction. Based on the presumptive diagnosis of biliary sepsis he was given piperacillin-tazobactam. However, his WBC count did not show any improvement. On the 8th day of his admission, Leptospira antibody report came back as strongly positive and he was commenced on ampicillin 1 g four times/day. Over the next few weeks he made a steady recovery and after spending 4 weeks in the hospital, he was sent back to Assam in a stable condition. On discharge his bilirubin level was 2.1 mg% and renal function had returned back to normal.*

DIAGNOSIS: Leptospirosis presenting with jaundice and renal impairment.

Leptospirosis should be considered in any patient with febrile jaundice with renal impairment and conjunctival congestion if there is a history of exposure to contaminated water (mainly standing water such as lakes, ponds, sewage water *etc.*). The antibody test may be negative initially and in suspected cases empirical antibiotics should be commenced (doxycycline, ampicillin, penicillin). There may be isolated bilirubinaemia and the CPK level may be high. Steroids may be needed in some cases (Weil's syndrome).

CASE: *A 48 years old patient presented with repeated attacks of abdominal pain. Investigations in each time did not reveal anything specific, except for evidence of old duodenal scar on gastroscopy. His LFT, amylase, lipase, USG abdomen, CT abdomen were all within normal range. Urine for porphobilinogen was negative and he was diagnosed to have abdominal pain of psychosomatic origin and was started on antidepressant medication. During the fourth admission within a span of 6 months, we decided to do an ERCP. The test was reported to be technically difficult and only* *pancreatogram could be performed. The next day before discharge, he was reported to have passed yellow coloured urine. His discharge was deferred and a liver function test showed bilirubin of 4.2 mg%, alkaline phosphatase was also raised. The patient got very worried. Clinical examination did not reveal any surgical problem like perforation. MRCP revealed mildly dilated CBD with a small stone near the sphincter. A repeat ERCP was successful in cannulating the CBD and the stone was extracted uneventfully along with sphincterotomy. Both patient's relatives and the medical team heaved a sigh of relief and the patient did not complain of abdominal pain thereafter.*

DIAGNOSIS: Jaundice due to obstruction of CBD due to a small unidentified stone.

This patient was getting a biliary colic by a small stone unidentified by the standard tests. The first ERCP perhaps inadvertently dislodged the stone from its critical position which caused obstruction to the biliary tract and caused jaundice thereby making the disease spectrum clinically obvious. The message of this case is that biliary colic may sometimes evade detection even with standard methods and the clinician needs to be cautious about it and repeat test including MRCP or ERCP may be needed before diagnosing it to be due to functional in origin.

CASE: *A 29 years old diabetic patient was admitted with a history of drowsiness and jaundice. Clinical examination revealed grade 3 hepatic encephalopathy. His hepatitis A, B, C and E profile were negative. There was no relevant drug history. Past medical history suggested recurrent jaundice from his adolescent period. He went to another city 10 years back where investigations revealed increased 24 hour urinary copper excretion and low serum ceruloplasmin level consistent with Wilson's disease. He was prescribed penicillamine but was not taking it over last one year. The patient responded to conservative management and before discharge an ophthalmological consultation ruled out any Kayser- Fleischer ring (KF ring) which is a hallmark of neurological involvement in Wilson's disease. On recovery, the confirmatory tests for Wilson's disease were repeated which showed reduced serum ceruloplasmin level and increased 24 hours urinary copper excretion. He was recommenced on penicillamine and for the last 3 years on regular follow up has been doing reasonably well.*

DIAGNOSIS: Wilson's disease presenting with recurrent jaundice and hepatic failure.

Although very rare, the clinician should think of this condition in young patients with recurrent jaundice, anaemia and neurological features like Parkinson's disease and when other common causes are adequately eliminated by appropriate tests.

Wilson's disease:

DIAGNOSTIC CRITERIA:

- Clinical features of chronic active hepatitis
- Neuropsychiatric manifestation
- Presence of Kayser-Fleischer ring on slit lamp examination.
- Ceruloplasmin level less than 20 mg%

MANAGEMENT:

- Zinc- in mild cases without hepatitis and neuropsychiatric manifestation.
- Penicillamine- particularly in patients with neuropsychiatric manifestation (as a chelating agent).
- Trientine hydrochloride (a chelating agent)- it may worsen neuropsychiatric manifestation.

CASE: *A 15 years old boy, son of our hospital staff who hails from tribal areas of Orissa was admitted with high fever, joint pain, deep jaundice and drowsiness. Clinical examination revealed deep jaundice, anaemia, swollen tender interphalangeal joints on his right hand and breathlessness. His bilirubin was 38 mg% (mostly unconjugated), WBC-18000, Hb- 6.1 g%, reticulocyte count 15%, Coomb's test negative, hepatitis B and hepatitis C were negative. His electrophoresis report was pending. A sickling test was performed which was positive.*

DIAGNOSIS: Sickle cell anaemia presenting with haemolytic crisis with severe jaundice.

He was treated with fluid resuscitation, correction of anaemia and acidosis. He received broad spectrum antibiotics and folic acid supplementations. The treatment was carried out with the help of a haematologist. He eventually made an uneventful recovery but remained mildly icteric. He needs hospital admission from time to time due to flare up of his jaundice which usually occurs following any intercurrent infection. Again this is a rare condition restricted to the population in certain parts of India; nevertheless the reason for presenting this rare case is that during evaluation of any patient with jaundice haemolytic causes like haemoglobinopathies, haemolytic anaemias etc should be borne in mind.

CASE: *A 51 years old lady presented with chronic low grade fever, arthralgia, weakness and mild jaundice. Investigations revealed Hb- 8.5 g%, WBC- 3900, ESR- 72 mm in 1st hour, bilirubin- 3.1 mg%, AST- 87, ALT- 93, Albumin- 2.4 mg% (low) globulin- 4.6 mg% (high). Virological screening negative, ANF +ve, anti-smooth muscle antibody +ve, antimitochondrial antibody was negative. She refused to undergo liver biopsy.*

DIAGNOSIS: Autoimmune hepatitis (chronic active hepatitis)

She was treated with steroids with improvement of her clinical condition. At present she remains asymptomatic on low dose of steroids. Although abnormal LFTs are more commonly found to be due to chronic viral hepatitis or alcoholic hepatitis, auto-immune screening should be done in selected cases in order to detect occasional autoimmune hepatitis.

CASE: *A 75 years old diabetic gentleman was admitted with a history of weight loss, anorexia, abdominal pain and jaundice. Investigations revealed bilirubin 11.2 mg% (mostly conjugated), alkaline phosphatase very high, AST and ALT moderately raised, USG dilated CBD and hypoechoic shadow over the head of pancreas. Alpha fetoprotein marginally raised, CEA-normal, CA 19.9 very high. CT scan of abdomen was suggestive of space occupying lesion of head of pancreas. In view of age and other co-morbid condition, he underwent biliary stenting with temporary improvement of his symptoms. He lived for another 6 months and died of severe biliary sepsis and massive gastrointestinal haemorrhage.*

DIAGNOSIS: Jaundice due to carcinoma head of pancreas.

CASE: *A 96 years old patient with ITP was getting repeated admission due to thrombocytopenia not responding to the usual medication like steroid. Although IV immunoglobulin was successful in bringing up the platelet count, the effect could not be sustained for more than 2 weeks. After failed attempt by different agents to maintain the platelet count, finally dapsone was started after checking Glucose-6-PD level. Within 10 days of commencement his Hb dropped to 6.1 g%, bilirubin 2.3 mg%, reticulocyte count- 8% and oxygen saturation to 86%. Dapsone was immediately discontinued. He was given oxygen therapy. He was not breathless however methaemoglobin level was checked and was found to be 10%. He was given blood transfusion and over a period of 1 week, the biochemical and haematological parameters became normal. Methaemoglobin level felt down to less than 2%.*

DIAGNOSIS: Anaemia, jaundice and falling oxygen carrying capacity due to oxidative damage of RBC caused by dapsone in a patient with normal G-6-PD level.

DISCUSSION:

Jaundice is a clinical manifestation of myriad of divergent clinical conditions and sometimes baffles the clinician. A systematic approach in investigation will enable the clinician to arrive at a correct diagnosis. While dealing with jaundice the clinician should consider the following conditions:

- **Infections:** Hepatitis, malaria, leptospirosis
- **Autoimmune:** Chronic active hepatitis, primary biliary cirrhosis.
- **Alcoholic liver disease**
- **Cirrhosis of liver due to various causes**
- **Obstruction**:

  Intrahepatic cholestasis *e.g.* certain drugs, jaundice of pregnancy, liver disease.

  Extrahepatic- biliary stricture, stone, pancreatic mass, biliary sepsis with cholangitis.
- **Mitotic lesions in the liver**: both primary and metastatic.
- **Metabolic jaundice due to haemolysis:** Wilson's disease, haemoglobinopathies, haemolytic anaemia due to various causes.
- **Microangiopathic anaemias**: HUS and TTP.
- **Jaundice due to drugs**: (discussed previously).

Finally a common cause of jaundice is a benign condition known as Gilbert's syndrome which presents with mild unconjugated hyperbilirubinaemia without any other abnormality. This is usually a diagnosis by exclusion and the patients should be reassured about it with the caution that the jaundice might increase slightly in the event of any intercurrent illness.

INVESTIGATIONS:

- Full blood count including reticulocyte count, malaria parasite
- RBC morphology
- Coomb's test

- LDH
- Hb electrophoresis
- Sickling test if clinically suspected
- G6PD
- LFT: AST higher than ALT in alcoholic liver disease, ALP is high in obstruction, gamma GT is high in obstruction, high in liver disease, high with enzyme inducing drugs.
- Virological studies: Hep A, Hep B, Hep C, Hep E, CMV- particularly in immunocompromised host.
- Leptospira antibody if clinically indicated
- Autoimmune screening: ANF, antimitochondrial antibody, anti-smooth muscle antibody.
- Metabolic: ferritin (to exclude haemochromatosis), ceruloplasmin level (to exclude Wilson's disease).
- Radio imaging: USG, CT abdomen, MRCP, ERCP.

The numbers of tests are huge and of course the clinician needs to exercise his clinical judgement before requesting the test particularly in India where resource limitation is a problem.

CASE: *A 79 years old lady presented with nonspecific abdominal pain of abdomen, her bilirubin level was 1.3 mg%, AST- 67, ALT- 61, alkaline phosphatase slightly raised, hepatitis B and C screening were negative, ultrasound and CT scan of abdomen revealed fatty liver, she was initially diagnosed to have hepatic steatosis and irritable bowel syndrome and was discharged with an advice to follow up in two weeks with repeat LFT which she failed. She again presented with features of jaundice and abdominal pain after three months. This time USG- abdomen revealed dilated CBD, ERCP revealed stricture of distal CBD and her CA 19.9 was very high, she was assessed for Whipple's procedure and was found unfit to undergo that operation. She was treated with stenting of CBD and was explained about the poor prognosis.*

DIAGNOSIS: Stricture of CBD due to cholangiocarcinoma of CBD.

The diagnosis may be missed in early stages and in patients with abdominal pain, with altered LFT, close follow up may be needed and MRCP should be done early.

: KEY POINTS :

- Jaundice is very common in clinical practice.
- Jaundice is a sign and not a disease which has got various divergent causes.
- History, occupation, travel and drug therapy will give important clues to the diagnosis.

FURTHER REFERENCES:

- NEJM- 2014; 371-1238-1247 Sept. 25.
- Harrison's Principle of Internal Medicine – 17th edition
- Oxford Textbook of Medicine – 5th edition.

65 A PATIENT WITH BRADYCARDIA

CASE: *A 46 years old male was transferred from a district hospital with a history of convulsion on two occasions. Clinical examination and ECG done later on did not reveal anything specific. During examination, he was found to be in sinus rhythm with a regular heart rate of 64/min, normal BP, no carotid bruit, CT brain scan was normal. X-ray cervical spine showed mild spondylosis. Echo and carotid Doppler did not reveal anything specific. He was normoglycaemic and his electrolytes were normal. EEG was normal as well. He was diagnosed to have adult onset idiopathic epilepsy and was commenced on phenytoin. The day before discharge, he again had an episode of convulsion when his heart rate dropped to 24/min with ECG showing complete heart block. He underwent urgent temporary pacemaker insertion followed by a permanent pacemaker implantation the very next day. One month at follow up, he was doing well.*

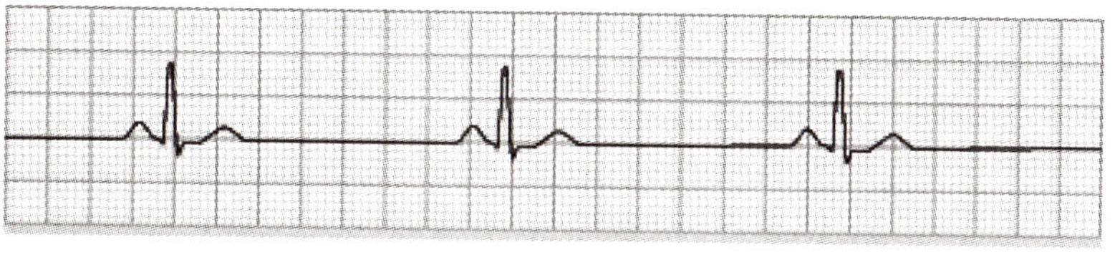

DIAGNOSIS: Stokes-Adams syndrome presenting with convulsion with normal ECG findings-possibly sick sinus syndrome.

Carotid sinus massage and tilt table test were not done in this patient.

CASE: *A 69 years old lady presented with a history of repeated syncope for last 6 months. Repeated neuro-cardiological consultation did not reveal any specific clue. Her ECG on several occasions were normal, CT and MRI brain scan were normal. Echo, Carotid Doppler scan and EEG were normal. 24 hours Holter monitoring on one occasion was normal. During her stay in ITU, she had one episode of syncope and her heart rate was noticed to be as low as 20/min. A repeat Holter monitoring showed evidence of prolonged sinus arrest on several occasions along with occasional bradycardia and episodes of several supraventricular ectopics. She was diagnosed to have sick sinus syndrome and was suggested to have urgent permanent pacemaker implantation.*

DIAGNOSIS: Sick sinus syndrome presenting with repeated syncope due to prolonged sinus arrest.

CASE: *A 56 years old gentleman was admitted with repeated attacks of syncope which eluded the clinicians for last few years even after detailed neuro-cardiac evaluation. Finally, while on a tilt table test at 30 minutes, his BP dropped to 70 mmHg with* *reproduction of similar symptoms. He was diagnosed to have neuro-cardiogenic syncope of vasodepressor type. He was prescribed fludrocortisones, elastic stocking of both legs and cautioned that the treatment might not offer a guaranteed relief of his symptoms and even a permanent pacemaker implantation will have limited beneficial role.*

DIAGNOSIS: Neuro-cardiogenic syncope of vasodepressor type.

CASE: *A 74 years old diabetic gentleman was admitted with dizziness. His heart rate was 36/minute and ECG showed nodal rhythm with absence of P wave. Temporary pacemaker was inserted urgently. Blood reports which was available later on showed urea 64 mg%, creatinine 1.9 mg%, Na 130 mmol/l, K 6.6 mmol/l (high) and random glucose 184 mg%. He was on a combination of ACE inhibitor and* AT_2 *receptor blocker. The drug was discontinued. Hyperkalaemia was treated with IV calcium gluconate, glucose-insulin infusion and IV* HCO_3. *His K normalized within next 24 hours and his rhythm returned back to normal sinus rhythm. He did not need any permanent pacemaker implantation.*

DIAGNOSIS: Severe bradycardia with escape nodal rhythm due to drug induced hyperkalemia in a diabetic patient with mild renal impairment.

DISCUSSION: Bradycardia and heart block is a common presentation in hospital practice. Bradycardia with nodal rhythm may be caused by reversible causes like hyperkalaemia, severe acidosis and drugs. Before considering for permanent pacemaker implantation such causes must be excluded.

COMMON CAUSES OF SINUS BRADYCARDIA:

- Young athletes
- Drugs- β blockers, digoxin and other anti-arrhythmic drugs
- Hypothyroidism
- Electrolyte imbalance- hyperkalaemia, severe acidosis (ACE inhibitors, AT2 receptor blockers, spironolactone can cause hyperkalaemia).
- Ischemic- myocardial infarction
- As a part of sick-sinus syndrome
- Carotid sinus hypersensitivity

CAUSES OF NODAL RHYTHM:

Aforementioned causes also can cause escape nodal rhythm.

CAUSES OF HEART BLOCK:

- Congenital- in children.
- Ischemic- following MI.
- Due to degenerative disease of the conducting system- mainly seen in the elderly population.

HYPERSENSITIVE CAROTID SINUS SYNDROME:

There are two varieties:

- **Cardio-inhibitory:** pressure over the carotid sinus causes asystole of more than 3 seconds. This is particularly common in the elderly population.
- **Vasodepressor:** Fall of systolic BP of more than 50 mmHg on carotid sinus massage.

While evaluating syncope, one should perform carotid sinus massage over the right and left side sequentially to note its presence. Tilt table test is also an important test to exclude carotid sinus hypersensitivity in the evaluation of patients with syncope. The condition is treated with permanent pacemaker implantation. The vasodepressor variety is particularly difficult to treat. Elastic stockings, sodium retaining drugs (fludrocortisone) and α stimulant like- midodrine may be partially helpful.

Sick-sinus syndrome comprises of several components:

- Sinus bradycardia
- Sinus arrest
- Combination of sinus arrest and AV block
- Episodic tachycardia-sinus as well as supraventricular (Tachycardia- bradycardia syndrome).

These patients usually present with intermittent palpitation and syncope and the diagnosis may elude the physician if the ECG during testing is normal. Repeated Holter monitoring may be needed to make a final diagnosis. It is treated with permanent pacemaker implantation with or without antiarrhythmic medication.

HEART BLOCK: This conduction abnormality is classified into 3 categories:

- First degree block: with prolongation of P-R interval. However all sinus impulses are conducted to the ventricles.

- Second degree block: This is of two types-

    i) **Mobitz type I:** There is progressive prolongation of P-R interval with subsequent loss of conduction of sinus node impulse to the ventricle (Wenckebach phenomenon).

    ii) **Mobitz type II:** Sudden block of conduction of sinus node impulse without any prior prolongation of P-R interval.

- Complete heart block: In this type of block no impulse is propagated to the ventricle and as a result both the atrium and ventricle show independent activity. This is usually treated with permanent pacemaker implantation.

In patients with acute MI, Type- I block usually occurs in patients with inferior wall MI (particularly right ventricular infarction) and usually does not require temporary trans-venous pacing. Type-II block, on the other hand usually accompanies acute anterior wall MI, may need temporary pacing or even permanent pacing in the long term and has a high mortality rate.

INDICATIONS OF PACEMAKER:

Although it falls in the domain of cardiologists, in India, the patients invariably take multiple opinions from clinicians before they actually undergo pacemaker insertion. Hence a brief discussion has been done in this regard.

- Acquired AV block: Mainly due to idiopathic or degenerative cause. (Mainly in the 2nd and 3rd degree block).

- Congenital complete heart block: Although it is usually occurs with narrow QRS complex of < 0.12 second with less chance of syncope, pacing is still indicated, if the heart rate is < 50/min or there is history of syncope or exercise intolerance.

- Chronic bifascicular block (Commonly right bundle branch block with left anterior hemiblock): With this background, if there is any history of syncope which cannot be explained by any other cause.

- Sick-sinus syndrome: If there is persistent symptomatic bradycardia of heart rate less than 40/min in awake state or if there is sinus pause of more than 3 seconds.

- Carotid sinus syncope: Particularly in the cardio-inhibitory type. (For details ACC guideline for permanent pacing should be consulted).

PACEMAKER CODE:

Revised NASPE/BPEG Generic Code for Anti-bradycardia Pacing					
Position	I	II	III	IV	V
Category	**Chamber (s) Paced** O = None A = Atrium V = ventricle D = Dual (A+V)	**Chamber (s) Sensed** O = None A = Atrium V = Ventricle D = Dual (A+V)	**Response To sensing** O = None A = Triggered V = Inhibited D = Dual (T+I)	**Rate modulation** O = None R = Rate modulation	**Multisite pacing** O = None A = Atrium V = Ventricle D = Dual (A+V)
Manufacturers' designation only	S = Single (A or V)	S = Single (A or V)			

SELECTION OF APPROPRIATE PACING MODE:

Single chamber pacing:

Ventricle Inhibited pacing (VVI): It is most commonly used pacing mode worldwide. It senses the ventricle, paces the ventricle and inhibits the ventricle on sensing the impulse. It is not physiological as the AV synchrony is absent. Due to absence of atrial contribution, adverse haemodynamic consequence in the form of pacemaker syndrome (palpitation, fall of BP *etc.*) may occur. This mode of pacemaker is used in presence of atrial fibrillation with slow heart rate as DDD pacing is not suitable in the presence of atrial fibrillation.

Atrial Inhibited pacing (AAI): This mode of pacemaker senses and paces the atrium. This mode of pacemaker is indicated in sinus node dysfunction. AV conduction must be normal in order to use this mode. This should be checked by increasing the atrial rate during pacing and look for any AV conduction block. If AV block is present, this mode of pacing is contraindicated.

Dual chamber pacing:

Atrial Synchronous pacing (VDD): In this pacing mode a single lead electrode is used. In the presence of normal sinus node function and AV block, it senses the atrium and paces the ventricle. In the absence of any sinus node function, it paces the ventricle (*e.g.* works as VVI). Because of sequential pacing, it is more physiological. It is cheaper than DDD pacemaker. This mode of pacing is indicated in patients with normal sinus node function with AV block.

Dual chamber pacing (DDD): DDD pacing is most appropriate in patients with normal sinus mode function and AV block. It is also indicated in carotid sinus hypersensitivity. It should be avoided in patients with sinus node dysfunction and atrial fibrillation.

Rate Responsive Pacing (VVI-R, AAI-R, DDD-R): Rate responsive pacing can increase the pacing rate according to the physiological demand of the body *e.g.* during exercise, running *etc.* This is done through sensors which monitor physiological processes like minute ventilation and activity. This is a more physiological kind of pacing as it adapts to the body's physiological demand.

Advantage of DDD over VVI pacemaker: A sizable number of patients on VVI pacemaker experiences pacemaker syndrome, in the form of palpitation, sweating, unusual sensation in the pericardium and presyncope, due to asynchrony of contraction between atrium and ventricle. DDD pacemaker being more physiological by way of synchronizing atrial and ventricular contraction and it reduces the incidence of pacemaker syndrome significantly.

Triple-chambered pacemakers:

Here typically have one lead in the right atrium, one to stimulate the right ventricle, and one to stimulate the left ventricle. These devices are inserted in patients who have weakened heart muscle (which results in heart failure). These pacemakers "resynchronize" the ventricles and may improve the efficiency of the contraction of the heart, improving its blood flow.

OTHER INDICATIONS OF PACING:

Hypertrophic obstructive cardiomyopathy (HOCM): AV sequential pacing has been used in patients with HOCM where medical treatment has failed. It works by altering the interventricular septal wall motion abnormality thereby reducing the LV outflow tract gradient. Three trials have addressed this issue with conflicting results (Mayo-Pacing in HCM, PIC and M-Pathy).

Cardiac resynchronization therapy (Biventricular pacing): It is indicated in cardiac failure in following situations:

- NHYA class III/IV
- LVEF < 35 %
- QRS duration >130 mili-seconds in ECG
- Normal sinus rhythm

It causes symptomatic improvement in patients with cardiac failure. Newer modes are available in combination with ICD device which has been shown to be useful in patients with cardiac failure and recurrent VT.

In SVT and AF: In addition, pacemaker may also be indicated in prevention of atrial fibrillation and supraventricular tachycardia. However, they are not commonly used in the Indian scenario.

In sick sinus syndrome, dual chamber pacing has been shown to reduce the incidence of atrial fibrillation in the future. In atrioventricular block particularly in elderly population, it has not shown to reduce atrial fibrillation or over-all mortality. (In dual chamber pacing, right ventricular activation can cause ventricular septal wall dyssynergia with its adverse effects on cardiac output thereby nullifying the beneficial effects of AV synchrony. This may indicate that the definition of physiological pacing may be changing in future). Biventricular pacing may be the best form of physiological pacing.

Precaution in patients with pacemaker:

This is a frequently asked question by the patients. Few points should be remembered in patients with pacemaker in situ.

- MRI scan should be avoided. Large magnetic fields such as power generation sites as industrial sites should be avoided however new pacemakers are now a day's available which are MRI compatible.
- Electrocautery / diathermy should be used with caution, during surgery as it may interfere with the pacemaker. Magnet should be used during the use of electrocautery.
- Cell phones of less than 3 watts of output do not seem to affect the pacemaker. As a precautionary method it should be kept at least six inches away from the pacemaker.
- Airport security detectors are generally safe for pacemakers, however the security personnel should know about the pacemaker as hand held. Detectors should not be held on the pacemaker.

Items which can be used safely:

- Electric toothbrush
- Hair dryers
- Electric razors
- Heating pads
- Electric blankets

- Microwave ovens
- Cordless phone- safe if not placed upon the pacemaker
- Television sets, CD players, radios
- Lawnmowers, weed eaters, electric drills or saws
- Hand held massagers- safe if not held over the pacemaker device

Items to be avoided:

- Magnetic mattresses or chairs
- Electrolysis (hair removal)

: KEY POINTS :

- Bradycardia is a common presentation in clinical practice.
- In the evaluation of syncope, thorough cardiac investigations are needed to rule out any bradyarrhythmias.
- Sick sinus syndrome and carotid sinus hypersensitivity sometimes elude clinician as to the cause of syncope.
- ACC guideline should be followed during pacemaker implantation.
- AV sequential pacing and rate responsive pacing are more physiological ways of pacing although they are most expensive.

FURTHER REFERENCES:

- Braunwald's Text Book of Cardiovascular Medicine: 7th edition.
- Changing Definition of Physiological Pacing: Editorial, NEJM, 2005.
- Harrison's Principle of Internal Medicine – 17th edition.
- Oxford Text Book of Medicine- 5th edition.
- Cardiac Pacing and Device Therapy; may 23: 2012, p-215-221

66 A PATIENT WITH BACK PAIN DUE TO ANKYLOSING SPONDYLITIS

CASE: *A 27 years old medical graduate attended the clinic due to increasing low back pain for last three months. Of late he had been experiencing morning stiffness and painful knee joints. Examination failed to reveal any significant abnormality except for some restricted moment of the lumbosacral spine. Investigations were unremarkable except for slightly raised CRP. ASO titre, rheumatoid factor, uric-acid were within normal range. X-ray lumbosacral spine also could not give any definite clue to the diagnosis. A subsequent MRI scan showed evidence of bilateral sacroiliitis. Radio isotope bone scan also showed increased uptake in both sacroiliac joints indicating bilateral sacroiliitis. Blood test for HLA-B27 which was sent early, come back as positive for HLA-B27.*

DIAGNOSIS: Ankylosing Spondylitis (AS).

DISCUSSION: Ankylosing Spondylitis (AS) is occasionally encountered in clinical practice where the patients present with low back pain. The diagnosis is sometimes delayed as initial radiographic findings do not show much change and classical radiological changes take some time to develop.

This condition predominantly involves young males in their 20's and 30's and 90% of cases are associated with HLA-B27 antigen. The primary site of pathology is in the enthesis, the site of ligamentous attachment to the bone where there is inflammation. Associated synovitis in the adjacent joints is also an additional feature. The brunt of the disease is in the axial spine mainly sacroiliac joints. However, peripheral joints may also be involved in the 10% of cases. The mechanism of the disease process is cytokine mediated which makes anti cytokine therapy and effective means of treatment.

CLINICAL FEATURES:

- Predominantly in males in 20's and 30's.
- Low back pain
- Morning stiffness
- Asymmetric peripheral arthritis in 10% of cases.
- HLA-B27 positive in more than 90% of cases.

EXTRA ARTICULAR MANIFESTATIONS:

- Uveitis
- Pulmonary upper lobe fibrosis
- Aortic regurgitation.
- Cauda equina syndrome.
- Increased incidence of prostatitis.
- Increased incidence of amyloidosis.

Modified New York criteria 1984 for AS clinical features

- Low back pain and stiffness for > 3 months which improves with exercise but not with rest.
- Restriction of motion of lumbar spine in both sagittal and frontal planes.
- Restriction of chest expansion.
- Radiological criteria- Sacroiliitis ⇒ bilateral or unilateral.

DIAGNOSIS: In addition to the clinical features there are tests to show reduced spinal mobility.

Schober's test- This test indicates spinal flexion moment. The patient stands on his heal. A point is identified over the spine corresponding to the line joining the two postero-superior iliac spine. Another point is demarcated 10 cm above the point. Now the patient is asked to bend as much possible. In case of normal mobility the distance between the two marks would increase by 5 cm, while in ankylosing spondylitis, it would be less than 4 cm.

Similarly chest expansion is measured which should be > 5 cm in a normal person and less in patient with ankylosing spondylitis. Lateral compression over iliac bones from both sides will cause tenderness over sacroiliac (SI) joint and direct percussion over the SI joint will also cause local tenderness.

DIFFERENTIAL DIAGNOSIS:

i) Trauma
ii) Lumbar spondylosis
iii) Lumbar disc disease
iv) Tuberculosis of spine and other infections
v) Metastatic bone disease

Tuberculosis of lumbar vertebrae is not uncommon in India and may present with low-back pain. Radiological investigations with X-rays and MRI scan will clinch the diagnosis. Although uncommon in young the generation, I have come across few cases of metastatic bone disease mainly arising from lower gastrointestinal tract. DISH (Diffuse Idiopathic Skeletal Hyperostosis) is a degenerative bone disease of the elderly which may mimic AS radiologically by the way of extensive calcification of anterior longitudinal ligaments. However in this condition SI joints are clear.

INVESTIGATIONS:

In advanced case except findings are characteristics with squaring of vertebral bodies, presence of anterior longitudinal ligament giving rise to typical bamboo spine.

MRI scan and radioisotope bone scan are also helpful adjuvant in making the diagnosis.

TREATMENT: Physical exercise is a very important facet to the treatment of AS. Certain exercise like swimming is helpful.

Drugs:

1) NSAIDs- These are helpful in symptomatic relief. Both COX1 & COX2 inhibitors may be used. One needs to be aware of cardiovascular side effects of long-term COX2 use. Nocturnal use of the retard preparation of indomethacin will help alleviate morning stiffness.
2) Sulphasalazine- Sulphasalazine in the dose of 2-3 g/day may help stiffness and been but not spinal mobility. There is a suggestion that use of sulphasalazine might reduce the attack rates of anterior uveitis.
3) Methotrexate- One cohort study and 3 case series found mixed results with methotrexate.
4) Bisphosphonates- It may have possible role on disease activity and physical function but not on spinal mortality
5) Thalidomide- Thalidomide may also have some beneficial effect in improving the symptoms.
6) Steroids- Both pulsed methylprednisolone for 3 days and short course of oral prednisolone may improve the symptoms of AS.
7) Anti TNF-α blockade- These drugs have dramatic effect on the symptoms and they also improve spinal motility. Patients with long standing disease also have shown to respond symptomatically. However it is yet to be known that whether these drugs can finally prevent ankylosis and bony ossification. Infliximab is more potent than etanercept. In the issue of concomitant inflammatory bowel disease (IBD), Infliximab is the preferred agent as etanercept does not work will in IBD.

Dose:

Infliximab- 5 mg/kg IV, repeated at 2 weeks and 6 weeks and then at 8 weeks interval. Etanercept- 25 mg SC thrice/week.

Side effects:

Reactivation of TB
Positive dsDNA antibody
Rarely demyelinating disease
Pancytopenia

CASE-II: *A 37 years old patient from Bangladesh presented with low back pain, pain and swelling of small joints of hands the hand and other joints. Investigations show normal rheumatoid factor, ASO titre and uric acid levels. On careful examination there was onycholysis with pitting of the nails in his hands. There was a scalp lesion resembling psoriasis and a small psoriatic patch at the exterior surface of his right elbow.*

DIAGNOSIS: Reactive arthropathy due to psoriasis with symptoms suggestive of sacroiliitis.

CASE-III: *A 48 years old diabetic male with past history of pulmonary tuberculosis, presented with low back pain and painful swollen joints in his lower extremities. He also gave a history of intermittent bowel irregularity and occasional bloody diarrhea which his GP ascribed as amoebic colitis and successfully treated with recurrent courses of ciprofloxacin and metronidazole. Investigations revealed normal ASO titre, rheumatoid factor and uric acid levels. A colonoscopic examination revealed extensive ulcerative colitis which was biopsy proven.*

DIAGNOSIS: Reactive arthropathy with sacroiliitis (as per symptoms) due to ulcerative colitis.

Other causes of reactive arthritis and sacroiliitis.

- Reiter's syndrome (urinary tract infection, uveitis, keratoderma blenorrhagica)
- Post yersinia (diarrhea)
- Behcet's syndrome (oral aphthous ulcer, scrotal ulcer, DVT, meningitis).
- Whipple's disease (fever, lymphadenopathy, serositis, CNS manifestation)

Treatment of psoriatic arthropathy:

Following drugs have been found to be of moderate benefit in psoriatic arthopathy-

1) Sulphasalazine
2) Methotrexate

3) Cyclosporin
4) Antimalarials but it may flare up the skin manifestation.
5) TNF-α blockers have also been found useful and particularly in the regard etanercept perhaps had an edge over others in as much as it's proven beneficial effects on both articular any skin manifestations.

Treatment of Reiter's disease:

1) Prolonged use of antibiotics in early stage (Ciprofloxacin, Doxycycline)
2) Sulphasalazine, methotrexate, azathioprine- may have some beneficial effects.

Treatment of IBD related arthritis:

Anecdotal evidence suggests that sulphasalazine, steroids and other immunosuppressive drugs are effective in IBD related arthritis. In Crohn's disease related arthritis infliximab works both for arthritis and Crohn's disease.

FURTHER REFERENCES:

- J. Braun *et al.* - Ankylosing Spondylitis. Lancet 2007: 369, page 1379-90.
- Harrison's Principle of Internal Medicine 17th edition.
- Oxford Text Book of Medicine 5th edition.

67 A PATIENT WITH ACUTE GOUT

CASE: *A 51 years old obese, hypertensive patient attended the clinic with increasing pain and swelling of the knee joints and ankle joints. The most severe pain and swelling was over the left metatarsal joints. He was a smoker and drank alcohol regularly. Examination revealed mild fever, right knee joint was hot, red and tender and so was the dorsum of the right foot. Interventions revealed WBC- 13 000, CRP high, ASO titer normal, rheumatoid factor negative, uric acid- 7.4 mg%, creatinine- normal, triglyceride- 400 mg%.*

DIAGNOSIS: Acute Gouty Arthritis.

DISCUSSION: Gout commonly involves middle aged male population with history of hypertension, hyperlipidaemia and frequent history of increased alcohol intake. It is distinctly uncommon in young premenstrual females but can occur in post-menopausal population. It usually presents with acute monoarticular joint pain mainly involving knee joints, ankle joints but characteristically the metatarsal joints particularly the first one. It can present with polyarticular joint pain resembling rheumatoid arthritis. The common precipitating events are –

- Alcohol intake
- High protein diet
- Trauma
- Diuretic therapy
- Following treatment of myeloproliferative disorders
- Serious medical illness like myocardial infarction and stroke

After many acute attacks it may eventually cause chronic synovitis leading to asymmetric chronic polyarthritis. With deposition of uric acid crystals as chronic tophaceous gout may happen.

How to diagnose?

ii) Increased uric acid level, however during acute attack serum uric acid level may also be normal.

iii) Aspiration of joint fluid would show-

a. Elevated cell count.

b. Presence of strongly birefringent needle shaped MSU crystals.

c. 24 hours urine uric acid excretion - This would not alter the acute management. This test may be helpful for long term management.

How to treat an acute attack?

- Application of ice pack has shown to reduce symptoms of pain and this has been borne out in randomized controlled trial.
- Diet- low purine diet and avoidance of alcohol may help in chronic cases.
- Drugs-

  a. **Colchicine-** Colchicine is a very effective drug but associated with frequent gastrointestinal adverse effects [dose 1 mg stat then 0.5 mg 2 hourly until complete response or toxicity]. The side effects are diarrhea and vomiting. IV colchicine can be also used. However this is a toxic substance.

  b. **NSAID-** This group of drugs is equally effective particularly the short acting ones like indomethacin, ibuprofen, diclofenac *etc*. Gastric side effects are major concern. COX-2 inhibitor has better side effect profile but fraught with increased cardiovascular risk if used long term.

  c. **Steroids-** Prednisolone in the dose of 30 mg for 7-10 days, single IV dose of methylprednisolone or IM injection of ACTH- 40-80 units IM thrice daily for 2-3 days may be equally effective for control of symptoms.

Long term treatment:

- Once the acute attack is under control, only then one should contemplate long term hypouricaemic therapy. Diet restriction and avoidance of alcohol also play an important role.

Choosing the right drugs-

Allopurinol:

- If there is uric acid overproduction
- During treatment of myeloproliferative disorder
- If 24 hours urinary uric acid excretion is > 800 mg.

Side effects are common in the form of a local skin reaction, vasculitis and occasionally toxic epidermal necrolysis, bone marrow suppression.

In this regard a new drug febuxostat, a xanthine oxidase inhibitor, but structurally distinct from allopurinol has been found to be useful with lesser side effect profile.

Allopurinol should not be started during acute attack and once started should be continued under cover of NSAID or colchicine until the patient is completely symptom free and normo-uricaemic. If the patient develops acute gout while on long term allopurinol, the drug maybe continued.

Probenecid:

- In the presence of normal renal function
- If 24 hours urinary uric acid excretion is < 600 mg.
- In elderly hypertensive and on thiazide diuretics.

However, if the excretion of uric acid is more than 800 mg/day, then uricosuric drug like probenecid would not be helpful and hyperuricaemia is primarily due to uric acid overproduction. Allopurinol or febuxostat would be the drug of choice.

How long to treat?

Treatment should be continued until the target uric acid level reaches below 6 mg%. Intermittent treatment 'Allopurinol Holidays' has shown to cause recurrent attack. So it is generally agreed that the treatment should be continued for indefinite period with the dose of 100–300 mg/day (in renal failure 100 mg/day). Febuxostat 40 mg daily is increasingly used for this purpose.

Is Aspirin contraindicated in gout?

Aspirin in high dose is uricosuric while in low dose (commonly used in clinical practice for preventive purpose) can cause uric acid retention. However for practical purpose, aspirin can be used in hyperuricaemic patient if there are compelling indications to do so.

FURTHER REFERENCES:

- Harrison's Principle of Internal Medicine – 17th Edition.
- Oxford Text Book of Medicine – 5th Edition.

68 EYE PROBLEM IN CLINICAL PRACTICE

CASE: *A 37 years old male patient was referred from the ophthalmology clinic for a medical opinion regarding anterior uveitis that the patient was suffering from. The reason of the referral was to exclude any undergoing medical condition that might have been causing his eye condition. The patient's ESR and CRP were high, Calcium high normal, serum ACE level was high, HLA-B27 negative, ANF negative, γ-interferon was normal,* Mantoux test *was negative, X Ray chest normal, X Ray lumbosacral spine was normal.*

DIAGNOSIS: Provisional diagnosis of Sarcoidosis causing anterior *uveitis was made.*

DISCUSSION: Ophthalmological examination frequently gives useful clues toward a diagnosis of an underlying medical condition attributing towards the cause and through investigation is mandatory in such cases. U*veitis* is one such condition which needs an internist impact and such patients are occasionally referred by ophthalmologists for opinion.

CAUSES OF UVEITIS:

- HLA-B27 related spondyloarthropathies like- Ankylosing Spondylitis.
- Granulomatous disorders like- Sarcoidosis.
- Infection- Tuberculosis
- Behcet's disease- a complex of recurrent oral aphthous ulcers, genital ulcers, and uveitis.
- Juvenile idiopathic arthritis- positive ANF

Appropriate tests need to be done to make a proper diagnosis. In India tuberculosis is a distinct possibility and when long term steroid therapy is contemplated for the treatment of uveitis. Anti-tuberculosis therapy should be strongly considered in suspected cases.

Other ophthalmological conditions related to medical diseases:

1. Rheumatological conditions:

- Episcleritis and scleritis- In Rheumatoid arthritis, Wegener's granulomatosis.

  Treatment: Immunosuppressive therapy using steroids may be indicated.
- Dry eyes - In Rheumatoid arthritis, primary Sjögren's syndrome.

2. Haematological conditions:

- Retinal vein occlusion – in hyper-viscosity syndrome.
- Proliferative retinopathy – in sickle cell disease.
- Retinal haemorrhage as in leukaemia, thrombocytopenia.

- Retinopathy as in diabetes.

3. **Renal diseases:**

- Von Hippel-Lindau disease (VHL)- presence of capillary hemangioblastoma.
- Alport syndrome– with presence of lenticonus along with renal failure and sensorineural deafness.
- WARG syndrome – Presence of Wilm's tumour, sporadic aniridia (absence of the iris) and mental retardation.

4. **Neuro-ophthalmic manifestations of phacomatosis:**

- **Tuberous sclerosis-** Retinal hamartomas along with neurological manifestations, and dermatological manifestations.
- **Ataxia telangiectasia**– conjunctival vessel telangiectasia along with cerebellar ataxia.
- **Sturge Weber's syndrome**– Choroidal haemangioma along with hemifacial haemangioma along with angiomas of meninges.
- **Von Hippel–Lindau syndrome**– retinal angioma, CNS hemangioblastoma, renal cell carcinoma.

5. **Infections and eye:**

- Herpes simplex keratitis, acute retinal necrosis
- Cytomegalovirus retinitis
- HIV retinitis
- Candida endophthalmitis

6. **Drugs and eye:**

- Vincristine – optic atrophy
- Cyclosporine – retinal toxicity
- Steroids – cataract, glaucoma
- Hydroxychloroquine
- Ethambutol
- Amiodarone – corneal microdeposits

FURTHER REFERENCES:

- Free British Journal of Hospital Medicine, Vol-72-Nov 12 Dec 2011.
- Oxford Text Book of Medicine- 5th edition.
- Harrison's Principle of Internal Medicine 17th edition.

69

A PATIENT WITH UNDIAGNOSED ATRIAL SEPTAL DEFECTS (ASD)

CASE: *A 47 years old patient presented with a history of repeated cough and cold of late he was getting shortness of breath on exertion. His GP found a systolic murmur in the precordium and referred to the clinic. Examination revealed systolic murmur best heard in the left mid sternal region. ECG showed RBBB pattern with right atrial and right ventricular hypertrophy. X-ray chest showed prominent pulmonary arteries and right atrial enlargement. Echocardiography showed presence of ASD of secundum type with presence of mild pulmonary hypertension.*

DIAGNOSIS: Secundum type ASD with pulmonary hypertension.

DISCUSSION: Undiagnosed atrial septal defect (ASD) is occasionally encountered in clinical practice either during routine check up for recent cold and breathlessness or during routine echocardiographic screening during other conditions like pre-operative checkup before a routine non-cardiac surgery. Sometimes the clinician and the patients are at a dilemma regarding the best course of action in such patients who are otherwise asymptomatic.

ASD accounts of 25-30% of congenital heart defects that are diagnosis in adulthood. Anatomically there are three types of lesions-

- Ostium Secundum type ASD (near fossa ovalis) - 75%
- Ostium Primum type ASD (near lower portion of atrial septum) - 15%
- Sinus Venous type ASD (near the orifice of superior vena cava) - 10%

How to diagnose?

- ECG - RBBB, RVH, Right atrial enlargement
- X-ray chest- Shows characteristic finding
- Echo- Diagnostic

How to treat?

In symptomatic patients operative closure will reduce long-term morbidity and mortality and sooner the treatment is done the better. It has been shown that best results are obtained if surgery is done between the ages of 25 to 40. However impressive results are obtained in patients over 40 years of age with somewhat increased attendant risk of the perioperative atrial tachyarrhythmia.

In asymptomatic adults with ASD, operative closure improves the morbidity but not the mortality.

Which method?

Surgical closure of ASD had been the gold standard since mid sixties with very few post-operative mortality and morbidity.

Since the early 80's trans-catheter closer of ASD has also be increasingly used in selected cases of Secundum type ASD. The criteria for the successful use of trans-catheter closer of ASD are-

- Secundum type ASD.
- ASD size less than 35 mm [measured by stretched balloon diameter].
- A rim of surrounding atrial tissue of 5 mm for better anchorage of the balloon.

How does it compare with conventional surgical closure?

In properly selected cases, it is equally effective in terms of symptomatic relief and prevention of long term problems. Immediate post-procedural complications are much less compared to the surgical procedure.

What are the complications?

Complications are more in the form of catheter embolization, cardiac perforation and transient arrhythmia. In properly selected cases they are rare. Percutaneous technique has become the procedure of choice in treating ASD in adulthood.

Following treatment it is recommended to give aspirin for the six months and clopidogrel for one month to prevent thrombosis of the device. Routine prophylaxis for infections endocarditis should also be provided in appropriate situations.

FURTHER REFERENCE:

- Harrison's Principle of Internal Medicine – 17th Edition.
- Oxford Text Book of Medicine – 5th Edition.

70 A PATIENT WITH INCREASED BLEEDING FOLLOWING CARDIAC BYPASS SURGERY

CASE: *A 51 years old diabetic patient, who underwent cardiac bypass surgery (CABG) and eventually extubated, was reported to have increasing amount of blood loss through thoracotomy drainage tube. His coagulation profile was normal. He was on aspirin which was stopped 24 hours before the surgery. Before going for the reopening procedure it was decided to go for conservative measures first. With this view in mind, the medical team was consulted and it was decided to commence him on IV aprotinin infusion. 24 hours after commencement of aprotinin, his bleeding eventually stopped and thus another invasive surgical procedure was avoided.*

DIAGNOSIS: Post CABG bleeding responding to aprotinin.

DISCUSSION:

Increased bleeding is a common problem encountered in hospital practice. Majority of the patients are post surgical. However acute medical cases are also equally frequently encountered like bleeding in uremia, chronic liver disease, DIC and other coagulation abnormalities, cerebral hemorrhage *etc.*

While blood transfusion is the initial treatment of choice, it is fraught with dangers like transfusion reaction, mismatched transfusion, transmission of diseases and sometimes non availability.

In these situations the drugs, those can be helpful to reduce the bleeding by their haemostatic action and may circumvent the necessity of re-exploration of surgical procedure are-

1) Aprotinin
2) Antifibrinolytics
3) Desmopressin
4) Recombinant factor VII

Aprotinin has been evaluated in randomized controlled trials and was found to be helpful in controlling post surgical bleeding. This was particularly noticeable in post CABG patients where its use has been associated with significantly reduced use of blood transfusion.

DOSE: 700 mg total, loading dose 280 mg then 70 mg/hour.

Tranexamic acid (dose 3-10 g) and **epsilon aminocaproic acid** (does 10-30 g) have also been found to be useful albeit to a lesser degree.

PROBLEMS:

Aprotinin may cause- a) post operative renal dysfunction, b) increases the risk of stroke and other cerebrovascular events. Side effect profile is less with the other two fibrinolytics.

CLINICAL USE:

Aprotinin is used in post CABG and other post operative bleeding, particularly those who have been on aspirin. However risk-benefit ratio needs to be judged before its use.

Recombinant factor VII- Initially licensed for use in haemophilia with antibodies to factor VIII or IX, this drug is increasingly finding its place in the other conditions with success. The condition where it has been found to reduce bleeding significantly are-

1) Major hemorrhage from surgery
2) Following open prostatectomy
3) Trauma
4) Intracerebral hemorrhage (if used early)
5) Following the liver transplant

DOSE: 80 -100 μg/kg of body wt. In trauma the dose may be increased.

Like other haemostatic agents, it can also increase the risk of thromboembolic events like stroke and myocardial infarction. In clinical practice, jury is still out regarding its beneficial role in the treatment of bleeding.

Desmopressin- This drug by way of releasing Von Willebrand factors the endothelium and associated factor VIII may be a useful haemostatic agent in certain clinical situations:

1) Mild Hemophilia A.
2) Von Willebrand disease.
3) Bleeding in cirrhosis.
4) Inherited platelet disorders.
5) Uremic bleeding.

[Although, since the advent of erythropoietin which improves homeostasis by increasing red cell mass, its role as haemostatic in uremia has declined.]

DOSE: 0.3 μg/kg, IV/SC or 300 μg for body wt > 50 kg (1 spray in each nostril).

SIDE EFFECTS: Flushing and hyponatraemia.

In conclusion, haemostatic drugs if carefully chosen can reduce bleeding and reduce the necessity of blood transfusion in many clinical situations. However, there is no panacea and other basic principle of homeostasis should be taken care of in order to stop bleeding.

What is Von Willebrand factor (VWF)?

VWF is a complex multimeric glycoprotein with two important roles in haemostasis. It binds to the platelet receptors bridging them to other platelets and sub endothelial tissue. It also acts as carrier protein for factor VIII, thus preventing its proteolytic inactivation in plasma. The absence of these multimers leads to defect in platelet adhesion thereby leading to increased bleeding. Ristocetin, an antibiotic increases the interaction between VWF and platelet, on the basis of which ristocetin co-factor activity test is used as a surrogate marker of the functional activity of the VWF. The absence of VWF leads to Von Willebrand disease, a coagulation disorder characterized by bleeding. Type-I Von Willebrand disease is the most common form of inherited coagulation disorder affecting 1% of the general population. Desmopressin is effective in this condition in type-III Von Willebrand disease, there is near total absence of VWF and desmopressin will not be effective. In type-II Von Willebrand disease where there is qualitative defect of VWF, desmopressin would probably also not effective in this condition.

FURTHER REFERENCES:

- Pior. M. Mannucci *et al.* Prevention and treatment of major blood loss. NEJM-2007 the: 356-2301-II.
- Harrison's Principle of Internal Medicine – 17th edition.
- Oxford Text Book of Medicine – 5th edition.

INFECTIONS IN DIABETES MELLITUS

CASE: *A 32 years old lady presented with high fever and diffused abdominal pain. She looked very toxic with right upper abdominal tenderness. Her blood glucose was very high with ketone bodies in the urine. There were numerous pus cells in the urine. Ultrasound examination revealed enlarged right kidney. Her urea and creatinine were high. CT abdomen showed right sided perinephric abscess.*

DIAGNOSIS: Right perinephric abscess with diabetic ketoacidosis.

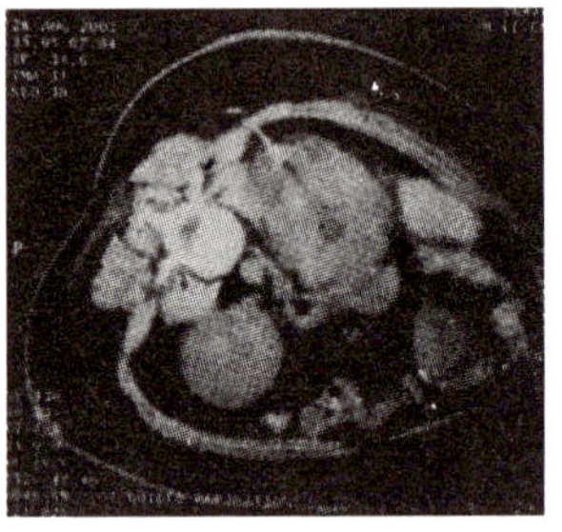

She was treated with IV insulin via infusion pump, IV antibiotics (cefepime) and CT guided percutaneous drainage of the pus on couple of occasions. Blood culture, urine culture and culture of the pus grew ESBL producing *E. coli,* sensitive to cefepime. She made a good recovery.

CASE: *A 56 years old diabetic gentleman presented with severe abdominal pain on vomiting and right hypochondrial tenderness. He was very toxic looking and was haemodynamically unstable. WBC count was 26,000. Liver function test was slightly deranged, amylase was normal. Ultrasound examination revealed hugely distended gall bladder without any calculus.*

DIAGNOSIS: Acute emphysematous acalculous cholecystitis.

He underwent laparotomy and a necrosed, gangrenous gall bladder was removed. After a stormy post operative course, he was finally discharged home.

CASE: *A 56 years old diabetic patient with steroid dependant nephrotic syndrome was referred to us with nasal discharge and gradually increasing proptosis. He complained of severe pain over the right eyeball with evidence of proptosis. There was external ophthalmoplegia and the maxillary sinus was tender. His vision was deteriorating rapidly. After an ENT consultation, he underwent MRI brain and paranasal sinus scan which showed invasive lesion in the right maxillary sinus, right orbit extending into sphenoidal region of the skull. He underwent urgent enucleation of the right eye and curettage of the paranasal sinus. Biopsy and fungal staining showed evidence of mucormycosis.*

DIAGNOSIS: Mucormycosis of orbit and paranasal sinus in a steroid requiring diabetic patient.

He was treated with IV amphotericin for 4 weeks. He had a turbulent course with development of renal failure, cerebrovascular accident and nosocomial infection. Fortunately he made a reasonably good recovery but remained dialysis dependent.

CASE: *A 72 years old diabetic gentleman presented to ITU because of suspected aspiration pneumonia which was due to recently developed bulbar palsy. 2 months before admission he was seen by an ENT specialist for left ear discharge. A polypoid mass was detected which on biopsy showed granulomatous lesion and culture from the lesion grew Pseudomonas. Over the next 2 months he developed left sided lower motor neurone facial palsy followed by gradual involvement of lower cranial nerves. MRI brain scan showed bony involvement of the mastoid and the base of the skull with evidence of bony destruction.*

DIAGNOSIS: Malignant otitis externa with involvement of the base of skull.

CASE: *A 42 years old diabetic lady was admitted from a remote village with history of fever, drowsiness and severely swollen right leg. She was very toxic and examination revealed crepitations in the right leg which was excruciatingly tender. X-ray of the hip and thigh showed evidence of gas in the subcutaneous tissue. CT scan also confirmed presence of gas. CPK was elevated.*

DIAGNOSIS: Necrotising fasciitis of right leg in a diabetic patient.

She received anti-gas gangrene serum (as gas gangrene was in the differential diagnosis) and broad spectrum antibiotics with anaerobic cover (penicillin, clindamycin and a 3rd generation cephalosporin). Unfortunately she went into multiorgan failure and finally expired.

DISCUSSION: I have presented five cases of specific infection that occur in diabetic patients. Most of these infections are rare but very characteristic in diabetic patients. In addition to these specific infections, it is well known that any infection occurring in a diabetic patient takes a particularly severe course and the treating clinicians should be aware of it and choose appropriate broad spectrum antibiotics to treat them. Diabetes causes an immunosuppressive state as well as alters leukocyte function. This in turn causes increased propensity and severity of infection in diabetic patients.

Some common infections in diabetes:

➢ Urinary tract infection:

Ascending UTI with pyelonephritis occurs more commonly in diabetics. Persistent pain and fever along with increased toxicity indicates complication like:

- Perinephric abscess
- Papillary necrosis

Ultrasound and CT scan will help in the diagnosis. In case of perinephric abscess surgical or percutaneous drainage will be needed in most of the cases. *E. coli* is the most common organism. However, *Staphylococcus* is the organism if the source is haematogenous. There may be emphysematous pyelonephritis by gas producing organism (like *E. coli*).

Cystitis is a common infection and candiduria should be treated if it is associated with presence of pus cells. Oral fluconazole may be used. Amphotericin irrigation has also been recommended.

➢ Chest infection:

Chest infection in diabetes takes a particularly severe course and chances of having bacteraemia is more common in diabetes particularly with Streptococcal and Staphylococcal infection. In our country tuberculosis should always be thought of in cases of unresolving pneumonia not responding to prolonged antibiotics.

➢ Emphysematous cholecystitis:

Diabetic patients are more prone to develop emphysematous cholecystitis due to gas producing organisms. Mortality is high if the diagnosis is delayed. Few points to be remembered in treating cholecystitis in a diabetic patient –

- Male preponderance
- Frequently it is acalculous
- Presence of gas may be present
- Delay in treatment may lead to gangrene or perforation with high mortality.

➢ Soft tissue infection:

Soft tissue infection like cellulitis, carbuncle *etc.* are commonly found in diabetes. Moreover diabetic foot disease occurs in patients with poorly controlled diabetes along with vasculopathy and neuropathy.

Necrotising fasciitis is a characteristic infection of soft tissue, occurs in diabetic patients. It is usually caused by anaerobic organisms (type I). However it can also be due to *Streptococcus and Staphylococcus* (type II). It should be treated with penicillin, clindamycin and a broad spectrum 3rd generation cephalosporin. Local debridement of the necrotic tissue will also be required. Mortality is high in case of delay.

- Malignant otitis externa:

  A rare condition usually caused by *Pseudomonas* with history of aural discharge, formation of granulomatous lesion in the ear cavity. This may invade the cranial bones and base of skull with resultant osteomyelitis and multiple cranial nerve palsies. The treatment is with prolonged anti-pseudomonal antibiotics (for 6 weeks) along with local curettage. Untreated, it has a high mortality rate.

- Rhinocerebral mucormycosis:

  This is a rare but characteristic infection occurring in insulin requiring diabetic patients. It is caused by fungus *Mucor* which usually invades the nasal sinus, orbit and spread intracranially to involve cavernous sinus. Bloody nasal discharge, proptosis, fungating growth over the orbital region in a diabetic patient should prompt the clinician to think of mucormycosis. The treatment is surgical debridement and with prolonged amphotericin treatment. Fluconazole and itraconazole do not work in this condition.

: KEY POINTS :

- Infection in diabetic patients takes a more severe course.
- Associated bacteraemia is common.
- Tuberculosis should be considered in case of unresolving pneumonia.
- Ascending infection causing pyelonephritis is common.
- Persistent pain and fever indicate complications like perinephric abscess or papillary necrosis.
- In a male patient with right hypochondrial pain, distended gall bladder, acute acalculous cholecystitis should be considered and surgical intervention should be done early.
- There are some rare but specific infection occurs in diabetes such as necrotising fasciitis, rhino cerebral mucormycosis and malignant otitis externa.

72 A PATIENT WITH FUNCTIONAL SOMATIC SYMPTOMS

DISCUSSION: "Functional Somatic Symptoms" also known as "Medically Unexplained Symptoms" are very common in outpatients' office practice and it is very frustrating for the patients and the treating doctors alike. With consumption of lot of resources, this umbrella term includes various bodily complaints affecting different parts of body without any definite structural or other specific pathology. It should be differentiated from malingering which has scored some gainful purposes. Broadly there are 3 main categories of symptoms-

a) Pain in different locations as- Fibromyalgia, nonspecific chest pain, low back pain.

b) Functional disturbance of different organs as in irritable bowel syndrome, dizziness.

c) Complaints centering on fatigue as in chronic fatigue syndrome.

Although not exactly known, some factors like adverse childhood experience, personality disorder and various socio-cultural factors have been attributed as to the cause of FSS.

MANAGEMENT:

While dealing with such patients, a thorough history, clinical examination and appropriate investigations should be done to rule out any organic pathology. Once excluded, the treatment needs to be individualized depending upon the situation. The main thrust of treatment would be to control bodily symptoms, either with analgesics or centrally acting antidepressants and non-pharmacological therapy like different forms of psychotherapy. Communication skills of the doctor also play an important role.

TREATMENT PLAN:

- Pharmacological-
  - Peripheral
  - Central.
- Non-pharmacological-
  - Different types of psychotherapy.
- Others-
  - Different types of physical involvements.

TREATMENT OF DIFFERENT FUNCTIONAL SOMATIC SYMPTOMS:

- Irritable Bowel Syndrome: the helpful drugs are-
  - Peripheral- Tegaserod- for management of constipation-predominant IBS.
    Alosetron- for diarrhea-predominant IBS, bulking agents.
    Mebeverine- in IBS associated abdominal cramping, spasmolytic agents.
  - Central- Tricyclic Antidepressants
- Fibromyalgia:
  - Peripheral- Steroids
    NSAIDs
    Inj of steroids at trigger points
  - Central- Tricyclic Antidepressants
    SSRIs
    Aerobic exercise
    Acupuncture
- Tension Headache:
  - Peripheral- Botulinum toxin
  - Central- Tricyclic Antidepressants
    SSRI
    Acupuncture
- Non-Ulcer dyspepsia:
  - Peripheral- Proton Pump Inhibitors
    H. pylori eradication
    H_2 blockers
    Prokinetics
- Chronic low back pain:
  - Peripheral- NSAID
    Muscle relaxants
  - Central- Tricyclic Antidepressants
    Acupunctures
    Spinal manipulation

- ❖ Premenstrual Syndrome:
  - Peripheral- GnRH
    Progestogen
  - Central- SSRI
- ❖ Chronic Fatigue Syndrome:
  - Peripheral- Immunoglobulins
  - Central- Antidepressants
    Assertive exercise

In conclusion FSSs are common condition in clinical practice and successful outcome depends upon the clinician's communication skills along with some therapeutic help from pharmacological and non-pharmacological means.

FURTHER REFERENCES:

- Peter Henningsen *et al.*, Management of Functional Somatic Symptoms, Lancet-2007- 369: 946-55.
- Harrison's Principle of Internal Medicine – 17th edition.
- Oxford Text Book of Medicine – 5th edition.

73 A PATIENT WITH SYNDROME- X

CASE: *A 56 years old lady, presented with recurrent chest pain classical of angina. ECG showed ST changes in inferolateral wall, exercise stress test was positive for provocable ischemia. Coronary angiogram was found to be normal.*

DIAGNOSIS: Syndrome-X.

DISCUSSION:

Cardiac syndrome-X is defined as the typical angina like chest pain without any evidence of obstructive coronary artery disease. This is not an uncommon condition encountered in clinical practice and sometimes in spite of treatment the patient continues to have symptoms. Although initially it was thought to be a benign disease, recent studies suggest it may not be as innocuous as presently thought. The basic mechanism is generalized endothelial dysfunction in the coronary arteries and new modalities of treatment have been proposed on the basis of this pathogenesis.

DIAGNOSTIC CRITERIA:

- Typical chest pain.
- Normal ECG or abnormal ECG during pain.
- Positive Exercise Stress Test.
- Perfusion scanning with Thallium may be positive.
- Coronary angiogram normal.

It usually affects middle aged females in their perimenopausal period. A definitive diagnosis would need a positive test for endothelial dysfunction. However these tests are not routinely available in the day to day clinical practice.

PROGNOSIS: This condition is not entirely benign and long term follow up is needed. Some studies have shown that these patients are prone to develop cardiovascular morbidity in the long run (acute coronary events, cardiac failure etc.).

TREATMENTS: Beta-blockers and to some extent calcium channel blockers and nitrates can be used with success. Some of these patients may have increased pain sensitivity. Treatment with imipramine has been a Class-II b recommendation by the American College of Cardiology guidelines, in patients who are not responding to conventional treatment.

However, recently the major thrust has been given to the treatment of endothelial dysfunction with statins and ACE inhibitors. Estrogen deficient women may benefit from transdermal oestrogen therapy. In addition, lifestyle modification should also be advised in order to improve endothelial dysfunction.

KEY POINTS: In premenopausal women, syndrome-x should be considered in the differential diagnosis of angina like chest pain.

CASE: *A 40 years old male attended the clinic with increasing obesity, joint pain and hypertension. Examination revealed an obese gentleman with a BP of 170/110 mm of Hg. His obesity was mainly confined to the abdomen with abdominal girth measurement of around 112 cm. Investigations revealed, triglycerides- 464 mg% (high), HDL- 29 mg% (low), LDL- 136 mg% (high), TSH- normal, glucose(F)- 137 mg% (borderline high), creatinine- normal, LFT- mildly raised AST and ALT, uric acid- 7.4 mg%, urine routine- Normal; USG abdomen-fatty liver; X-ray chest- LVH; ECG- LVH.*

DIAGNOSIS: Metabolic Syndrome with impaired glucose tolerance, hypertension and fatty liver.

DISCUSSION:

Metabolic Syndrome-X was first described by Dr. Reaven in the 80's where he had shown that presence of abdominal obesity was associated with insulin resistance diabetes mellitus, hypertension, low HDL and high triglyceride level. This syndrome is presently known as metabolic syndrome-X, has been associated with increased cardiovascular risk and mortality.

MECHANISM:

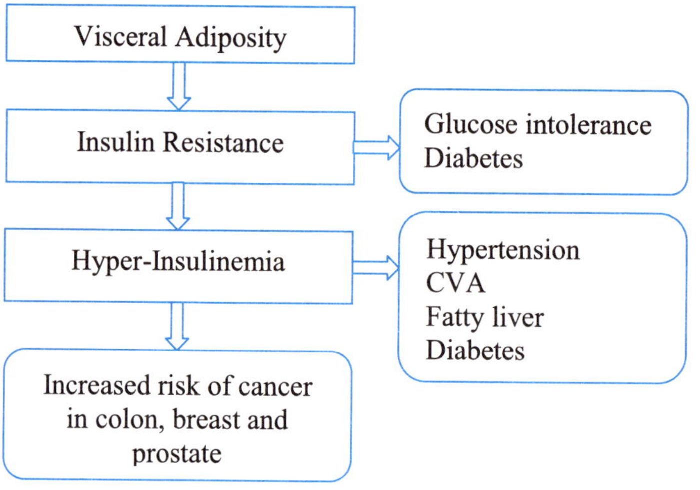

This condition is frequently associated with non-alcoholic fatty liver and hyperuricaemia is also an association.

In Indian scenario, this condition is seen very frequently. Aggressive treatment is warranted as it predisposes to myriad of cardiovascular and non-cardiac condition with attendant risk of increased mortality and morbidity.

The main goal of treatment is weight reduction with lifestyle modification, appropriate diet and regular exercise, control of hypertension, diabetes and hyperlipidaemia with drug therapy.

TREATMENT PROTOCOL OF METABOLIC SYNDROME:

Adult Treatment Panel-III
National Cholesterol Education Program (NCEP)

Risk Factors:		Male	Female
Abdominal obesity (cm)	:	>102	>88
Triglycerides (mg %)	:	>150	>150
HDL-Cholesterol (mg %)	:	<40	<50
Fasting Glucose (mg%)	:	>110	>110
Blood Pressure	:	$^{130}/_{85}$	$^{130}/_{85}$

TREATMENT SUMMARY:

- Lifestyle modification- weight reduction with vigorous exercise.
- Antihypertensive mainly Angiotensin Receptor Blockers (ARBs) or ACE inhibitors (can delay development of diabetes).
- Statins- treating to the target HDL, LDL and triglyceride levels.
- Control of blood glucose- particularly with the use of insulin sensitizing agents like pioglitazone.

FURTHER REFERENCES:

- A Galassi- Metabolic syndrome and risk of cardiovascular disease- A Meta Analysis, AJM- 2006-11.

- Louis J Aronne- Targeting Abdominal Obesity to reduce cardiovascular risk in patient with type-II diabetes mellitus- Ani J need Feb 2007, 120 (2A).
- E Ritz et al.- A new dawn in cardiovascular protection-III-, The Am but J Med- May 2006, vol.-II 9 (5A).
- Endothelial Dysfunction- New Concept in Prognosis and Treatment- Am J Med- 2006. 119, 560-566.
- Harrison's Principle of Internal Medicine – 17th edition.
- Oxford Text Book of Medicine – 5th edition.

74

A PATIENT WITH MULTIPLE MYELOMA

CASE: *A 61 years old gentleman presented with recurrent chest infection over last few months. He had increasing joint pain which was ascribed to increased uric acid level. On the third occasion, when he was readmitted with fever and cough, empirical anti-TB medication was started in view of a suspicious shadow in the X-ray chest. Sputum for AFB was negative however. His urea and creatinine level was raised, Hb was low, and LFT showed raised globulin and low albumin, calcium level was high normal. His ESR was persistently high. Serum immunoglobulin electrophoresis report, which came back later on showed 'M' band, suggestive of multiple myeloma. Bone-marrow examination showed more that 30% of plasma cells consistent with multiple myeloma.*

DIAGNOSIS: Multiple myeloma with renal impairment.

DISCUSSION:

Multiple myeloma is a variety of paraproteinemia arising as a result of clonal proliferation of mature B-cells. Monoclonal gammopathy of undetermined significance (MGUS) on the other hand, on the other side of the spectrum, generally asymptomatic albeit with a propensity to progress of multiple myeloma in certain percentage of patients needing regular follow up.

CAUSES OF PARAPROTEINAEMIA:

A. Malignant B-cell disorders-

- Multiple myeloma (IgG, IgA, IgD, IgE, alpha and delta free high chains)
- Lymphoproliferative disorders like chronic lymphatic leukemia, Hodgkin's disease, Waldenstrom's macroglobulinemia.
- Amyloidosis.
- POEMS Syndrome.

B. MGUS

C. Non-malignant conditions-

- Rheumatoid arthritis
- Autoimmune diseases
- Hepatic cirrhosis
- Mycobacterium tuberculosis.

What is POEMS syndrome?

It is associated with the following conditions:

- Polyneuropathy
- Organomegaly
- Endocrinopathy
- M-protein
- Skin change

What is Waldenstrom's macroglobulinaemia?

It is associated with the following conditions:

- It is a lymphoproliferative disorder
- Happens at the median age- 72 years
- Associated with IgM paraprotein
- Hyper-viscosity is common e.g. visual disturbance
- CNS disturbance
- May present with hepatosplenomegaly
- Cells resembling plasma cells and lymphocytes are present in bone marrow and lymph nodes.
- Treated with plasmapheresis

CLINICAL PRESENTATIONS:

The usual presenting features to a clinician are-

- Fever of unknown origin with malaise
- Bone pain
- Recurrent chest infection
- Features of peripheral neuropathy and renal failure
- High calcium level, anaemia with high ESR.

The clinician should suspect multiple myeloma and ask for immunoglobulin electrophoresis if confronted with the above symptoms. In clinical practice multiple myeloma is sometimes diagnosed late by the primary care physicians.

CAUSES OF RENAL IMPLEMENTS IN MULTIPLE MYELOMA:

- Hypercalcaemia
- Amyloidosis
- Use of NSAIDs
- Precipitation of Benz Jones proteins in renal tubules.
- Infection

INVESTIGATIONS:

- Full blood count- shows normocytic normochromic anaemia with high ESR.
- Renal function test- shows renal impairment.
- Hypercalcaemia in 30% of cases.
- Liver function test shows low albumin and globulin (this feature may raise the suspicion of multiple myeloma in appropriate clinical situation).
- Presence of M-band in immunoglobulin electrophoresis.
- Urine for light chain- determination of urinary light chain (α or γ) is important as in 15% of multiple myeloma, that will be the only abnormality with normal blood paraprotein levels.
- Bone-marrow examination- more than 30% increase of plasma cells.
- β_2 micro globulin levels (for prognostic purpose).
- X-ray for skeletal survey- to show typical punched out lesion in the skull.

Prognostic markers in multiple myeloma:

It has been shown that β_2 micro globulin and albumin levels are the useful prognostic markers with β_2 micro globulin level of < 3.5 mg/liter and albumin level of > 35 g/liter increasing survival of more than 5 years while β_2 micro globulin level of > 3.5 mg/liter would signify a survival of approximately 2.5 years.

How to differentiate between multiple myeloma and MGUS?

MGUS is usually symptomatic. The paraprotein levels are less than 30 g/litre, bone-marrow plasma cells is typically $< 10\%$ (in multiple myeloma $> 30\%$). In plasmapheresis immunoparesis is unlikely and associated features of fever, anaemia and hypercalcaemia are not present. Although benign they should be carefully followed up as the rate of transformation to multiple myeloma is approximately 1% per year.

TREATMENT:

Supportive treatment consists of-

- Management of bone pain and hypercalcaemia- bisphosphonates, pamidronate, zoledronic acid.
- Anaemia- erythropoietin is a helpful adjuvant.
- Renal impairment- to ensure adequate fluid intake, avoidance of nephrotoxic drugs.
- Hyperviscosity- needs plasma exchange.

Specific therapy-

- Autologous stem cells transplantation- for young patients.
- High dose therapy (HDT) with autologous stem cell transplant- for patients of less than 65 years of age.
  [The chemotherapy regime includes vincristine, doxorubicin and dexamethasone]
- Oral therapy for patients ineligible for HDT. Regime used are-
  - Melphalan + Prednisolone
  - Thalidomide + Dexamethasone
  - Lenalidomide (a derivative of thalidomide) + Dexamethasone
  - Bortezomib (in relapsed cases)

Thalidomide is a preferred agent and current practice is to use thalidomide following relapse after oral chemotherapy. It has a 60% remission rate. Lenalidomide, a newer generation of drug with cytokine and anticancer activity and devoid of the side effects like-

- Teratogenicity,
- Constipation,
- Peripheral neuropathy,
- Sedation.

CASE: *A 56 years old lady presented with severe back pain. On investigation, she was found to be severely anaemic with Hb of 5 g%, WBC- 3100, platelets- 1,10,000, calcium- 11.1 mg% (high), low albumin and high globulin. X-ray lumbosacral spine showed osteoporotic collapse of lumbar vertebrae. A bone scan revealed multiple hot sports. Immunoglobulin electrophoresis and bone marrow examination was consistent with multiple myeloma.*

CASE: *A 65 years old lady presented with fever of unknown origin. Except for bone pain which was thought to be due to osteoarthritis. She did not have any localizing symptom. She was anaemic with Hb of 7 g%. She also had high ESR of 116 mm/hr. Her albumin and globulin ratio was altered. Bone-marrow and immunoglobulin electrophoresis confirmed the diagnosis of multiple myeloma.*

CASE: *A 78 years old gentleman presented with acute visual disturbance. Of late he has been complaining of a headache, intermittent fever and weakness. Examination revealed hepatosplenomegaly and lymphadenopathy. Ophthalmoscopy revealed retinal vein occlusion on the right. Immunoglobulin electrophoresis revealed pretense of paraproteins (M-band) and serum IgM level was very high. Bone-marrow examination was consistent with hyperviscosity syndrome (Waldenstrom's macroglobulinemia). He was referred to the haematologist, unfortunately he developed septicemia and multi organ failure from which he did not recover.*

When to think of multiple myeloma and other macroglobulinemia:

- Fever of unknown origin
- Bone pain
- Osteoporosis with vertebral collapse
- Presence of anemia, High ESR
- Presence of rouleaux formation in blood film
- Low albumin, high globulin, high calcium.
- Unexplained renal failure
- Retinal vein thrombosis

In this Background's the clinician must always check serum electrophoresis for M-band.

FURTHER REFERENCES:

- Lvey Cook *et al*. Management of Paraproteinemia. Postgraduate Medicine J-2007:83:217-223.
- A Mehta, V Hoffbrand: Haematology at a glance-2002.
- Harrison's Principle of Internal Medicine – 17th Edition.
- Oxford Text Book of Medicine – 5th Edition.

75 A PATIENT PRESENTING WITH DIABETIC RETINOPATHY

CASE: *A 56 years old insulin requiring Type II diabetic patient presented with rapid onset deteriorating vision of his right eye. He has been diabetic for last 12 years and was on insulin for last 2 years. His sugar and BP was not very well controlled.*

Recent blood tests showed his HbA_1C was > 8.5% and both LDL and triglyceride level were elevated. His BP was 170/100 mmHg. Ophthalmoscopic examination of the left eye showed presence of proliferative retinopathy with haemorrhage and exudates while the right retina could not be visualized properly. He was urgently referred to the ophthalmologist who diagnosed it to be a case of vitreous haemorrhage in the right eye.

DIAGNOSIS: Diabetic retinopathy with vitreous haemorrhage of the right eye.

DISCUSSION:

Visual problem is a common complaint faced by the primary care physicians. Although the patients are finally referred to the ophthalmologists, the initial assessment and management are done by the physicians and a working knowledge of the condition is very much essential in order to give appropriate consultation to the patients.

While examining such a patient, a physician needs to evaluate quickly following points-

a) Visual acuity by finger counting method

b) Visual field by confrontation method- papillitis

c) Ocular movement - cranial nerve palsy

d) Pupil reaction and size - *e.g.* trauma, drugs

e) Anterior chamber - conjunctiva, cornea, iris - infection *etc.*

f) Posterior chamber - retina by an ophthalmoscope diabetic retinopathy.

Before proceeding any further, non-pathological causes of deteriorating vision like refractive error should be considered and tested. Common causes of diminished vision are-

A. Acute unilateral painless -

- Vitreous haemorrhage - history of diabetes
- Retinal detachment
- Retinal vein occlusion
- Retinal artery occlusion
- Retinal artery embolism - Amaurosis fugax

B. Acute unilateral painful -

- Trauma
- Infection *e.g.* corneal ulcer due to herpetic infection
- Papillitis *e.g.* in multiple sclerosis
- Glaucoma - headache, vomiting.
- Cranial arteritis - headache, high ESR

C. Acute bilateral painless -

- In patient with poorly controlled DM resulting swelling of the lens.
- Some anticholinergic agents may cause acute onset bilateral blurred vision.

D. Acute bilateral painful -

- Rarely infection, trauma, glaucoma

E. Gradual unilateral painless -

- As in cataract, senile macular degeneration.

F. Gradual, unilateral painful

- Neoplastic lesion like retro orbital tumours.
- Inflammatory lesion like granuloma.
- CT or MRI scan may be helpful.

G. Gradual bilateral painless -

- *e.g.* cataract, macular degeneration
- Drugs- hydroxychloroquine, ethambutol

H. Gradual bilateral painful

- Inflammatory conditions like sarcoidosis, collagen vascular disorders.

This patient was clinically diagnosed to have proliferative retinopathy with probable vitreous haemorrhage. He was urgently referred to ophthalmologist for treatment.

DISCUSSION:

Diabetic retinopathy is one of the leading causes of vision loss in adults. Patients with Type I diabetes are at a higher risk of developing more severe retinopathy. Patients with Type II diabetes has a lower prevalence of retinopathy and tends to have less severe disease. However, Type II diabetes comprises 90% of the population with diabetes and thus comprises a larger proportion of those affected with diabetic retinopathy.

Risk factors:

Modifiable risk factors:

1. Diabetes mellitus:

The results of DCCT and UKPDS show that although intensive therapy of blood glucose control does not prevent retinopathy completely, it does reduce the risk of development and progression of diabetic retinopathy. This may be translated clinically to both preservation of vision and reduction in therapies *e.g.* laser photocoagulation.

	Decreased in HbA1C	Reduction in progression of retinopathy
DCCT	8% to 7.2%	35-40%
UKPDS	Every point decrease (9 to 8%)	35%

2. Hypertension:

In UKPDS study, tight BP control was associated with a 37% reduction of micro-vascular diseases, predominantly reduced risk of retinal photocoagulation. Beta blockers and ACE inhibitors were equally effective.

3. Serum lipid levels:

Raised triglyceride and LDL levels were associated with increased incidence of proliferative diabetic retinopathy.

4. Other risk factors:

a) Diabetic neuropathy- the risk of diabetic retinopathy is 5 times more common in patients with neuropathy.

b) Presence of anaemia and hypoalbuminaemia also increase the risk of retinopathy.

MANAGEMENT:

Although management is done by an ophthalmologist, primary prevention remains the most effective way to treat diabetic retinopathy and involves limiting modifiable risk associated with glucose control, BP and lipid control.

Both DCCT and UKPDS demonstrated that the importance of maintaining good metabolic control to prevent worsening or development of retinopathy. UKPDS clearly showed that controlled BP substantially reduces the risk of progression of diabetic retinopathy and visual loss. Tight BP control (Mean 144/82) resulted in 35% reduction of retinal photocoagulation and a 34% reduction in progression of diabetic retinopathy.

Diabetic nephropathy is a strong predictor of diabetic eye disease. Patients with early nephropathy should be aggressively treated with diet and ACE inhibitors in order to reduce the incidence of retinopathy.

Although increased lipids are associated with worsening of retinopathy, there is no conclusive evidence that lowering the level improves retinopathy. However, from cardiovascular point of view, aggressive lipid lowering strategy should be taken.

Physical exercise which can cause sudden rise in systolic BP should be discouraged as this may worsen vitreous haemorrhage. Low risk exercise like cycling, swimming and walking should be encouraged. Close watch should be done during pregnancy, as it might worsen retinopathy.

From this discussion it is evident that primary care physician has a big role to play in the primary prevention of diabetic retinopathy.

This patient had vitreous haemorrhage and after proper evaluation by the ophthalmologist, underwent vitrectomy and laser photocoagulation. Unfortunately the recovery of the vision of his right eye was suboptimal.

: KEY POINTS :

- Deteriorating vision is a common clinical presentation in primary care practice.
- Primary care physician should attempt to make a clinical diagnosis before referring to an ophthalmologist.
- Diabetic retinopathy is a common condition for deteriorating vision.
- At primary care level meticulous management of blood glucose, BP and lipid levels are the best way of preventing diabetic eye disease.

FURTHER REFERENCES:

- Diabetic retinopathy - medical management and assessment- M Deli *et al.* -Hospital medicine, Vol. 64 NO.7 July 2003, Page P 400-403.
- Epidemiology of diabetic retinopathy- Emily Chew, Hospital medicine – vol. 64, NO.7 July 2003, 396 - 399.
- Blurred vision- J Bradford *et al.* NEJM vol. 343 No.8 August 24-2002, P 556-562.

76 AMIODARONE INDUCED THYROTOXICOSIS

CASE: *A 59 years old patient with dilated cardiomyopathy recurrent ventricular tachycardia needing frequent hospital admission attends the clinic on monthly basis for follow up. He has been remaining stable with cardiac medications and amiodarone for last 3 years. Of late during his visit he has been complaining of weakness, tiredness, unwell being etc. Cardiac investigations were satisfactory. However, the routine T_3, T_4, TSH revealed he had overt thyrotoxicosis with very high T_3, T_4 and very low TSH (checked from two sources). There was no obvious thyroid swelling.*

DIAGNOSIS: Thyrotoxicosis probably amiodarone induced.

DISCUSSION:

Amiodarone is a very common and popular drug prescribed in cardiac practice mainly for recurrent atrial fibrillation and also in ventricular arrhythmias in patients with cardiac failure (in view of paucity of use of ICD's in our country). Although user-friendly, it has got a host of side effect profile and the use should be followed up by regular monitoring of certain biochemical parameters-LFT, T3, T4 &TSH *etc.*

Amiodarone causes thyroid dysfunction in approximately 4% of patients. Hypothyroidism is common but occasional patients also develop thyrotoxicosis. They may not have specific symptoms of thyrotoxicosis but may cause worsening of the original disease like cardiac failure.

Amiodarone inhibits the 5-deiodinase activity and prevents thyroid hormone entry in the peripheral tissues. This results in slight increase in T4, decrease in T3 and increase in TSH. This may be a transient phenomenon and may not need any treatment.

In drug induced thyrotoxicosis, it has got two mechanism of action. In Type I, the patients usually have a latent thyroid disease or multinodular goitre. The iodine load associated with amiodarone triggers off thyrotoxicosis in such cases (Jod-Basedow effect). In type II, there is destructive thyroiditis with consequent leakage of thyroxine into the circulation. In the second variety, the thyroid gland may be entirely normal.

MANAGEMENT:

In type I, in view large intra thyroidal accumulation of iodine, large dose of carbimazole (40-60 mg) may be needed. In addition, potassium perchlorate may be added to inhibit iodine uptake thus contributing to the depletion of intra-thyroidal iodine stores. AIT often recurs following discontinuation of treatment and radioactive iodine therapy may sometimes be needed. Type II variety occurs with normal thyroid. It is due to thyroiditis and leakage of thyroid hormone from the gland. In type II variety, carbimazole may not be effective. Corticosteroids (prednisolone 15-80 mg) may be required. This works by its membrane stabilizing and anti-inflammatory property. Sometimes combination therapy may be needed.

The main question arises whether amiodarone could be continued or resumed following successful treatment of thyrotoxicosis. If the use of amiodarone is optional, it may be discontinued. However, in the absence of appropriate anti arrhythmic drugs, amiodarone can be continued or resumed as it has been shown that this approach does not influence the clinical outcome in amiodarone induced thyrotoxicosis.

Mildly elevated TSH does not need anything specific except for careful follow up. In case there is development of overt hypothyroidism with low T3, T4 and high TSH, thyroxine supplementation will be needed along with continuation of amiodarone therapy. It is mandatory that patients on amiodarone therapy should have a *protocol based check up of* 6 *monthly* T_3,T_4, *TSH, liver function test and yearly X-ray chest (to detect amiodarone induced lung damage).*

This patient did not respond to high dose of carbimazole (6 weeks therapy) and prednisolone was added (which normalized the thyroid function test). The treatment was eventually stopped. Unfortunately within another 2 months, he was admitted with acute LVF because of septicemia needing artificial ventilation and had recurrence of ventricular arrhythmia. Amiodarone was resumed. He was discharged home with amiodarone with an advice to check his LFT and thyroid function test in next 3 months time. In 3 months at follow up, he was doing well with normal thyroid function test.

Common side effects of amiodarone:

- Corneal microdeposits
- Pigmentation of skin
- Thyroid dysfunction
- Liver dysfunction
- Pulmonary fibrosis.
- Drug interaction with -
    - i) Oral anticoagulants (potentiates the action).
    - ii) Digoxin (increases the level).

: KEY POINTS :

- Amiodarone is a commonly used drug in clinical practice.
- Although very effective, it has a number of side effects.
- It can cause both hypothyroidism and thyrotoxicosis without any obvious clinical features.
- Steroids may be needed to treat thyrotoxicosis.
- Amiodarone can be resumed following successful treatment with proper supervision.
- A protocol based investigation will detect complications early.

FURTHER REFERENCES:

- Thyrotoxicosis: Lazarus JH (1997)- Hyperthyroidism, Lancet 349: 339 - 343.
- Goodman and Gilman- The pharmacological basis of therapeutics. 9th edition (1996), Philadelphia.

77 A PATIENT WITH PSORIASIS

CASE: *A 27 years old gentleman presented with skin lesions over his knees, elbows, legs, scalp and back of his ear lobes. These lesions were itchy, affected his nails and caused psychological embarrassment. He also complained of joint pain in the hands and the knees. Examination revealed erythrosquamous skin lesions over the extensor surface of the knee joints and the legs, elbows and scalp. The lesions were shiny, scaly and had a silver colour. The fingernails were also affected with evidence of pitting, ridging and onycholysis. Investigation did not reveal any abnormality.*

PROVISIONAL DIAGNOSIS: Chronic plaque psoriasis with possible arthropathy.

DISCUSSION:

Presented in the classical form as above, it does not cause any difficulty in the diagnosis. Initially they present to the primary care physician for advice who has to differentiate it from eczematous skin lesion in the extremities and seborrheic dermatitis if the lesion is in the scalp. If confidently diagnosed, the physician can take responsibility to treat it provided the lesion is not too extensive. In my personal experience, the clearance of the lesion is good and very swift with the modern regime. However in difficult cases dermatological assistance will be required.

The disease is characterized by increase in dermal blood flow finally leading to scaling and thickening due to hyperkeratinization of stratum corneum, thickening of the entire epidermis, dermal oedema and inflammatory dermal infiltrate. It appears to be at the site of trauma, a characteristic known as Koebner's phenomenon. Drug history is important as certain drugs can aggravate psoriasis like-

- Chloroquine
- Lithium
- β blocker

Different Varieties:

- Acute guttate psoriasis - large number of small lesions often following streptococcal infection.
- Chronic plaque psoriasis - mainly affecting extensor surface, most common presenting features to the GPs.
- Generalized pustular psoriasis.
- Palmoplantar pustulosis
- Erythrodermic psoriasis - presenting with generalized erythroderma. It may cause difficulty in diagnosis initially.

Sometimes it is associated with arthritis which might resemble rheumatoid arthritis. However, distal interphalangeal involvement is characteristic as opposed to proximal found in rheumatoid. In addition mono-articular and sacroiliac joint involvement might also occur.

MANAGEMENT:

- Topical therapy:
    - Tar + Dithranol
    - Steroids + Keratolytics
    - PUVA
- Systemic therapy

TOPICAL THERAPY:

1. **Salicylic acid** ointment and potent steroid (topical application). Keratolytic ointment softens the scales and addition of potent steroid in combination (betamethasone or clobetasol) helps in disappearance of the lesion. The lesions become less scaly as well. However discontinuation of treatment causes quick reappearance of the lesion. They should be used as a short term measure.
2. Application of vitamin D analogue *e.g.* **calcipotriol**, can cause partial clearance and render the plaque lesions soft and less thick.

The keratolytic, steroids and vitamin D analogues can be used by the primary care physicians.

In more severe cases, topical preparation like **dithranol** and tar may be used and they can cause complete clearance. Dermatological help should be needed for their use. Similarly photo chemotherapy using **psoralen and ultra-violet-A** radiation is very helpful in psoriasis (PUVA). Again it should fall in the domain of dermatologists rather than the internists. 70-80% of psoriatic patients can be treated adequately by topical agents.

SYSTEMIC THERAPY:

This has revolutionized the management of psoriasis with disappearance of lesions within 6-8 weeks, the agents most commonly used are:

1. **Methotrexate**- on weekly basis upto 25 mg/week. The response rate is good with quick disappearance of the lesion, 2 monthly follow up with LFT is essential as it can cause cirrhosis. Weekly folic acid supplementation reduces the gastrointestinal side effects.

2. In patients who cannot tolerate methotrexate, **cyclosporine** (2.5-5 mg/kg) may be used with similar degree of effectiveness. Renal function should be monitored regularly. It can also cause hypertension.

3. **Acitretin** - It is a retinoid which may be effective in psoriasis. Specialist's advice will be required. It is teratogenic.

The index patient also responded to methotrexate and arthritic symptoms (psoriatic arthopathy) had responded very well. He is under regular follow up with routine blood tests. After 2 years of use, he developed abnormal LFT and methotrexate was discontinued. He had flare up of her psoriasis. He was finally treated with cyclosporine, acitretin and topical application of calcipotriol and steroid. He is doing well now. Dermatological help was needed before commencement of acitretin.

ROLE OF BIOLOGICAL THERAPY IN PSORIASIS:

Biologic therapies are designed to target specific components of the immune system and pathways such as antibodies against cytokines or cell surface receptors. The structure of biological therapies is as follows:

1. Ximab: chimeric monoclonal antibody
2. Zumab: humanized monoclonal antibody
3. Umab: human monoclonal antibody
4. Cept: receptor blocker protein

Biologic therapies targeting tumour necrosis factor:

- Infliximab
- Adalimumab
- Galiximab
- Etanercept
- Certolizumab Pegol

Role in psoriasis:

Infliximab: It is highly effective. The dose is 5 mg/Kg IV infusion at weeks 0-2-6 and then every weeks.

Etenercept: The onset is slower. The dose is 25 mg thrice/week sc injection.

Adalimumab: Quick acting. The dose is 80 mg sc at week '0', 40 mg at week 1 and 40 mg every other week.

Methotrexate may be combined with these drugs.

Ustekinumab, human IgG monoclonal antibody which inhibits the action of interleukin (IL-12 and IL-23), has been found very effective in treatment of psoriasis.

Use of biologics in other dermatological conditions:

Infliximab	• Psoriasis • Sarcoidosis • Pyoderma gangrenosum • Hidradenitis suppurativa • Behcet's syndrome • Wegner's granulomatous • Microscopic polyangiitis
Etanercept	• Psoriasis • Behcet's syndrome
Adalimumab	• Psoriasis • Sarcoidosis • Hidradenitis suppurativa
Ustekinumab	• Psoriasis
Rituximab (targeting B cells)	• Autoimmune blistering disorder • SLE • Cryoglobulinaemia • Wegner's syndrome

Side effects of biologic therapies:

- Upper respiratory tract infection, sinusitis, headaches
- Increased incidence of non-melanoma skin cancer

- Reactivation of latent TB
- Should be avoided in patients with personal or family history of demyelinating diseases, heart failure or cancer.

IMMUNOLOGICAL MEASURE:

Cytokine dysregulation may be an important mechanism for perpetration of psoriatic skin lesion and biological agents like etanercept, alefacept and efalizumab are currently approved by FDA for the treatment of psoriasis. Infliximab is under consideration for approval.

: KEY POINTS :

- Psoriasis is a common condition in clinical practice.
- It should be differentiated from eczematous condition and seborrheic dermatitis (in scalp).
- With modern regime the clearance of lesion is good and primary care physicians can take patients with uncomplicated psoriasis.

FURTHER REFERENCES:

- Psoriasis and its management, L-Naysmith *et al.*-JR Col physicians Edinb 2003, 33: 104-113.
- BHJM. –Biological therapy in dermatology, vol.-74, no 1 January 2013-p12-17.
- Clinical Medicine- Arif Aslam- Drug Therapies in dermatology, vol-14, No. 1- Feb 2014, 47-53.

78 A PATIENT WITH PNEUMOTHORAX

CASE: *A 36 years old diabetic and hypertensive gentleman was admitted with recent onset of chest pain and breathlessness. Chest pain started few days back while travelling in a train. It started with a sudden bout of cough. He was admitted to a local hospital where myocardial infarction was ruled out with appropriate tests. He did not have an X-ray chest however. He was readmitted to this hospital, this time with shortness of breath. Examination revealed pulse rate of 120/min, BP- 100/60 mmHg and breath sound diminished over the right side. ECG showed sinus tachycardia. X-ray chest showed right sided pneumothorax. He underwent intercostal water seal drainage with immediate symptomatic improvement.*

However in view of persistence of air leak, he also received slow suction of the water seal drainage. Finally on the 6th day, the tube was taken out following complete expansion of the lungs. During his stay, he received supportive therapy with oxygen, antibiotics and chest physiotherapy.

DIAGNOSIS: Spontaneous pneumothorax following a bout of severe cough.

DISCUSSION:

In acute onset chest pain, in addition to ruling out MI with appropriate tests, X-ray chest should be routinely done. We have found few cases where patients presenting with such problems underwent full cardiac work up and discharged, only be readmitted with dyspnea, with X-ray chest showing pneumothorax.

CAUSES OF PNEUMOTHORAX:

Primary or spontaneous: due to rupture of apical blebs mainly in COPD, occasionally in asthma, tubercular lesion (in India), cystic lung disease, carcinoma of lung, rupture of lung abscess with bronchopleural fistula, rarely in connective tissue disorders, Marfan's syndrome, Ehler Danlos syndrome *etc.*

Secondary: following trauma, following procedures like CVP line insertion, barotrauma, during mechanical ventilation.

DIAGNOSIS: X-ray chest may miss a small pneumothorax and CT thorax can detect.

MANAGEMENT:

A rim of air < 2 cm on the inspiratory film usually indicates small pneumothorax. Anything more than this should be considered as a large pneumothorax. If the patient has a small primary pneumothorax without any history of COPD, one can pursue conservative management with rest, avoidance of strenuous activities and avoidance of flying in an aircraft for next 8 weeks. However, regular radiological surveillance will be needed. If the patient has a large primary pneumothorax, the initial management should be with aspiration, failing which intercostal water seal drainage should be done. Suction should be applied only after 48 hours if there is non-resolution of the air leak. Surgical consultation will be required at this point.

Secondary pneumothorax should be treated with intercostals tube drainage (unless the pneumothorax is very small).

Indications of surgery:

- A contralateral pneumothorax
- Second ipsilateral pneumothorax
- Bilateral spontaneous pneumothorax
- Persistent air leak for more than 5 days.

General advices:

- The patient should stop smoking (as it increases recurrence rate of pneumothorax).
- Underlining tuberculosis should be ruled out.
- High flow oxygen therapy during intercostal drainage (as it increases reabsorption of air from the pleural space).

CASE: *A 71 year old patient was admitted with breathlessness and the swelling of the subcutaneous tissue of this neck. 24 hour before admission, he underwent gastroscopy for evaluation of dysphagia and biopsy specimen was taken from a lesion in the mid oesophageal region. On examination, he had subcutaneous emphysema over the chest wall and neck. X-ray of chest showed mediastinal emphysema along with subcutaneous emphysema and left sided plural effusion.*

DIAGNOSIS: Mediastinitis along with mediastinal emphysema due to esophageal perforation.

DISCUSSIONS:

Mediastinal air leak may be due to similar causes that lead to pneumothorax particularly barotrauma due to mechanical ventilation. Oesophageal rupture leak due to any cause may be a causative factor. Median sternotomy may occasionally cause it. X-ray chest showing air shadow along the left border of the heart gives useful clue toward the diagnosis. Conservative measurers like needle aspiration along with supportive therapy may suffice in majority of cases. In cases of esophageal rupture due to any cause (trauma, malignancy, insertion of Sengstaken-Blakemore tube), should be referred to the surgeon for consideration of surgical repair. High concentration of oxygen therapy may sometimes helps in absorption mediastinal air.

CHRONIC MEDIASTINITIS:

It is not an uncommon presentation in clinical practice. The patients usually presented with shortness of breath and features of superior venacaval syndrome with engorged jugular vein X-ray chest is indicative of fibrotic lung disease. It frequently poses a diagnostic dilemma and these patients land up with antitubercular treatment; however other causes like histoplasmosis and sarcoidosis should also be borne in mind.

Causes of chronic mediastinitis:

- Tuberculosis
- Fungal infection (histoplasmosis)
- Sarcoidosis
- Silicosis

CASE: *A 34 years old patient with sepsis underwent central venous line insertion via subclavian route. A routine X-ray chest was not done due to an oversight. 2 hours later, patient developed severe breathlessness with oxygen saturation dropping to below 50%. While awaiting an urgent portable chest X-ray, RMO made a clinical diagnosis of pneumothorax and immediately put an intravenous needle blindly which drained out the air with improvement of oxygen saturation and haemodynamic stability. X ray chest later on confirmed pneumothorax and intercostal drainage tube was electively inserted later on with further stabilization of patient's condition.*

DIAGNOSIS: Pneumothorax as complication of subclavian line insertion.

DISCUSSION: Presently in our unit, we are looking at the feasibility of doing all the subclavian line under ultrasound guidance which has shown to reduce complication rate of all subclavian line insertions.

Similarly a patient on mechanical ventilation, if develops sudden breathlessness or the machine shows high pressure alarm, one needs to do an urgent chest X-ray to rule out barotrauma (other causes of high pressure alarm are ventilator-tube block and severe bronchospasm).

: KEY POINTS :

- Pneumothorax is a common in clinical practice particularly in ITU setting.
- Pneumothorax should be considered in any person with sudden onset of breathlessness or chest pain.
- Chest X-ray is mandatory in evaluation of patients with chest pain and following insertion of central venous line.
- Pneumothorax should be considered if there is sudden onset of desaturation or increase in peak airway pressure in a ventilated patient.

FURTHER REFERENCES:

- Management of spontaneous pneumothorax- M. H. Baumann *et al.* An American college of chest physicians, Delphi consensus Statement; chest 2001-119; 590-602.
- BTS guidelines for the management of spontaneous pneumothorax. M. Henry *et al.* Thorax 2003, 58, Suppl.11, P-39 - 52.
- What is new in respiratory disease medicine, vol. 32:5, 2004, P 1-4.
- Harrisons Principle of Internal Medicine 17th edition.

79 A PATIENT WITH MOTOR NEURON DISEASE

CASE: *A 67 years old gentleman attended the clinic with progressive weakness of both upper and lower extremities. Examination revealed bilateral small muscle wasting of hands. There was prominent fasciculation in the thigh muscles. Deep reflexes in the upper extremities were diminished while in the legs these were brisk. There was no sensory involvement, however. Plantar response was upgoing bilaterally. Haematological and biochemical parameters were normal CPK,* T_3, T_4, *TSH, liver function test, renal function test were normal. CT brain and MRI cervical spine were normal. EMG study of both extremities confirmed the diagnosis of amyotrophic lateral sclerosis. He was referred to a neurologist for further management.*

DIAGNOSIS: Amyotrophic lateral sclerosis.

DISCUSSION:

Weakness and wasting of the small muscle of the hands is an uncommon presentation in clinical practice. Although finally these patients are managed by the neurologist, initial assessment and diagnosis is often done by the internist and knowledge about the approach, differential diagnosis and treatment of such condition would be helpful.

Causes of small muscle wasting of hand along with spasticity of legs and upgoing planters:

- Cervical myelopathy
- Amyotrophic lateral sclerosis
- Syringomyelia
- Spinal cord compression by tumour at cervical region (neurofibroma, meningioma)
- Rarely multiple sclerosis (subacute cord compression type)
- Radiation myelopathy

Causes of upgoing planter response (upper motor neuron sign) with loss of reflexes in legs (sensory movement):

- Subacute combined degeneration of spinal cord
- Tabes dorsalis
- Friedreich's ataxia

In these conditions there is variable involvement of upper motor neurons and sensory tracts which causes loss of tendon reflexes in spite of upper motor involvement.

Generalized small muscle wasting of hands without any upper motor neuron signs in legs:

- Motor neuron disease (MND)
- Myasthenia gravis (MG)
- Inflammatory myopathies
- Peripheral neuropathies due to various causes
- History of poliomyelitis in childhood

Unilateral small muscle wasting of hands without involvement of any other parts of the body:

C_8T_1 root lesion due to:

- Cervical radiculopathy
- Pancoast tumour
- Thoracic outlet syndrome
- Cervical rib

Individual nerve lesion:

- Ulnar nerve palsy
- Median nerve lesion

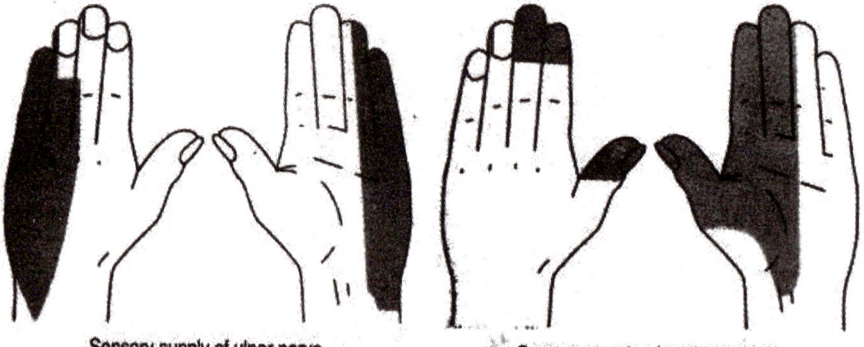

Sensory supply of ulnar nerve   Sensory supply of median nerve

History and thorough clinical examination is very important. Presence of speech problem indicates bulbar involvement as may occur in syringobulbia, motor neuron disease with bulbar involvement, polymyositis *etc.*

Presence of fasciculation in the muscles may indicate MND whereas presence of sensory deficit rules out MND. Loss of pain and temperature sensation in the affected extremity may indicate syringomyelia; presence of sensory level may indicate cord compression. Early involvement of bladder and bowel usually goes in favour of cord compression due to any cause rather than MND. Hereditary neuropathies usually present at a younger age.

Initial investigations:

- CPK (myopathies)
- Anti acetylcholine ester antibody titre (myasthenia gravis)
- MRI cervical spine - helpful in syringomyelia, tumours, multiple sclerosis.
- EMG and nerve conduction studies helpful in MND, MG, neuropathies.

In MND, motor nerve conduction velocity is normal (slow conduction suggests a neuropathy), sensory studies are normal and EMG shows diffuse fibrillation and fasciculation.

A neurologist's input is essential as there are treatable conditions like multifocal motor neuropathy with conduction block and pure motor chronic demyelinating neuropathy which mimic MND. They have characteristic changes in nerve conduction study. Before stamping a diagnosis of MND, these two treatable conditions must be excluded.

- Lumbar puncture: It is usually not needed. However in special circumstances where one needs to exclude primary progressive multiple sclerosis, suspected demyelinating polyneuropathy or paraneoplastic syndrome.
- Test for urinary porphobilinogen: This will exclude the rare cause of porphyria presenting as peripheral neuropathy and wasting of hand muscles.

This patient's clinical features and EMG findings were consistent with amyotrophic sclerosis. He was treated with the help of a neurologist. The family members were apprised of the poor prognosis of the condition.

MOTOR NEURON DISEASE (MND): MND and amyotrophic lateral sclerosis is a neurodegenerative disorder of unknown etiology with a bad prognosis. No definitive treatment is available for this condition and till date the treatment is mainly symptomatic.

It usually presents in 3 forms:

- **Amyotrophic lateral sclerosis (ALS)** with evidence of spinal & cortical involvement. There is usually small muscle wasting of hands with brisk reflexes in the legs.
- **Pure lower motor neuron syndromes (progressive muscular atrophy):** typically there is generalized wasting without any evidence of upper motor lesion.

A group of inherited conditions called spinal muscular atrophy may present at an early age and progress very slowly. These disorders may be inherited either as X-linked, autosomal dominant and recessive trait.

- **Pure upper motor syndrome (primary lateral sclerosis):** This is a rare variety. It usually presents as spastic paraplegia and should be differentiated from hereditary spastic paraparesis, Vitamin B_{12} deficiency, primary progressive multiple sclerosis *etc.*

Bulbar involvement may be a feature of any variety of motor neuron disease.

MANAGEMENT: Management is frustrating as till date no specific therapy is available for this condition.

- Riluzole, a glutamate antagonist has been shown to increase tracheostomy free survival by 3-6 months in ALS variety of MND. It does not improve the symptoms of ALS however. It causes gastrointestinal side effects.
- Supportive therapy is the most important part of the treatment. This is carried out by giving chest physiotherapy, making provisions for noninvasive ventilation, maintenance of nutrition by percutaneous endoscopic gastrostomy (PEG). Muscle cramps can be treated with baclofen or tizanidine. Botulinum toxin can be used for excessive drooling of saliva. These patients are frequently depressed, so treating depression and psychological counseling might be helpful for them.

ULNAR NERVE LEISON: Usually occurs at the elbow occasionally can occur in the hand as the nerve passes, the hook of hamate in Guyon's canal. Bone deformity at the elbow and external pressure are the causes. Other causes that one should exclude are:

- Vasculitis
- Diabetes mellitus
- Leprosy (In Indian subcontinent)

Palpable thick ulnar nerve in the elbow may indicate:

- Hereditary neuropathies
- Leprosy

FEATURES: Tingling and numbness in the little and ring fingers.

- Weakness of hand. Finally wasting of the small muscles of the hand giving rise to claw hand deformity.
- Examination reveals weakness of interossei and weakness of the long flexor of little and ring fingers. Sensory loss will be noted in the ulnar nerve distribution.

MEDIAN NERVE LESION: (Discussed in carpal tunnel syndrome chapter). The wasting is noted predominantly over the thenar eminence. Sensory changes are noticed over 3½ fingers (thumb index, middle and half of the ring finger).

C_8T_1 ROOT LESION:

- Motor deficit - all small muscles of the hand, finger flexors, finger extensors.
- Sensory deficit - medial forearm to include little finger, axilla down to the olecranon. (This differentiates the condition from ulnar nerve lesion).

RADIAL NERVE LESION:

- It is usually involved in the upper arm in the radial groove.
- As a part of mononeuritis multiplex in vasculitis or diabetes mellitus.
- Lead poisoning.
- There is weakness of wrist and finger extensors, giving rise to wrist drop.
- Sensory loss is over a small area over the dorsum of the hand.
- Triceps reflex may be occasionally impaired.

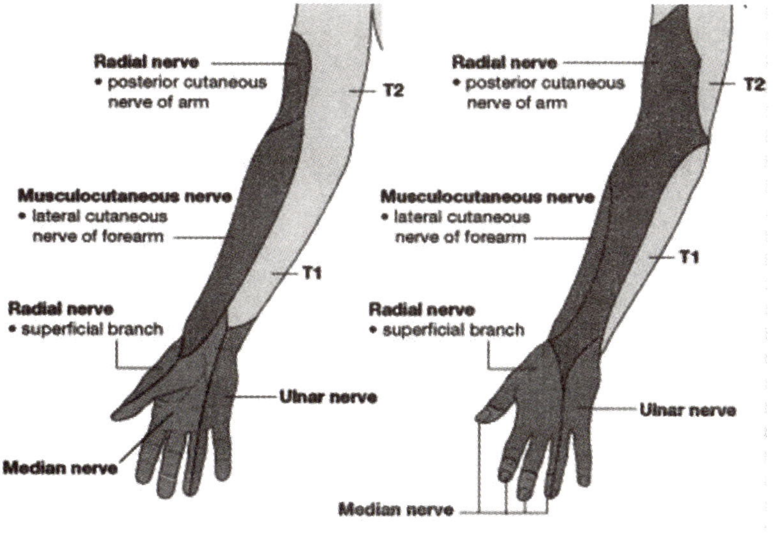

CASE: *A 37 years old car mechanic attended the clinic complaining of loss of power in his left hand. He first noticed it in the morning following waking up from a deep sleep during Bishwakarma puja festival (Bishwakarma is the God of industry and technology in Hindu mythology). He was very worried and tense as he thought that he had a brain stroke. Examination revealed presence of left sided wrist drop. Functions of the other muscle groups in that hand were intact. He was reassured and sent to the physiotherapist for local electrical nerve stimulation. He recovered completely in the next 7 days.*

DIAGNOSIS: Saturday night palsy.

: KEY POINTS :

- Small muscle wasting of hands is an uncommon presentation in clinical practice. Motor neuron disease has a uniformly bad prognosis.
- Before stamping MND other treatable condition must be excluded with appropriate tests.
- In unilateral wasting of hands, differentiation between nerve lesion and root lesion should be made.

FURTHER REFERENCES:

- Motor neurone disease—K. Talbat, Post grad med journal, 2002, 78: 513-519.
- Neurology - an illustrated textbook- Geraint Fuller, Mark Man fold.
- Neurological differential diagnosis- John Patten.

80

A PATIENT WITH PORPHYRIA

CASE: *A 30 years old lady, wife of registered medical practitioner was admitted with history of abdominal pain and vomiting. Examination revealed slightly confused lady with abdominal distension. Investigations showed FBG- normal, Na- 122 mg%, K- 3.1 mg%, urea- 35 mg%, liver functional test mildly abnormal with raised AST and ALT. Amylase and lipase was normal. In USG NAD, X-ray abdomen showed distended bowel loops and distended stomach but no fluid levels. A working diagnosis of severe gastritis with vomiting induced hyponatraemia with mild grade encephalopathy was made. Supportive therapy failed to give symptomatic relief. CT abdomen showed distended stomach and small bowel loops. Surgical consultation ruled out any surgical abdomen, gastroscopy also failed to show any definite abnormality. On the 5th day, she showed some symptomatic improvement and she was discharged on request.*

She was readmitted after a week, this time utterly confused and with quadriparesis. Examination revealed muscle power 1/5 upper and lower extremities, loss of reflexes and intact sensory system. Acute demyelinating polyneuropathy was considered as a possibility. Her lumbar puncture was normal and nerve conduction study was consistent with axonal neuropathy. Urine examination at this point revealed strongly positive porphobilinogen which confirmed the diagnosis of acute intermittent porphyria.

DIAGNOSIS: Acute intermittent porphyria.

DISCUSSION: Porphyria is rarely encountered in primary care although in secondary care hospital practice, one occasionally comes across acute intermittent porphyria mainly presenting with abdominal pain, neuropsychiatric symptoms or peripheral neuropathy. Porphyria is disorder of haeme synthesis and classified erythropoietic and hepatic. Of the different varieties, acute intermittent porphyria most commonly presents to the clinicians.

In mild enzymatic deficiency, the disease may not manifest throughout the life time or present with intermittent mild symptoms thereby escaping the notice of the patients and the attending doctor.

Pathophysiology and mechanism of symptoms:

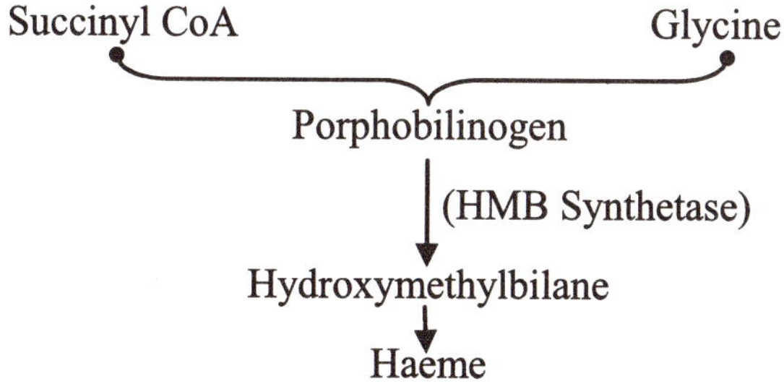

In acute intermittent porphyria there is deficiency of HMB Synthetase with resultant accumulation of precursor porphobilinogen. Enzyme inducing drugs may precipitate an acute attack by stimulating the already deficient enzymatic system.

The main presenting features are:

1) Intermittent acute colicky abdominal pain with vomiting.

2) Neuropsychiatric symptoms.

3) Autonomic disturbance like tachycardia, labile hypertension, sweating.

4) Seizures, peripheral motor neuropathy.

5) Investigations- Low Na^+ (due to SIADH), abnormal liver function test, change of colour of urine on prolonged standing, presence of porphobilinogen in urine.

CASE: *A 15 years old boy was admitted with history of intermittent palpitation along with episodic rise of BP and constipation. He was seen as an outpatient and underwent investigations like CT adrenal, 24 hours urine for VMA along with other routine tests which were all normal. The reason of his admission was history of seizure on two occasions during one of the episodes of hypertension. CT brain and EEG were normal. He was started on phenytoin and admitted to HDU for observation. In the ward he was noticed to be confused which was thought to be due to postictal confusional state and he was also increasingly constipated with abdominal distension. Colonoscopy did not reveal anything specific. Soon after he came from endoscopy unit, he was noticed to be restless with a distended urinary bladder due to retention. Catheterization was done and after one hour the attending nurse informed that he was having haematuria. Examination revealed very high coloured dark urine which was, though unlikely, to be due to blood. Urgent urine examination from three sources confirmed the presence of porphobilinogen.*

DIAGNOSIS: Acute intermittent porphyria.

DISCUSSIONS:

This patient had features of autonomic disturbance and seizure. Phenytoin aggravated porphyria further and he developed neuropsychiatric symptoms, increasing constipation and urinary retention. The catheterized urine quickly changed colour in the uro-bag which helped in the diagnosis. Unfortunately, he deteriorated acutely with development of quadriparesis with respiratory failure needing ventilatory support. His heart rate and BP fluctuated widely and his Na^+ fell down to 110 mg%. He was treated with temporary pacemaker insertion, IV glucose infusion, sodium supplementation. Intravenous haematin which is a very expensive specific therapy for porphyria was arranged from outside. Unfortunately he had an episode of cardiac arrest from which he could not be resuscitated.

The first patient described here, is doing reasonably well, however. She was treated with IV glucose, sodium supplementation and physiotherapy. Specific therapy, haematin could not be organized for her. Although disabled from her neuropathy, she became independently mobile. She needs intermittent admission, for her abdominal pain which settles with IV dextrose. Meanwhile she has developed dilated cardiomyopathy for which she is on specific treatment.

So far we have diagnosed five cases of acute intermittent porphyria, with single mortality, described above. The main presenting features were intermittent acute abdominal pain and neuropsychiatric symptoms or peripheral neuropathy. I think that before stamping patients with functional abdominal pain, in patients with undiagnosed acute and chronic peripheral neuropathy and in young patients with features of autonomic disturbance, urine for porphobilinogen should be checked routinely which will enable us to diagnose this rare disorder. One should also remember that lead toxicity which is prevalent in certain industries can also present with abdominal pain, constipation and positive urinary test for porphobilinogen. Relevant history and checking serum lead level will resolve the issue.

One of the most common causes of precipitation of acute attack of porphyria is certain drug therapy which induce liver enzyme and thus aggravate the symptoms. Common drugs that might precipitate an acute attack are -

- Phenytoin,
- Barbiturate,
- Rifampicin,
- Oestrogen etc.

A full list of drugs including anaesthetic agents should be available in the ITU for emergency purposes. While treating patients with porphyria, we faced tremendous difficulty in getting hold of haematin which was finally arranged from abroad. Although it is not expected to get rare and uncommon medicines through the general pharmacy, we feel that such medicines for uncommon and rare disorders should be available in the central drug store run by the State Government to cater to the need of the patients of that particular state.

: KEY POINTS :

- Acute intermittent porphyria is a rare disorder of haeme synthesis.
- Clinicians should think of this condition in any patient with undiagnosed intermittent abdominal pain, neuro-psychiatric symptoms, neuropathy or autonomic disturbance.
- The diagnosis is done by urine examination of porphobilinogen which is a simple and inexpensive test.
- Lead toxicity should be considered in differential diagnosis.
- A full list of drugs and anaesthetic agents should be available in ITU.
- Medicines for rare and uncommon diseases should be made available in the central drug store run by the State Government.

FURTHER REFERENCES:

- Oxford Text Book of Medicine.
- Harrison's Principle of Internal Medicine- 15th edition.
- Kumar and Clark- Clinical medicine- 5th edition.

81 ACUTE CORONARY SYNDROME

CASE: *A 53 years old gentleman with history of hypertension and smoking, presented with a history of chest pain of 6 hours duration. Initially, it was thought to be due to hyperacidity. In spite of taking antacids, the pain persisted. He was immediately admitted to ICCU. Examination revealed a pulse rate of 96 m/min, BP 120/80 mmHg and chest was clear. Rest of the examination was satisfactory. ECG showed T wave inversion in the lateral leads. CPK, CPKMB were normal, X-ray chest normal, CRP was elevated. Rest of the biochemical and haematological parameters were within normal limits. Troponin-T test was weakly positive.*

DIAGNOSIS: Acute coronary syndrome - non ST segment elevation MI.

DISCUSSION: Acute coronary syndrome is a common presentation in clinical practice mainly those who deal with acutely ill patients. Recently there have been a lot of changes in nomenclature of acute coronary syndromes as well as their management. Those presenting with ST segment elevation are termed acute ST segment elevation MI and the treatment is fairly well protocolized with thrombolysis or primary angioplasty along with aspirin, low molecular wt. heparin, beta blocker, ACE inhibitors etc. Those presenting with normal ECG or ST segment depression or T wave inversion were until now variously called unstable angina, crescendo angina or non Q wave MI. Now-a-days, with the availability of troponin, many of these patients with normal CPK with afore-mentioned ECG changes and positive troponin are called non-ST segment elevation MI. Newer management protocols are gradually evolving for these conditions. The significance of these conditions is that although the initial prognosis during hospital admission is better in comparison to ST segment elevation MI, the long term prognosis is much the same indicating increased number of out of hospital adverse events in these conditions.

MANAGEMENT:

- **Nitrates** - IV nitrates should be titrated according to the symptoms, BP response and side effects like headache.
- **Aspirin** - 150 mg should be given immediately.
- **Clopidogrel** - 75 mg can be added as recent trial suggested that addition of clopidogrel improves the outcome in a small albeit statistically significant number of patients (CURE STUDY).
- **β blockers and / or calcium channel blockers** (diltiazem) - should be added to the regime.
- **Thrombolysis is not indicated**. It increases the mortality and should be avoided.

- **Heparin or low molecular weight heparin** - heparin was the initial treatment of choice. Since the availability of low molecular weight heparin, they are being used more frequently. Although initial study did not show any significant difference in outcome with heparin, subsequent studies (ESSENCE study, where enoxaparin was used) showed results in favour of low molecular weight heparin both in short term and long term outcome of acute coronary syndrome.

- **Early invasive vs. early conservative therapy** - The physicians are sometimes in dilemma whether to intervene with coronary angiography followed by angioplasty or CABG. Initial studies in early 1990's gave the verdict in favour of conservative measures during the initial admission and only to proceed for angiography in patients with persistent angina in spite of conservative treatment (VANQUISH study). More recent studies favour early intervention (FRISC II, TACTICS, TIM I 18). Even in these studies, the benefits were observed only in that subset of patients who had troponin positively (Non-ST segment elevation MI). So depending upon the facilities available one can proceed for early intervention in troponin positive non ST segment elevation MI, given the late adverse outcome in that group of patients.

- **GP-IIb-IIIa inhibitors** - (*e.g.* reopro, tirofiban) these drugs are particularly helpful in those patients undergoing coronary intervention like PCI with stenting (along with aspirin and weight adjusted heparin). They have been shown to reduce the incidence of post procedural complication including the closure of the artery. Orally available GP-IIb-IIIa blockers have also been tried. However, meta-analysis of the studies using these agents has shown increased mortality and hence at the present time not recommended for use.

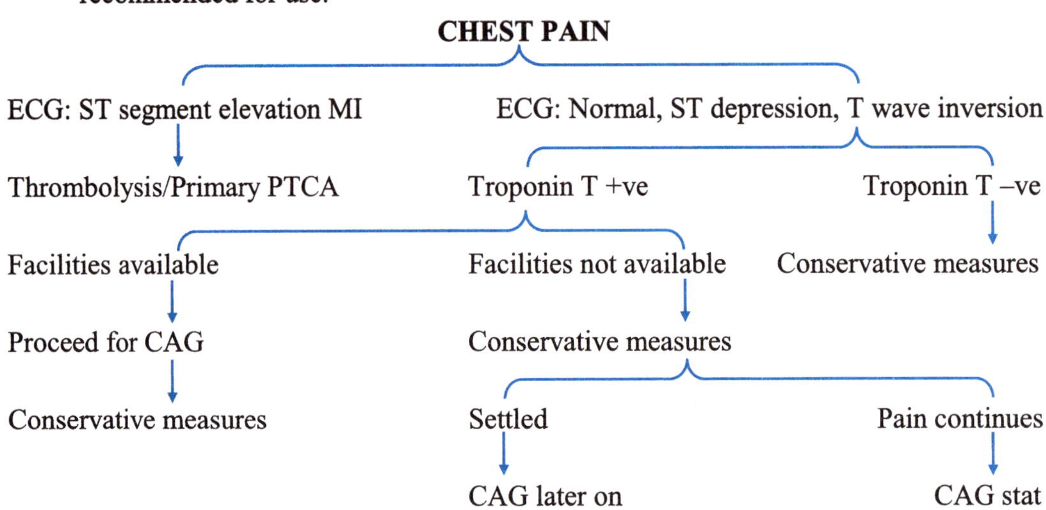

: KEY POINTS :

- Chest pain is a common presentation both in hospital and primary care practice.
- Acidity and heart burn in a high risk patient should be dealt with caution in primary care practice.
- Troponin helps establish the diagnosis of non-ST elevation MI in patients presenting with non-specific ST changes.
- Thrombolysis is not indicated in non ST segment elevation MI but low molecular weight heparin is.
- Early invasive strategy is indicated in non ST segment elevation MI because of the increased incidence of late adverse outcome in this group of patients.
- GP IIb/ IIIa inhibitors are useful adjunctive to coronary intervention procedure (PCI).

FURTHER REFERENCES:

- Braunwald's heart disease- 6th Ed.
- Harrison's principle of internal medicine- 15th Ed.

82 A PATIENT WITH OSTEOARTHRITIS OF KNEE JOINTS

CASE: *A 51 years old obese lady presented with history of joint pain mainly in the knees, wrists along with neck pain and low back pain. The pain interfered with her day to day activities. Examination revealed crepitated painful knee joints, no joint deformity. Investigations showed normal FBC, ESR and CRP. ASO titre, rheumatoid factor and ANF were negative. Uric acid was normal. X-ray of knee joints showed joint space narrowing with presence of osteophytes. X-ray cervical spine and lumbar spine showed spondylotic changes.*

DIAGNOSIS: Generalized osteoarthritis with involvement of knee joints.

DISCUSSION:

Generalized aches and pains in the joints are a very common presentation in clinical practice. Although the case described above had classical features of OA, it is sometimes difficult to differentiate between the causes. This is important as some inflammatory arthropathies have specific treatment.

Common causes of joint pain and swelling in clinical practice:

Generalized pain:

- **Rheumatoid arthritis**: Symmetrical, involves small joints of the hands, early morning stiffness is characteristic, high ESR, high CRP and positive rheumatoid factor (rheumatoid factor may be negative).

- **Osteoarthritis:** Usually big joints especially knee, 1st metacarpophalangeal joint is characteristically involved. Lumbar pain and cervical pain are common.

  Heberden's node in distal interphalangeal (DIP) joint may be present, obesity is a common association, *stiffness of joint is transient (unlike rheumatoid),* CRP, ESR are usually normal.

- **Gouty arthritis:**

  Although usually monoarticular, may present with generalized joint pain as well.
  Axial skeleton is not usually involved.
  Tenosynovitis may be present.
  Associated with obesity, hyperlipidaemia, HTN, diuretic therapy or alcohol intake.
  Uric acid will be high.
  CPPD (Calcium Pyrophosphate Deposition) arthropathy is classically associated with shoulder joint involvement.

➢ Seronegative inflammatory arthropathy:

Usually there is history of preceding skin problems like psoriasis, bowel problems like ulcerative colitis or acute diarrhoea and urinary infection.

Usually asymmetrical, with big joint involvement in the lower extremities (knee joint and ankle joint are commonly involved).

Enthesitis (inflammation of the entheses, the sites where tendons or ligaments insert into the bone) may be present.

Axial spine involvement like sacroiliitis may be present. HLA B_{27} may be positive in sacroiliitis.

CRP and ESR may be elevated.

➢ Rheumatic fever:

Usually found in childhood or young age.

Preceded by sore throat and high ASO titre.

Arthritis is fleeting in character associated with fever.

While diagnosing rheumatic fever Jones criteria should be followed. Mere fever, sore throat with raised ASO titre is not sufficient enough to diagnose acute rheumatic fever.

Jones criteria-
Presence of two major or one major and two minor criteria establishes diagnosis.

Major criteria	Minor criteria
Carditis	Fever
Arthritis- migratory polyarthritis	Polyarthralgia
Sydenham's chorea	ECG changes- ↑ PR interval
Erythema marginatum	Acute phase reaction- ↑ ESR, ↑CRP,
Subcutaneous nodule	Leukocytosis
	History- previous episode of rheumatic fever or inactive heart disease

- **Fibromyalgia:**

  It is very common in clinical practice. Often associated with depression and anxiety.

  Inflammatory parameters like ESR, CRP are normal.

  There are specific trigger points which can be elicited during examination (occipital, cervical, gluteal *etc.*).

In addition to these common conditions, other causes like muscles problems- polymyalgia, generalized metabolic disorders like osteomalacia, haematological problems like acute leukemia in children and multiple myeloma in adults should also be considered if appropriate. A common cause of generalized joint pain is post viral reactive arthritis which is usually transient.

Monoarticular involvement:

- **Osteoarthritis**- commonly knee joints.
- **Acute gout**- commonly 1st MTP joint and knee joints.
- **CPPD arthropathy**- usually elderly, characteristically shoulder joint is involved, knee joint may also be involved.
- **Seronegative reactive** arthritis - may involve knee joint only.
- **Ankylosing spondylitis** with peripheral joint involvement. Big joints of lower extremity are usually involved.
- **Septic arthritis** - associated with pain, fever and swelling.
- **Infections**- Tubercular arthritis (occasionally seen in India), Gonococcal arthritis (associated with tenosynovitis and skin rash).
- **Haemarthrosis**- Usually there is history of trauma. Coagulation abnormalities like haemophilia or Vitamin C deficiency mainly in children. Synovioma or pigmented villonodular synovitis in adults (rare in clinical practice).

In monoarthritis it is necessary to examine the joint fluid and look for viscosity and cell count. Normal joint fluid has a very high viscosity, clear in appearance with a cell count of < 200 (poly < 25%). Non-inflammatory condition (like OA) will not cause any appreciable change. In inflammatory arthropathy, the viscosity will be low, opalescent in colour with a high cell count (poly > 75%). Gram stain and culture will be helpful. Joint fluid can also help to diagnose gout and CPPD arthropathy.

CASE: *A 16 years old boy was admitted with severe bloody diarrhoea. He was treated with IV fluids, antibiotics like metronidazole and ciprofloxacin. The stool culture report which came after 72 hours showed growth of Shigella group of organism. 3 days following discharge, he was readmitted with pain and swelling of the right knee joint. He was treated with NSAID. Joint aspiration excluded septic arthritis and he received intra articular injection of steroid. He took nearly 6 weeks for complete recovery.*

DIAGNOSIS: Reactive arthritis following Shigella diarrhoea.

CASE: *A 56 years old lady with known rheumatoid arthritis was admitted with increasing pain and swelling of her left knee joint. Examination revealed swollen tender left knee jt. Her ESR, CRP and WBC counts were high. Before proceeding to IV methyl prednisolone for disease flare up, joint aspiration was done which showed opalescent fluid with low viscosity and high cell count (Poly > 75%). Staphylococcus was grown from the fluid. She was treated with IV linezolid followed by oral linezolid with good response.*

DIAGNOSIS: Septic arthritis of left knee joint in a patient with rheumatoid arthritis.

MANAGEMENT OF OA:

Since this is a very common day to day problem, it will be worthwhile to discuss few salient points in its management, particularly because there is a great deal of pessimism in patients suffering from OA. Many of them spend years of inactive life either bed bound or housebound thinking that there is no effective treatment. While cure is certainly not a possibility, with proper management, pain and quality of life can certainly be improved.

Few salient points in the management are:

- Reduction of weight by diet and if necessary with drugs like orlistat and sibutramine.
- Analgesics - Simple analgesics like paracetamol may be tried.
- NSAIDs - They certainly reduce pain. Gastrointestinal bleeding and renal problems may be encountered in long term use. Nowadays with the availability of COX2 inhibitors (which are equipotent) the gastrointestinal side effects have reduced considerably. In one study comparison between COX2 inhibitor rofecoxib and naproxen, showed that the gastric bleeding was significantly less with COX2 inhibitors, but the incidence of MI was significantly high in the COX2 inhibitor group (probably due to selective COX2 inhibition). In another study, combination with aspirin caused loss of gastrointestinal protective effect of COX2 inhibitors.

- Diacerein an agent hypothesized to inhibit H-1 activation and encourage cartilage preservation has been shown to reduce pain thereby having a NSAID sparing effect.
- Topical therapy - Application of topical capsaicin ointment may be helpful in pain relief, although there is no evidence that local application NSAID helps.
- Glucosamine sulphate and chondroitin sulphate: Long term use of glucosamine sulphate and chondroitin sulphate over a period of 3 years has been shown to reduce pain and progression of the disease (mainly in OA knee joints).
- Often suggested treatment options are tetracyclines which have demonstrated to inactivate collagenase and gelatinase which are responsible for joint degeneration. Use of doxycycline for more than 3 months has been shown to reduce joint space narrowing but without any significant reduction of pain.
- Regular exercise is a very helpful part in the management.
- Different kinds of support, foot wear and walking aids and appliances along with physiotherapy can make a lot of difference in the symptoms and daily living activities.
- In spite of medical therapy, the pain still continues and in these situations, local steroids injection (upto 2-3 times a year) may give symptomatic relief. It works better if there is joint effusion and post injection rest is a mandatory. Physicians trained in joint injection can easily give it.
- Intra articular injection of hyaluronic acid (with or without steroid) - Hyaluronic acid is a natural joint replacement fluid. Injection of hyaluronic acid on weekly basis for 3 to 5 courses has been shown to reduce pain compared to steroids with much more durability. The first injection may be combined with steroid.

With this line of management, many of the patients will lead a reasonably comfortable life. If still symptoms persist, one should take an orthopaedic opinion regarding further management like:

- Arthroscopic clearance of the knee joint this procedure may sometimes be helpful in the treatment of knee joint arthritis.
- Joint replacement surgery, whenever possible and feasible this option should be explored, before abandoning the patient to fate. By Indian standards, indeed cost is a limiting constraint but one should remember that successful joint replacement may improve the quality of life enormously.

: KEY POINTS :

- Joint pain and swelling is a common presentation in clinical practice.
- A systemic approach would help us to find out a definitive cause.
- In patients with acutely swollen and painful joints, septic arthritis should be excluded before prescribing steroids.
- Asymmetrical lower arthropathy with enthesitis usually indicates seronegative arthritis.
- Quality of life can be improved with treatment in patients with osteoarthritis.

FURTHER REFERENCES:

- Schumacher HR JR- Arthritis of recent onset- A guide to evaluation and initial therapy for primary care physician, Post Grad Med. 97: 52, 1995.
- Circuttini F M *et al.* (1998).
- Osteoarthritis, Medicine 26 (6).
- Creamer P. *et al.* (1997).
- Osteoarthritis Lancet 500-508.
- Harrison's Principle of Internal Medicine - 17th edition.
- Oxford Textbook of Medicine - 5th edition.

83 A PATIENT WITH POLYMYOSITIS

CASE: *A 56 years old gentleman presented with difficulty in walking and standing up from sitting posture. He could not lift his hands above his shoulder. He was also complaining of difficulty in swallowing. He was increasingly getting bedbound. Examination revealed marked proximal muscle weakness. Investigation revealed normal glucose, thyroid function test, CPK was raised upto 12,000 unit (normal 195 units), Autoantibody screening was normal. X-ray chest and USG abdomen was normal. EMG findings consistent with myositis, muscle biopsy showed presence of fibrosis and fatty tissue (non-contributory).*

DIAGNOSIS: Polymyositis.

DISCUSSION:

Although rare, inflammatory myopathic conditions are occasionally encountered in the clinical practice. The condition includes:

- Polymyositis (PM)
- Dermatomyositis (DM)
- Inclusion body myositis (IBM)

The first two conditions are immune mediated whereas inclusion body myositis is not and does not respond to immune suppression.

EPIDEMIOLOGY:

Both PM and DM are more common in women. While PM is a disease of adults, DM affects both children and adults. IBM is a disease predominantly of older men (male & female ratio 3 : 1).

There is an association with malignancy with PM and adult DM. So in patients with PM and adult DM, one should look for an occult malignancy particularly of breast, lungs, pelvic organs and abdomen.

Overlap syndromes:

In some cases myositis is seen as a part of wider autoimmune conditions like SLE, rheumatoid arthritis. In Sjogren's syndrome, myositis is particularly associated with interstitial lung disease and anti Jo-1 antibody.

PRESENTATION:

- Muscle aches, pain and weakness- inability to stand up from squatting position or difficulty in combing.
- In DM- heliotropic skin rash around the periorbital region or raised scaly lesions over the knuckles (Gottron's patches).
- Cardiac abnormalities
- Pulmonary involvement
- In childhood DM, vasculitis, subcutaneous calcification along with contracture.
- In IBM, preferential involvement of quadriceps ilio-psoas biceps and triceps.
- Mild facial weakness (not a feature of PM) is seen in 60% of cases resulting dysphagia.

DIAGNOSIS:

- Raised **CPK** which may be > 50 times the normal value. However, CPK may be normal. In IBM, CPK is either normal or mildly elevated.
- **EMG** may be indistinguishable between PM, DM and IBM. It shows spontaneous insertional activity and fibrillation.
- **Muscle biopsy** shows inflammatory infiltrates (mainly endomysial) along with necrosis of muscle fibres. As the findings are patchy, small sample will miss the characteristic features.

TREATMENT:

Immunosuppression with steroid is the main stay of treatment. Usual regime is IV methyl prednisolone 1 g for 3 days followed by prednisolone 60 mg daily. This dose is continued for 4 weeks or until CPK becomes normal. Then the dose in quickly tapered off to 20 mg daily and any further reduction is made very slowly. It should be given in once daily dose. Prophylaxis for osteoporosis should be given.

Azathioprine has a steroid sparing effect and it should be started early (1.5-3 mg/kg). IBM does not respond to steroids.

Other immunosuppressive agents:

- IV gammaglobulin has been tried with mixed results in steroid resistant PM or DM without any significant benefit.
- Methotrexate (weekly oral) has a role in steroid resistant cases. The usual dose is 7.5 mg weekly initially followed by increment upto 20 mg weekly if needed.

In non-responsive cases, chlorambucil, cyclophosphamide and cyclosporine have been tried with varying results.

When patients fail to respond to steroid, steroid myopathy should be considered. This can only be resolved by a repeat muscle biopsy.

CASE: *A 56 years old lady presented with non-specific aches, pain and stiffness of proximal part of upper and lower extremities. Autoimmune screening was negative. TSH, CPK were normal and her ESR and CRP were very high. NSAID was not helping her much. She was diagnosed to have polymyalgia rheumatica and responded well to low dose steroid therapy.*

Although uncommon in India, polymyalgia rheumatica should be considered if there is symptom of predominant stiffness of proximal muscles along with pain. ESR and CRP are characteristically high whereas CPK is normal and they respond very well to low dose steroid (starting dose 15 mg of prednisolone per day). Inflammatory arthropathy like rheumatoid arthritis should be ruled out, however as they can cause early morning stiffness along with other evidence of arthropathy. Associated headache in polymyalgia rheumatica may indicate giant cell arteritis which is a common association.

CASE: *A 48 years old male presented in the clinic with muscle pain and stiffness mainly of the calf muscles. He also complained of generalized muscle cramp. In addition he had facial puffiness which he ascribed to allergy to certain foods. He also had a broken hoarse voice which he thought to be due to recurrent cold with laryngitis. Investigations revealed TSH of > 50 and CPK 3500 mg% (very high). Diagnosis of hypothyroidism with myopathy was made and he responded very well to thyroxine replacement therapy.*

I have found hypothyroidism with myopathy is a rather common condition in clinical practice. Any patient presenting with muscle cramp and stiffness along with hoarseness of voice, facial puffiness and generalized weakness, blood for T_3, T_4, TSH and CPK should be checked.

: KEY POINTS :

- Polymyositis is an uncommon condition in clinical practice.
- Muscle pain and weakness are the two characteristic features.
- Raised CPK is very characteristic.
- PM and adult DM may be associated with malignancy.
- Childhood DM may be associated with vasculitis and subcutaneous calcification.
- Steroid is the treatment of choice.
- Non-responder to steroid may be due to IBM or steroid myopathy.

FURTHER REFERENCES:

- Inflammatory Muscle Disease- S. Hall, ACNR Vol. 2, May/June - 2002 P 14-15.
- Myositis Diagnosis and Management, G. Cheurel *et al.*, 2, P 4-11. Practical Neurology 2002.

84

A PATIENT WITH IRRITABLE BOWEL SYNDROME

CASE: *A 19 years old girl attended the clinic with her parents with altered bowel habit which was interfering with her day to day activities. She had intermittent abdominal pain and bloating. She had periods of severe watery diarrhoea interspersed with constipation with passage of hard pellet like stool. She was very much stressed and anxious. There was no history of weight loss or blood in the stool. On examination NAD. Investigations normal stool examination, normal CRP and ESR. Normal haematological and biochemical parameters. Thyroid function was normal. The X-ray chest and ultrasound of abdomen were also normal.*

DIAGNOSIS: Irritable bowel syndrome.

DISCUSSION:

Irritable bowel syndrome is a very common problem in primary care affecting nearly all sections of the population. Although it is a functional bowel disorder, it significantly affects the day to day activity with morbidity. It usually presents in three forms –

1. Abdominal pain and bloating relieved by defecation.
2. Predominant diarrhoea.
3. Predominant constipation.

The revised ROME II criteria for IBS are-

1. Minimum twelve weeks of symptoms in previous one year of abdominal pain and bloating.
2. Altered frequency of stool.
3. Altered consistency of stool.

While dealing with IBS, one should exclude more serious organic causes of altered bowel habits.

1. **Infective diarrhoea** - It is very common in India. Chronic amoebiasis and amoebic colitis can cause similar symptoms. There may be history of bloody diarrhoea, tenesmus and *increased mucus* in the stool. Stool examination may not reveal cysts of amoeba. A course of *ciprofloxacin* and *metronidazole* may be tried as therapeutic measure.

2. **Inflammatory bowel disease** - This condition is increasingly being detected since the use of colonoscopy in investigation of chronic diarrhoea. Usually there is *weight loss, blood in stool, nutritional deficiency.* Markers of inflammation like *ESR* and *CRP are markedly raised.*

3. **Bowel malignancy** - In elderly patients presenting with altered bowel habits, loss of weight - and blood in the stool, malignancy of the large gut needs to be excluded. Haemoglobin will be low. ESR and CRP will be elevated.

In addition, other conditions that should also be considered in differential diagnosis are –

1. **Lactose intolerance** - It is relatively common in certain parts of India. A trial of exclusion of milk should be tried if suspected. However, lactose intolerance only becomes symptomatic if more than 280 ml of milk is consumed.
2. **Malabsorption** due to any cause should also be excluded by doing appropriate stool tests and blood tests. Coeliac disease although uncommon in India, should be considered in western population. Antigliadin and antiendomysial antibodies should be requested for if clinically suspected. Chronic pancreatitis with abdominal pain and malabsorption can cause diagnostic confusion.
3. **Medical disease** like thyrotoxicosis can cause diarrhoea and should be excluded.

Alarm signals suspected in IBS are:

1. Weight loss.
2. Progressive anaemia.
3. Blood in the stool.
4. High ESR and CRP.

Investigation in suspected IBS:

- Stool for routine and culture and occult blood.
- Hb, TC, DC, Platelet, ESR, CRP.
- Liver function test.
- Amylase, Lipase.
- Thyroid function test.
- Antigliadin and antiendomysial antibodies (in selected population)
- Urea, electrolytes, calcium, folic acid, ferritin.

If there is weight loss with bloody diarrhoea or recent onset of constipation and weight loss in middle aged and elderly patient, colonoscopy should also be considered.

CASE: *24 years girl working as a dietician presented with a history of intermittent abdominal pain and diarrhoea. She was initially suspected to have amoebic colitis. She lost considerable amount of weight and repeated courses of metronidazole and quinolones only gave her partial relief. She was admitted for further investigations. She also gave history of passage of blood with mucous. Her Hb was 8 g%, WBC 16,000, ESR 76, low albumin, stool- RBC++, pus cells++. Colonoscopic examination revealed left sided ulcerative colitis. Biopsy confirmed the colonoscopic findings. In addition to supportive therapy, she received oral steroid, mesalazine and antibiotics. She is in remission now. She has regained weight and her Hb has gone upto 12 g%.*

DIAGNOSIS: Inflammatory bowel disease.

MANAGEMENT OF IBS:

Constipation predominant -

High fibre diet along with increasing dose of isabgol husk will be needed. Osmotic laxative may also be added. One should try to avoid stimulant laxatives.

Diarrhoea predominant -

Infection should be excluded and treated with appropriate antibiotics. *Loperamide* and *diphenoxylate* may be used to control diarrhoea. Morphine containing preparations may be used but they can cause rebound constipation.

Abdominal pain and bloating -

Prokinetic agents will be helpful. Cisapride but not metoclopramide or domperidone decrease colonic transition time. Unfortunately, the use of cisapride has been stopped following reports of fatal cardiac arrhythmia. Anticholinergic like mebeverine is a commonly used drug with some beneficial effects.

Treatment of depression and anxiety -

This is very important and SSRIs are perhaps better than tricyclics in view of the later's constipating effect. Psychiatric counseling may be required. The patient must be reassured that although chronic and persistent, it does not have any effect on mortality and should be given an optimistic picture.

: KEY POINTS :

- Bowel irregularity is a very common problem in primary care.
- One needs to differentiate between functional and organic bowel disorders by history and simple blood and stool tests.
- Colonoscopic examination may be needed in middle aged, elderly and in patients with suggestive symptoms.
- Lactose intolerance is common in certain parts of India.
- IBS may need psychiatric input along with medical therapy.

FURTHER REFERENCES:

- Talley NJ, *Evaluation of drug treatment for irritable bowel syndrome*- Br J. Clin. Pharmacol. 56: 362, 2003.
- American gastroenterological Association, medical position statement- Irritable bowel syndrome. Gastroenterology 112: 2118, 1997.

85 A PATIENT WITH PLEURAL EFFUSION

CASE: *A 31 years old nonsmoker gentleman was admitted for investigation of weight loss, low grade fever and persistent cough for last 2 months. Examination revealed a thin emaciated man with evidence of diminished breath sound over the right base. There were few supraclavicular matted lymph nodes over the right side. ESR was 110 mm 1st hour, Hb 10.2 g%, WBC- 4800, biochemical parameters were normal. X-ray chest showed moderately large right pleural effusion. Mantoux test was strongly positive. Sputum for, AFB was negative. Aspiration of pleural fluid showed pH- 7.2, LDH- raised, protein- 56 g%, glucose- 44 mg%, AFB stain negative, gram stain negative, PAP stain- NAD, pleural fluid adenine deaminase (ADA) level marked raised.*

DIAGNOSIS: Exudative pleural effusion, possibly of tubercular origin.

He was treated with 4 drugs antitubercular regime and 3 months at follow up, he was afebrile, gained weight and X-ray chest showed resolution of the pleural effusion.

CASE: *A 59 years old diabetic gentleman was admitted with fever, chest pain and breathlessness which were found to be due to right lower lobe pneumonia. Although he responded to antibiotic therapy, he had persistent low grade fever and right sided chest pain. Repeated X-ray showed right sided pleural effusion which was aspirated and the fluid analysis showed a pH of 7.1, LDH- very high, WBC > 8000, with predominant lymphocytes, there was presence of pus cells.*

DIAGNOSIS: Complicated parapneumonic effusion with empyema thoracis. He was treated with intercostal tube drainage along with prolonged antibiotic therapy to which he responded satisfactorily.

CASE: *A 61 years old lady with past history of malignant parotid tumour 4 years back was admitted with breathlessness. X-ray chest showed massive left pleural effusion. In spite of repeated aspiration she developed recurrent rapid re-accumulation of fluid. Pleural fluid analysis showed exudative nature of fluid (high protein, high LDH), AFB negative, PAP stain negative on two occasions. CT thorax and fiber optic bronchoscopy showed no focal lesion. Biopsy from a cervical lymph node confirmed metastatic adenocarcinoma.*

DIAGNOSIS: Malignant pleural effusion due to recurrence of malignant parotid tumour.

DISCUSSION: Pleural effusion is a very common presentation in clinical practice.

CASE: *A 31 years old Bangladeshi lady presented with arthralgia and shortness of breath. Examination revealed facial rash, X-ray chest showed bilateral pleural effusion and echocardiography showed moderate pericardial effusion. Her ANF was strongly positive. She underwent bilateral pleural aspiration and was commenced on steroids and HCQS with symptomatic relief. She had recurrent pleural effusion on both sides needing intercostal drainage in spite of being on steroids and mycophenolate mofetil necessitating use of 5 % povidone iodine for pleurodesis. Fortunately her effusion did not recur but unfortunately she presented with bilateral hip-joint pain found to be due to avascular necrosis of hip joints. She underwent bilateral sequential total hip joint replacement and 6 months on follow up was doing well.*

DIAGNOSIS: Recurrent pleural effusion due to polyserositis due to SLE.

Common causes encountered are:

Exudative:

- Tuberculosis (common in India)
- Parapneumonic
- Malignancy – primary, metastatic, lymphoma
- Pulmonary embolism
- Connective tissue disorder like SLE

Transudative:

- Congestive heart failure
- Cirrhosis.
- Hypoalbuminaemia
- Nephrotic syndrome
- Peritoneal dialysis

While dealing with a case of pleural effusion, proper history and clinical examination is important. History of smoking, occupational exposure to asbestos, past history of any malignancy will have an important bearing to the diagnosis. Presence of a small cervical lymph node might give important histological clues. X-ray chest may indicate tuberculosis or bronchogenic carcinoma. However, examination of the pleural fluid provides the most important information regarding the aetiology.

Presence of RBC is non-specific and cannot differentiate between exudates and transudate.

Gold standard tests for exudative effusion:

- A ratio of pleural fluid protein to blood protein more than 0.5 (traditionally pleural fluid protein of more than 3.5 g% is used as the cut off value).
- A ratio of LDH in pleural fluid & blood > 0.6.
- Pleural fluid LDH more than two thirds the upper limit of normal for blood LDH.

With the above criteria there is only 10-20% chance of misdiagnosis of transudative pleural effusion as exudative, particularly in cardiac failure who are receiving diuretics. In such patients, pleural fluid cholesterol level of less than 55 mg% or a pleural fluid to plasma cholesterol ratio of less than 0.3 suggests transudate.

Physical characteristics: Normal appearance of pleural fluid is usually clear light yellow.

- Milky appearance may point to lymphatic system involvement.
- Reddish pleural fluid may indicate the presence of blood as in trauma, malignancy, or pulmonary infarction.
- Cloudy, thick pleural fluid may indicate the presence of microorganisms and/or white blood cells.

Other tests:

- Glucose level is lower than blood indicates rheumatoid arthritis, infection.
- Lactate levels increases in infectious pleuritis, either bacterial or tuberculosis.
- Low complement levels in SLE.
- High amylase level in pancreatitis.
- Low pH (less than 7.1), very high leukocyte count, LDH more than 1000 u/*l*, glucose less than 40 mg% and presence of pus indicates complicated parapneumonic effusion and is an indication of intercostal tube drainage.
- Presence of very high number of leukocytes (> 10,000/ mm^3) usually indicates infection.
- An increased number of neutrophils is found in bacterial infections and increased number of lymphocytes indicates cancers and tuberculosis.

- Pleural fluid culture for AFB has a low sensitivity (24%) but a high specificity.
- Pleural fluid cytological examination has got a reasonably good sensitivity.
- High pleural fluid ADA level is very characteristic of tuberculosis.
- Tumor markers can be detected in different cancers.
- High triglyceride level in pleural fluid indicates chylous effusion due to malignant obstruction of the lymphatic vessels.
- Pleural biopsy can sometimes make the final diagnosis (gives the diagnosis in 50-60% of cases).
- Other ancillary tests like bronchoscopy or CT scan of thorax will give some useful clues.
- Non-diagnostic exudative pleural effusion in a smoker should be carefully followed up as the probability of developing a malignancy at a later date is at least 30%.

: KEY POINTS :

- Pleural effusion is common in clinical practice.
- Tuberculosis, pneumonia and malignancy are the common causes.
- Examination of pleural fluid will give important diagnostic clues.
- A low pH in pleural fluid along with brisk leukocytosis is an indication of insertion of intercostal tube drainage.
- The chance of malignancy in a non-diagnostic pleural effusion in a smoker is approximately 30%.
- Although biochemical tests can reliably differentiate between transudative and exudative pleural effusion, diagnostic dilemma may occur in cases of transudative effusion caused by cardiac failure.

FURTHER REFERENCES:

- Dermatology in practice- Anthony Villeor.
- Clinical dermatology- 4th ed. - Rona M Mackie.

86 A PATIENT WITH HAEMOPTYSIS

CASE: *A 44 years old gentleman attended the clinic with 2 months history of low grade fever and painful subcutaneous nodules. His Hb was 9.2 g%, WBC- 8200, ESR-110, CRP-high, ANF, ANCA, rheumatoid factor, HIV antibody negative. Serum angiotensin converting enzyme levels were normal, urea, creatinine normal, urine examination normal, serum calcium normal, initial X-ray chest normal, biopsy from the subcutaneous nodule showed no evidence of granuloma, there was evidence of necrotic tissue. CT scan of thorax, done later on, showed multiple nodular shadows in both lung fields. While awaiting a CT guided FNAC, he was admitted acutely with nasal bleeding and while in hospital he developed massive haemoptysis and in spite of all resuscitative measures, he exsanguinated to death. A repeat ANCA sent during his last admission came back to be positive for cANCA in low titre. Cancer markers like alpha feto-protein and CEA were reported to be normal.*

PROVISIONAL DIAGNOSIS: Massive haemoptysis due to vasculitis (?).

The diagnosis could not be confirmed because of inability to perform a post mortem examination. Possibilities that were strongly considered besides vasculitis were-

- Granulomatous disorder like sarcoidosis
- Malignancy (metastatic)
- Infections like fungus

DISCUSSION: Haemoptysis is a common cause for medical consultation and can be life threatening. Upper respiratory tract infection can cause expectoration of blood tinged sputum, which causes a great deal of concern and anxiety to the patients. It usually settles on its own and perhaps does not need any special investigation except for a routine X-ray chest (in non-smokers). Recurrent haemoptysis or massive haemoptysis always indicates serious underlying pathology and should be thoroughly investigated.

In haemoptysis the expectorated blood usually originates from:

- Bronchial circulation *e.g.* in bronchitis, bronchiectasis, pneumonia, lung cancer and tuberculosis.
- In 10% of cases the blood originates from pulmonary circulation *e.g.* lung abscess, pulmonary infarct, necrotising pneumonia, AV malformation.
- Rarely haemoptysis is the manifestation of diffuse alveolar hemorrhage as may be found in vasculitis due to Wegener's granulomatosis, Good Pasture's syndrome and small vessel vasculitis or Idiopathic pulmonary haemosiderosis.

List of differential diagnosis of haemoptysis is long. Some causes have been enumerated here:

Due to endobronchial lesions:

- Carcinoma (primary)
- Metastatic- renal cell / ovarian / thyroid carcinoma, melanoma.
- Vasculitis due to different causes
- Tuberculosis
- Sarcoidosis
- Fungal infections like aspergilloma, histoplasmosis
- Acute necrotising pneumonia
- Bronchiectasis
- Endobronchial endometriosis

Most of the cases can be diagnosed from the history and initial investigation like X-ray chest and CT scan of thorax.

X-ray chest may show pneumonia, tubercular lesions, bronchiectasis, fungal ball as in Aspergilloma, calcified lesion in the hilar region usually indicates old tubercular lesion, fungal infections like histoplasmosis or certain occupational lung disease like silicosis, cavitating lesion may indicate tuberculosis, carcinoma, acute necrotising infection or vasculitis. Nodular lesion may indicate vasculitis, sarcoidosis or metastatic disease.

Presence of active urinary sediments along with altered renal function usually suggests vasculitis lesions. In suspected causes, vasculitis and autoimmune screening should be done (ANF, ANCA, anti glomerular basement antibody *etc.*). Mantoux test, sputum examination for C/S, AFB and cytology should also be done. Old tuberculosis with scarring and traction bronchiectasis is a very common cause of haemoptysis in India. Fungal infection due to *Histoplasmosis* is also a common cause of lung calcification and haemoptysis (It can also cause broncholithiasis and granulomatous mediastinitis).

Fiber optic bronchoscopy should be done in patients with recurrent haemoptysis (particularly in smokers).

In selected cases lung biopsy or CT guided FNAC from the pulmonary nodules will yield the diagnosis of vasculitis, idiopathic pulmonary haemosiderosis, mitotic lesion *etc.*

In idiopathic pulmonary haemosiderosis (a rare disorder), lung function test will show increased CO diffusing capacity and sputum examination may show increased number of haemosiderin laden macrophages.

MANAGEMENT OF MASSIVE HAEMOPTYSIS:

It is a life threatening condition and the patient must be managed in ITU. Brief outline of management is given below:

- The patient should be placed with the bleeding side down to prevent aspiration in the contralateral lung. Airways should be protected by endotracheal intubation.
- Mild sedation may be given to allay anxiety.
- Cough suppressant may be used however aggressive cough suppressant should be avoided.
- Coagulation abnormalities should be corrected.
- Early bronchoscopic evaluation will be needed to locate the bleeding site and find out the cause. Saline lavage during bronchoscopy may be helpful.
- Unilateral lung ventilation- The non bleeding lung may be selectively ventilated. Collapse of the non-ventilating lung is a complication.
- Ventilation with double lumen endotracheal tube, if available may be tried.
- Since majority of life threatening bleeding is from the bronchial artery circulation, bronchial artery embolization may be used in recalcitrant cases.
- Often non surgical interventions like laser coagulation; electro-coagulation *etc*. may be tried depending upon the availability.
- Surgical intervention- surgical intervention in the form of segmental or lobar resections is indicated in massive haemoptysis or recurrent haemoptysis in following circumstances- localized bronchiectasis, aspergilloma, resectable carcinoma.

CASE: *A 29 yrs old woman attended the clinic with history of recurrent haemoptysis for last 8 months. She was seen in the periphery and was commenced on antitubercular therapy on the basis of a cavitating lesion in the right lung field without any clinical improvement. She had a past history of childhood pulmonary tuberculosis however. Examination did not reveal anything specific. Sputum for AFB on three occasions was negative. Sputum for fungal stain was positive and fungal culture grew Aspergillus group of organism. X-ray chest showed evidence of cavitations with a ball along with a radiolucent crescentic shadow over the ball, a classical feature of Aspergilloma. In view of recurrent massive haemoptysis, she was treated with lobectomy followed by a course of itraconazole. (Fluconazole is not effective against Aspergillosis). Biopsy specimen confirmed presence of Aspergillosis. At present she is symptom free.*

DIAGNOSIS: Haemoptysis due to Aspergilloma in a tubercular cavity.

CASE: *A 62 years old gentleman was admitted with history of haemoptysis of one day duration. He was recently seen in the clinic with a big unresolving pneumonia of the left side of the lung over last 2 weeks. In view of delayed resolution of the pneumonia, he underwent bronchoscopy and CT guided FNAC, which failed to show any mitotic lesion. There was evidence of inflammatory necrosis. In the ITU he was treated with piperacillin-tazobactam and vancomycin, needed urgent endotracheal intubation for massive haemoptysis and underwent repeat bronchoscopic evaluation which located the site of bleeding but failed to show any endobronchial lesion. He also received 4 units of blood transfusion. Fortunately over next few days, his condition stabilized and the X-ray chest started to show improvement. He was finally extubated and a sputum culture grew Klebsiella pneumonia. One month following discharge, his X-ray chest showed almost complete resolution of the lung lesion.*

DIAGNOSIS: Severe haemoptysis due to necrotising pneumonia due to *Klebsiella* infection.

CASE: *A 31 years old gentleman was transferred from another medical facility where he was initially admitted with severe thrombophlebitis and cellulitis of the right hand. While in the hospital, he continued to have high fever, developed breathlessness and a couple of episodes of haemoptysis. He was hypoxic with a* PaO_2/FiO_2 *ratio of* < 300. *X-ray chest showed bilateral cavitating and nodular shadow. The reason of transfer was further management of the acute lung injury following septicaemia. On examination, he was very toxic, breathless and hypoxic. The right hand was marked swollen and tender to touch. His pulse rate was 140/min, BP- 100/70 mmHg. CT scan of the thorax showed bilateral nodular cavitating lesions on both sides of the lungs. The WBC count was 23,000. Blood culture did not grow any organism.*

DIAGNOSIS: Metastatic multiple septic pulmonary emboli following thrombophlebitis of right upper extremity.

DISCUSSIONS:

He was treated with meropenem, teicoplanin and supportive care for acute lung injury. He also underwent surgical debridement of the cellulitis of his right hand. After a turbulent course of three weeks in hospital, he went home without any residual problem. Repeat CT scan following discharge showed almost complete resolution of the cavitating lesion.

Septic pulmonary embolism is a complication of severe thrombophlebitis and should be suspected in any patient with thrombophlebitis developing characteristic. X-ray lesion with cavitation and necrosis along with high fever, breathlessness, haemoptysis and features of acute lung injury.

Lemierre's disease is one such condition that occurs following infection in the tonsillar and peritonsillar region with invasion of infection to the jugular vein which is complicated with distant spread of infection including septic pulmonary emboli. Although, it is rare now-a-days, any patient with unresolving sore throat with evidence of increasing toxicity and spreading septicaemia and characteristic X-ray findings, Lemierre's disease should be strongly suspected.

: KEY POINTS :

- Haemoptysis is a common presentation in clinical practice.
- Massive haemoptysis is a life threatening condition.
- Infection, bronchiectasis, vasculitis and malignancy are the common differential diagnosis.

FURTHER REFERENCES:

- Case records- A 32 yrs old man with haemoptysis of nearly 3 decades duration. E.G. Silverman *et al., NEJM* Vol. 347, N - 21, Nov 21, 2002, 1693-1702.
- Case records- An eight year old girl with fever haemoptysis and pulmonary consolidation. BPO. Sullivan *et al., NEJM* -Vol. 347, Sept. 26, 2002, N-13, 1009-1018.
- Case records- A 51 yrs old woman with recurrent haemoptysis - J.S. Daly *et al. NEJM* – Vol. 346, Nov. 9, 2002, IN 19, 1475 - 1483.

87 A PATIENT ON MECHANICAL VENTILATION

CASE: *A 68 years old patient with COPD was admitted with the evidence of chest infection and drowsiness. He was clinically cyanosed with the evidence of widespread crepitations and rhonchi in the lung fields. He was tachycardic with a rate of 136/m with a bounding pulse and a BP of 130/68 mmHg. Investigations revealed PaO_2- 51 mmHg, $PaCO_2$- 62 mmHg, HCO_3- 36, pH- 7.3, WBC- 19,000, with slightly raised urea and creatinine level. ECG showed sinus tachycardia and X-ray chest showed emphysematous chest with right lower lobe infection. He was treated with antibiotics, chest physiotherapy and adjuvant therapy. However, he became drowsier and a repeat blood gas analysis showed PaO_2- 48 mmHg, $PaCO_2$- 71 mmHg, and pH-7.21. In view of profound acidosis, it was deemed that noninvasive ventilation would not be helpful and it was decided to intubate him and put him on mechanical ventilation. After 48 hours of mechanical ventilation, his condition became stabilized and he was successfully weaned off from mechanical ventilation.*

DIAGNOSIS: Acute respiratory failure needing mechanical ventilation.

DISCUSSION:

Mechanical ventilation is needed in critical care practice in the following clinical conditions:

- Hypoxaemic respiratory failure.
- Hypercapnoeic respiratory failure.
- Neuromuscular respiratory failure.
- Post surgical for requirement of therapeutic muscle paralysis.

Positive pressure mechanical ventilation is provided in following modes:

1. **Volume Controlled Mechanical Ventilation:** Pre-sets are respiratory rate, tidal volume or inspiratory pressure, inspiratory flow rate. Volume controlled mode is not the patient triggered mode and it does not encourage patient's normal breathing effort. So sedation is needed. It is of two types-
    a. Volume cycled- Here inspiration normally ends when a pre-set tidal (inspiratory) volume is delivered. It may cause barotrauma.
    b. Pressure cycled- Inspiration normally ends when preset inspiratory pressure is reached. This may cause delivery of low tidal volume and auto PEEP because of air trapping due to diminished expiratory volume.

2. **Assist Controlled Ventilation:** Respiratory rate and tidal volume are preset. Although time triggered, the patient can trigger additional breath above the pre-fixed rate with delivery of pre-fixed tidal volume. This is the most common form of ventilation in ITU.

3. **Synchronized Intermittent Mandatory Ventilation (SIMV):** In this mode there is mandatory pre-fixed respiratory rate and tidal volume. Mandatory breaths are time triggered but can synchronize with patients breathing effort near the trigger interval to deliver the pre-fixed tidal volume. In addition, in between the mandatory breaths, spontaneous breaths are allowed without any positive pressure ventilatory assistance. This is commonly used mode for weaning.

4. **Pressure Support:** The patient takes spontaneous breath and the tidal volume depends upon the preset inspiratory pressure. There is back up respiratory rate or tidal volume. (Some machine gives backup support in the event of apnea).

HOW TO PROCEED:

The ventilatory mode is to be selected first → then tidal volume is to be selected (ideally 5-12 ml/kg) → then respiratory rate is to be selected to achieve minute ventilation of 8-14 ml/kg → then inspiratory flow rate needs to be selected to adjust the inspiratory-expiratory ratio (typically 40-60 ml/m). In some ventilator I:E ratio is adjusted independently. Then FiO_2 needs to be selected. Finally PEEP needs to be selected.

[Ventilatory mode → Tidal volume → Respiratory rate → Inspiratory flow rate → FiO_2 → PEEP]

Selection of trigger mechanism:

- Pressure trigger- Patient generates negative airway pressure below a preset threshold (typically between 0.05 and 3 cm of H_2O) to initiate mechanical breath.
- Flow trigger- Constant gas flow is maintained across the ventilatory circuit, inspiratory effort causes differential flow between inspiratory and expiratory limbs of the circuit which triggers a mechanical breath.
  Incorrect setting of trigger modes will cause patient-ventilator dyssynchrony.

OBSERVATIONS TO BE MADE:

- Peak inspiratory pressure.
- Plateau pressure.

- Blood gas analysis at 15 minutes and 1 hour following commencement of ventilation and readjust the ventilatory settings and FiO_2 according to PaO_2 and $PaCO_2$ values.
- Hemodynamic status needs to be monitored.

VENTILATOR ALARM SYSTEM: THIS INCLUDES:

- Threshold minimum and maximum values of respiratory rate.
- Airway Pressure.
- I : E and exhaled tidal volume.

In volume controlled mode 'peak pressure' alarm will identify the risk for barotrauma.

In pressure controlled mode alarms for 'minimum and maximum tidal volume' will alert the clinician for inadequate ventilation.

Apnoea alarm will indicate 'ventilator disconnection or leak' of patient triggering.

MONITORING OF PATIENT-VENTILATOR INTERACTION:

- Peak airway pressure- reflects both lung compliance and airway resistance. High peak airway pressure will indicate-
    a. tube blockage
    b. bronchospasm
    c. pneumothorax
    d. secretion
- Plateau pressure, on the other hand is a static airway pressure obtained during end-expiratory hold up maneuver, allowing equilibration of pressure within the airway.

Elevated peak airway pressure + normal plateau pressure is due to increased airway resistance like tube blockage, secretions, bronchospasm but due to normal lung compliance.

Elevated peak pressure + elevated plateau pressure is due to decreased lung compliance as in ARDS.

During ventilation, the goal should be to keep the plateau pressure below 35 cm H_2O without much difference with the peak airway pressure.

Management of plateau pressure:

1. Manually occluding the exhalation port at end inspiration and observing plateau pressure from the airway pressure reading.
2. In assist control mode- Setting up of inspiratory pause of (0.5-1 s) and observing the inspiratory pressure at the end of the pause.

Application of PEEP:

Positive end expiratory pressure refers to pressure in the airway at the end of expiration that exceeds atmospheric pressure. The term is applicable for the patients for receiving mechanical ventilation. For spontaneously breathing patients, the term CPAP is used when inspiratory and expiratory circuits are pressurized about atmospheric level.

What does it do?

- It improves oxygenation by recruiting lung units improving lung compliance and preventing alveolar collapse.
- It reduces ventilator associated lung injury.

What are the problems of PEEP?

- It can cause fall of cardiac output and BP.
- It can cause barotrauma.

When to use PEEP?

- ARDS.
- Cardiogenic pulmonary oedema.
- Diffuse pneumonia requiring mechanical ventilation.

Where not to use PEEP?

- Pneumothorax.
- Broncho-pleural fistula.
- Haemodynamic compromise with low cardiac output state (unless concomitantly treated).

Ideally the PEEP should be started at 5 cm of H_2O and gradually titrated upwards. Alternatively PEEP is set at 2 cm H_2O above the lower inflection point of the inspiratory pressure-volume curve.

Complications of mechanical ventilation:

- Infection- ventilator associated pneumonia.
- Ventilator induced lung injury.
- Barotrauma.
- Haemodynamic instability.
- Patient-ventilation dyssynchrony.

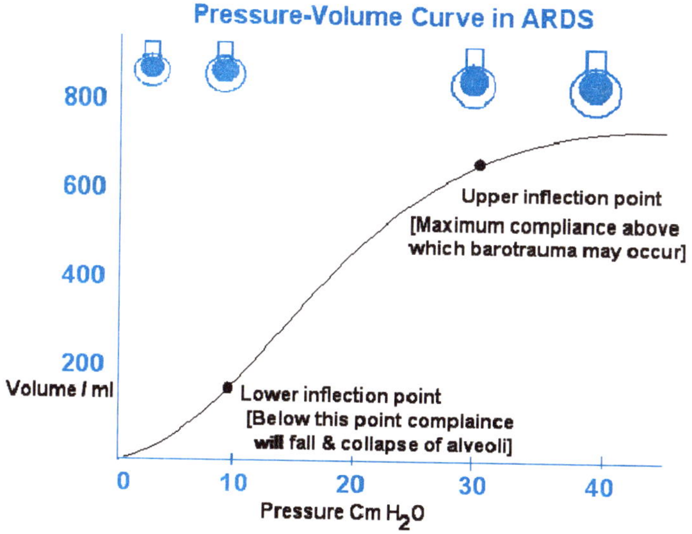

To select PEEP just above lower inflection point and maximum plateau pressure below upper inflection point.

Weaning from mechanical ventilation:

Before attempting to wean from mechanical ventilation, following criteria should be satisfied-

- Resolution of the primary condition
- The patient must be alert and not on any sedative
- Haemodynamically stable
- PaO_2 / FiO_2 should be > 200 on PEEP of < 5 cm.
- Acceptable $PaCO_2$.
- Good nutritional status
- Electrolytes, haemoglobin, albumin, CPK, TSH should be reasonably satisfactory.

After the above mentioned criteria are met, the ventilatory parameters should be checked e.g. respiratory rate should be less than 30/ minute. Tidal volume generated by the patient should be more than 5 ml/Kg.

Rapid shallow breathing index- It is calculated as frequency divided by tidal volume is the single best method of assessment regarding suitability of weaning. If the value is less than 105, it usually predicts weaning success. Other methods like measurement of vital capacity, minute ventilation, maximum inspiratory pressure, airway occlusion pressure may be helpful to indicate successful weaning.

What are the different methods of weaning?

Spontaneous breathing trial via T-piece → if tolerated for 30 minutes to 2 hours, extubation can be done.

SIMV mode of ventilation- gradual reduction of respiratory rate of SIMV. If the patient tolerates at a rate of 6-8/ minute, extubation can be done. This method may be continued with using pressure support.

Pressure support- pressure support is applied at 15 cm of H_2O and slowly reduced to 5-6 cm H_2O. If tolerated well, the patient can be extubated.

During weaning trial respiratory adjuvant therapy should be continued. In spite of best efforts the reintubation rate following a successful weaning is approximately 20%.

To identify patients who can be considered for a trial of spontaneous breathing:

Respiratory criteria:

- $PaO_2 > 60$ mm Hg on FiO_2 of 40-50% and PEEP < 5-8 cm of H_2O.
- $PaCO_2$ normal or baseline

Cardiovascular:

- Heart rate < 140 bpm.
- BP maintained with minimum vasopressor.

Others:

- The patient is arousable
- Afebrile
- No significant electrolyte abnormalities

	Net range in adults	Threshold for successful SBT
Tidal volume	5-7 ml/kg	4-6 ml/kg
Respiratory rate	10-18/min	30-38/min
Tidal volume	5-6 litre/min	10-15 litre/min
RR/V_T ratio	40-50/litre	60-105/litre
Maximum inspiratory pressure	90-120 cm H_2O	15 -30 cm H_2O

Rapid shallow breathing index:

This is provided by the ratio of respiratory rate to tidal volume (RR/V_T) which is also known as a rapid-shallow breathing index. This is normally 40-50/*l* and is often above 100/*l* who do not tolerate spontaneous breathing trial.

Failure of spontaneous breathing trial:

This indicates that the patient needs ventilatory support for some more time.

- **Causes:**

➢ Low cardiac output state

➢ Myocardial ischemia

➢ Over feeding – leading to increased CO_2 production

➢ Respiratory muscle weakness (critical illness polyneuropathy and myopathy)

➢ Repletion of magnesium, phosphorous and hypokalaemia

After successfully weaning the next step would be tracheal de-cannulation (removal of tracheal tube).

- **Issues:**

➢ Protection of the airways from secretion– to check gag reflex.

➢ Laryngeal oedema– particularly in patients with prolonged intubation

Cuff leak test:

This test is designed to identify patients with severe laryngeal oedema. This test is performed while the patient is on volume cycle ventilation and it involves measurement of the volume of gas exhaled through the endotracheal tube before and after deflating the cuff. A decrease in exhalation volume after cuff deflation is used as evidence against the pressure of significant distension at the level of larynx.

Post extubation:

- Steroid for laryngeal oedema
- Aerosolized epinephrine (2.5 ml of 1 % epinephrine) mainly in children
- Chest physiotherapy
- BiPAP

Other newer methods of ventilation:

- High frequency positive pressure ventilation.
- High frequency jet ventilation.
- High frequency oscillation.
- Inverse ratio ventilation instead of 1:1 ratio of 1:2 → to as high as 4% → increases mean alveolar pressure without increasing peak airway pressure → to improve PO_2 which causes auto PEEP due to less expiration → can cause barotrauma in volume control mode.
- Liquid ventilation.
- Proportional assist ventilation.
- Airway pressure release ventilation.

Role of tracheostomy:

It is followed in case of prolonged ventilation for more than two weeks. Nowadays tracheostomy is done early if it is deemed that the projected ventilatory period would be prolonged. It is a useful method to expedite weaning by reducing the dead space. Presently percutaneous tracheostomy is the method of choice.

Use of non-invasive ventilator in clinical practice:

NIPPV is a recent therapeutic tool in our armamentarium over last one decade that has made for management of ventilatory failure in certain group of patients greatly reducing the rate of intubation and ventilation.

In non-invasive positive pressure ventilation (NIPPV), the higher inspiratory pressure that is set is called inspiratory positive pressure (IPAP) which is kept approximately at a level of 12-16 cm H_2O and lower pressure that is set, is termed as expiratory positive pressure (EPAP) which is typically set in between 4-8 cm H_2O. This is in contrast to continuous positive pressure (CPAP) ventilation where a continuous pressure is maintained throughout the inspiration and expiration as in type-I respiratory failure, NIPPV is mainly used for decompensated type-II respiratory failure.

What are the indications?

- Acute exacerbation of COPD.
- Cardiogenic pulmonary oedema.
- Obesity-hypoventilation Syndrome.
- Acute severe asthma.
- Acute pneumonia.
- Respiratory failure in myasthenia and GB syndrome.

The main use of NIPPV is in acute exacerbation of COPD which are associated with acidosis and hypercapnia. It has been shown that it works best at a pH between 7.25 and 7.30 and it reduces intubation rate to less than 50% in such situation. In lower pH values it may be associated with failure. In appropriate situations, it can even be safely used in general wards. In case of cardiogenic pulmonary oedema, NIPPV has been shown to reduce intubation rate and reduced mortality. The number needed to treat (NNT) was 4 to avoid one intubation. However, due to unstable nature of the condition, the treatment needs to be closely supervised in ITU.

Contraindications:

1. Should be avoided in patients with increased retained secretion.
2. Facial trauma.
3. Vomiting.
4. Impaired consciousness.

Complications:

1. Ulceration over the bridge of nose.
2. Claustrophobia.
3. Excessive air leakage.
4. Gastric insufflations.

NIPPV is carried out with a well-fitted nasal or facial mask under close supervision. However, it is not a panacea for respiratory failure. To use successfully it should be used early and continuous assessment needs to be done to see whether 'stepping up' of treatment is needed with intubation and invasive ventilation.

Extracorporeal life support (ECLS) for respiratory failure:

ECLS technique like ECMO (Extra-corporeal membrane oxygenation) ECCOR or $ECCO_2R$ (extracorporeal CO_2 removal) are frequently used in patient with respiratory failure with persistent hypoxemia or high CO_2 level. These techniques may become more popular in treatment of patients with ARDS.

FURTHER REFERENCES:

- Janes A. Kruse *et al.* - Saunders manual of critical care.
- Conventional Mechanical ventilation- 2003.
- Newer Modes of Mechanical ventilation – PEEP
- Discontinuing Mechanical ventilation. P-808-822.
- Chakroborty B *et al.*: Management of acute ventilatory failure.
- Postgraduate Medical Journal- 2006: 82: 438-445
- Harrison's Principle of Internal Medicine- 17th edition
- Oxford Book of Medicine- 5th edition.

88

A PATIENT WITH ALOPECIA

CASE: *A 47 years old lady presented in the clinic with a history of increasing hair fall leading to thinning of the hair line. She was very depressed and wanted some remedy for it. A battery of tests including thyroid function test, liver function test, full blood count and renal function test were requested. Apart from total hypothyroidism, other tests were within normal limits. She was reassured and in addition to prescribing vitamin E, thyroxin, she was advised to apply 2% minoxidil lotion over the scalp for a prolonged period.*

DIAGNOSIS: Female pattern hair loss.

DISCUSSION:

Hair loss disorders are common presentations in the clinical practice which is a cause of worry and anxiety and frequently the patient consults their primary care physicians rather than dermatologists initially for advice.

HOW TO APPROACH:

A thorough examination to rule out any endocrinological problem, hormonal dysfunction, a thorough drug history, and investigation routine and special blood tests should be carried out to find out the exact cause. Before discussing the cause, it is pertinent to discuss about the 'hair cycle' which consists of three phases-

1) Anagen – The acute growth phase.
2) Catagen – a short transition phase lasting for about two weeks.
3) Telogen – a resting phase lasting for approximately 3 months awaiting due to shed and replaced by new hair growth.

CAUSES:

1. TELOGEN EFFLUVIUM (telogen phase means the resting phase of hair follicle)

Common trigger:

- Child birth
- Psychological stress
- Acute febrile illness
- Malnutrition : Iron deficiency, Vitamin D deficiency
- Drugs: oral retinoids, β blockers, antidepressants, anticoagulants, OCP.
- Chronic diseases: thyroid disorders, chronic kidney diseases, liver disorders, connective disorders, malignancy.

TREATMENTS: Underlying causes should be treated. Application of 2 % minoxidil lotion over the scalp may be helpful.

2. ANAGEN EFFLUVIUM (pathologic loss of anagen or growth-phase hairs)

This is more widespread with universal hair loss. It is mainly caused by chemotherapeutic agents.

TREATMENTS: It is treated by psychological support and use of wig. 2 % minoxidil lotion application over the scalp may fasten recovery.

3. ALOPECIA AREATA: It may be –

- Diffuse alopecia areata.
- Alopecia totalis – with complete loss of scalp hair.
- Alopecia universalis - associated loss of body hair.

Nail dystrophy is present in 10% of cases. It is associated with other autoimmune diseases.

TREATMENTS:

- Local application of potent steroid.
- Intralesional injection of steroid.
- Contact immunotherapy with diphencyprone for large area of hair loss.
- Doubtful value- oral steroids, minoxidil and psoralens with ultraviolet A.

4. FEMALE PATTERN HAIRLOSS:

It is characterised by diffuse thinning of frontal and mid areas of scalp as opposed to recession of frontal hair line. It is treated with twice daily application of 2% minoxidil lotion or once daily application of 5 % minoxidil lotion application.

5. INFECTIVE CAUSES OF ALOPECIA:

- ***Tinea capitis:***

  Oral terbinafine is more efficacious than oral griseofulvin in its treatment.

- ***Alopecia syphilitica:***

  It may be a presentation of secondary syphilis.

❖ *Cicatricial alopecia:*

This condition is caused due to scarring of the scalp *e.g.*

- **Primary**: By *Lichen planopilaris.*

It is treated by:

1) Topical steroid
2) Intralesional steroid

- **Secondary:** By *Chronic cutaneous lupus erythematosus.*

It is treated with:

1) Topical steroid
2) Intralesional steroid
3) Topical tacrolimus
4) Antimalarials
5) Thalidomide
6) Oral retinoids. *e.g.* acitretin

❖ Folliculitis decalvans:

May presents as local hair loss of the scalp. Local culture frequently grows *Staphylococcus aureus*. It is treated with 10 weeks course of rifampicin 300 mg twice daily and clindamycin 300 mg thrice daily in combination.

GENERAL MANAGEMENT:

Approximate investigations should be carried out and iron deficiency, vitamin deficiency or hypothyroidism, if found, should be treated accordingly.

Finally, when no remedial causes are identified, wigs and hair transplantation should be considered. Hair transplantation should be considered when sufficient occipital scalp hair is present and other methods of treatment are failing.

FURTHER REFERENCES:

- Harrison's Principle of Internal Medicine- 17th edition.
- Oxford Text Book of Medicine- 5th edition.
- Dr. A. Macbeth- Hair loss in Hospital Medicine: A practical guide- JHM July 2012, vol 73, No 7: p-372-379.

89 A CANCER PATIENT WITH INTRACTABLE ABDOMINAL PAIN

CASE: *A 72 years old male patient with severe abdominal pain which was found to be due to pancreatic cancer which was thought to be inoperable and a decision of palliative care was taken. His pain remained intractable in spite of conventional analgesics and morphine patch. He was referred to a pain specialist who finally performed coeliac plexus block with relief of the symptoms.*

DIAGNOSIS: Cancer related pain needing regional blockade.

DISCUSSION:

Pain is one of the most common presenting symptoms in clinical practice and an adequate relief of pain is a basic pre-requisite that is expected from a clinician. The century old adage of Dr. William Osler 'We can cure little, alleviate some and solace every one', still holds true even in the modern day clinical practice.

Different varieties of pain:

- Acute pain
- Chronic pain
- Neuropathic pain
- Pain of psychogenic origin

Pain management is a basic fundamental human right. As per as the WHO guideline comprises of **Three Step Analgesic Ladder** starts with non-opioid analgesic, the second step comprises of usage of weak acting opioid analgesics and finally 'strong opioids' comprises the last step of the ladder. While using analgesics, the right dose at the right interval should be used.

NON-OPIOD ANALGESICS	WEAK OPIOIDS ANALGESICS	STRONG OPIOIDS ANALGESICS
Paracetamol Aspirin NSAIDS	Codeine Tramadol Oxycodone	Morphine

Since perception of pain may vary and a similar situation can both enhance or reduce the magnitude of the pain sensation by way of activation of pain modulating circuit through secretion of endogenous opioids such as encephalins and β-endorphins which work through μ receptors. In these regards the pain modulator drugs are helpful particularly in chronic pain.

Pain modulators are helpful in:

- Fibromyalgia
- Tension headache
- Post herpetic neuralgia
- Diabetic neuropathy
- Cancer

PAIN MODULATORS (Antidepressants)	ANTICONVULSANTS AND OTHER DRUGS IN NEUROPATHIC PAIN
➢ Doxepin	➢ Gabapentin
➢ Amitriptyline	➢ Pregabalin
➢ Duloxetine	➢ Phenytoin
	➢ Carbamazepine

Sometimes combination of different group of medication may be needed. In cancer pain adequate dose of morphine should be used to get an adequate effect.

Other drugs that may be helpful:

- **Muscle relaxants**
  - Diazepam
  - Chlorzoxazone
  - Methocarbamol
  - Baclofen
- **Steroids**
  - Oral steroids
  - Local injection of steroid at the trigger point or nerve root

(Oral steroids may be helpful by reducing swelling in cases of cervical root pain. However, specialist's opinion needs to be taken in this regard.)

Interventional therapy in the management of pain: Interventional procedures are getting increasingly popular in the management of main persistent pain syndrome.

Lumbar pain:

- Epidural injection of steroid.

- Facet block with local anaesthetics and steroids.
- Pulsed radiofrequency at the dorsal root ganglion.
- Trigger point injection
- Botox injection in myofascial pain

Other nerve block procedures:

- Trigeminal nerve block
- Glossopharyngeal nerve block
- Cervical nerve block
- Celiac block as in pancreatic cancer pain
- Hypogastric nerve block as in pelvic tumour related pain
- Sphenopalatine ganglion blockade in intractable facial pain

Other advanced techniques in pain management:

- Spinal cord stimulation
- Intradiscal radiofrequency
- Ozone discectomy
- Kyphoplasty / vertebroplasty- as an alternative to surgery with adequate pain relief.

Since many of the facilities are now available and with the emergence of 'pain' as a speciality with many postgraduate training programmes with certificate course have been introduced with availability of expert pain specialists, their help is frequently needed in clinical practice to offer a total pain management for the patients suffering from intractable pain.

Pain and sedation in critical care units:

Frequently the patients in ICUs suffer from pain and sleep related problem particularly in patients who are undergoing mechanical ventilation or other invasive interventions in the unit. Opioids like fentanyl, morphine and hydromorphone remains the drug of choice for management of pain in ICUs. Remifentanil, in view of its rapid onset of action is getting increasingly popular. Ketamine although not popularly used in ICU, has shown to reduce post operative pain score.

The ideal goal of use of analgesia and sedation is not only symptomatic relief but also to prevent delirium in ICU and prevention of long term PTSD (Post traumatic stress disorder). To achieve these goals now-a-days use of analgo-sedatives rather than pure sedative based regimes are preferred.

Comparative study between benzodiazepine with propofol, remifentanil and dexmedetomidine has shown the superiority of the last 3 drugs over benzodiazepine as sedatives in ICU.

SEDATION IN ICUs
➢ Midazolam infusion
➢ Propofol infusion
➢ Dexmedetomidine infusion

Sedation scale in ICU:

- Patients anxious and agitated
- Patients cooperative, oriented and tranquil
- Patient responds to combat only
- Patient is asleep with brisk response to glabellar tap.
- Patient is asleep with sluggish response to glabellar tap.
- Patient is asleep and no response to glabellar taps.

General recommendations:

- To use light sedative
- To use analgesic first than sedative.
- To prefer non-benzodiazepine based regime e.g. propofol or dexmedetomidine
- Haloperidol has not shown to reduce the incidence of delirium. However atypical anti-psychotics may do so.

FURTHER REFERENCES:

- Harrison's Principle of Internal Medicine 17th edition
- Oxford Text book of medicine- 5th edition.
- Editor E. Welesly, selected articles from respiratory and critical care medicine, Vol-34: 2, April 2013 ISSN 1069-3424.
- World pain symposium Kolkata 2013. Conference Book.

90 A PATIENT WITH MOOD SWINGS

CASE: *A 32 years old male patient was brought by his relatives in the outpatient clinic for abnormal behavioural problem which was hampering his daily activities. Episodically he was excited with loss of sleep and lavish expenditure and having skirmishes with his colleagues and his boss while on often occasions he was withdrawn from the family, not communicating with any one with loss of appetite and sleep disturbances. His wife was unable to cope with this mood swings and the family members thought that they should first discuss with an internist before seeking advice from a psychiatrist.*

DIAGNOSIS: Bipolar disorder.

DISCUSSION:

Bipolar disorder is a medical condition associated with recurrent mania (bipolar I disorder) or hypomania (bipolar II disorder) which are characterised by elevated mood along with functional disability and one or more episodes of depressive spell with symptoms similar to that of major unipolar depressive disorder.

This disorder is frequently associated with history of substance abuse, premature death and increased risk of suicide. Moreover significant working days are lost compounding the problem further.

Bipolar disorders are occasionally encountered in clinical practice by the physician and before psychiatric consultation, the relatives frequently request their primary care doctors to deal with such problem.

HOW TO TREAT:

➢ **Atypical antipsychotics**

- Quetiapine monotherapy, with a dose going upto 600 mg has been found to be helpful in this condition particularly in manic and hypomanic phase.
- Olanzapine, alone or in combination of fluoxetine, has also been found to be effective in this condition with combination being more effective than monotherapy. Weight gain, tardive dyskinesia and increased incidence of diabetes are the usual side effects.

The anti-depressant effect of quetiapine or olanzapine and fluoxetine combination is not a class effect as similar beneficial effects have not been observed by other atypical antipsychotics like aripiprazole or ziprasidone (both are approved for the treatment of manic episode) in reducing the episode of depressive spells.

➢ Antiepileptics

- Lamotrigine (dose 50 to 200 mg) has been found to be effective in bipolar disorder with significant improvement of depressive symptoms.
- Sodium valproate monotherapy has also been shown to be effective in bipolar disorders.

➢ Antidepressants

This is a controversial area as there is always a risk of precipitation of mania with antidepressants if used as monotherapy without co-administration of mood stabilizers. However, use of antidepressants like paroxetine or fluoxetine may be considered in the depressive phase along with a mood stabilizer. Specialist psychiatric opinion needs to be taken in this regard.

➢ Other drugs:

- Lithium has been traditionally used for this condition for long. However one needs to aware of side effect profile like renal impairment, tremor, hypercalcaemia, *etc.*
- For associated sleep - wakeful related problems modafinil may be tried. Pramipexole, an antiparkinsonian drug has also been shown to be helpful for the treatment of depression in bipolar disorders.
- Patients with bipolar disorders should also be assessed for suicidal risk and psychiatric input is essential in this regard.

: KEY POINTS :

- ☞ Bipolar disorders are occasionally encountered in clinical practice.
- ☞ They are frequently associated with substance abuse & increased suicidal risks.
- ☞ Atypical antipsychotics with or without SSRIs are the usual method of treatment.
- ☞ Psychiatric input is frequently needed.

FURTHER REFERENCES:

- Harrison's Principle of Internal Medicine 17th edition.
- Oxford Text Book of Medicine- 5th edition.
- M.A. Frye, Bipolar disorder. NEJM 2011: 364: 51-59.

91 A PATIENT WITH HYPERCALCAEMIA

CASE: *An 83 years old lady (my mother) was admitted with history of joint pain, generalized body ache and mild confusional state. Investigations revealed normal full blood count, CRP was normal, Uric acid 6.1 mg% (borderline high), negative rheumatoid factor and ANF, normal creatinine and LFT. Her calcium was found to be 12.8 mg% (normal is < 10 mg% in that laboratory), normal sodium, potassium and high chloride. Her vitamin* D_3 *level was normal; Ig electrophoresis for M-band was negative, Parathyroid hormone 265 μg/dl (normal < 60 in that laboratory). X-ray lumbosacral spine- osteoporotic bones, ultrasound examination of abdomen, X-ray chest, breast screening and other tumour markers like CA-125, CA-19.9, CEA and α-fetoprotein were all normal. CT scan of neck showed enlarged diffuse parathyroid glands.*

DIAGNOSIS: Hypercalcaemia due to primary hyperparathyroidism.

DISCUSSION:

Although hypercalcaemia is not a common problem in clinical practice, occasionally it is accidentally detected while screening for bone and joint pain, screening for dementia and acute care while dealing with acute confusional state.

While dealing with calcium metabolism, it needs to be realised that 50% of calcium is in ionised form and the rest is protein bound (mainly albumin or immunoglobulin). Therefore while dealing with serum calcium level, serum albumin level should also be measured and the corrected calcium level should be adjusted accordingly.

Since the ionised calcium level needs to be maintained within a narrow range in the body, a homeostatic mechanism exists in the body involving the parathyroid hormone and vitamin D levels and the kidneys, intestinal tract and the skeletal system takes an active part in maintaining the homeostasis. PTH usually maintains the serum calcium level by mobilizing it from the skeletal system and increasing calcium absorption from the renal tubules while vitamin D acts mainly through increasing the absorption of calcium from the intestine.

CAUSES OF HYPERCALCAEMIA:

- With high parathyroid hormone level:
  - Primary hyperparathyroidism
    (adenoma, carcinoma or hyperplasia)
  - Ectopic parathormone secretion by tumour

- With low or normal parathyroid levels:
  - Malignancy with skeletal metastasis
  - Multiple myeloma
  - Hypervitaminosis D
  - Granulomatous disease like sarcoidosis
  - Osteoporosis with prolonged immobilization
  - Paget's disease
  - Addison's disease
  - Thyrotoxicosis

DRUGS:

- Lithium
- Thiazide
- Vitamin A intoxication

SYMPTOMS:

Hypercalcaemia (> 12.5 mg%) is a medical emergency and the patients frequently present with comatose state. Mild hypercalcaemia usually does not cause any symptoms except for anorexia, constipation, nausea, depression etc. QT interval may be shortened.

CASE: *An 81 years old patient presented with comatose state which developed over a period of few days, initially starting with obtundation, confusion and apathy. He looked dehydrated. Hyponatraemia was suspected. However, his Na^+ level was normal. His creatinine was 3.2 mg%, urea 168 mg% and calcium was 13.8 mg%, Hb 8.4 g%, alkaline phosphatase was 484 mg% (high), albumin was 2.5 g%, bilirubin was normal. His corrected albumin level was calculated to be even higher. With active resuscitation his calcium level came down to 9.6 mg% over next few days. His X-ray showed evidence of an SOL which later on proved to be due to small cell carcinoma of lung and bone scan showed multiple hotspots all over the skeleton which is consistent with disseminated bony metastasis.*

DIAGNOSIS: metastatic bone disease causing severe hypercalcaemia.

MANAGEMENT:

- Vigorous hydration with normal saline along with frusemide.
- Zoledronic acid (4 mg) or pamidronate (60-90 mg) as a single infusion.
- Steroids are helpful in multiple myeloma or 1,25-dihydroxyvitamin D_3 mediated hypercalcaemia like sarcoidosis or hypervitaminosis-D but not in hyperparathyroidism.
- Dialysis using low calcium dialysate is the final option.
- Calcitonin, mithramycin or gallium nitrate used in the past, are rarely used now a days.

DISCUSSION ON HYPERPARATHYROIDISM:

CAUSES:

<table>
<tr><td>A) Primary</td><td>➢ Hyperplasia, adenoma, carcinoma
➢ Associated with multiple endocrine neoplasia
- MEN I
• Gastrinoma
• Pituitary adenoma
- MEN II
• Medullary carcinoma of thyroid
• Pheochromocytoma</td></tr>
<tr><td>B) Secondary</td><td>➢ Due to persistent hypocalcemia as in vitamin D deficiency or chronic renal failure.</td></tr>
<tr><td>C) Tertiary</td><td>➢ As in secondary where the gland becomes autonomous.</td></tr>
</table>

MANIFESTATIONS:

Anorexia, depression, bone pain, and renal stones classically described as ***moans, pains and groans*** are the classical presentation. However finding of high calcium in routine examination is the commonest way of diagnosing hyperparathyroidism.

INVESTIGATIONS:

- High Ca^{++}, low phosphate, low HCO_3 and high chloride (hyperchloremic acidosis).
- Osteoporosis of bones, subperiosteal resorption of phalanges.
- High PTH hormone level in the face of high calcium.
- Localization of parathyroid gland with CT scan, MRI scan.
- Isotope scanning with technetium-99m sestamibi scan.
- Invasive tests with selective angiography and selective venous sampling for PTH levels.

MANAGEMENT:

Ideally, following localization of the tumours parathyroidectomy should be done. However, in elderly patients who are asymptomatic conservative management with close follow up is all that is needed. Calcium intake needs to be restricted so is the intake of vitamin-D. Raloxifene (SERM) may prevent osteoporosis but has no effect on calcium level.

Cinacalcet, a drug which reduces the secretion of PTH by increasing calcium sensitivity of the gland, may be useful in reducing calcium level, if available.

CASE: *A 13 years old girl attended the clinic with history of profound weakness, mild ptosis, brittle nails and recurrent fungal infection of her toes. She was short statured for her age. Her TSH was 14 (high), Calcium 7.2 mg% (low), phosphate was high normal, Na^+ was 124 mg%, K was 5.1 mg%, and Hb was 9.4 g%. Her BP was low and she had frequent pre-syncope. Second line investigation showed her PTH was low, cortisol was low with inadequate response to ACTH injection, vitamin B_{12} level was low normal. A collective diagnosis of hypoparathyroidism, hypothyroidism, Addison's disease and associated recurrent fungal infection was made which could collectively be fitted in the syndrome based classification of '**Polyglandular failure type-I**'. She was treated with replacement therapy for thyroid and adrenal with thyroxin and steroids respectively. She also received calcium and vitamin D supplementation and a long course of terbinafine. She is under regular follow up in the clinic.*

DIAGNOSIS: Polyglandular failure type I with hypoparathyroidism hypothyroidism and Addison's disease.

CASE: *A 48 years old patient was admitted with diagnosis of acute necrotising pancreatitis. In the ward he developed an episode of convulsion which was preceded by tingling sensation in the body. His calcium was found to be 7.1 mg%. His symptoms were successfully treated with IV calcium gluconate injection.*

DIAGNOSIS: Acute hypocalcaemia due to acute severe pancreatitis.

CASE: *A 21 years old girl presented with acute breathlessness. Asthma was excluded and a diagnosis of hyperventilation syndrome was made. In the ITU while checking her BP, she developed severe carpopedal spasm, which was found to be due to a low calcium level. She was treated with IV calcium gluconate and was made to breathe in a plastic bag.*

DIAGNOSIS: Hyperventilation syndrome causing hypocalcaemia due to respiratory alkalosis.

CAUSES OF HYPOCALCAEMIA IN CLINICAL PRACTICE:

- ❖ Hypoparathyroidism with low PTH level:
  - Primary
  - Secondary– due to thyroidectomy, radiation
  - Hypomagnesaemia
- ❖ Vitamin D deficiency with high PTH level:
  - Rickets, Osteomalacia
  - Vitamin resistant states like Fanconi's syndrome
  - Vitamin D resistant rickets

OTHER CAUSES:

- Acute pancreatitis
- Acute rhabdomyolysis
- Massive blood transfusion
- Hyperventilation

DRUGS:

- Phenytoin

- Bisphosphonates
- Calcitonin

MANIFESTATIONS OF HYPOCALCAEMIA:

Symptoms are due to neuromuscular irritability and are manifested by

- Paraesthesia
- Tetany
- Seizures
- Prolonged QT interval in ECG
- Presence of classical signs like Chvostek's sign and Trousseau's sign

MANAGEMENT:

In symptomatic patients it is treated with IV injection of 10 ml of 10% calcium gluconate which should be given slowly and can be repeated if needed. Concurrent hypomagnesaemia, if present, should also be corrected, simultaneously.

DISCUSSION ON HYPOPARATHYROIDISM:

- It can be idiopathic- Presenting with short stature, skeletal abnormalities like short metacarpal bones and basal ganglion calcification.
- Secondary- Due to thyroidectomy and parathyroidectomy, radiation and hypomagnesaemia.
- Due to ineffective PTH action- As in pseudohypoparathyroidism where the clinical features will be that of hypoparathyroidism but with a high serum PTH level.
- In another variety called pseudo pseudohypoparathyroidism inherited as an autosomal dominant trait, presents with clinical features of hypoparathyroidism with a normal PTH level. There are different varieties of disorders which are outside the scope of discussion in this book.

Other inherited conditions associated with hypoparathyroidism:

- DiGeorge's syndrome: Neonatal hypoparathyroidism with thymic aplasia and T-cell immune deficiency, congenital heart disease.
- Kenny-Caffey syndrome: Hypoparathyroidism and skeletal abnormalities.

- Blomstrand disease: Hypoparathyroidism with chondrodysplasia.
- Polyglandular autoimmune (Type I) hypoparathyroidism, which is associated with Addison's disease, autoimmune thyroid disease, diabetes mellitus, pernicious anaemia, candidiasis, ectodermal dystrophy *etc.*

(A case has been discussed).

In polyglandular autoimmune failure type II, hypoparathyroidism is not a presenting feature.

MANAGEMENT:

In hypoparathyroidism it will need calcium and vitamin supplementation. Associated conditions should be treated accordingly.

FURTHER REFERENCES:

- Harrison's Principle of Internal Medicine 17th edition.
- Oxford Text Book of Medicine- 5th edition.

92

A PATIENT WITH MIXED CONNECTIVE TISSUE DISEASE

CASE: *A 29 years old British lady, visiting Kolkata, presented with a history of tingling and numbness of her left hand and numbness over the right facial region. She has been complaining of joint pain and swelling for last 6 months and was awaiting rheumatological consultation before she left for India. Rheumatoid factor checked while she was in the UK was positive in low titre. She gave history of Raynaud's phenomenon over a period of last 2 years. Examination revealed swollen MCP joints of both hands. Skin over both forearms was pigmented thick and indurated. Subcutaneous tissue over her right thigh was swollen and indurated. There was no neuro deficit. Initial investigations revealed normal haematological and biochemical parameters ESR was 60 in the 1st hour. MRI Scan of cervical spine and brain ruled out any demyelinating or ischemic lesions. Her rheumatoid factor was positive in moderately strong dilution. In view of the skin lesions and history of Raynaud's phenomenon, she underwent routine rheumatological screenings which were as follow:*

- *X-Ray chest, ECG and lung function test were within normal range.*
- *ANF (immunofluorescent technique) - +ve in 1 : 1000 dilution (speckled pattern).*
- *Anti Scl70 - negative.*
- *Anticentromere antibody - negative.*
- *ANCA - negative.*
- *Anticardiolipin antibody - negative.*
- *Anti RNP antibody - strongly positive.*
- *CPK - normal.*
- *T_3, T_4, TSH - normal.*
- *Rheumatoid factor - positive.*

DIAGNOSIS: Mixed connective tissue disease (MCTD).

DISCUSSION:

MCTD is a rare presentation in clinical practice in the Indian setting, although systemic sclerosis do present occasionally to the primary care physicians with various clinical manifestations. Main presenting symptoms relate to dermatological problems with Raynaud's phenomenon, tight and thickened skin, sclerodactyly *etc.* Patients may present with dry cough, shortness of breath and other features of *fibrosing alveolitis, rheumatological symptoms* with joint pain and swelling may be the main presenting feature. *Gastroenterological symptoms* include features of gastro-oesophageal reflux.

At a later stage, the patients present with accelerated hypertension, renal impairment and cardiac involvement. In its full blown form, it is easy to diagnose a case of systemic sclerosis. In its early stage, the physician needs to be vigilant and request for relevant tests not only for early diagnosis but also for sub-classification of the disease which has got prognostic value.

The patient described above was given a course of steroid for her arthritic symptoms. She was also prescribed penicillamine at a low dose. She was also advised to check her pulmonary function test and X-ray chest on a yearly basis.

CLASSIFICATION:

- **Diffuse cutaneous scleroderma-**

Involvement of kidney and other viscera are common. (**ANF**, **Anti Scl70** +ve)

- **Limited cutaneous scleroderma-**

Skin thickening is limited to the distal extremities and face. One subset of this type is known as CREST syndrome (calcinosis, Raynaud's phenomenon, oesophageal dysmotility, sclerodactyly and telangiectasia) the prognosis is generally better except for a subset of patients who may develop pulmonary hypertension in the long run **(Anticentromere antibody** +ve).

Scleroderma can also occur in localized form without systemic involvement. One such variety is known as morphea.

Scleroderma can also occur in association of other connective tissue disorders like SLE, rheumatoid arthritis, and polymyositis. This is known as *MCTD (mixed connective tissue disorder)*. Characteristically they have high titre of anti RNP antibody. They have a better prognosis although a subset of these patients will develop pulmonary hypertension in the long run **(Anti RNP antibody** +ve).

There are many scleroderma like clinical conditions such as scleromyxedema, eosinophilic fasciitis, eosinophilia myalgia syndrome etc. They are rarely encountered in day to day clinical practice and usually present to the dermatologist.

Immunological investigations:

- ANF - mainly speckled pattern (homogenous pattern in SLE).
- Anticentromere antibody- usually in CREST (60-80%) syndrome.

- Anti Scl70 - in diffuse systemic sclerosis (40%).
- Anti RNP antibody - in MCTD (95 - 100%).
- Anti SS-A and Anti SS-B antibodies - overlap between systemic sclerosis and Sjogren's syndrome.

These tests are important not only for diagnosis and sub-classification of the disease but also for prognostication.

MANAGEMENT:

1. **Penicillamine** (250-1000 mg) has been reported to reduce the skin thickening. It should be started in a low dose with gradual increment over months. It is a toxic drug with lot of side effects, like leukopenia, thrombocytopenia, rashes, loss of taste and features of myasthenia gravis. Appropriate monitoring should be done during therapy.
2. **Azathioprine and cyclophosphamide** may be used in more severe cases with organ involvement like fibrosing alveolitis.
3. **Antiplatelet** agents like aspirin, has also been tried (because of the role of platelet in its pathogenesis) with limited success.
4. **Steroid** may be helpful in MCTD with predominant myositis or arthritis.
5. *Raynaud's phenomenon* is treated with physical methods like keep the extremities warm. Vasodilators like nifedipine and prazosin may be tried. Ketanserin, an oral serotonin antagonist has also been shown to be effective. In acute situations, short course of iloprost, a prostacyclin analogue may decrease the severity of Raynaud's phenomenon and healing of digital ulcers. They are not routinely available in this country. Moreover they are expensive. In difficult cases, cervical sympathectomy may produce temporary relief of pain.
6. Oesophageal reflux is treated with dietary manipulation, H2 blockers, proton pump inhibitors and metoclopramide.
7. Hypertension is treated with ACE inhibitors for pulmonary hypertension; nifedipine may be used to reduce pulmonary artery pressure albeit on a temporary basis.

: KEY POINTS :

- MCTD is an uncommon presentation in clinical practice while scleroderma is not so uncommon.
- Limited variety of scleroderma has a better prognosis than the diffuse variety.
- Autoimmune screening helps in diagnosis, sub-classification and prognostication of the disease.
- Speckled pattern positive ANF is suggestive of scleroderma or MCTD.
- Antibody to RNP is high titre is present in majority of patients with MCTD.

FURTHER REFERENCES:

- Dentol CP *et al.* (2000), Scleroderma and related disorders: therapeutic aspects-Baillier's clinical Rheumatology 14 (1), 17-35.
- Harrison's Principle of Clinical Medicine- 17th ed.
- Kumar and Clark- Clinical medicine- 5th ed.

93 A PATIENT ON HAEMODIALYSIS

Frequently, patient with chronic renal failure on maintenance haemodialysis consults their internist for various medical problems and in many dialysis centres of India a nephrologist is not readily available. Therefore the primary consultant needs to be aware of the basic day to day management issues in such patients. This brief discussion is for the benefit of such doctors who confront such patients in clinical practice.

PERSISTENT ISSUES:

- **Vascular access:** This is either by AV fistula or polytetrafluoroethylene grafts, the former being better because of its longer life span.

  Problems encountered are:

  a) Infection – mainly by *Staphylococcus aureus*.

  b) Blockage – this can be treated by thrombolysis, angioplasty or surgical correction.

- **Nutrition:** The so called renal diet is inadequate for patients on maintenance haemodialysis and the diet should include at least 1.5 g/kg of protein with a caloric intake of 35 Kcal/Kg as dialysis is a catabolic state. Strict K^+ restricted diet is usually not necessary as K^+ clearance is adequate in haemodialysis.

- **IHD, HTN and CCF:** Both PTCA and CABG may be performed in patients with HD. However, the rate of re-stenosis following PTCA is high. Modifiable risk factors need to be treated vigorously.

  Hypertension is usually controlled by adequate fluid removal through HD. However, antihypertensive medication, either single or in combination, may be used if necessary. Associated cardiac failure should be treated in the usual line. Antilipidaemic drugs should be used with a target LDL level of < 70 mg%.

- **Haematological problems:** This is due to erythropoietin deficiency state and should be treated with erythropoietin injection once or twice per week. Iron deficiency, if present should be corrected by parental iron as it may cause resistance to the action of erythropoietin.

  If haemoglobin fails to rise with adequate dose of erythropoietin, one needs to consider iron deficiency, occult blood loss, inadequate dialysis, occult cancer, haemoglobinopathies or rarely antibody to erythropoietin.

  Increased tendency to bleeding may be treated with heparin free dialysis and injection of DDAVP (desmopressin).

INFECTIONS:

Being in an immunocompromised state, patients with CRF on HD are prone to infections. In patients with fever of unknown origin, tuberculosis, particularly extra-pulmonary tuberculosis should be ruled out. Dose adjustment is not needed for the 1st line anti TB medication. However, they should be given following dialysis. The patients should be vaccinated with Influenza, Pneumonia and Hepatitis B vaccination.

BONE METABOLISM:

Secondary hyperparathyroidism is common in renal osteodystrophy and serum PTH level should be monitored. Calcitriol (0.25 microgram) should be administered orally. Phosphate levels should be monitored and if more than 7 mg% it should be temporarily withheld and phosphate binders to be used. Rarely, parathyroidectomy may be needed. In chronic haemodialysis for prolonged period, β_2-microglobulin amyloidosis may develop which manifests as carpal tunnel syndrome, diffuse arthropathy and soft tissue or bone cyst.

ENDOCRINOLOGICAL AND REPRODUCTIVE PROBLEMS:

Sexual dysfunction is common. Sildenafil may be used for erectile dysfunction. Although vast majority of patients are outside the child bearing age, if pregnancy occurs, its outcome may be improved with good monitoring, adequate haemodialysis, correction of anaemia and control of BP. Preeclampsia, abortion are common events and the patients should be cautioned about if before planning for conception.

MISCELLANEOUS PROBLEMS:

- Peripheral neuropathy needs treating with tricyclic antidepressant, pregabalin or gabapentin.
- Anorexia, nausea usually improves with adequate dialysis. Symptomatic relief may be achieved with H_2 blockers, proton pump inhibitors and domperidone.
- In diabetic patients, the dose of insulin needs to be reduced frequently because of decreased catabolism of insulin.
- Depression is common and the conventional antidepressants may be given in the usual dosage.
- Preoperative management: Patients undergoing surgery should receive dialysis before any surgical procedure. Use of heparin or low molecular weight heparin should be minimised during perioperative period.

Indication of inadequate dialysis:

- Anorexia, nausea, vomiting
- Peripheral neuropathy
- Drowsiness
- Fluid retention
- Ascites
- Presence of anaemia in spite of erythropoietin
- Low serum albumin.

FURTHER REFERENCES:

- Harrison's Principle of Internal Medicine 17th edition.
- Oxford Text Book of Medicine- 5th edition.
- O. Isfedu.- Care of patients undergoing haemodialysis N.E.J.M- vol. 339-15, 1998, 1054-62.

94 A PATIENT WITH COPD

CASE: *A 62 years male with history of smoking presented in the clinic with a history of chronic cough with mucoid expectoration for 6 months duration. He also complained of shortness of breath on climbing stairs along with generalized weakness. He was a company executive and did not have any significant past medical history. There was no family history of asthma.*

Examination revealed occasional rhonchi in the chest. He was normotensive. Rest of the examination was satisfactory. Haematological and biochemical profile was normal, ECG- normal, X-ray chest hyper inflated chest, echo- slightly enlarged RV, lung function test: FEV_1- 80% of the predicted value, FEV_1/FVC- 70% of the predicted value. Pre and post bronchodilator (salbutamol- 5 mg nebulisation) FEV_1 measurement- showed 10% increase of FEV_1- 15 minutes following bronchodilator therapy.

DIAGNOSIS: Early COPD.

DISCUSSION:

COPD is a major cause of morbidity with frequent encounter of both GP and hospital services. Usually a history of more than 20 packets/year smoking history is obtained although it can rarely occur in non-smokers. Dusty environment aggravates it and deficiency of α1-antitrypsin is associated with emphysema in non-smoker but the risks are greatly magnified in those who are smokers.

INVESTIGATIONS:

Lung function test:

FEV1- < 80% of predicted

FEV1/FVC- < 70% of predicted

Peak flow variability < 20%

Bronchodilator reversibility testing - before & after 2.5 mg salbutamol
- before & after 5-10 mg terbutaline.

[15% increase of FEV_1) following bronchodilator indicates reversibility and these patients are more likely to respond favourably to a trial of oral or inhaled steroids].

X-ray chest: shows hyperinflation.

Other tests like **pulse oximetry** for O_2 saturation may be done on outpatient basis.

MANAGEMENT:

Differentiation from asthma is sometimes difficult but it is important to differentiate as the management strategies are different in those two conditions (Asthma needs anti inflammatory treatment with steroid inhalers to start with). Helpful points are variability of symptoms throughout the day, history of allergy and atopy, family history of asthma and a positive bronchodilator reversibility test [Improvement of FEV1 of > 15% following salbutamol or terbutaline nebulisation therapy] are generally indicative of asthma rather than COPD. Marked diurnal peak flow variability also favours asthma.

Bronchodilator therapy: The treatment should be started with either a short acting β2 agonist (salbutamol or terbutaline) or inhaled anticholinergics like ipratropium thrice or four times a day. Recently a long acting anticholinergic (tiotropium) has also been launched which can be used as once daily dosage. If individual drug therapy is causing inadequate response, consideration should be given to combination therapy. In non-responders, inhalation technique should be reassessed as it is a common cause of drug failure. There are different delivery systems which are simple and improve drug delivery to the lungs in spite of poor coordination. In difficult case; home nebulisation therapy may be instituted.

Theophylline: The British Thoracic Society guidelines suggest it to use only when inhaler therapy fails. However, in our country, we tend to use early as it is cheap and readily available. Apart from its bronchodilator properties it also has anti-inflammatory properties and the western literature is reviewing its status in the management of COPD in the light of its other helpful properties.

Steroids: Although generally not indicated as a first line therapy, occasional patients respond to inhaled steroids. A trial of oral steroid for 2 weeks may be prescribed to predict the response of long term inhaled steroids. Those who show subjective and objective improvement in their symptoms can be prescribed inhaled steroid on long term basis. Oral steroids should be used as short term for acute exacerbation.

Other medications: Like sodium cromoglycate, nedocromil, leukotriene antagonists have no role in the treatment of COPD.

In patients not responding to treatment, careful check up of other medications like β-blockers for heart disease, β-blocker eye drop (timolol) for glaucoma should be done as they can aggravate COPD.

Other measures:

Regular exercise to increase exercise tolerance and good nutritious diet should be advised.

The main thrust should be given to smoking cessation as it reduces the rate of decline of FEV1. Counseling should be done and in a willing patient it should be aided by other methods like - nicotine patch, nicotine gum and drug therapy with bupropion (zyban- 150 mg) twice daily for 8 weeks might help. It should not be used in epileptic. It is also helpful in alcohol dependence.

Long Term Oxygen Therapy (LTOT):

LTOT for 15 hours of oxygen therapy per day has been shown to improve survival in MRC study in the UK (5 years survival improved from 25% to 41%.).

The study showed:-

- Less secondary polycythaemia
- Prevention of progression of pulmonary hypertension
- An improvement in neuropsychological health.

The indication for LTOT in COPD is:

- Persistent hypoxia with or without hypercapnia.
- $FEV_1 < 1.5$ litre
- Evidence of peripheral oedema
- Nocturnal hypoxemia
- The patient must stop smoking before commencing on LTOT.

The patient should be admitted and base line blood gas checked. After starting the oxygen 2 *l*/min, blood gas should be repeated to see whether there is any CO_2 accumulation and the oxygen flow rate adjusted accordingly, on discharge. The oxygen should be delivered via an oxygen concentrator. However in India many patients cannot afford it and hence oxygen through cylinder is commonly prescribed.

Air travel:

In patients with severe hypoxemia and hypercapnia air travel even in modern pressurized air craft may be risky. Provision should be made for supplemental oxygen therapy in case of an emergency. The patients with bullous emphysema with recurrent pneumothorax should also be careful as there may be further risk of pneumothorax particularly during descent.

Acute Exacerbation of COPD:

The commonest precipitating case is lower respiratory tract infection. This may lead to acute respiratory failure or acute on chronic respiratory failure. This is one of the most common causes of hospital admission in COPD patients.

Common precipitants of acute on chronic respiratory failure:

- Viral or bacterial infection
- Pneumonia
- Pulmonary emboli
- Pulmonary oedema
- Pneumothorax
- Uncontrolled Oxygen therapy
- Retained secretions
- Post operative

Other causes of respiratory failure:

- Chest wall problems *e.g.* kyphoscoliosis
- Neuromuscular– myasthenia gravis, motor neuron disease
- CNS disorder- Brain stem CVA

Others- Obstructive Sleep Apnea syndrome.

Respiratory failure is a syndrome in which the respiratory system fails in one or both of its gas exchange functions: oxygenation (hypoxemic or Type-I) and carbon dioxide elimination (hypercapnic or Type-II).

Type-I failure (hypoxemic respiratory failure)- With PaO_2 of less than 60 mmHg and $PaCO_2$ may remain normal or even low because of hyperventilation. It is of usual Type and due to Ventilation/perfusion (V/O) mismatch in airways disorder. Common causes -

- Pneumonia
- Pulmonary oedema
- Pulmonary embolus

- Pulmonary hemorrhage
- Interstitial lung disease
- Right to left shunting

Type II respiratory failure is due to respiratory pump failure with PaO_2 less than 60 mmHg and $PaCO_2$ more than 50 mmHg. The causes are -

- drug overdose,
- chest wall abnormalities,
- Respiratory muscle fatigue due to any cause
- Neuromuscular and thoracic wall disorder
- Severe airway disorders (e.g. asthma and COPD)
- Late stage of airway diseases.

Management of acute exacerbation of COPD leading to respiratory failure:

- Oxygen therapy with a target oxygen saturation of 88% to 92%.
- Antibiotics- usually covering *H. influenzae*, *M. catarrhalis* and *Streptococcus pneumoniae*.
- Nebulisation with Salbutamol and ipratropium.
- Systemic steroids- can marginally affect the outcome favourably. Prolonged use may cause critical care myopathy.
- Intravenous aminophylline is not generally being recommended.
- Doxapram infusion- may be helpful if non-invasive ventilation is not avoidable. However, one comparative study has shown that it is inferior to non-invasive ventilation.

Indications of Non-invasive ventilation:

The pH should be less than 7.35 and $PaCO_2$ more than 6 KPa (44.77 mmHg) and the patient should be tachypnoeic. Although in the past coma and severe acidosis were considered as contraindications recent evidence suggests that they can be tried successfully in such conditions.

Practical guide:

- Nasal mask or face mask may be used although facial mask may cause claustrophobia in some patients.
- Oxygen should be entrained to attain oxygen saturation of around 88% to 92% (usually 1-2 *l*/min).
- For pressure preset bi-Level ventilator, an initial IPAP of 12 cm of H_2O and EPAP at 4 cm of H_2O should be selected. A back up rate of 12/minute should be set. If inspiratory time needs to be set, it should be set 2–3 seconds or < 50% of the respiratory cycle. IPAP trigger should be set at 0.5 cm of H_2O.
- IPAP may be titrated upto 20 cm of H_2O according to the blood gas response and EPAP titrated maximum upto 10 cm of H_2O above which it does not produce any beneficial effect and may reduce the venous return.
- Blood gas should be checked at one hour, upto 30% of patient would not benefit from noninvasive ventilation.
- Weaning should be done slowly initially keeping nocturnal ventilation on and reducing the day time ventilation and the process may last for 3 to 4 days.
- Non-invasive ventilation may also be successfully applied during weaning from invasive mechanical ventilation. A proportion of patients with chronic respiratory failure would also benefit from non-invasive ventilation on domiciliary basis.

Relative Contraindications:

- Imminent cardio-respiratory arrest.
- Vomiting
- Increasing pulmonary secretion
- Undrained pneumothorax
- Orofacial abnormality

Other conditions when non-invasive ventilation is useful are-

- Type I respiratory failure as in pneumonia
- Very useful for acute left ventricular failure
- Sometimes restricts neuro-muscular disorders causing respiratory failure

For patients with non-invasive ventilation, constant vigilance should be kept with blood gas analysis and clinical examination, if any deterioration is noticed prompt clinical judgement would be required to switch over to invasive ventilatory support. A trial may be useful but if needed intubation and ventilation should be done early.

ASTHMA:

Whereas COPD is characterized by destruction of smaller airways along with enlargement of areole which is by and large irreversible, asthma is an inflammatory disorder of airways which may be reversible.

Risk Factors:

- Genetic pre disposition
- Atopy
- Indoor or outdoor allergens
- Passive smoking
- Respiratory infection
- Occupational exposure (sensitizing agents)

Lung spirometry in asthma:

There is reduced FEV_1, FEV_1/FVC ratio and peak expiratory flow. Reversibility is demonstrated by a 12 % increase of FEV_1, 15 minutes after inhaled short acting β2 agonist measurement PEF twice/day confirms the diurnal variation. Flow volume loops show reduced peak flow and reduced maximum expiratory flow. Gas diffusion is usually normal.

Management of chronic asthma:

Mild intermittent: Short acting β2 agonist intermittently for symptomatic relief.

Mild persistent: Low dose inhaled corticosteroid.

Moderate persistent:

- Long acting bronchodilator
- Low dose inhaled corticosteroid

Severe persistent:

- Long acting bronchodilator
- High dose inhaled corticosteroid

Very severe persistent:

- Oral corticosteroid
- Long acting bronchodilators
- High dose inhaled corticosteroids

In each variety, short acting β_2 agonists may be required on 'as and when' required basis.

Role of anti-leukotrienes:

Montelukast and zafirlukast may be used as an add-on therapy of inhaled steroids, are not very effective.

Anti-IgE:

Omalizumab has been shown to reduce the number of exacerbation of asthma attack. It is given by subcutaneous route every 2-4 weeks. It is only useful in a selected group of patients with high IgE level.

Drug interaction of Theophylline:

Increased clearance	Decreased clearance
• Enzyme inducers • Rifampicin • phenobarbitone • Ethanol • Smoking	• Enzyme inhibitors • Erythromycin • Allopurinol • Ciprofloxacin

: KEY POINTS :

- COPD is an important cause of morbidity seen in clinical practice.
- Smoking is the most important cause and smoking cessation is the major part in the management of COPD.
- It should be differentiated from asthma as line of management in these two conditions will be different.
- Anticholinergics are more effective than β stimulants and should be started early.
- Tiotropium is long-acting anticholinergic with specific to muscarinic m2 receptors.
- Home oxygen therapy has a role in the management of severe emphysema.
- BiPAP therapy has made revolution in the management of respiratory failure.

FURTHER REFERENCES:

- J.J.P Goldring *et al.*-BJHM - Managing acute on chronic respiratory failure- Vol.69, No.-8-August 2008 P 444 – 449.
- Harrison's Principle of Internal Medicine- 17th edition.

95 A PATIENT WITH HAEMOLYTIC ANAEMIA

CASE I: *A 20 years old person diagnosed to be a case of SLE for last 3 years presented in the clinic with mild fever and feeling of unwell being. SLE was diagnosed 3 years back when he presented with fever of unknown origin. During that time he had a. stormy course and had every possible complications of SLE including cerebral infarction along with status epilepticus, cardiac tamponade due to pericardial effusion, prolonged sepsis and spent nearly four months in the hospital. Fortunately everything ended in a happy tone and he was discharged home on maintenance dose of steroid and azathioprine. At the end of 18 months he was doing perfectly well on prednisolone (5 mg) every alternate day and azathioprine (50 mg) twice daily with periodic check up of Hb, TC, DC, platelet, creatinine and LFT.*

While stable on treatment, one day he presented in the clinic with history of fever for few days, weakness and tiredness.

An urgent test for Hb, TC, DC, platelet and MP and blood culture urine were sent. Hb was dropping (8.6 g%), WBC- 3,800 and platelet count was 90,000. Thinking it to be due to azathioprine effect, the drug was immediately withdrawn and he was started on a broad spectrum oral antibiotic. Unfortunately he came back in 4 days time without any relief of his symptoms and he was feeling very weak. Repeat tests showed Hb- 6 g%, WBC- 4,700, platelet-50,000, bilirubin was 4.6 mg (mainly unconjugated). He was urgently admitted, repeat MP test was negative and LDH was very high, direct Coomb's test was strongly positive with a strongly positive ANF and raised dsDNA titres.

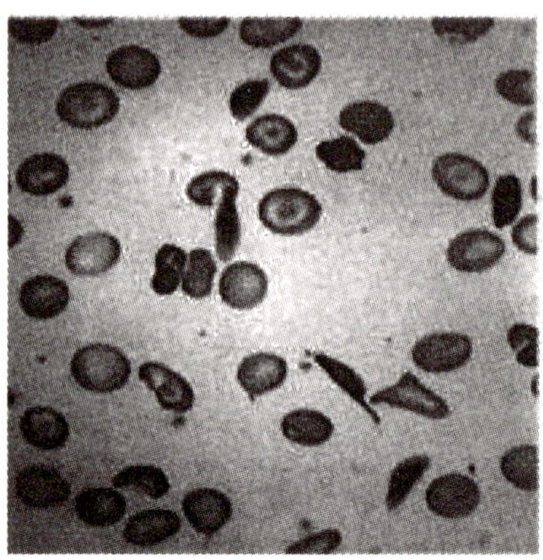

DIAGNOSIS: Auto immune haemolytic anaemia with thrombocytopenia (Evan's syndrome) in a patient with SLE.

He was managed with IV gamma globulin for 5 days, pulsed methyl prednisolone for 5 days followed by high dose of oral prednisolone. He also needed blood transfusion. At present, he remains well and on 10 mg of prednisolone. Azathioprine was not resumed in view of persistent mild neutropenia.

CASE II: *A 61 years old gentleman presented with unilateral swelling of his left leg. He was treated outside for suspected lymphatic oedema due to filariasis. Examination revealed swollen left leg but no clinical evidence of DVT, bilateral moderate sized inguinal lymphadenopathy, presence of left iliac fossa mass. Urgent CT scan of abdomen revealed multiple retroperitoneal lymphadenopathies along with hepatosplenomegaly. Appropriate biopsy specimen taken from the lymph nodes confirmed the diagnosis of Hodgkin's lymphoma.*

Haematologist was involved and after appropriate investigation, he was started on chemotherapy. While in the hospital, he became progressively anaemic. This was initially thought to be due to chemotherapy side effect. However in view of rising bilirubin, LDH and high reticulocyte count, a direct Coomb's test was performed which was strongly positive. He was treated with high dose of IV methyl prednisolone for 5 days to which he responded favourably. He is under regular follow up. His lymphoma remains under remission and he did not have any further recurrence of haemolytic anaemia.

DIAGNOSIS: Auto immune haemolytic anaemia in a case of Hodgkin's lymphoma.

DISCUSSIONS: Unilateral swelling of leg is a common presentation in clinical practice. Common conditions causing unilateral oedema are- thrombophlebitis, cellulitis, lymphangitis with lymphoedema and deep vein thrombosis. All these conditions have evidence of inflammation on local examination. Appropriate test like venous duplex scan, venogram etc. will help in making a proper diagnosis. However when unilateral, painful swelling not associated with any evidence of local inflammation is present, the clinician should also exclude an intra abdominal compressive pathology causing venous obstruction. In last 4 years we have come across 6 such cases- 4 lymphomas and 2 ovarian neoplasms. Early abdominal scanning will help in early diagnosis in such cases.

CASE III: *A 46 years old lady presented in the clinic with history of progressive anaemia and jaundice. Examination revealed moderate splenomegaly. Investigations showed Hb- 6 g%, Bilirubin- 7.8 mg% (mostly indirect) strongly '+ve' direct Coomb's test, negative ANF, LDH was high. She was admitted and treated with IV steroids and blood* *transfusion. Over the next 1 year she needed several admissions needing IV methyl prednisolone and blood transfusion. She was also started on azathioprine therapy. She was not responding adequately to conservative therapy, the pros and cons of splenectomy was discussed with her and after taking appropriate, precautions (like vaccination against Haemophilus, Meningococcus and Pneumococcus) she underwent splenectomy. She is under regular follow up and remains in remission on a very low dose of steroid and azathioprine. She has developed diabetes mellitus however.*

DIAGNOSIS: Idiopathic auto immune haemolytic anaemia requiring splenectomy.

CASE IV: *A 41 years old patient suffering from benign tertian malaria was successfully treated with chloroquine outside. Following treatment he was given a course of primaquine as a part of eradication therapy. Glucose-6-PD level was not checked due to an oversight. The reason for his admission was vomiting, weakness and mild fever. Investigations revealed severe anaemia (6.4 g%), jaundice (bilirubin 6.3 mg%, mostly unconjugated) reticulocyte count was high. Coomb's test was negative. He was treated with hydration and supportive care and finally recovered. Couple of weeks following his discharge, G-6-PD level was checked and was found to be very low.*

DIAGNOSIS: Drug induced haemolytic anaemia due to glucose-6-PD deficiency.

DISCUSSION: Haemolytic anaemia, though not very common in primary care clinical practice, one occasionally encounters while evaluating patients with anaemia, one should include following screening tests in order to detect the condition early (particularly if the blood film show evidence of macrocytosis, normoblastemia, spherocytosis). In thalassemia, haemolytic anaemia typically presents with hypochromic microcytic anaemia, target cells, normoblast in peripheral smear.

The tests should include haemogram, reticulocyte count, liver function test, renal function test, Hb electrophoresis, glucose-6-PD, LDH, Coomb's test *etc*. If clinically indicated ANF should also be done. A thorough drug history should also be taken. In patients with febrile illness, infective causes like malaria should be excluded. In patients presenting with renal dysfunction, microangiopathic haemolytic anaemias should be considered. Patients with musculoskeletal symptoms, connective tissue disorders, lymphoproliferative disorders *etc.* should also be considered and appropriately tested.

CASE V: (From the UK experience): *A 46 years old male presented in the OPD with recurrent history of passage of blood in the urine. One day he got admitted with severe abdominal pain and investigations showed mild pancytopenia, unconjugated hyperbilirubinaemia, presence of hepatomegaly with dilated IVC and ascites. LDH was high. Sucrose lysis test and acid haemolysin (Ham) test was positive and a diagnosis of paroxysmal nocturnal haemoglobinuria was made leading to intravascular haemolysis along with hepatic vein thrombosis leading to Budd Chiari syndrome.*

DIAGNOSIS: Paroxysmal nocturnal haemoglobinuria (PNH) with hepatic vein thrombosis.

DISCUSSION: Although in clinical practice it is a very rare condition. I have mentioned my experience because in the event of any history of early morning blood in urine along with features of ascites simulating cirrhosis of liver with the background of haemolytic jaundice and evidence of intravascular haemolysis like high LDH, PNH should be suspected.

COMMON CAUSES OF HAEMOLYTIC ANAEMIA IN CLINICAL PRACTICE	
Infective causes	Malaria, bacterial sepsis, virus infection
Auto immune causes	**Warm antibody mediated:** Idiopathic, lymphoma, SLE, chronic lymphatic leukemia. **Cold agglutinin syndrome:** Idiopathic, viral infections, *Mycoplasma pneumoniae*.
RBC enzyme deficiency	Glucose 6-PD deficiency
Haemoglobinopathies	Thalassemia, sickle cell disease
Mechanical haemolytic anaemia	HUS, DIC, cardiac prosthetic valve
Drugs	Methyldopa: membrane modification (Coombs positive) Penicillin: Hapten mechanism (drug adsorption) Rifampicin : Immune complex Quinine : Immune mechanism (Innocent bystander) Dapsone : Oxidative intravascular haemolysis

Clinical features:

- Evidence of intravascular haemolysis (increased bilirubin, increased LDH and presence of haemoglobin in urine)
- Haemoglobinuria (red urine)
- Pancytopenia
- Thrombosis of hepatic vein

Diagnosis:

- Sucrose Lysis test
- Acid HAM test
- More recently flow cytometry

Mechanism:

The haemolysis is complement mediated.

Treatment:

- Folic acid supplementation
- Transfusion of filtered blood
- More recently with monoclonal antibody eculizumab which is directed against the complement.

: KEY POINTS :

- Screening for haemolytic anaemia should be done in diagnostic work up for anaemias.
- Macrocytosis, hypochromia, microcytosis, stippled cell, target cell, sickle cells, normoblastemia, spherocytosis *etc.* in peripheral blood film give an important clue to differentiate between congenital and acquired haemolytic anaemia.
- Reticulocyte count LDH, Coomb's test, bilirubin, ANF, Hb electrophoresis will help in the diagnosis of haemolytic anaemias.
- Patients with febrile illness, malaria should be excluded.
- Thorough drug history along with status of glucose-6-PD level should also be evaluated in patients with haemolytic anaemia.

FURTHER REFERENCES:

- Hillman RS, Aulk KA, Haematology in Clinical Practice, New York Mc Graw Hill 2002.
- Harrison's Principle of Internal Medicine - 17th edition.

HEALTH INSURANCE AND THE DOCTOR

Since independence, the health care system in India has been expanded and modernized considerably with dramatic improvement in life expectancy and the availability of the health care facilities and better training of medical personnel. In spite of this, the guiding principle of Bhore Committee in 1946 that no individual should fail to secure adequate health care because of inability to pay for it, looks unreachable still, after more than 50 years of independence. In spite of development in the health care sector we are still lagging behind than that of many developing countries in terms of health outcome. Over the years the 'consumers' have become more knowledgeable about what is available in the market and for more demanding regarding the quality and services.

What went wrong?

The situation is due to poor performance in three dimensions of health care system-coverage, purchasing and delivery.

Coverage: Coverage or prepayment for needs is poor. Almost two-third of spending is out of pocket which is inefficient and inequitable. Private insurance, social insurance, community insurance and employer's cover under reimbursement scheme cater to only 14% of the population. In addition, government provides its cover through its own infrastructure. As a result of low insurance cover, majority of the health spending is out of pocket in our country.

Purchase: Purchasing of health care is inefficient with over 60% of the health care delivery being financed through out of pocket spending; the purchase of health care is inefficient. Individuals are unable to negotiate with the providers on the cost and quality of care because of their limited bargaining power. This leads to compromise in medical care, to the extent of abrupt withdrawal or termination of care midway through because of lack of funds, with its harmful effect on quality of health care.

Delivery: The quality of health care delivery is suboptimal at both public and private sectors. The public infrastructure is large in both rural and urban areas. It is often of low quality in rural areas and inequitable in urban areas. The private sector comprises large number of private practitioners, private hospitals and nursing homes. The private providers are unregulated and fragmented. Consequently provision is of substandard quality.

The combination of limited coverage inefficient purchase and poor delivery has led to poor health outcome in our country.

In India there is preference for private sector medical facilities because of perceived qualities in private care. The private sector delivers the care through a three-tier system- **tertiary care facility** (super speciality hospitals), **secondary care facility** (general hospitals) and **primary care facilities** (like outpatients' clinics, polyclinics *etc.*). Many of the private providers are unregulated and practice without minimum standards. The standards vary widely and there is no uniformity of care. On many occasions, the treatment is not protocol or guideline based leading to wide fluctuation of standards.

With the advent of industrializing and economic development, the spectrum of disease is also changing in India. In addition to the usual medical problems like infection, communicable diseases, malnutrition the incidence of life style related diseases is also increasing exponentially, thereby causing double burden of disease of communicable and non-communicable diseases. This is compared with burgeoning spiraling health cost and high financial burden on the poor. Around 24% of the Indian population falls below poverty lines in each year due to hospitalization. India being a country of sharp contrast, the affordable can bear the cost of highly sophisticated private health care, while the marginalized needs to sell their assets for hospitalization. This is a big hindrance to the vision of health for all in an affordable and equitable manner. In India the public health spending in health is dismally low which has compounded the problem further.

Under this backdrop the role of health insurance becomes of paramount importance in order to provide basic health care facility to all section of population particularly the vulnerable sector.

Different health insurance schemes in India:

- Voluntary health insurance schemes on private for profit schemes in public sector, general insurance corporation (GIC) and its four subsidiary companies (National Insurance Corporation, New India Assurance Company, Oriental Insurance Company & United Insurance Company) as well as Life Insurance Corporation of India (LICI) provide voluntary insurance scheme. Mediclaim is the prime insurance product of GIC either by reimbursement or through cashless scheme. There is exclusion of pre-existing disease.

  In 1999 the insurance sector was opened to the private and foreign players can hold upto 26% of the capital in an Indian company provided they have a capital of Rs. 100 crore.

- Insurance offered by NGOs: Community based insurance schemes provided by NGOs are mainly targeted towards the economically marginalised population.

- Social insurance or mandatory health insurance schemes or Government run schemes:

  - ESIS: For the power or non power using factors using 20 or more employees there is a monthly waged limit (Rs 6500/month) with a nominal pre payment contribution.

  - CGHS: Mainly for the central govt employees, treatment facilities in the govt hospitals and in approved private hospitals are offered. This scheme is mainly founded by the central govt funds with a premium ranging from Rs. 15 to Rs. 150 per month.

- Other community based insurance scheme:

  - In 2003-2004 budget another community based insurance scheme was announced (Universal Insurance Scheme) for economically disadvantaged population with a premium of Re. 1/day for one person (total 365/366 per year), Rs. 1.50/day per person for a family composed of five (Rs. 548 per year) and Rs. 2/day for a family composed of seven (total Rs. 730 per year) with the govt contributing Rs. 100 per year towards the yearly premium for the people below poverty line. The total coverage is of Rs. 30,000 per year for the hospitalization.

  - RSBY (Rashtriya Swasthya Bima Yojona) Scheme consuming Rs. 30000 per annum for hospitalisation also runs in nearly similar fashion. RSBY card holders are using facilities both in private hospitals as well as public hospitals which is helping to make the public sector hospital financially stronger in an already financially depleted and cash strapped coffer of the state govt budgets.

Unless the whole of the Indian population is brought under the health insurance scheme the goal of affordable and equitable health care for all will remain a distant future.

In my opinion the public sector hospitals should also gradually come under the ambit of public or private for profit insurance schemes mainly consuming the paying beds and cabins which will not only boost up the public sector hospitals but also encourage a healthy competition between private and public sector facilities and eventually will help to check unrealistic escalation of expenditure which is presently prevalent in India recognizing that this is a service oriented industry where the patients are not just a customer but at the very centre stage of the service delivery.

Changing demographics and disease profile and rising treatment cost will cause the spending on health care delivery to more than double over the next 10 years and the private health care will continue to be the largest component of health care spending in the next decade. To meet up with the increasing demand, minimum standards should be set for all health care providers.

Minimum standards should be set on following dimensions:

1. Infrastructural:

- Location of medical establishment in non-residential buildings (to prevent infection).

- List of equipment required by the department should be kept.

2. Personnel:

- Medical establishment should be manned by trained personnel at different levels of care.

3. Information:

- Record keeping of patient data.

- Reporting on sanitation, hygiene and public health data.

- Display the room tariffs and service charge *etc.*

Continuous endeavour should be made to improve upon the standard of care by the service provider through regular internal auditing. The statistics on death rate, discharge rates and duration of hospital stay should be analyzed regularly and compared with national and international standards from time to time. Cost-effectiveness analysis should be done to ensure that best quality of care is given at an affordable price. Regular appraisal of customer satisfaction scores should be done to improve upon customer satisfaction. Treatment should be protocol based and regular communication with customer should be done regarding different treatment options and the prognosis of the disease.

There should be regulatory or enforcing bodies to ensure that minimum standards are maintained and quality care delivered, standards of medical personnel like doctors should also be monitored through some kind of updating or revalidation programmes (like activities of GMC in the UK).

No doubt the provision of such a standardized protocol driven; uniform health care delivery system would be expensive and non-affordable for most of the Indian population. With the present state of limited capability of the public sector, it is implied that the majority of the share of the burden has to be borne by the private health care providers. It will be impossible to provide such a care through out of pocket expenditure only which will lead to suboptimal delivery of care and the government should stimulate the growth of private, social and community insurance to improve affordability. The insurance cover should be comprehensive so that it can cover outpatients (60% of the medical spend), inpatients and domiciliary treatment. Ways and means are to be found to cover some chronic diseases and some infectious diseases which are going to be prevalent in India in next one or two decades with appropriate premium adjustments. Low premium based insurance schemes should be introduced for the economically weaker section of the population so that certain basic diseases are covered.

I work in a private hospital which usually caters to the needs of middle and upper middle class of the population. Even then; I feel the necessity of proper insurance cover as many times investigation and treatment have to be curtailed on financial ground resulting in premature discharge and haphazard treatment.

By a coordinated effort between the public, private and the insurance sector with the provision of insurance cover with cashless benefit for the common and basic diseases prevalent in India, we can provide the fruits of modern medicine to the door step of millions in our country.

: KEY POINTS :

- In India, majority of the health care spend is out of pocket expenditure.
- Only a small proportion of Indian population is under some form of insurance cover.
- Out of pocket expenditure is the major limiting factor in delivering appropriate medical care to the vast majority of Indian population.
- Ways and means need to be found to provide insurance cover to the majority of Indian population either through Government or private insurance schemes.
- Insurance cover should include common chronic diseases prevalent in India and it should cover both outpatients as well as inpatient population.
- Standardization of medical care both in private and public sector along with strict quality control is the need of the hour.

97 ETHICAL AND MEDICOLEGAL ASPECTS IN TERMINALLY ILL

Since in India, critical care medicine has progressed at a rapid pace leading to prolongation of life with mechanical support in patients with irrecoverable conditions in many cases which in turn not only increases unnecessary cost of such futile treatment but also causes emotional distress to the family members and the patients as well. While in western countries there are specific guidelines in such situations, in India such guidelines and definite legal position is ambiguous in many issues making the doctor vulnerable to offer a definite opinion in such cases. Under this background, this consensus statement may shed some light to many of the grey areas confronted by the doctors in day to day clinical practice.

- Communication to the relatives regarding the prognosis of the patient in simple terms.
- The communication should be informative discussing not only about the prognosis but also the available therapy and cost of therapy and should be with sympathy and empathy.
- The primary care physician should discuss about the options available at terminal situation, such as-
    - Do not resuscitate
    - Withholding of medical treatment or life support system
    - Withdrawal of life support system

It should be remembered that euthanasia and physician assisted suicide is not permitted by Indian law.

The physician should also discuss and can pronounce brain death if indicated as Indian law, in a recent judgement (Aruna Sambagh case), has pronounced that brain death is equivalent to cessation of life. Thus overruling the previous judgement in 1994 which proclaimed brain death can only be accepted in the context of organ transplantation only.

- Family member should be assured that every effort will be taken for comfort care, for relief of distress, rather than a futile technical care which would lead to prolongation of the suffering only.
- The decision of the physician should not be imposed in a manner of command and control; rather it should be a joint decision. Another senior physician may be involved in the decision-making discussion.
- Proper documentation of the discussion must be done.

- ❖ In the event of withdrawal of care, the physician has to be extremely careful as there is no proper legal guideline in this regard and even with informed consent legal problems may crop up *post hoc.* Gradual de-escalation or non-escalation of therapy may be a better option in such events.
- ❖ If the family members are insistent to take discharge, it should be properly documented, transport should be arranged and extubation should be done at home. The physician and the medical team should be available for consultation or counselling. Analgesics and sedatives may be used in therapeutic dosage. A tracheostomy tube may remain *in situ* and oxygen therapy may be optional.
- ❖ Patient's family members should be allowed to visit the patient beyond the normal visiting norms.
- ❖ Whenever possible a second opinion should be taken to discuss the futility of treatment. If needed, mental counselling may be requested for. In extreme cases like patients with metastatic cancer with poor prognostic status, dementia, chronic vegetative state, decision of withdrawal may be taken although remembering that there is no clear cut verdict in the Indian law regarding taking such unilateral decision. Any unilateral decision needs to be avoided. However, the physician needs to discuss with the relatives and get a formal written consent from them before unilaterally deciding upon "DO NOT RESUSCITATE" status on that patient.
- ❖ Clearly these issues should be dealt with early during the admission. Otherwise, there may be unnecessary intervention with expensive treatment, like intubation and ventilation with prolongation of suffering much to the dislike of the relatives.

CASE: *An 83 years old male was admitted with history of severe respiratory distress. He was gasping for breath. Examination revealed pulse rate of 152/min., BP- 100/70 mmHg, bilateral crepitations and rhonchi in lung fields, abdomen soft, no focal neurological signs. He was a known patient with diabetes mellitus with renal impairment. He was also suffering from dementia and was home bound for last one year. He was being looked after well by his family members with the help of domiciliary nursing support. His Hb was 10.1 g%, WBC- 21,000, urea-164 mg%, creatinine- 4.8 mg%, random glucose- 336 mg%, X-ray chest showed bilateral pneumonitis, blood gas showed severe metabolic acidosis.*

DIAGNOSIS: Bronchopneumonia with respiratory failure in a patient with diabetes mellitus, renal impairment and dementia.

After explaining the prognosis to the relatives, he was intubated and ventilated, started on antibiotics, inotropic and vasopressor support along with other supportive measures. Active intervention was only started after consultation with the family members and following a telephonic consultation with his eldest son settled in the USA who wanted full resuscitative measures to be taken in his father's case. On the 4th day, he still remained semi-conscious, ventilator dependant, needed haemodialysis, inotropic support TPN and combination of expensive antibiotic therapies. On the 6th day, the family members expressed their concern about the expenses of ITU management and judging the ultimate poor outcome of this patient, requested for withdrawal of ventilatory support. The patient was not under any insurance cover or any kind of reimbursement scheme and it was an out of pocket expenditure in his case. The medical team was reluctant to withdraw life support unless the family members were willing to give written consent regarding the withdrawal. The family members were divided in opinion and wanted his eldest son, living in the USA, to take the decision. Unfortunately, the eldest son could not come immediately because of his official commitment. The futile attempt to rescue him continued till the 11th day, when he had a cardiac arrest and expired.

DISCUSSION:

Ethical and medico-legal aspect of medical care is an important aspect yet often a neglected part in the management in clinical practice. Primary care physicians are frequently involved in difficult decision makings during the end-of-life events. If not properly dealt with, the physician can be unnecessarily dragged into legal controversies.

In the presence of an advanced directive by the patient, where the patient clearly states in advance, his wishes regarding the management during his terminal illness (*e.g.* not to resuscitate or not to ventilate), the problem would be straight forward. However, in our country, rarely such advanced directives regarding the medical matters are available and the responsibility of difficult decision making naturally falls on the shoulders of the next of kin of the patient (surrogates) and the treating medical team.

Other examples:

- In an elderly demented patient with a suspicious malignant looking shadow in X-ray chest, the physician can withhold further tests like CT guided biopsy, if the family members are convinced that confirmation of malignancy is not going to improve the ultimate outcome of the patient.

- While treating a hospitalized patient with multiple CVAs with poor quality of life, the treating physician might feel the futility of any resuscitative measures in the event of cardio respiratory arrest.

Withdrawal of life support system:

Once the treatment is initiated, withdrawal is very difficult decision to make. This is the most common problem the physicians in India now-a-days are facing. Most commonly the emotionally charged relatives take a decision to go all out for their dear ones and once it becomes evident to them that expensive life support system is not going to give any positive fruitful outcome in the long run, they usually take a fresh look and request the treating medical team for withdrawal of expensive life support measures.

In view of lack of proper legal protection, the doctors are also reluctant to take a unilateral decision on their own in the absence of proper signed consent from the surrogates. This is a major reason of unhappiness, discontent and mistrust on the medical team by the relatives while treating such terminally ill patients with expensive medicines and devices. Withdrawal of treatment (left against medical advice) is another common scenario in the Indian context mainly for economic reason. Again, this has to be done with properly signed document.

Finally, physician assisted suicide (PAS) or euthanasia does not have any legal sanction in our country. It is usually practiced in Netherlands (The Netherlands never had legal sanctions but because of a 'tolerable judiciary' the practice of euthanasia is common among Dutch physicians). In Oregon in the USA, Death with Dignity Act was passed allowing PAS. However, even in this state, the practice is not wide spread.

While treating terminally ill patients, counseling and regular communication with the relatives are the most important factors. Lots of misgivings can be allayed through proper counseling. Planning regarding the withholding of resuscitative measures should be taken well in advance so that unnecessary futile intervention can be avoided in many cases with terminal illness.

Moribund terminally ill patients should be managed in special areas of the hospital like 'High Dependency Units' with better nurse-patient ratio. The relatives will feel happy and reasonably satisfied if they find that their terminally ill dear ones are properly attended by the nursing staff for terminal loving care at the time of distress. Most of the mistrust and misgivings between the doctors and the relatives occur in this area and proper counseling will help avert many of these situations.

CASE: *A 71 years old gentleman suffering from metastatic prostate cancer on hormone therapy along with history of orchidectomy was admitted in a drowsy state. His Na^+ was 114 mg% which was treated accordingly. In ICU, he had three episodes of ventricular fibrillation related cardiac arrest and needed defibrillation (in spite of being on amiodarone, $MgSO_4$ and potassium supplementation). The relative was very keen to offer any form of therapy that was available in spite of being aware of the prognosis. He underwent ICD implantation and coronary angiogram showed severe 3 vessel disease with an ejection fraction of 35%. Anti-anginal therapy was maximised. Since PTCA was not feasible, the relatives were insisting for CABG. However the medical team along with the cardiothoracic surgeon had to go against the relative's wishes as it was judged that the overall chance of survival of this patient was limited and CABG may actually shorten the life span. While in the hospital patient had several episodes of VT which was controlled by ICD. Fortunately, the patient attended clinic for follow up after one month following ICD implantation.*

BRAIN DEATH:

Since Indian law has accepted 'Brain death' to be equivalent to the cessation of life, it is important that all Indian ICUs should declare it whenever such incidence occurs not only for the organ donation purpose but also it saves lot of families from being penniless to meet up with the cost of unnecessary treatment which is futile. It must be remembered that the daily cost of ICU treatment may amount to Rs. 40,000 to 50,000 per day, and many times this is 'out of pocket expenditure'. This will not only save many families from becoming financially ruined but also address the issue of alleged unfair practice by many Indian ICUs leading to increase discontent and disillusionment amongst the lay public.

The Transplantation of Human Organ Act (1994) defines brain death and withdrawal of life support in patients with brain death in the context of organ transplantation is perfectly justifiable. However, in situations other than organ transplantation, the clinicians have to be careful regarding the withdrawal of life support even in the brain dead patients particularly if the relatives are not willing to accept the concept of 'brain death' with ongoing cardiac activities. This contrasting attitude is sometimes evident in minority of affordable patient population from affluent section of Indian Community who would like to continue with this kind of futile life sustaining measures till the last moment. Because of lack of definite legal guidelines in these matters in our country, the clinician has to be careful in these situations and disconnect the ventilatory support only after obtaining formal consent from the relatives of the patient.

DETERMINATION OF BRAIN DEATH:

To exclude reversible causes of coma
• Shock • Hypothermia • Sedative drugs • Metabolic encephalopathy • Encephalitis • Irreversible coma after excluding reversible causes • Absence of motor responses to pain

Assessment of brain stem reflex
• Loss of pupillary reflex • Loss of oculo-cephalic reflex • No deviation of eyes to irrigation of ears with 50 ml of cold water • No corneal reflex • No jaw reflex • No cough response following pharyngeal stimulation.

Absence of respiratory effort following hypercapnia
Following disconnection from ventilator if respiratory movements are absent and arterial PO_2 is more than 60 mmHg, the apnoea test is positive.

The diagnosis of brain death is clinical:

Two assessments of brainstem reflexes (at six hours interval) and a single apnoea test are conclusive of brain death.

Brain death should be certified by two separate physicians at 6 hours interval and in the case of organ donations, the doctors should not be involved in the transplant team. After confirming brain death, ventilation may be withdrawn after discussing sympathetically with the family members. In the event of organ donation, ventilation should be continued till the organ has been retrieved.

In rare instances other confirmatory tests may be needed like EEG, cerebral angiography, nuclear brain scanning, transcranial Doppler ultrasonography.

'Do not resuscitate' order, a personal experience: A six month retrospective analysis of palliative care in critically ill terminal patients in two level-III ITU's of Kolkata.

Total no of deaths- 53 Palliative care discussed on- 41 Age range: 20-90 years Sex: M-38, F-15	
Causes of death	counseling done
CVA- 10	08
Dementia with acute infection- 8	07
Road traffic accident- 3	01
Post resuscitation- 4	03
Sepsis with MODS- 16	13
Acute chronic respiratory failure of ventilator- 5	04
Hepato-pulmonary syndrome- 2	01
Malignancy withy metastasis- 5	04

Counseling successful	35 no of patients (85%)
Withholding of treatment including ventricular support	21
Withdrawal of support (mainly driven by relatives)- unilateral decision	4
DNR	5
Intubate but not ventilate	2
Continue ventilation but withhold and withdraw other forms of resuscitative and curative treatment	3

Counseling unsuccessful	6 no of patients (15%)

Barriers identified	
Fight till last attitude	3
Next of kin residing abroad	1
Third party payment issue	1
VIP syndrome	1

Effects of successful counseling:

- Shortening of duration painful suffering
- Cutting down of expenses

[Presented as poster presentation in the national ISCCM conference held at Kolkata in 2013]

: KEY POINTS :

- Ethical and medico-legal aspects form an important part in clinical practice particularly while dealing with terminally ill and critically ill patients.
- Withholding of life support in cases of terminally ill patients is justifiable in many cases.
- Withholding of life support may reduce unnecessary prolongation of suffering in many instances.
- DNR decision should be taken well in advance with proper consent from the relatives.
- Withdrawal of life support no doubt is a difficult decision to make in the Indian context. The Indian psyche and the economic factor should be taken into consideration.
- PAS has got no legal sanction in our country.

- Proper communication and counseling with the relatives will allay many of the misgivings between the doctors and the relatives of patients.

FURTHER REFERENCES:

- Jean Carlet *et al.*- Challenges in end of life care in ICU, statement of the 5th International consensus conference in critical care Brussels, Belgium, April 2003.
- Intensive Care Medicine- (2004) 30, 770-784.
- Mani RK- limitations of life support in ICU; Ethical issues relating to relating to end of life care- Indian Journal of Critical Care Medicine (2003, 7: 112 -117).
- R. K. Mui *et al.*- Guidelines For End of Life and Palliative Care in Indian ICUs
- ISCCM, Consensus ethical position statement-Indian Journal of Critical Care Medicine 2012, 16 (3): 166-181.
- Oxford Text Book of Medicine- 5th edition
- Harrison's Principle of Internal Medicine 17th edition.

98 A PATIENT WITH LACTIC ACIDOSIS

CASE: *A 46 years old gentleman with high risk behaviour was admitted with severe breathlessness. He was known to be HIV positive and was on combination therapy (HAART) regime for it. The regime included 2 NRTIs and one PI. Examination revealed pulse rate of 130/min, BP 100/70 mmHg, cold extremities and clear chest. Investigations revealed normal glucose, urea and creatinine slightly raised, mildly altered LFT, Hb was 9.4 %g, WBC- 15,000. MP- negative, in X-Ray chest NAD, ECG showed sinus tachycardia. Blood gas showed-*

PO_2	: 86 mm/Hg
PCO_2	: 23 mm/Hg
HCO_3	: 9
pH	: 7.10
Base Excess	: -15
Na	: 140 mmol/l
K	: 3.6 mmol/litre
Cl	: 100 mmol/litre
Serum Lactate	: 20 mmol/litre (normal < 2)

DISCUSSION: There is severe metabolic acidosis due to raised lactate level (lactic acidosis). There is also high anion gap acidosis as calculated by serum Na^+, K^+, Cl^- and HCO_3^- levels. The normal value is 12-14, whereas in this patient the value is very high (>30).

$$\text{Anion gap} = (Na^+ + K^+) - (HCO_3^- + Cl^-)$$

Accumulation of lactate has caused the increase in the unmeasured anion in this case.

FINAL DIAGNOSIS: Drug induced lactic acidosis.

Antiretroviral therapy, mainly NRTI can sometimes cause severe fatal lactic acidosis. In our unit we had so far come across two such cases both of which ended up in fatality.

Lactic acidosis is a problem mainly encountered in critical care unit where many patients with sepsis and organ dysfunction get admitted. Common causes are:

- ***Tissue hypoperfusion*** (*Type* A) - *shock of any kind, severe sepsis.*
- ***Inadequate uptake and utilization*** (*Type* B)
  - Chronic leukemia
  - Adrenalin therapy
  - Biguanide therapy
  - Chronic liver disease

Anion Gap:

Measuring anion gap gives an important clue to the diagnosis of metabolic acidosis. Normally the anion gap is 12-14. The reason for the apparent difference of cations and anions is that there are certain unmeasured anions in the body which accounts for this anion gap. [cations: Na^+ & K^+] - [anions: HCO_3^- & Cl^-].

However, in certain conditions the amount of unmeasured anions increase tremendously thereby giving rise to high anion gap. In the given case lactate was the unmeasured anion accounting for the high anion gap. While dealing with metabolic acidosis, measuring anion gap helps in the differential diagnosis.

Increased anion gap acidosis	Normal anion gap acidosis
DKA Lactic acidosis Renal failure Salicylate poisoning Ethylene Glycol toxicity	Severe diarrhoea Acetazolamide Renal tubular acidosis

In normal anion gap acidosis is usually the loss of HCO_3^- (measured anion) provokes increased absorption of Cl^- (measured anion) thereby the anion gap remains within normal limits.

CASE: *An 8 years old boy was referred to the clinic for increasing shortness of breath. He did not improve with a course of antibiotic and it has thought to be due to acute asthmatic attack. The boy had a pulse rate of 140/min respiratory rate- 40/min, chest auscultation was surprisingly clear, X-ray chest normal, Na^+- 149 mmol/l, K^+- 5.2 mmol/l, Cl-100,HCO_3^-- 12 mmol/l. He had an acidosis with high anion gap= 32. His urine was positive for ketone body and glucose++++, blood glucose was 412 mg%.*

DIAGNOSIS: Diabetes ketoacidosis with high anion gap.

DISCUSIONS:

Sometimes, as in this case IDDM may present for the first time with ketoacidosis. His breathlessness initially misinterpreted as asthma was due to hyperventilation caused by severe acidosis.

CASE: *A 57 years old patient was admitted in the ITU with severe breathlessness. Examination: BP- 210/110 mmHg, pulse rate 40/min. Chest relatively clear. ECG- LVH with nodal rhythm. Although LVF was initially thought of, the clinical picture did not clearly fit in with the diagnosis.* Na^+*- 146 mmol/l,* K^+*- 6.8 mmol/l,* Cl^-*- 102 mmol/l,* HCO_3^-*- 5 mmol/l, Hb- 5.2 g%,* PaO_2 *- 64 mmHg,* $PaCO_2$*- 24 mmHg. He had very high anion gap acidosis. Later on his urea was found to be 240 mg% and creatinine- 12.2 mg%.*

DIAGNOSIS: Chronic renal failure with high anion gap acidosis with hyperkalaemia induced nodal rhythm.

IV bicarbonate therapy improved his breathlessness very quickly. Hyperkalaemia was treated with IV calcium gluconate and glucose insulin infusion. He was urgently seen by the nephrological team and underwent peritoneal dialysis in the same evening.

DISCUSSION:

The reason of discussing these cases was to discuss the basic and preliminary aspects of blood gas analysis which every physician should be able to understand and interpret. To understand the basic aspects of blood gas analysis we should first discuss the preliminary aspects of it.

- Hydrogen ions are only present in the body in very low concentration.
- As the hydrogen ion concentration increases, the pH falls
- As the hydrogen ion concentration falls, the pH rises.
- An acidaemia occurs when the pH is below 7.36.
- An alkalaemia occurs when the pH is above 7.44

Normally, the body produces huge amount of water, acid and CO_2 every day. Their accumulation in the body is prevented by compensatory buffering mechanism. CO_2 is released from the cells are transported to the lungs and finally removed from the body during expiration. If the removal is impaired due to lung pathology, CO_2 will accumulate. It will finally react with H_2O to produce H^+ and HCO_3.

$$CO_2 + H_2O = H_2CO_3$$
$$H_2CO_3 = H^+ + HCO_3^-$$

Greater the CO_2 is accumulated the higher the H^+ ion concentration will be with resultant acidaemia. This condition is known as respiratory acidosis.

RESPIRATORY ACIDOSIS		
	Normal	**Respiratory acidosis**
pH	7.36 - 7.44	↓↓
$PaCO_2$	35 - 40 mmHg	↑↑↑
HCO_3^-	21 - 27 mmol/l	↑

Here, the HCO_3 will also increase but the net increase will be small.

In certain conditions there is production of huge amount of acids (like DKA) where the body's protein buffers and HCO_3^- cannot cope with it. Because of H^+ accumulation the pH falls and the condition is known as metabolic acidosis.

METABOLIC ACIDOSIS		
	Normal	Metabolic acidosis
pH	7.36 - 7.44	↓↓
$PaCO_2$	35 - 40 mmHg	36 - 40 mmHg
HCO_3	21 - 27 mmol/l	↓↓

The metabolic and respiratory components are interlinked and can compensate for each other. As in COPD and respiratory failure there will be accumulation of CO_2 and the kidneys start producing excess HCO_3^-. Using the carbonic acid link, it will enable to remove some of the excess CO_2 produced and restoration of pH towards normal. However this takes several days to become effective. Moreover, this mechanism will only partially compensate the respiratory acidosis.

RESPIRATORY ACIDOSIS WITH METABOLIC COMPENSATION			
	Normal	Respiratory acidosis	Metabolic compensation
pH	7.36 - 7.44	↓↓	↓
$PaCO_2$	35 - 40 mmHg	↑	↑
HCO_3	21 - 27 mmol/l	↑	↑↑

In DKA there is accumulation of excess acid. Although kidneys will try to increase HCO_3 production, it will take several days. Instead increased H^+ will cause stimulation of respiratory centre and increase CO_2 elimination. Lowering of CO_2 stimulates further free acid to be converted to H_2CO_3 and eventually CO_2 production.

Again the respiratory compensation for the metabolic acidosis will be only partial.

METABOLIC ACIDOSIS WITH RESPIRATORY COMPENSATION			
	Normal	Metabolic acidosis	Respiratory compensation
pH	7.36 - 7.44	↓↓	↓
$PaCO_2$	35 - 40 mmHg	35-40 mmHg	↓
HCO_3	21 - 27 mmol/l	↓↓	↓

Combined metabolic and respiratory acidosis:

This will happen in a case of cardiorespiratory arrest. There is severe lactic acidosis because of severe tissue hypoxia which will not be compensated by hyperventilation due to respiratory arrest resulting in accumulation of CO_2. The blood gas picture will be:

pH	-	↓↓
$PaCO_2$	-	↑↑↑
HCO_3	-	↓↓↓

Base Excess:

It is number of mmol of HCO_3 which must be added to the equivalent of one litre of patient's blood so that a PH of 7.4 is produced. Respiratory elements are removed by keeping the partial pressure of CO_2 constant at 40 mm/Hg. The value is '0' but varies from +2 to -2 mEq/L.

Base excess is helpful in calculating the amount of HCO_3 that should be given to a patient with metabolic acidosis.

Multiple or combined acid base disturbance:

Sometimes the patient may have combined acid base disturbance. For this we need to consider how much $PaCO_2$ (for metabolic compensation) and HCO_3 (for respiratory compensation) has changed. If they fall within certain limits then a single acid base disturbance is present otherwise there is possibly a presence of combined acid base disturbance.

There are two methods of assessing their changes:

1. Graphical method *e.g.* Finley's graph.
2. Arithmetic method.

Acute respiratory acidaemia: 1 mmHg rise of $PaCO_2$ produces a 0.1 mmol/l rise in HCO_3.

Chronic respiratory acidaemia: 1 mmHg rise of $PaCO_2$ produces a 0.5 mmol/l rise in HCO_3.

[If HCO3 rise is more than these expected ranges then the possibility of concomitant metabolic alkalosis is high.]

Chronic respiratory alkalaemia: 1 mmHg fall of $PaCO_2$ will produce 0.4 mmol/l fall in HCO_3

Metabolic acidaemia: A 1.0 mmol/l fall in HCO_3^- will cause 1 mmHg fall in $PaCO_2$ [Rise in $PaCO_2$ will indicate associated respiratory acidosis and greater degree of fall in $PaCO_2$ will indicate respiratory alkalosis].

Metabolic alkalaemia: 1 mm/lit rise in HCO_3 will cause 0.6 mmHg rise in $PaCO_2$.

[Greater rise of $PaCO_2$ will indicate associated respiratory acidosis].

: KEY POINTS :

- Severe metabolic acidosis can cause hyperventilation which may be confused with asthma, LVF and chest infection in clinical practice.
- In patients with severe shortness of breath but paucity of clinical findings on auscultation, metabolic acidosis along with psychogenic hyperventilation and pulmonary embolism should be considered in the differential diagnosis.
- The concept of anion gap helps in the differential diagnosis of metabolic acidosis.
- A good understanding of the blood gas analysis will help the clinician to diagnose primary metabolic and respiratory acid base disorder with or without compensation and treat them appropriately.

A PATIENT WITH METABOLIC ACIDOSIS

Practical approach in day to day practice:

Arterial blood gas tells us about two systems, respiratory and metabolic. If one system is disturbed the other tries to restore the balance to keep the pH in the normal range. Among these the respiratory system is a quick and efficient system than metabolic system to maintain the pH of blood. $PaCO_2$ is the main stimulator of the respiratory system although hypoxia may also play a role in regulating the respiratory centre.

How to approach: In practical terms arterial blood gas presents 6 steps which need to interpret to make a clinical diagram.

1) **First look for the pH** - Is there acidosis or alkalosis?

2) **Second to look at the $PaCO_2$.**

If for example, the pH is low and $PaCO_2$ is also low, then clearly the respiratory system is involved to compensate for the acidosis. Thus by looking at these two values numbers (pH and $PaCO_2$) majority of the interpretation can be done.

3) **Third - to look for 'base' picture.**

Actual bicarbonate ($aHCO_3^-$) vs. standard bicarbonate ($SHCO_3^-$): Actual bicarbonate is the actual measured HCO_3^- in the blood. It depends upon $PaCO_2$ which if high will also drag the $aHCO_3^-$ high. Standard HCO_3^- on the other hand denotes the value of HCO_3^- that is expected if the $PaCO_2$ were within the normal range. This value tells us about the metabolic compensation that might have taken place.

4) **Fourth - What is base excess?**

It not only denotes the HCO_3^- but also other bases as well. It's significance is like that of HCO3. The normal value would be '0' with a range from '+3 to –3'.

5) **Fifth - What does base excess tell us?**

If the pH and $PaCO_2$ tell us that the problem is primarily metabolic, HCO_3^- or BE will just merely confirm it, with $SHCO_3^-$ being high in alkalosis and low in acidosis.

If the problem is respiratory, then the $SHCO_3^-$ and BE will tell us about the duration of the problem.

Example: If in respiratory acidosis the $SHCO_3^-$ is within the normal range, it will signify that the problem is acute as there was no time for compensation. In respiratory acidosis, on the other hand if $SHCO_3^-$ is high it will signify that the acidosis is chronic (the pH will also be low). It must be remembered that a grossly deranged pH cannot be chronic as it is incompatible with life.

6) Sixth - To look for oxygen.

PaO_2 helps in differentiating type-I respiratory failure which is due to certain structural lung disease of VQ mismatch with ventilatory failure with near normal lung parenchyma. In the first instance, PaO_2 is low and $PaCO_2$ is near normal whereas in the later case PaO_2 is low while $PaCO_2$ is high. However, in clinical practice, very frequently these two types of failure may co-exist and one needs to differentiate between them for rational management.

In this regard, measurement of alveolar-arterial gradient (difference between alveolar partial pressure of oxygen PAO_2 and PaO_2). PaO_2 is measured from blood gas analyzers and PAO_2 needs to be calculated from alveolar gas equation.

$$PAO_2 = 150 - 1.25 \times PaCO_2.$$

If alveolar-arterial gradient is high then it implies type-I respiratory failure with VQ mismatch due to either any problem with lung parenchyma or VQ mismatch. In healthy young person PAO_2 - PaO_2 is approx 15 ml/kg and in elderly it may be as high as 30 ml/kg. High PAO_2 - PaO_2 would indicate either shunt due to alveolar collapse, pneumonia, pulmonary embolism or VQ mismatch due to interstitial lung disease, COPD *etc.*

Example: A young lady presented with acute shortness of breath. The blood gas analysis shows-

pH - 7.55 - alkalosis
$PaCO_2$ - 24 mmHg - contributing respiratory alkalosis
$SHCO_3$ - 22 - acute
$aHCO_3$ - 16
BE - 2

The picture is that of acute respiratory alkalosis. This picture might well be due to hyperventilation syndrome or acute pulmonary embolism.

If AQ gradient is normal, the diagram would be hyperventilation syndrome where as high AQ gradient would indicate VQ mismatch either due to pneumonia or pulmonary embolism.

FURTHER REFERENCES:

- Fall P.J.- A stepwise approach to acid base disorders, Post Grad. Med. 107:249, 2000.
- Dubose T.D. Jr.- Acid base disorders- Brenner's and Rector's, The kidney, 7th edition, philadelphia, Sunders 2004, p 921-996.
- Acute medical emergencies- The practical approach- BMJ Book.
- Sraham P Bums- Arterial blood gases made easy Clinical Medicine 2014 Vol. 14

99 A PATIENT WITH AORTIC STENOSIS

CASE: *A 79 years old male patient was admitted with breathlessness. His echocardiogram showed aortic stenosis, X-ray chest showed enlarged heart, ECG showed LVH with strain pattern.*

DIAGNOSIS: Aortic stenosis with breathlessness for evaluation.

DISCUSSION:

Aortic stenosis / sclerosis is a common problem in clinical practice and physicians need to opine regarding the treatment of such a condition. Aortic stenosis is sometimes detected during routine clinical examination. Occasionally it is detected during evaluation of patients with chest pain and shortness of breath.

Causes of aortic stenosis / sclerosis:

- Age related degenerative changes
- Rheumatic conditions
- Congenital bicuspid valve

Associations:

- Hypercholesterolemia
- Hypercalcaemia (as a part of William's syndrome- hypercalcaemia, mental retardation and aortic stenosis).
- Hypertension, diabetes mellitus
- Renal failure
- Metabolic syndrome
- Heyde's syndrome– association of colonic angiodysplasia with propensity for lower gastrointestinal bleeding which gets cured following successful aortic valve replacement.

How to approach:

Echocardiography is the sheet anchor of all the investigation and it gives a very useful clue as to the timing of aortic valve replacement. Coronary angiogram should be performed prior to contemplation of surgery to rule out associated coronary artery disease. The asymptomatic patients should be regularly followed up clinically. Prophylaxis for infective endocarditis should be provided in the appropriate background.

While performing echo, 3 main criteria should be looked for viz.

i) Aortic valve orifice

ii) Flow-velocity across the valve

iii) Ejection fraction

Indications for surgery:

- If flow velocity is more than 4 m/sec with a mean DP > 40 mmHg.
- If aortic valve orifice is < 1 cm^2.
- In case of ejection fraction of less than 50 %, the flow velocity may be falsely low, and in that event dobutamine echocardiography should be performed to increase the stroke volume which may reveal the true velocity across the aortic valve.
- Exercise stress test should be performed to evaluate exercise tolerance.

Which operation?

- **Mechanical valve replacement** – It should be used in patients below 65 years of age and it needs life-long anticoagulants.
- **Bio-prosthesis** – It should be used in elderly patients where risk of anticoagulants is high. It should also be used during pregnancy to avoid anticoagulants.
- **Trans Catheter Aortic Valve Replacement (TAVR)** should be considered in very old symptomatic patients where surgical risks are very high.
- **Balloon valve dilation** provides only limited haemodynamic benefit with high evidence of recurrence
- Associated coronary artery disease, if present should also be treated and cardiologist's view point should also be taken for formulating a definite treatment planning.
- In rheumatic conditions, due to frequent presence of mitral valve involvements decision taking may be different as double valve replacement is associated with increased morbidity and mortality.

FURTHER REFERENCES:

- Harrison's Principle of Internal Medicine 17th edition
- Oxford Text Book of Medicine- 5th edition
- C.M. oho *et al.* Aortic Valve Stenosis- NEJM-2014-371 : 744-756, August 21, 2014.

100 A PATIENT WITH DYSTONIC MOVEMENT

CASE: *An 18 years old girl presented with 1 year history of abnormal movement involving her left hand in the form of episodic jerky movement along with abnormal posture. This interrupted her day to day activities, causing sleep disturbance and interfered with her schooling activities. The movement was aggravated while she was observed. She received a course of propranolol followed by anticholinergic medication as well as clonazepam without any effect. She was admitted for observation and further management; routine tests were within normal range. CT brain was normal. Functional element was also considered and she was given a course of SSRI without any effect.*

PROVISIONAL DIAGNOSIS: Dystonia with a pronounced functional element.

PROGRESS AND TREATMENT:

Since she did not respond to the medication, further assessment of her neurological status was made. It was decided to treat her with local injection of botulinum toxin-A to the intrinsic muscles of her left hand. She was referred to a neurological expert in this field. Following injection, she showed significant improvement of her abnormal hand movements, could write and was finally discharged with an advice to repeat the injection in next 3 to 4 months time.

FINAL DIAGNOSIS: Adult onset idiopathic dystonia.

DISCUSSION:

Tremor and abnormal movement of hands are frequent presentation in clinical practice. Although most of the cases are due to benign essential tremor, occasionally clinicians come across unusual case such as described above.

CASE: *A 63 years old hypertensive and diabetic lady presented with drowsiness and confusional state along with slow dancing rhythmic movement of her right side of the body along with facial dyskinetic movement. Her haematological and biochemical parameters were normal. MRI Brain Scan revealed bilateral ischaemic changes in both basal ganglion regions. She was provisionally diagnosed as a case of ischaemic cerebrovascular disease and treated accordingly. Additionally she received Clonazepam and tetrabenazine. Eventually her abnormal movements stopped and before discharge she was fully conscious with independent mobility.*

WORKING DIAGNOSIS: Acute choreoathetotic movement following acute ischaemic involvement of the basal ganglion.

DISCUSSION: Movement disorders other than tremors are also a common problem in clinical practice and in many cases such internists have to deal with the problem before referring to a Neurologist.

CASE: *A 71 years old male patient suffering from Parkinson's disease presented with abnormal facial movement along with visual hallucination. He was on levodopa therapy. Investigations did not reveal anything specific. It was thought to be due to levodopa therapy which was temporarily discontinued. Olanzapine 5 mg at bed time was started. The dystonic movement stopped within 72 hours and levodopa was reinstituted continuously at a lower dose. Olanzapine was eventually withdrawn in a month's time after subsidence of her hallucination.*

DIAGNOSIS: Levodopa induced dystonia and hallucination

Drugs causing dystonia:

- Neuroleptics – May cause rigidity, may develop at mouth.
- Atypical antipsychotics e.g. clozapine, risperidone.
- Olanzapine have lesser risk compared to traditional antipsychotics like haloperidol.
- Metoclopramide.

TREATMENT: Parenteral administrations of anticholinergics like benztropine or benzodiazepines like diazepam or lorazepam are very effective.

CASE: *A 68 years old hypertensive lady presented with violent movement of left side of her body along with mild weakness on the same side. CT scan revealed small putaminal haemorrhage on the right side of her brain. She was treated with clonazepam and tetrabenazine and her violent movement eventually subsided.*

DIAGNOSIS: Hemiballismus due to putamen haemorrhage.

While dealing with such patients, one should take a detailed drug history. Common iatrogenic causes of tremor include:

- Bronchodilators
- Lithium
- SSRI's
- Valproate
- Excess dose of thyroxine

In addition, excessive smoking and coffee intake can-also cause tremor. Next one should notice the type of tremor:

I. Action tremor:

a) Essential tremor: Fine tremor observed in outstretched hands, pronounced on action, progressive, and family history is present. Although called benign it may cause major disruption in the day to day activity including loss of job or career.

b) Enhanced physiologic tremor: Fine tremor in outstretched hands and legs more pronounced on action, associated features like exophthalmos may be present. Thyroid function should be tested.

II. Resting tremor:

c) Parkinson's tremor: Slow pill rolling type mainly in resting condition but may be present during action. Other features of Parkinsonism may be present.

III. Resting and action tremor:

d) Intention tremor: Coarse terminal tremor that occurs as the limbs approach the target *e.g.,* finger-nose testing. If accompanied by other neurological features like ataxia, dysarthria, nystagmus *etc.* central cerebellar causes should be excluded and a brain imaging is a must.

IV. Other varieties of tremor:

e) Adult onset idiopathic dystonia: The tremor is of jerky type, abnormal movement of extension and flexion of the wrist and fingers may be present. Other features of dystonia *e.g.* torticollis may be present.

f) Wilson's disease- wing beating: Other features of Wilson's disease will help in the diagnosis *e.g.* (dysarthria, Parkinson like features). Blood tests like low ceruloplasmin level will be diagnostic.

On the whole in clinical practice, vast majority of the patients will have either benign essential tremor, Parkinson's disease or iatrogenic.

Management of essential tremor:

- The most commonly used drug is non-selective β blocker like propranolol in the dose of 40 mg thrice daily. Selective β blocker like atenolol is less effective.
- If β blocker is contraindicated because of asthma, heart block *etc.*, antiepileptic primidone in the dose of 250 mg thrice daily may be tried. It is equally effective. Sedation may be a side effect.
- If the patient still does not respond, gabapentin in the dose of 300 mg thrice daily may be tried.
- Alprazolam and clonazepam, in view of their potentiating effect on GABA are helpful drugs. Drug dependence is a problem with the use of benzodiazepines.
- Calcium channel blocker, flunarizine 10 mg daily has also been shown to reduce tremor in selected group of patients.
- Injection of Botulinum toxin-A into the intrinsic muscles of the hands may reduce tremor. This therapy is particularly helpful in dystonia. (As in the case described above) the injection may need to be repeated.

  Uses of Botulinum toxin- 1) blepharospasm, 2) muscle spasticity 3) Excessive drooling of saliva following CVA *etc.*

Common movement disorders (in addition to tremor) encountered in clinical practice.

- Chorea: Huntington's Chorea (genetic), SLE.
- Chorea and athetosis: Polycythaemia rubra Vera, thyrotoxicosis, acute rheumatic fever.
- Dystonia / Dyskinesia: i) Primary dystonia – Blepharospasm, cervical, drug induced (Levodopa). ii) Focal dystonia.
- Myoclonus: Metabolic encephalopathy, anoxic encephalopathy, Prion disease (neurodegenerative conditions).
- Hemiballismus: Cerebrovascular accident.
- Tics or habit spasm: Tourette's syndrome.

TREATMENT:

- In dystonics, anticholinergic drugs may be helpful. Other drugs like baclofen, tetrabenazine and clonazepam may also be tried. Repeated dose of botulinum toxin is helpful. Deep brain stimulation may also be tried if available.
- In Chorea, clonazepam, tetrabenazine, propranolol and baclofen may be tried.
- In hemiballismus also, above mentioned drugs along with haloperidol may be helpful.
- In Tourette syndrome (a neurobehavioral disorder with tics) may be treated with alpha agonists like clonidine, quetiapine and atypical neuroleptics.

CASE: *A 58 years old lady presented with recurrent fall and in-coordinated during walking. Examination revealed finger nose in-coordination and ataxic gait. Thyroid function test was normal. Vitamin B_{12} level was normal. Electrolytes were normal. MRI scan showed mild cerebellar degeneration. Nerve Conduction Study of lower extremities revealed mild sensorimotor neuropathy. She also gave history of regular intake of alcohol. Later on she revealed that she was on phenytoin for many years for her epilepsy and never had any follow up for last 2 years. Phenytoin level was checked which was very high. The drug was stopped temporarily and resumed at a lower dose after her ataxia was under control.*

DIAGNOSIS: Drug induced ataxia. Other contributing features are mild cerebellar degeneration, alcoholism with peripheral neuropathy.

Causes of ataxia:

<table>
<tr><td colspan="2">Inherited ataxias</td><td>Friedreich ataxia
Olivo-ponto-cerebellar degeneration
Ataxia telangiectasia</td></tr>
<tr><td rowspan="2">Cerebellar disorders</td><td>Bilateral</td><td>Hereditary ataxias, metabolic, hypothyroidism, alcoholism, hyponatraemia
Vitamin B_{12} deficiency
Chicken pox cerebellitis</td></tr>
<tr><td>Unilateral</td><td>Cerebellar infarction
Metastatic
Cerebellar haemangioma (Von Hippel Lindau disease)</td></tr>
</table>

CASE: *A 38 years old patient with schizophrenia on atypical antipsychotics was transferred from another hospital with history of high fever and severe hypertension following a hernia repair surgery. Although initially it was thought to be due to sepsis, broad spectrum antibiotic therapy did not help. Moreover, procalcitonin level was normal. He was treated with intravenous fluids, antipyretics and antihypertensives. Dantrolene could not be given because of the non-availability. His temperature hovered between 105° to 106°F. He was treated with Levodopa. In spite of all efforts, he could not be resuscitated.*

DIAGNOSIS: Malignant neuroleptic syndrome in a patient on antipsychotics following a surgical procedure

This is a dreadful condition in patients on antipsychotics. It presents with malignant hyperthermia and high BP. It is treated with dantrolene, levodopa, diazepam, antipyretics and supportive therapy. It has got a high mortality rate.

: KEY POINTS :

- Tremor is a common presentation is clinical practice.
- Benign essential tremor in young and middle aged and Parkinsonism in elderly population are the most common causes.
- Benign essential tremor may be disabling and may interfere with career prospect.
- While dealing with tremor, drug history should be taken meticulously.
- Non selective β blockers are helpful in the management of benign tremors.
- Botulinum toxin A is an effective, new mode of therapy available for dystonia.
- Other forms of therapy like unilateral implantation of a deep brain thalamic stimulator contralateral to the more disabled arm, is not generally available in our country.

FURTHER REFERENCES:

- Marsden CD *et al.* (1994), Movement disorders- Oxford Butterworth-Heinemann.
- Pahwa R Lyon's K- Differential diagnosis and current therapy. Am J Med 115:134, 2003.
- Harrison's Principle of Internal Medicine- 17th edition.

101 A HIV POSITIVE PATIENT WITH CEREBRAL TOXOPLASMOSIS

CASE: *A 46 years old housewife presented with a history of vomiting. Examination did not reveal any specific clue. She was cachectic and slightly obtunded which was thought to be due to mild hyponatraemia that she had. Her Hb was low (7.2 g%), LFT- normal, renal status normal. X-ray chest suggestive of old tuberculosis and she was recently treated with empirical anti-TB medication in view of prolonged pyrexia. Her vomiting was not responding to the usual management and she underwent gastroscopy which was normal. USG of whole abdomen was also normal.*

Since her sensorium was deteriorating she underwent CT brain scan which showed multiple ring enhancing lesions in the brain with gross cerebral oedema. The radiologist suggested that the lesion could be due to either Koch's or metastatic brain disease. Other possibilities like cerebral toxoplasmosis were also considered. In view of the possibility of toxoplasmosis, HIV antibody tests were requested. She was found to be HIV positive (ELISA and Western Blot). Toxoplasma antibody IgM was also positive. On enquiry her husband was found to have high risk behaviour and the source of her infection.

She was treated with IV co-trimoxazole and trimethoprim for 3 weeks, anti Koch's therapy was continued. Anti cerebral oedema measures like mannitol and steroids were given. She also needed mechanical ventilatory support for a while. She was transfused with 6 units of blood. She was seen by infectious disease consultant and was started with anti-retroviral 'HAART' therapy (highly active anti retroviral therapy) with a combination of lamivudine, AZT and nelfinavir. After 6 weeks of hospital stay she was finally sent home with a tracheostomy in situ. Serial CT brain scans done in the ward showed remarkable improvement of the lesions. Her CD4 count before commencement of treatment was 84 and she had a very high viral load.

DIAGNOSIS: Cerebral toxoplasmosis in a patient with AIDS.

DISCUSSION:

Although first described in 1981, this disease has already affected millions of people in the world. Initially described in homosexuals the disease started spreading among the heterosexuals with high risk behaviour. Blood transfusion and IV drugs abuses are the other major risk factors. This disease is spreading rapid and fast in India and sooner or later the internists will have to deal with this problem regularly in their day to day practice and a working knowledge about this condition will become essential in no time.

AIDS should be suspected in any patient presenting with-

- Profound weight loss
- Prolonged pyrexia
- Generalized lymphadenopathy.
- Unusual infections like persistent oral candidiasis, oral leukoplakia, recurrent viral infection like herpes *etc.* AIDS should be considered in the differential diagnosis particularly in the at risk population and after proper consent, HIV test should be requested for. If positive, (ELISA, Western Blot), other tests like CD4 count and viral load should also be done.
- Patient diagnosed to have lymphoproliferative malignancy at an unusual age.

Once diagnosis has been made, treatment should be started urgently. The idea is to hit hard with combination of anti retroviral drug therapy with a view to restoring the immune function as much as possible and reduce the viral load to the minimum possible levels. With this in mind HAART therapy was proposed in 1996 and it has already had a big impact in reducing the morbidity and mortality in patients with AIDS. Although cure is not possible, the patients remain asymptomatic with reduction of incidence of secondary infection. Mere positivity of HIV antibody is not an indication for commencement of treatment. The treatment is usually commenced with the CD4 count falls below a certain limit goals.

CD4 count > 350 - **any viral load, no treatment necessary.**

200-350 - **may need treatment if a) symptomatic b) high viral load**

< 200 - **needs treatment**

What is CD4 count?

CD4 cells are part of the body's infection fighting system. HIV can destroy entire 'families' of CD4 cells. That's when opportunistic infections are likely to develop. HIV binding to the surface of CD4 cells and enters to it. As CD4 cells multiply to fight infection, they also make more copies of HIV only and families of healthy CD4 cells decline. Thus the immune system gets weaker and weaker. Acute illnesses such as pneumonia, pyelonephritis, influenza, herpes simplex virus, mononucleosis, cellulitis, injuries and burns and even chemotherapy or sepsis can cause low CD4 counts temporarily. Unexplained low CD4 counts may also be found in "Idiopathic CD4 T Lymphopenia".

CASE: *A 23 years old young man was admitted with right lower lobe pneumonia and was treated with broad spectrum antibiotics with improvement. Within one week he was readmitted with severe pneumonia in right lower lobe with partial improvement with antibiotic therapy. HIV test was negative.*

He was again readmitted with severe pneumonia involving both lungs. Fibre-optic bronchoscopy did not reveal any endobronchial lesion, AFB, cytology was repeatedly sent. Once specimen revealed scanty growth of Aspergillosis. He was treated with voriconazole, meropenem, empirical anti TB and steroid. Without any response, his CD4 count was reported to be low. He went to another hospital (CMC Vellore) in another state and received treatment. He developed features of ARDS in X-ray and blood gas analysis and finally underwent repeated bronchoalveolar lavage- no abnormal cells were found. After 4 weeks of therapy finally his fever subsided. The second time he underwent transbronchial biopsy which revealed histopathological features suggestive of sarcoidosis.

DIAGNOSIS: Recurrent bilateral pneumonia with features of ARDS and low CD4 count and HIV negativity, which was due to sarcoidosis which is known to cause altered CD4 and CD8 ratio.

Idiopathic CD4 low count although rare has been described in literature as well. However a transbronchial biopsy was done at CMC Vellore, the report was consistent with Sarcoidosis. Sarcoidosis is also well known to cause CD4 and CD8 ratio alteration. Final diagnosis was Sarcoidosis.

DRUGS TO TREAT HIV:

There are 3 classes of antiretroviral drugs that are available:

NRTI Nucleoside Reverse Transcriptase Inhibitors	**NNRTI** Non-Nucleotide Reverse Transcriptase Inhibitors	**PI** Protease Inhibitors
Zidovudine Stavudine Lamivudine	Nevirapine Efavirenz	Ritonavir Nelfinavir Indinavir

In 'HAART' therapy commonly a combination of 2 NRTI with one PI or 2 NRTI with one NNRTI or 3 NRTI are used. The idea of combination therapy is to suppress the viral load as quickly as possible as well as prevention of drug resistance. Using 3 drugs of the same class is also aimed at preventing drug resistance.

Monitoring therapy:

The treatment should be monitored by checking the CD4 count and viral load periodically. With successful treatment CD4 count should come up and viral load should decrease at a very low level (less than 50 copies). The patients' well being is also improved with reduction of morbidity. Failure to improve in aforementioned parameters would indicate either

- Non adherence to therapy or
- Drug resistance.

Side effects of the medication:

Side effects are common and the drug therapy should be monitored carefully. The common side effects are:

- Lipodystrophy and abnormalities in lipid metabolism- common with NRTI, can also occur with PI. Hyperlipidaemia should be treated appropriately (statins).
- Lactic acidosis- It is a serious complication and if not detected early has a very high mortality. It usually occurs with NRTI. We had two patients presenting with lactic acidosis following treatment with NRTI. Both of them died.
- Hyperglycemia- may occur with PI.
- Skin rash- 5% of the patients treated with NNRTI develop rash.
- Neuropsychiatric- Vivid dream mainly occurs with efavirenz (NNRTI).
- Drug interactions- Most problematic drug interactions occur between rifampicin and PIs or NNRTIs. As rifabutin interaction is less pronounced, it can be considered as an alternative to rifampicin. Clinical judgement is required as rifabutin is less effective than rifampicin.

2 NRTI+ PI	2 NRTI + NNRTI	3NRTI
Lipodystrophy Lactic acidosis	Rash (5%) Vivid dreams (in efavirenz)	Lipodystrophy Increased glucose

CASE: *A known patient with AIDS on HAART presented with mild jaundice. Initial investigations showed she was positive for HCV antibody. She developed severe breathlessness. Her cardiac and respiratory parameters were normal. Blood gas showed severe metabolic acidosis with a large anion gap. Plasma lactate level was very high- more than 9 mg% (normal < 2 mg%). She died in spite of all resuscitative measures.*

CASE: *A 43 years old male was admitted with collapse and respiratory distress. Since he was recently bed bound for a spell of gastroenteritis, a provisional diagnosis of pulmonary embolism was made. However, the test results were inconclusive. A blood gas analysis showed severe metabolic acidosis with a high anion gap. Lactate level was > 20 mg%. Meanwhile a history HAART therapy for last 6 months for HIV positivity was obtained. Drug induced lactic acidosis was diagnosed. He did not respond to resuscitative measures.*

: KEY POINTS :

- The incidence of HIV infection is on the rise.
- Primary care physician should be aware of this condition and have a low threshold for requesting for HIV test if clinically indicated.
- CD4 count is an important determinant for the requirement of drug therapy.
- HAART therapy is very effective in keeping patient's symptom free.
- Clinicians should be aware of side effects and drug interactions.

FURTHER REFERENCES:

- AIDS 2000 a year in review (2000) - AIDS 14 (Supply 3).
- Carpenter CC *et al.* (2000) Anti retroviral therapy in adults, JAMA 283; 381-391.
- Harrison's Principle of Internal Medicine- 15th edition.

102 A DIABETIC PATIENT WITH HYPERTENSION

CASE: *A 54 years old male suffering from Type-II diabetes mellitus, attended the clinic for routine checkup. He gave a history of hypertension detected 1 year back. He was taking oral anti-diabetic medication regularly, he used to skip his blood pressure tablet and he felt that high BP was not causing any problem to him. Examination revealed BP of 166/100 mmHg, rest of the examination was satisfactory. Haematological and biochemical parameters were satisfactory, random glucose was 186 mg% with an HbA1C of 7.1%. His lipids were satisfactory. Urine examination showed trace of protein.*

DIAGNOSIS: uncontrolled hypertension in Type II diabetes mellitus.

DISCUSSION:

Hypertension is a common accompaniment of Type II diabetes mellitus and a cause of significant morbidity and mortality. 80% of the diabetics die of macro vascular disease (MI and CVA) and hypertension is a significant risk factor. Trials like DCCT and UKPDS have shown that strict control of diabetes mellitus can reduce micro vascular complications like retinopathy, nephropathy etc. but has negligible effect on macro vascular complications whereas control of hypertension can reduce it. So it is very important that clinicians should pay meticulous attention in controlling BP in their Type II diabetic patients.

1. The question would arise whether control of BP helps in diabetes? In three trials on hypertension (SHEP, HDFP and SYST-Eur) where different antihypertensives were used; there was evidence of reduction of cardio-vascular mortality and morbidity in a subset of patients with diabetes mellitus.

2. The next question we need to answer what is the optimum BP in a diabetic patient? Results from the studies like HOT and UKPDS indicate that probably the target BP in diabetic patient is 135/80 mmHg at which level the patient will derive maximum benefit.

3. The choice of agent is also important. Three trials compared ACE inhibitors with calcium channel blockers (FACET, ABCD STOP II). In these trials-

   - ACE inhibitors fared better compared to calcium channel blockers.
   - *In UKPDS,* ACE inhibitors and β blocker were equipotent, although β blocker caused more weight gain.
   - *In INSIGHT,* calcium channel blocker nifedipine and diuretics were found to be the same.
   - *In NORDIL,* β blocker and calcium channel blocker were found to be equally effective.

- *In ALLHAT*- diuretic chlorthalidone, ACE inhibitor lisinopril and calcium channel blocker- amlodipine were equally effective although the incidence of heart failure was more with amlodipine. Chlorthalidone was particularly effective in Black Americans.
- In the diabetic subgroup of LIFE study, losartan treated patients had less event rates compared to β blocker (atenolol) treated patients.

Although so far ACE inhibitors and β blockers have been the drugs of choice, from the above discussion it is evident that one can extend the choice of drugs further depending on the clinical situation, like diuretics in African population, beta blockers and Ca^+ channel blockers in IHD, ACE inhibitors and or Angiotensin II receptor blockers in renal impairment, with other drugs suitably added to the regime depending on the BP level, Calcium channel blocker should be used as a third line agent. If needed, α blockers may also be added but they do not alter the prognosis in such patients.

It is important to remember that most of the patients are asymptomatic and would try to avoid medication. It is incumbent on the clinicians to stress on the importance of controlling the BP meticulously. On many occasions the patients might need combination of 2 to 3 antihypertensive medication to achieve the target BP. One should remember control of blood glucose will reduce the microvascular complication only, whereas simultaneous control of BP will reduce the macro vascular complication the main cause of morbidity and mortality in diabetic patients.

While treating hypertension without diabetes similar principle should be adopted. However, the target BP is slightly higher compared to diabetes. In patients of less than 50 years of age, ACE Inhibitor and or beta blocker should be tried first. In patients above 50 years, low dose diuretic and or calcium channel blockers should be the drugs of choice. In the event of poor control these group of drugs can be suitably added or substituted for one another.

In addition to drug therapy, life style modification, regular exercise, weight reduction, low salt intake, low alcohol intake, will also help the patient in controlling the BP.

ACE Inhibitors in diabetes, IHD, kidney disease, heart disease β blockers in IHD.

Combination of ACE inhibitor with AT-II receptor blocker in non-diabetic renal disease with proteinuria delays the progression of renal disease. [CO-OPERATE STUDY-Lancet 2003; 361, Page 117-24]

However, this combination may cause hyperkalaemia with increased complications.

While treating isolated systolic hypertension, calcium channel blocker has a special edge over the other agents. The recent guideline of the British Hypertension Society has been outlined below:

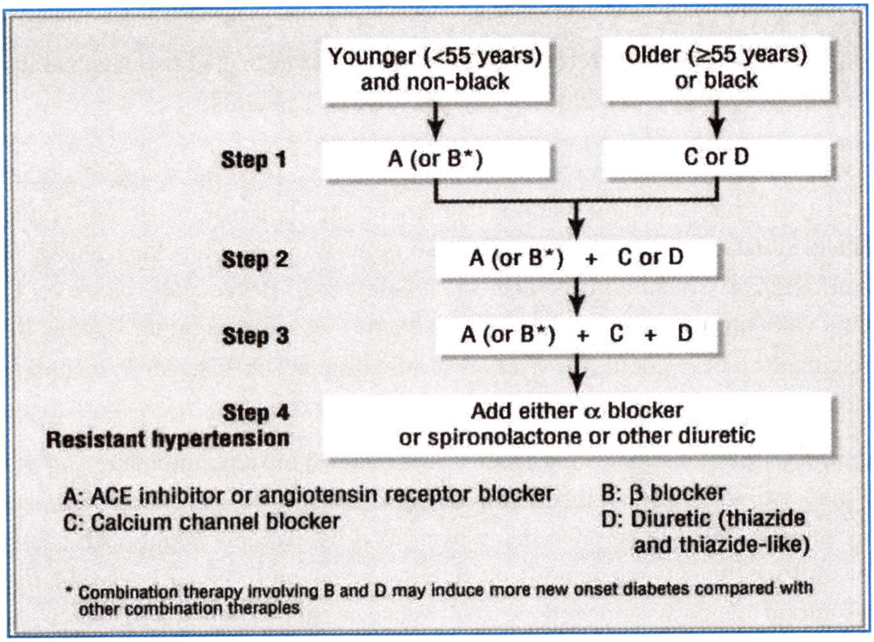

In clinical practice blood pressure control may sometimes be difficult.

Causes:

- Resistant hypertension
- Inappropriate commitment
- White coat effect
- Drug related side effects *e.g.* Steroids
- Inappropriate BP measurement.
- OSA
- Atherosclerotic disease
- NSAID
- Immunosuppressive in organ transplant.

: KEY POINTS :

- Hypertension is a common association with Type II diabetes mellitus.
- 80% mortality in diabetes occurs due to macrovascular complication.
- Meticulous control of diabetes reduces microvascular complications whereas control of hypertension reduces macrovascular complications.
- The target of BP control is 130/85 mmHg and one needs to use combination therapy to achieve the target.
- Although ACE inhibitors and β blockers are still the drugs of choice, one can extend the list depending upon the clinical situation.
- Since hypertension is asymptomatic in most patients, primary care physician should stress the need of tight BP control as a preventive strategy to the patients via individual consultation, group discussion and seminars.

FURTHER REFERENCES:

- The evidence base for tight BP control in the management of Type 2 DM- Snow *et al*.- Annals of internal medicine, 1 April 2003, Vol. 138, N-7: Page 587- 592.
- Essential hypertension- J. A. Gtaessen *et al.*, The Lancet Vol. 361 N 9369, 10th May 2003: P 1629-1641.

103 A PATIENT WITH MACROCYTIC ANAEMIA

CASE: *A 38 years old vegetarian woman had been complaining of tingling, numbness and paresthesia of her legs for last 6 months. Past medical history: she had history of subacute intestinal obstruction 5 years back and underwent laparotomy followed by intestinal resection of the terminal ileum and proximal colon. Biopsy was suggestive of granulomatous colitis although it could not be conclusively stamped as tuberculosis or Crohn's disease and she received a course of anti TB medication along with mesalazine. Investigations revealed Hb of 9.4 g%, MCV- 100, WBC- 3100, Platelets- 86,000, urea- and creatinine- normal, LFT showed bilirubin-1.2 mg%, AST- normal, CPK- normal, LDH slightly raised. Vitamin B_{12} level low, folate level- low normal, T_3, T_4, TSH- normal, bone marrow examination revealed megaloblastic changes. NCV study indicated mild degree of axonal neuropathy.*

DIAGNOSIS: Peripheral neuropathy due to vitamin B_{12} deficiency in a vegetarian lady undergoing intestinal resection due to granulomatous colitis.

She received vitamin B_{12} injection 1 mg daily for 5 days followed by at a 3 monthly interval. She also received folic acid supplementation 5 mg daily. At present she is doing well and her symptoms of neuropathy have disappeared.

DISCUSSION: Macrocytic anaemia is occasionally encountered in clinical practice. Although pernicious anaemia is distinctly uncommon in India compared to the European population, macrocytic anaemia due to vitamin B_{12} deficiency is occasionally encountered in vegetarian population. While dealing with anaemia due to macrocytosis, following causes should be kept in mind.

Causes of macrocytosis:

- Alcoholism vitamin B_{12} and folate deficiency
- Hypothyroidism
- Severe bleeding due to reticulocytosis
- Myelodysplastic syndrome
- Drugs- phenytoin, sulphonamides, methotrexate and other folate antagonist.

Appropriate history and relevant investigations will provide the clue to the correct diagnosis; vitamin B12 and folate levels should be checked to rule out their deficiency particularly in vegetarian, in patients with small intestinal resection and history of malabsorption.

Common causes of vitamin B_{12} and folate deficiency:

- Diminished intake of vitamin B_{12} – vegetarian diet.
- Due to deficiency of intrinsic factor (essential for vitamin B_{12} absorption from intestine) – gastrectomy, pernicious anaemia.
    - Blind loop syndrome
    - Intestinal malabsorption
    - Intestinal resection

Manifestation: Apart from symptoms of anaemia, there may be features of neuropathy.

INVESTIGATIONS: Preliminary investigations can suggest vitamin B_{12} deficiency *e.g.*

- Low WBC count, hypersegmented WBC
- Low platelet
- Raised LDH
- Mildly raised bilirubin
- Parietal cell antibody (95%)
- Intrinsic factor antibody (50%)

Specific tests:

- Vitamin B_{12} and folate levels.
- Schillings test- this test demonstrates deficient absorption of radioactive vitamin B_{12} from the gut which can be corrected by addition of intrinsic factor, indicating the diagnosis of pernicious anaemia. In case of malabsorption, addition of intrinsic factor would not correct the abnormality.
- Bone marrow examination will show active marrow with megaloblastic changes.

TREATMENT:

Injection vitamin B_{12} 1 mg daily for 7 days then monthly for 3 months. The marrow starts regenerating very rapidly and blood transfusion is usually not required.

FOLATE DEFICIENCY:

- Increased demand- pregnancy, haemolytic anaemia.

- Increased loss- dialysis.
- Decreased absorption- malabsorption due to various causes.
- Drugs- antifolate drugs.

Investigations: Serum and RBC folate level.

MANAGEMENT:

Folic acid supplements (5 mg daily). It should always be co-prescribed with vitamin B12, in vitamin B_{12} deficiency anaemia. In pregnancy, folic acid deficiency can cause neural tube defects. Hence folic acid supplementation should be given to all pregnant women during the initial period of gestation.

CASE: *A 58 years old vegetarian gentleman attended the clinic with weakness, oedematous legs and persistent diarrhoea. Investigations revealed Hb- 6 g%, MCV- 110, macrocytosis, WBC- normal, Platelet- normal, albumin- 2.2 g% (low), calcium- 6.1 mg% (low), Ferritin- normal, vitamin B_{12}- low, folate- low, urine for routine test- normal, stool examination- presence of fat globules, colonoscopy- NAD, Barium follow through- malabsorption pattern in small intestine,*

DIAGNOSIS: Vitamin B_{12} and folate deficiency due to small intestinal malabsorption.

He was treated with IV vitamin B_{12} and folic acid supplementation along with a prolonged course of tetracycline. He also received 2 units of blood. 8 weeks at follow up, his Hb was 10 g%, MCV- 91, albumin- 3.3 g% and oedema had disappeared.

Approach in patients with microcytic anaemia: Microcytic anaemia is a very common presentation in clinical practice. Most common cause encountered in clinical practice is iron deficiency anaemia.

Common causes of iron deficiency anaemia in clinical practice:

- Poor nutrition
- Increased loss
- Gastric- peptic ulcers- NSAID
- Intestinal- bleeding due to various causes like vascular ectasis, angiodysplasia haemorrhoids.
- Malignancy

- Increased menstrual blood loss
- Intestinal malabsorption
- Infection *e.g.* Hookworm infestation

Other causes of microcytic anaemia:

- Thalassemia (common in certain parts in India)
- Anaemia of chronic disorder
- Sideroblastic anaemia

INVESTIGATIONS:

- **Confirm iron deficiency *e.g.* Ferritin level-** It will be low in iron deficiency. However it can give misleading results in certain situation. Since it is an acute phase reactant, it can go up in any inflammation, malignancy, hepatic disorders and thereby mask iron deficiency. As for example in rheumatoid arthritis, ferritin may be high (acute phase response) in spite of iron deficiency due to NSAID induced blood loss.
- Soluble transferrin receptor (sTfR), a relatively new investigation may be helpful in such solution. It is high in iron deficiency only and it does not go up in the other condition.

Causes of high ferritin:

Non-haematological causes:

- Acute inflammation (acute phase response).
- Malignancy
- Hepatic disorder
- Haemochromatosis

Haematological causes:

- Sideroblastic anaemia

Other diagnostic workup:

- Hb electrophoresis- raised HbA2 will indicate thalassemia.
- Presence of target cells in peripheral blood film- in thalassemia.
- Bone marrow- increased iron stores with ring sideroblasts- in sideroblastic anaemia.

Differential diagnosis:

- **Iron deficiency:** low MCV, microcytosis, low ferritin, high soluble transferrin receptor molecule, marrow iron absent.
- **Thalassemia:** very low MCV, microcytosis, target cells, increased HbA2, normal ferritin, high soluble transferring receptor molecule, marrow iron present.
- **Sideroblastic anaemia:** low, normal or high MCV, microcytosis, (may be normo- or macrocytosis), high ferritin, normal soluble transferring receptor molecule, marrow iron present.
- **Anaemia of chronic disorder:** low or normal MCV, micro or normocytosis, high ferritin, normal soluble transferring receptor molecule, marrow iron present.

  Once iron deficiency is confirmed, investigations like stool test, gastroscopy, colonoscopy or ultrasound examination of abdomen will be needed to find out the cause.

TREATMENT:

Oral iron supplementation is sufficient in majority of the cases. In patients with malabsorption IM/IV iron may be substituted. IV iron can cause anaphylaxis and one should be careful about this. In renal failure patients, IV iron along with erythropoietin is a helpful combination in treating anaemia.

: KEY POINTS :

- Anaemia is very common in clinical practice. Complete haemogram with determination of MCV value will help to classify anaemia into macrocytic or microcytic which have completely different causes.
- Common causes of macrocytic anaemia are alcoholism, vitamin B_{12} or folate deficiency.
- Pernicious anemia is distinctly uncommon in India.
- Chronic blood loss and nutritional deficiency are the common causes of microcytic anaemia.
- Haemoglobinopathies should be ruled out in selected cases.
- Ferritin level may be helpful if differential diagnosis of microcytic anaemia.
- Ferritin level may be misleading in patients with associated inflammatory disease as it will increase as an acute phase response protein in spite of presence of iron deficiency.

FURTHER REFERENCES:

- ABC of clinical haematology- edited by D. Provan. BMJ Books. Iron deficiency anaemia, P 1-4. Macrocytic anaemia, P 5-8
- Haematology at a glance- A Mehta and V. Hoffbtrand Iron, Physiology and deficiency- P 32-22. Megaloblastic anaemia- P 36-41.

DIFFICULT WARD ROUND

INTRODUCTION:

In India an internist, consultant or primary care physician is a friend, philosopher and guide to the patients. In a country like India an internist's role is tremendous as maximum information gleaned from a single consultation from a doctor rather than multiple referrals because of logistic problems. With this in mind this chapter has been written for the upcoming consultants, internists and primary care physicians.

The ward full of patient is like a castle to a clinician and he guards the castle with a team of doctors. Many varieties of patients may be admitted under his care, which needs input from different sub-specialities. The physician should play the role of band master of this orchestra and the main grip should be in his hand.

STEM CELL THERAPY:

CASE: *A 61 years old patient post cardiac arrest survivor with persistent vegetative state with tracheotomy in situ for last 2 weeks was being treated in HDU with supportive care. One day a person claimed to be related to the patient, came to see and discuss with the treating physician. He was a resident of USA and came for 2 weeks holiday and was scrutinizing the treatment that was offered to the patient. In the discussion he mentioned that did the treating physician explore the possibilities of stem cell therapy as he has surfed the internet and gave reference to such treatment which has been tried in USA where it was a new development. Obviously the answer from the treating team was a 'No'. He urged to explore that option, as the patient did not have any problem of going to USA or to receive such treatment.*

DISCUSSION:

Regenerative medicine is a relatively new field in the horizon of clinical medicine and although still in the initial phase of development seems to have a wide scope in future particularly in many disease conditions where till date treatment options are limited. The basis of stem cell which is nothing but an undifferentiated pluripotent cell and being a progenitor cell may differentiate in unipotent cells having the potential to be used as a therapeutic option in different medical conditions. It must be mentioned the Hematopoietic Stem Cell Transplantation (SHCT) is already in clinical practice for long in different haematological conditions like multiple myeloma, leukaemia *etc.*

The sources of stem cell may be Embryonic Stem cells (ES cells), Embryogenic Germ cells etc. Umbilical cord blood progenitor may also be used for this purpose. Organ specific stem cells can also be obtained from the patient and may be amplified for the therapeutic application.

Therapeutic application

Possible areas where this new technology of regenerative medicine may be applied are in disorders involving skin, eye, kidney, cartilage and neurological disorders like Parkinson's disorder, stroke, traumatic brain disorders, diabetes mellitus and cardiac disorders like ischemic heart disorders and cardiomyopathy. Although not generally available in India, the caring physician should always discuss about this new field in appropriate background so that the informed relatives are aware that the clinician is aware of this new frontier as many of them have capacity to treat these patients outside India.

GENETICS:

CASE: *A 51 years old lady who recently underwent surgery for her breast cancer and was recuperating slowly from her surgery was visited in the ward by her younger sister who while routinely communicating with the doctors asked one of the doctor whether there are any tests for her which can predict the possibility of breast cancer in her case which might help her to take preventive measures. The informed doctor mentioned about testing for BRCA1 gene which may not only predict about breast cancer but also about ovarian cancer and advised to oncologist in this regard.*

DISCUSSION ON GENETIC TESTING IN CLINICAL PRACTICE:

Genetics is rapidly playing an important role in clinical medicine in present diagnosis and treatment for many disorders. Although the features are not wholly available in India as yet, in the era of globalization the internists need to be aware of the developments as he may be encountered with enquiries from the informed patient for guiding them or for purely educative purpose.

Traditionally genetics had been viewed in the past for single gene disorders like Mendelian inheritance, due to chromosomal aberration like Down's syndrome (Trisomy-21), to disorders arising from the mutation of the genes controlling growth, apoptosis and cellular differentiation. The human genome is estimated to contain 30,000 to 40,000 genes that are divided in 22 pairs of autosomes and pair of sex chromosomes or allosomes (X and Y).

Different methods of identifying genetic aberrations including mutation are cytogenic analysis (for simple chromosomal disorders), Fluorescent *in situ* Hybridization (FISH), Polymerase Chain Reaction (PCR), Reverse Transcriptase PCR (RT-PCR), DNA sequence and Restriction Fragment Length Polymorphism (RFLP). Newer methods now include are SNP (Single Nucleotide Polymorphism) and WAS (Whole Genome Sequencing).

MENDELIAN INHERITANCE

: **Autosomal dominant conditions** :

- Achondroplasia
- Huntington's disease
- Familial hypercholesterolemia
- Neurofibromatosis types I and II
- Marfan syndrome
- Acute intermittent porphyria (AIP)

These result from mutation of one copy (allele) of a gene carried on an autosome. All the offspring will have a 50 % chance of inheriting the mutation.

: **Autosomal recessive conditions** :

- Alkaptonuria
- Ataxia telangiectasia
- Glycogen storage disorders
- Wilson's disease
- Tay-sachs disease

These result from mutation in both copies (alleles) of autosomal genes. When both parents are affected there are 25% chances of the offspring being affected and 50% chance of being carrier.

: **X-linked recessive inheritance** :

- Haemophilia A and B
- Lesch-Nyhan syndrome
- Duchenne muscular dystrophy
- Glucose 6-PD deficiency (females are usually not affected)
- Becker's muscular dystrophy

: **X-linked dominant inheritance** :

- Vitamin D resistant rickets
- Rett syndrome
- Fragile- X syndrome
- Goltz syndrome

Clinical application of genetic testing:

1. In prenatal diagnosis

- Amniocentesis
- Chorionic villus sampling
- Foetal blood sampling

2. For multifactorial inheritance – To find out the susceptibility of the disease

This can be done for population screening or more commonly for family screening for certain diseases with multi-factorial origin like hypertension, diabetes or hyperlipidaemia or coronary artery disorders. Predictive genetic testing usually carried out in presymptomatic patients with family history like Huntington's disease. It may also be considered in patients with family history of breast cancer.

THERAPEUTIC APPLICATIONS:

IN-VITRO FERTILIZATION AND GENETIC ENGINEERING

A glaring example of in-vitro fertilization and genetic engineering is the treatment of mitochondrial diseases which affects one child in every 1 in 4000. Scientists hope to prevent it at conception by transferring a healthy nucleus of egg cell in place of the damaged mitochondria. Therefore, any child born as a result of such intervention will inherit genes from three sources (**3 parents' baby**). It is a germ line modification and thus irrevocable. Some ethical objections have been raised regarding this procedure but the good results which have come out outweigh the ethical objection of mitochondrial donation. The UK parliament has approved the procedure by thumping majority to be implemented. It is to note that Great Britain is also the land of the first test tube baby.

GENE THERAPY

This involves transfer of the missing gene to a physiologically relevant target cell. This may find its application in cancer diseases to prevent the uncontrolled growth of the primary tumour by prevention of tumour angiogenesis, vascular diseases like use of VEGF in patients with myocardial ischemia or cardiomyopathy who are not fit for operation or monogenic disorders.

When to council for genetic disorders:

- Advanced maternal age
- Previous history of birth defect
- Family history of genetic disorders
- Family history of cancer

Genetic tests helping in early intervention in cancer patients:

- Familial Adenomatous Polyposis
- Breast and ovarian cancers
- Familial melanosis

Other diseases where genetic predictability will help early intervention:

- Haemophilia A and B
- Polycystic kidney disease
- Multiple endocrine neoplasia type 2
- Wilson's disease
- Haemochromatosis

However gene therapy is still in its infancy and lots of questions relating to the long term safety and finally ethical issues are involved which need to be addressed before it becomes a common armamentarium in the day to day clinical practice.

FURTHER REFERENCES:

- Harrison's Principle of Internal Medicine 17th edition
- Oxford Text Book of Medicine- 5th edition.

MISCELLANEOUS

CASE: *A 90 years old terminally ill patient was decided by the relatives not for resuscitation (DNR) and for comfort care only. However at 5am in the morning the patient had a cardiac arrest and was intubated, which prolonged the life and suffering for another four days much to the annoyance to the relatives. This was in spite of written instruction in the bed head ticket.*

CASE: *A 40 years old lady was admitted with tuberculosis. One day in ward round, she complained that the nurses gave her anti-TB medicine on two occasions and forgot to give her the usual hypertensive medication.*

CASE: *A patient with known history of severe drug allergy to NSAID in the past was prescribed the same drug which caused a severe reaction, needing to transfer the patient to ITU.*

CASE: *A 71 years old lady admitted with OA in the ward fell on the floor while trying to go to the toilet independently, leading to fracture of her left femoral bone. She complained that in spite of calling the nursing bell for prolonged period no one responded and she had to go to the toilet independently.*

CASE: *A 74 years old patient with CVA was admitted in ITU. He was seen by a full team of doctors along with physiotherapists and speech therapists. One day the patient developed severe breathlessness and it was found that it was due to aspiration of food content. He needed intubation and ventilation and expensive medication. This was in spite of the speech therapist's recommendation that the patient had a swallowing problem and should not be fed orally until further direction. The physiotherapists repeatedly mentioned that the patient should be kept at 30° reclined position which was also ignored by the nurses. This lack of communication led to not only prolonged stay but also increased the cost tremendously much to the annoyance of the relatives.*

CASE: *A 31 years old patient was admitted with a history of weight loss. Initially screening test showed that his HIV antibody test was positive. The patient wanted to get discharged for financial reason. In the discharge summary the diagnosis of HIV positivity was mentioned without any advice to repeat the HIV test or confirming with western blot technique. An official complaint was lodged to the hospital administration by the relatives. Later on he underwent repeat HIV test with western block technique which was positive and later on he was referred to appropriate specialist for further management.*

CASE: *A 64 years old patient was admitted in ITU with sepsis and multi organ failure. He had a history of IHD, hypertension and diabetes mellitus. He was on ventilatory support. The caring primary care internist took multiple opinions. Cardiologist came and opined that the patient must be on aspirin/clopidogrel as the risk of further cardiac event was high. Gastroenterologist gave an opinion that aspirin/clopidogrel must be avoided as the risk of gastrointestinal bleeding was high. The nephrologist recommended that fluid challenge should be given to which the cardiologist vehemently opposed. The respiratory* *physician wanted to do prone ventilation to which the nursing staff vehemently objected in view of lack of man power support. The neurologist thought addition of modafinil might help to improve his drowsy state. A specialist then came from Delhi and opined that he should immediately have ECMO support.*

Needless to say that all the super specialist consultants spent only brief amount of time, never looking back at progress of the patient. The poor internist who was spending prolonged time with the patient and relatives and trying to coordinate with the whole team with so many conflicting opinions and attempting to streamline the whole process was really in a fix. As anticipated the patient finally did not survive this entire onslaught and expired due to multi organ failure in a case of sepsis. The relatives requested the hospital administration for some concession on the hospital bills which was regretted. The internist made a concession of 50% of his personal fees. Relatives were happy; the doctor also did not have any frustration for his financial loss. In this particular case the internist did an excellent job as a doctor as well as a member of the society. The medical fraternity needs this category of doctor called generalist or internist who not only works as a gate keeper but also plays in the mid-field and works holistically keeping in mind the socio-economic and cultural back ground of the patient. This group is fast dwindling due to the overgrowth of super specialist (which is also equally important) because of increased work burden and less financial compensation. In order to sustain and help to flourish these holistic doctors, in the bigger interest of the society.

DISCUSSION:

The cases described here are problems very frequently encountered in day to day clinical practice. Lack of communication amongst the hospital staff, or lack of coordination amongst the health care workers, lack of documentation in the medical charts on bed head tickets, absence of nurses in the ward rounds can lead to disastrous consequences not only on the patient's health but may also ruin the relationship between the patients and the doctors and with the medical administration and frequently may lead to legal complication. These are all preventable by practising certain norms in practice and by improving communication and coordination skills amongst the health care staff and the doctors' need to take a role as a manager and leaders in these regards. These lapses just mentioned about also occurs in hospitals with NABL accreditation indicating that personal skill development is more important rather than paper accreditation. In the UK in the Mid Staffordshire NHS Foundation Trust it was reported that over a prolonged period of time between 2005-2009, there had been excess amount of death, suffering of the patients in the way of diet, falls in hospital, increased incidence of bed sores and other medical related negligence because of all the factors that has just been described which led to formation of Francis Inquiry committee which published its report in 2010 after making a thorough inquiry with the help of huge number of witnesses, over a period of two years and the main recommendation that emerged was that it categorically stressed on the role of medical professionals on their role as a manager and overall as a leader beyond their usual call of duty as a clinician. It stressed the need for a patient centred care with a holistic approach with empathy and sympathy and develops a system which supports a delivery of that holistic care with the doctors taking the main leading role in delivery of complete health care.

Doctors must take leading responsibility for driving change in their organisations rather than blaming the management. The leadership should emerge by encouraging medical professionalism in regard to clinical practice, reflection and self awareness, responsibility for action, respect for patients, encouraging team work and showing social responsibility.

Communication skills should be improved; team work should be encouraged involving different team members such as physiotherapist, dietician, speech therapist and nursing staff. Documentation should be perfect, medical charts should be signed by the doctors. Handover mainly in the shift hours should be perfect which may avoid many disasters particularly increased accidents mainly in the early morning hours when majority of the adverse events usually happen. Any event that is happening like falls, wrong admission of medicine should be recorded in 'event recording' system and should be communicated to the relatives and thorough audits should be done to prevent further occurrence of such events.

Counselling mainly death counselling, breaking bad news counselling, futility of treatment and convincing the patients for agreeing them for DNR status in terminally ill patients, discussing about 'brain death' status should be done in appropriate situations. The leading doctor of the team should take the responsibility of training his junior staff in this regard.

Disclosing the HIV positive status of the patient is a tricky situation. If HIV test is positive, it needs to be repeated and if that test is positive it should be confirmed by Western block technique. It is absolutely strictly confidential and although approved authority should be informed about it, a positive test result should not be reflected in the prescription or discharge summary. A prior consent is essential before performing the test in a patient.

A physician should take a leading role in taking a holistic approach. He or she should remember that from admission till discharge, even for the minor complaints, the overall well being of the patient is his or her duty and any breech in this will be harmful for his goodwill.

CASE: *A 63 years old female patient was admitted with a history of mild TIA due to atrial fibrillation leading to a fall. Although she was fit for discharge within 5 days of her admission, her discharge was deferred because she developed fever due to thrombophlebitis in the IV site and a urinary tract infection related to urinary catheter. Her discharge was deferred by another 7 days during which she received expensive antibiotics and expensive investigations leading to not only extra stay in the hospital but also extra cost. The relatives applied to the management regarding concession and to allow them to procure medicines from outside pharmacy (fair-price medicine shops) to which the authority did not agree. Finally during discharge a meagre amount of concession was made on the bed charge only and the doctors also reduced their bill amount.*

DISCUSSION:

Nosocomial infection and hospital related problems, leading to increased stay in hospital with extra expenditure is an emerging problem throughout the world however it does not pinch so much in a developed countries where in majority of cases it is out of pocket expenditure rather than insurance based payment. In USA this problem leads to legal battles, in India in addition, it leads to violent outburst by the relatives which frequently become a good source of adverse publicity in the press.

This is true hospital acquired infections are a reality and it may not be avoided absolutely, every effort should be made to minimize its incidence and the onus is not only on the administration but also the nurses and the medical faculties as well. A doctor should take a leading role in this aspect rather than a hospital administrator as there will be conflict of interest particularly in a private hospital.

How a leading role of doctors may reduce the incidences of nosocomial infection? This is mainly by regular training, education and performance auditing of his or her units. Catheter and IV channel related problem, bedsore related problem may be reduced significantly by following standard protocols and doing regular ward round and examination of the patients; aspiration and bedsore related problem may be to a large extent prevented by following standard protocols in the hospital related to the treatment of bedridden and frail patients, simple procedures like 30° reclined position and frequent moving of patients will prevent these complications. Hand washing should be strictly monitored through regular auditing. Ward cleansing, equipment sterilization must be ensured regularly with regular bacteriological surveillance with proper documentation. To ensure all these efforts are bearing fruit monthly auditing must be done on monthly basis to ensure that the evidence of hospital related problems are really reducing in number, otherwise it will only become an eye washing theoretical excuse. If the doctors don't take a leading role in this matter the onslaught would come from the consumers. Before it comes, let us take initiatives from the medical professionals. It is ridiculous that from the second day of stay in the ITU, there were growths of MDR *Klebsiella*, which not only causes high cost but also causing organ problems like kidney failure again spiralling the cost of the therapy. Many times some of the enlightening people smell some nexus between the hospitals, pharmaceutical houses and the medical communities. The medical communities should come forward and break their wrong assumption.

It must be remembered a patient admitted in the hospital the doctor is fully responsible till the last day of his or her stay in the hospital not only for medical problems, but also for other administrative issues like food quality / nursing care / total care and his or her goodwill depends upon the entire package of care even in matters where hospital administration is responsible. An administrator in a private set up looks at the problem from a different angle, hence the doctor's role as a holistic leader is most important.

: KEY POINTS :

- Doctors are not only clinicians nor a meagre manager.
- He or she is a leader!
- He or she is the torch bearer to a new horizon in the health care!

FURTHER REFERENCES:

- Harrison's Principle of Internal Medicine 17th edition.
- Oxford Text Book of Medicine- 5th edition.
- Judy Mc Kimme, Medical Leadership From Policy To Practice BJIAM-Vol. 72, No. 5, May 2011
- Journal of Royal College of Physicians-Community Issue, April 2013.

OVARIAN HYPERSTIMULATION SYNDROME WHILE UNDERGOING TREATMENT FOR INFERTILITY:

CASE: *A 36 years old lady was admitted with abdominal pain while undergoing treatment for infertility with ovarian stimulation therapy. The patient was suspected to have ovarian hyperstimulation syndrome and gynaecologist decided her to admit the patient under the medical team for treatment.*

DIAGNOSIS: Possible ovarian hyperstimulation syndrome.

DISCUSSION: Infertility is a common problem in clinical practice and the primary care physicians and internists are frequently involved in the decision making.

CAUSES OF INFERTILITY:

30% male causes	30% female causes	30% no cause is detected
- Azoospermia	- Tubal blockage - Endometriosis - Ovarian problem	- Immunological causes

With newer technology and *in vitro* fertilization (IVF) technology and laparoscopy surgical techniques for tube blockage and endometriosis, the rate of fertility has increased along with ovarian stimulation therapy. Instillation of single sperm in the uterus during ovulation as determined by ultrasound techniques, many yield good results. In patients with tube blockage, the egg and sperm after retrieval may be fertilized outside the body and implantation in the uterus (IVF). This technique was first introduced by Patrick Steptoe and Robert Edwards in the UK. In India the first test tube baby was pioneered by Professor Subhash Mukhopadhay, however he did not receive due recognition by the medical faculty and finally committed suicide as he was criticized by the then medical community and was not allowed to attend the international conference to demonstrate his research.

In patients with azoospermia even with one single sperm which can be incorporated within the egg called ICSC technique; however it is an expensive technique.

In patients with uterine problem, surrogate motherhood is also a possibility where the fertilized egg may be implanted in another woman's uterus. The legal implications of surrogate motherhood are outside the scope of discussion in this book.

FURTHER REFERENCES:

- Harrison's Principle of Internal Medicine 17th edition.
- Oxford Text Book of Medicine- 5th edition.
- An article written by Dr. Gautam Khastagir Indian Express, Consultants' Pearls.

METASTATIC CANCER WITH UNKNOWN PRIMARY:

It is a frequently confronted situation by the clinicians and many times exhaustive tests may be elusive. In addition to an oncologist, an internist's opinion is frequently needed in such conditions.

TYPES OF HISTOLOGICAL OR CYTOLOGICAL DIAGNOSIS:

- Well differentiated adenocarcinoma (60%)
- Poorly differentiated adenocarcinoma (30%)
- Malignant undifferentiated neoplasm (5%)
- Squamous cell carcinoma (5%)

CLINICAL EVALUATION:

Focus investigations like gastroscopy, colonoscopy, bronchoscopy, MRI scan and CT scan of different organs.

- ➢ Tumour markers:
    - α fetoprotein
    - CEA
    - PSA
    - CA-199
    - CA-125
    - β HCG

They may be particularly helpful in monitoring the response to therapy.

- ➢ Immunohistochemistry and molecular profiling may be helpful in pinpointing the exact source of the primary cancer.

TREATMENT:

It is usually treated platinum based therapy with response rate of 25-35% with a survival rate ranging from 6-16 months. Visceral based diseases have a poorer prognosis (6-9 months) compared with nodal pleural or peritoneal disease (14-16 months).

FURTHER REFERENCES:

- NEJM- Cancer of unknown primary site- August, 21st 2014, Vardhacharya G.R., 371: 757-765.
- Harrison's Principle of Internal Medicine-17th edition.
- Oxford Text Book of Medicine- 5th edition.

ALTERNATIVE MEDICINE:

CASE: *While in the ward round a relative of an incurable cancer patient asked would I have any objection in the relatives trying homeopathy or Ayurveda medicine to treat the patient. I told them that I had no objection as with modern medicines I was unable to provide any relief.*

DISCUSSION:

I strongly feel that we should encourage alternative medicines in India. A glaring example on one hand is China. Its indigenous treatment like acupressure has yielded very good results. China encouraged indigenous medicine in their country which has helped treating many people at a low cost. In India we should also encourage alternative medicines like AYUSH (A – Ayurveda, Y – Yoga, U – Unani, S – Siddha and H – Homeopathy) as a complement to modern medicine which is costly and not affordable by a huge number of poor people who are below the poverty line.

Citing an example; a patient is infected with *Acinetobacter* infection which is a deadly bacterium. The drug of choice is colistin (maximum dose 3 million units thrice daily) the cost of which is around Rs. 6000 per day. Further research suggests addition of penems improves the cure rate. Cost of penems is around Rs. 6000 per day. Clinical research suggests the ideal duration of treatment should be for 14 days. The majority of the patients may need ventilator support and ITU support and regular investigations as these drugs are toxic. So taking all these into account the approximate cost per day comes to be around Rs. 30,000 and the total cost for 14 days will amount to Rs 4, 20,000. One cannot imagine a poor person without any insurance cover to afford this costly treatment. Only upper middle class patients and middle class patients with insurance cover can afford such treatment. If such a patient is admitted, the doctors are bound to follow this mode of treatment for 14 days as that is the approved protocol. If a socio-economically marginalized patient gets such an infection the doctors are in "Horns of Dilemma" as they know very well that the patient cannot afford the treatment but sometimes are forced to follow the guidelines being apprehensive of medico-legal hazard if something goes wrong with the patient. With this background it is easy to imagine why alternative medicine may play an important role in India where a huge chunk of the population is below the poverty line. We should encourage research in the field of alternative medicine.

I can site one example where patients who were symptomatic of severe neuropathic pain got relief by undergoing acupuncture and acupressure therapy. Both these alternative modes of treatment are affordable.

Modern medicine is bound to stay and flourish and provide miraculous cures for incurable diseases in the future with the advent of stem cell therapy, genetic engineering, modern gadgets etc. However, in India and other developing countries alternative medicine also have a role to play. Hence research in this field should be actively encouraged by the Indian government and I am sure with proper research the horizon of alternative medicine particularly Ayurveda medicine can be broadened.

CONFLICT OF INTEREST IN MEDICAL RESEARCH AND PRACTICE

While in the ward round a patient relative asked me regarding a reference made in two popular Bengali movies about various privileges granted to doctors by the pharmaceutical companies. These are very contentious issues frequently discussed and get a bad publicity against the doctor community. These relationships create conflicts of interest when physicians accept company gifts of various kinds including meals, drug samples, etc at the expense of the pharmaceutical companies. This is also reflected in the contemporary movies and it puts the whole community in a bad light. I remember during my initial training in the UK, the hospital academic weekly sessions used to be sponsored by the pharmaceutical companies. However since 1992 while going to work in NHS in UK as a house doctor, I found that there was a big change. For the weekly hospital meeting the doctors have to pay one pound for their lunch.

It is true that throughout the world the pharmaceutical companies play a big role for propagating, medical education among the doctors as a part of their corporate social responsibilities and for that a special monetary allotment is there from the pharmacy house as a part of continuous medical education. But, question arises whether the pharmaceutical companies can invite a doctor to attend the conference directly or not. Here, definitely a conflict of interest arises, as a doctor becomes obliged to prescribe the bounded medications promoted by the particular companies. How this problem can be circumvented?

The funds allocated to these pharmaceutical companies for educational purpose, in my opinion, can be utilized by the following ways:

- To create a corpus fund created by the pharmaceutical houses and involve different academic bodies like API, CSI, diabetic association etc to select the candidate to attend the conference in rotation so that everybody gets a chance to attend the conferences.

- The pharmaceutical houses may approach different hospitals of all levels for suitable candidates and different corporate hospitals management bodies may be involved in selecting the candidates who can avail the opportunity to attend the international conferences in rotation.
- Doctors attending the conference should be imparted with responsibility for CME at district level and rural level, a very useful way of revalidation without undergoing through the paraphernalia that the western countries have taken for revalidation.
- Pharmaceutical housings may directly sponsor those who are faculty members or paper presenters in the conference.

By this way direct conflict between pharmaceutical house and doctor can be avoided. At the same time a wide sector of doctors can get the opportunity to attend the conferences to enrich their knowledge. These doctors in turn may use to propagate their knowledge at a sub-centre level hospital through different seminars. Thus this process may be utilized to revalidate programs that the western countries have adopted.

This is very controversial topics; however I should ventilate the ideas to take opinion from the medical communities. However, those doctors attending for a paper presentation and faculty of the drug companies may directly sponsor from them.

105

ROLE OF PREVENTIVE MEDICINE IN LIFESTYLE DISEASE
A lecture delivered to general people in a Rotary meeting

INTRODUCTION:

India is a country with double burden. On the one hand we have the age old problems of infection, malnutrition (it still continues to be a major problem), on the other hand there is emergence of life style disease hitherto unique to the west due to rapid economic development in one sector of the population. These include 1) HTN, 2) DM, 3) Obesity, 4) IHD, 5) Dyslipidaemia, 6) Smoking related problems, 7) Cancer to some extent 8) New kind of infection called nosocomial and 9) environment related problems. Fortunately many of them are preventable, which is important and these life style diseases not only cause increased mortality and morbidity but also poses a huge financial burden.

- **HTN:** In India 10 million people are not aware that they are suffering from HTN, 25% of urban population and 10% of rural population are not aware of presence of HTN.

- **DM:** 7- 8% of the world population die due to direct or indirect effects of DM. It is major cause of blindness throughout the world. In India its incidence is increasing exponentially and it has been projected that, by 2025 about 50% of world diabetic population will come from India.

- **IHD:** Ischemic heart disease is also quite rampant in India with its unique prevalence in the younger population.

- **Cancer:** Nearly 2 million people of India suffer from cancer with a yearly death rate of more than 550,000 people. Some of them are preventable.

- **Asthma/COPD:** Increasing asthma/COPD incidence is directly related to environmental pollution which is increasing in India.

- With the advent of ITU/ICU there is emergence of novel kind of infection called 'Nosocomial infection'.

- In many of these instances, preventive approach with control of HTN, DM, smoking, obesity and exercise can prevent many of the life threatening dreadful conditions to a significant extent.

- Environment related problems: These can be kept away by preventing pollution and conservation of the nature and natural resources.

What is the evidence?

The evidence emerges from the '7 countries study' conducted during 1957-1962 with follow up upto 15 years in 7 countries including European countries, USA and Japan (the only Asian country included in this study). A lot of useful information emerged from this study which showed that those who have sedentary life style, should have DM, HTN, obesity, have high cholesterol and tend to suffer much from heart attack and/or brain attack.

Amongst these risk factors, high cholesterol was found to be the single most important factor as evidenced by the incidence of heart attack in Japan and Finland. In Japan smoking rate was high, but heart attack rate was low because Japanese people have a low level of cholesterol which is genetically determined. In contrast, in Finland, the patients used to exercise more, with less incidence of smoking. Still the heart attack rate was high .This was because; in general their cholesterol level was high, which superseded the protective effect of exercise and lack of smoking.

Let us take the issue of hypertension which is a silent killer. It usually does not cause symptom but strikes suddenly in the uncontrolled, with the devastating effect of cerebral haemorrhage, heart attack, kidney failure or haemorrhage in the eyes. So routine check-up of BP is mandatory for everyone after a certain age as a part of general check-up and if found high should be controlled with medication either one, two or sometimes combination of multiple anti-hypertensives. This is important as medical therapy alone will be fruitful when the target BP is achieved which is below 140/80 mmHg. There are certain situations where the target should be even lower.

Diabetes mellitus is another silent killer if not controlled adequately. Since it is an asymptomatic disease in the initial stages, the only way to detect it is by routine check up of blood glucose in high risk patients with family history of diabetes. Like hypertension, it also strikes suddenly– heart attack, brain attack, kidney failure, blindness etc. Any organ may be affected, if blood sugar is allowed to remain high. If oral medicines fail to control the blood glucose, insulin should be added sooner the better. Again achieving target is an essential part of treatment lest the desired benefits will be apparent. The targets are fasting glucose less than 120 mg%, postprandial glucose less than 180 mg% and HbA_1C value less than 7%. The last test is done to identify the errant patients who sometimes hoodwink doctors by producing satisfactory fasting and PP reports by meticulously taking medicines for few days prior to the blood tests. However HbA_1C reflects the overall control of glucose over last 3 months thereby detecting those patients who are actually cheating themselves.

Fortunately diabetes may actually be prevented. Studies have shown that regular exercise can prevent development of diabetes. In this study a number of population were divided in two groups– one group underwent vigorous exercise and the other group led sedentary lifestyle. After 5 years, it was found that those groups of people who underwent vigorous exercise had lesser number of patients who developed diabetes compared to the other group. Similarly, weight reduction, low salt intake and regular exercise also help control blood pressure to a significant extent.

Obesity is another risk factor affecting the Indian population. Obesity particularly the central obesity is dangerous in the sense that, the fat in the central abdomen inactivates body's endogenous insulin which in turn leads to hypertension, high cholesterol and myriad adverse effects which leads to diabetes, heart attack and high BP. This is known as **metabolic syndrome.** The only way to circumvent it is to regular exercise, walking and low caloric diet.

High cholesterol is another risk factor. As a matter of fact 3 types of fats are of clinical importance, like **LDL**- which is a bad cholesterol, the deposition of which in the vessel walls gives risk to blocking of arteries, **Triglycerides**- which has similar effects to some extent and **HDL** which is good cholesterol by virtue of its power of scavenging the fat deposits from the vessel wall by a reverse transport mechanism. The ideal value of LDL should be below 100 mg%, Triglyceride below 150 mg% and HDL above 45 mg%. Regular blood tests are very important in this regard as any deviation may be brought back to the target level by diet and medicines like statins.

Dietary use of oil is a very much discussed issue amongst the lay people. In simple terms, dietary fats can be divided into saturated fat which is invariably bad– like ghee, Vanaspati (solid fat at room temperature), butter etc. Unsaturated fats may be divided into– polyunsaturated fat, which is further subdivided into N3 and N6 and mono-unsaturated fats. None of these unsaturated fatty acids are singularly beneficial as all of them have a mixture of good fatty acids and bad fatty acids in them. So ideally one should use such oils which have varied combination of different fatty acids like vegetable oil, safflower oil, even occasionally mustard oil. It is of note that olive oil, rape seed oil contain good amount of mono-unsaturated fatty acids which is protective for the heart. However, I am not sure whether these oils would suite the palate of Indians particularly Bengalis who make *Hilsa* or *Pabda* fish.

Drugs may also be used for preventive purpose. Dain, the aphorism 'one aspirin a day really keeps the doctor away' is really true. It is a contention issue if used in low risk patient; perhaps it is not as the side effect of bleeds outweighs its beneficial effects. However in high risk patients' with hypertension, diabetes, high lipids it is worth taking the risk as the beneficial effect of preventing the stroke or heart attack is commendable. This I mentioned as a primary preventive strategy only. In cases of secondary prevention, meaning someone who has already had an event, it is a must in all cases. Similarly, cholesterol reducing drug statin has also been shown to prevent the first heart attack or brain attack, if used in middle aged population with high cholesterol level but without any prior history of any attack. This was brought out in an epidemiological study in Scotland where a subset of population was divided into two groups either receiving statin or placebo (dummy medicine). Like aspirin, statin is a must in all patients with an attack as a secondary preventive strategy.

Occasionally vitamins are also helpful in rare conditions like deficiency of homocysteine which is a hereditary disorder and predisposes one to heart or brain attacks at an early age. Otherwise they are not recommended for routine use. Similarly, role of fish oil is not firmly established. In post menopausal women hormone replacement therapy was popularly used for preventive purpose which has been recently found to be of no benefit, on the contrary it may do some harm.

Coming to cancer which is sometimes lifestyle related or occupation related. Smoking is the single most important culprit responsible not only for lung cancer but also the cancer of throat, stomach, oesophagus, urinary bladder etc. Obesity is also indirectly related to some cancers like colon cancer. In males, routine screening with PSA to detect prostate cancer or periodic X-ray chest in patients with chronic cough, haemoptysis should be done. For females, periodic mammography, PAP smear for cervical cancer screening should also be done. Any bleeding through rectum should be investigated with colonoscopy to detect early colon cancer.

With the advent of critical care units many lives have been saved by judicial use of life saving gadgets and interventions. However it has left one major problem while saving lives, it can create problem in the form of nosocomial infection. Hospital acquired infection is a dreadful condition affecting all critical care units globally with high mortality and morbidity. One of the major reasons of spread of infection is through the hands of doctors, nurses and relatives who visit the patients and touch them. Hand washing before survey of a patient is the way forward to prevent it.

Over the last few years the numbers of asthma and COPD patients are increasing exponentially. Apart from smoking, environmental pollution is an important contributing factor. Fumes, belching gases from the errant cars, buses and autos, emending construction of roads and bridges are one of the major factors towards it. Many of my young patients get apparently cured when they go for jobs or studies overseas where pollution is relatively less.

This summer there were unusual admissions of patients with pneumonia, undiagnosed fever with mortality. I am certain that these unusual cases were related to an unusual weather condition with temperature hovering around 41-43°C. Kolkata did not record this kind of dry heat in the past. Experts say that this is all due to climatic change - Global Warming. True we have been talking about this global warming as a part of past time gossip or intellectual discussion in seminars and talk shows or enjoy thriller movies about global warming, about rising water levels and melting glaciers. However, I feel it is not a matter of casual discussion but a very serious matter in our day to day life and we all have some positive role to play to prevent it. Rampant filling up of water bodies and construction of high rises, felling of trees, inviting more people and cars in an infrastructure which is not capable to handle it leading to overcrowding are some of the causes responsible for it. Moreover, emission of greenhouse gases due to use of fossil fuels are compounding the problem more. True India is progressing and power is needed, energy is needed. However, we must remember that the civilization is at cross roads.

On the one hand there is question of progress and advancement and on the other the mere existence of civilization is at stake. We need to reduce the use of coal, gas and oil and instead increase more renewable energy like solar, hydroelectric, atmosphere and perhaps nuclear energy in order to reduce greenhouse gases. In the environmental conferences, the developed and developing countries are bashing each other as to who is responsible towards the menace of 'carbon' emission and the concept of 'carbon' credit has been raised. While we may not have a lot of say in these issues, as a common man we should take a vow that in individual capacity we should maintain greenery, plant trees, protest against illegal closure of water bodies, make sure that cars and buses comply with the emission rules, consider green autos and maintain the East Kolkata wetlands for our buffer zone- which works as a ventilation lung for this polluted city. In London at its heart, an 11 sq-km forest has been maintained untouched to maintain the ecological balance. In Kolkata, we should resolve to do so as well for the sake of every dweller of the city. So, as a citizen while talking on lifestyle diseases I would also include environmental factors.

May we take this opportunity to vow that in addition to preventive aspects of conventional life style diseases we should also concentrate on environmental factors. We should protect the greenery, raise our voice against illegal filling of water bodies, create noise against air pollution by the erring vessels, press on early construction of roads and above all maintain East Kolkata wetlands. 'THE WORLD CONFERENCE OF PUBLIC HEALTH' held in Kolkata in Feb, 2015, we used this platform to raise these issues so that appropriate policies may be formulated.

EXPERIENCE OR EVIDENCE?

CASE: *An 84 years old diabetic, hypertensive patient was admitted with cerebrovascular accident. On examination, the patient was unconscious; there was evidence of gross left hemiplegia. His hospital stay was turbulent with development of nosocomial pneumonia needing ventilation and ultimately tracheostomy, renal failure needing dialysis support and development of a pressure sore. He underwent multiple medical consultations from neurologist, neurosurgeon, chest physician and nephrologist. Fortunately he could be transferred out of ITU to HDU and after 5 weeks of intensive therapy, he was discharged home with tracheostomy tube in situ with advice of domiciliary nursing support and advice for regular domiciliary physiotherapy and medical checkup.*

Although from medical point of view the nurses and medical team were very happy in sending this critically ill patient home which by any standard was thought to be a lost case. Many questions were being raised from the relatives, point in view mainly regarding the cost of treatment, occasional communication gaps in informing the exact clinical status of the patient, occasional lack of co-ordination particularly in carrying out the instructions from various specialists which were sometimes divergent in nature, occasional apathetic attitude from some of the medical and nursing staff and finally the formation of a pressure sore. A complaint letter written to the hospital administrator, made the entire medical and nursing team demoralized. Fortunately, things settled amicably following a prolonged conversation with the relatives and finally they left the hospital with a happy note.

DISCUSSION:

The aforementioned case depicts not so uncommon scenario in modern day clinical practice. Where, in spite of best efforts, application of modern technology the relatives feel far from happy about the overall approach in spite of apparently successful outcome following treatment. This again raises so many important issues which perhaps is pertinent to each and every country of the world as evidenced by enormous increase of litigation, complaints, media attention either in western country like USA or UK as well as in India. With the advancement of medical technology, better diagnosis and treatment facilities and above all much better overall treatment outcome with increased survival from any disease, this kind of discontent and disillusionment is indeed unfortunate and unwarranted.

What is going wrong?

We are perhaps getting too technical in dealing with our patients as an object rather than a human being. Perhaps we have become more precise but lost the humane and sympathetic touch so essential in treating ailing patients. Very frequently our predecessors drop names of famous physicians of yesteryears who had great healing powers and frequently compare with the present day degrading and degenerating standards.

But is it true? The great physicians of the bygone days were indeed great, they could diagnose without the help of any gadgets but while treating all they had had sympathy and empathy and most of their patients with MI, serious infections etc would die yet at the end of the day they were hailed as heroes while in spite of better treatment and survival, the present generation medicos are frequently dealt with suspicion and sometimes with contempt. I find similar scenario in the UK National Health Service, where the old generation patients were much happier with old system and values in spite of the sea change in the overall survival of the patients in last 2 decades. I feel we should offer sympathy, empathy and a humane approach as much as possible. In addition to our professional calling, we should also have some service orientation. During medical selection, this should be borne in mind and special points should be allocated for service orientation in addition to the academic brilliance. It reminds me of a famous saying from one of the great physicians which we read in the medical schools *"we can cure only* a *few, alleviate some but solace everybody"*.

Role of communication:

The second question that was raised in this case was communication gap. This is really a big issue and I have found it a very distressing issue particularly while dealing with patients having multiple divergent problems with input from different specialists. The communication to the relatives should be precise and at least twice a day by the resident doctors and once a day by the in-charge consultant. The communication from the nursing team should run in parallel and there should be coordination between the nursing and medical communication. Nurses should communicate regarding the development of the any pressure sores as many times the relatives are not aware of it till the discharge which usually has many adverse consequences. The pros and cons of the treatment plans should be communicated daily along with its cost implications. No doubt it is quite labour intensive and consumes a lot of hospital resources in appointing adequate number of nurses, doctors and other ancillary staff. Nevertheless, I feel this is absolutely essential in order to dispel the misgivings that are clouding the minds of patients group in recent times. Sudden unexpected death and natural death in elderly population are occasionally encountered in hospital practice. Medical team with the help of the nursing team should have the mechanism to deal with such events as it may lead to violent emotional outbursts from the relatives.

Who takes the charge?

Frequently patients with multifaceted problems get admitted in the hospital and doctors from multi-specialties are involved in the management. In such cases, the internists can take charge of the overall care of the patients although the primary problem may not be related to his specialty. His role is usually a band-master who orchestrates between the different subspecialists to give a well directed management goal after filtering informations from different circles. Failure of such a coordinator may lead to serious miscommunication which may adversely affect the outcome and may even cause serious medico legal problems. Internists can definitely play such role effectively. This is particularly important in critical care area where such kinds of patients are usually admitted.

When to take second opinion?

Frequently in hospital practice relatives ask for a second opinion. While working in hospital practice over the years, I found a second or third opinion is helpful in certain situations such as:

- At the request of the relatives, should never be denied and should be of their choice. If the primary physician disagrees with the choice and the relatives are insistent, it would be prudent to transfer the patients under that consultant following mutual agreement.
- In obscure, undiagnosed cases where the patient is chronically suffering without any definitive diagnosis. Undiagnosed prolonged fever is one such example.
- Where diagnosis has been confirmed but progress is not satisfactory, as in MI with prolonged chest pain, arrhythmias or cardiac failure in spite of treatment as protocol.
- When specific organ involvement is present. It is always prudent to consult a nephrologist in renal failure, or a chest physician if asthmatics when patients are not responding satisfactorily to the standard treatment or a neurologist in a stroke patient with delayed recovery or a surgeon in case of acute pancreatitis etc.
- In patients where a medico legal problem is anticipated it is always advisable to involve the senior most doctors for his opinion.

While taking second opinion, the views and opinion of that person should be communicated directly to the relatives and properly documented. Frequently in critically ill or terminally ill patients relatives request opinion from specialists of alternative medicine. The treating doctor, in my opinion should not object to it as long as there is not much to offer from his or her side.

CASE: *A 56 years old patient was admitted with a 5 days history of fever. The reason for admission was that his family members noticed his eye ball movement was intermittently abnormal. He had a long history of joint pain and swelling for which he had not had any investigations and was treated with painkillers on as and when required basis. Examination revealed synovial swelling of the small joints of the hands consistent with rheumatoid arthritis. There was evidence of bilateral VI nerve and VII nerve palsy. Rest of the examination was normal. His WBC count was 15,000. CRP high and RA factor was very high. CT brain scan was normal. LP revealed cell count 4, all lymphocytes, protein 120 mg% (↓), normal glucose, NCV study at this point did not reveal anything specific. Over the next 48 hours his condition deteriorated with increasing confusional state (Na^+- 122 mmol/l) and increasing retention of secretion in the oropharynx. He was transferred to HDU where he was intubated. MRI scan of brain with contrast revealed multiple small infarcts bilaterally.*

Neurological consultation could not give a specific diagnosis and suggested a differential diagnosis of atypical GB syndrome, viral encephalitis and rheumatoid vasculitis although the investigations did not classically fit with any of the aforementioned causes. After consultation with the neurologist the patient was empirically started on IV acyclovir for 10 days, IV gamma globulin (25 g/day) for 5 days, IV ceftriaxone. Steroid was recommended but withheld for initial few days and started from the 7th day when the CSF report for Herpes simplex DNA per report came back as negative. The patient was transferred to ITU.

On 8th day onwards I went for a scheduled study leave for a week to participate in a national conference, handing over the case to another physician colleague of mine. This was explained to the relatives adequately. So far the relatives were regularly communicated regarding the gravity of the situation, uncertainty of the diagnosis and possible outcome of the condition. Although very concerned, they were reasonably satisfied about the care given to the patient. On my return after 7 days, I found the patient was transferred to HDU and intubated; he was afebrile, on IV steroids, conscious but obtunded. On meeting the relatives I could see change in their attitude and expression, aggressiveness in their attitude and suspicious about the medical approach. My colleague had to face difficult situation and on the request of the relatives, took two opinions (one from another neurologist, another from a physician who had seen the reports only). The neurologist who saw on the 12th day thought atypical GB was unlikely and probably it was a case of viral encephalitis. The physician who also saw the report on the same time thought that atypical GB syndrome was unlikely and thought that IV gamma globulin was not indicated.

These two statements by two doctors who were not involved with the management in the initial turbulent phases of the illness ignited the anger and frustration among the relatives who thought that treatment with an expensive medicine was unwarranted and detrimental to the patient's health (the patient was not under insurance cover).

Fortunately the patient could be extubated in next few days and following intensive physiotherapy, left the hospital in an alert and conscious state walking with some help.

While dealing with this patient, prolonged discussion that used to take place with the relatives on daily basis has been narrated in the next few paragraphs.

QUESTION: We got our patient admitted under your care referred by our distant relative. Why did you go on leave requesting your colleague to look after?

ANSWER: It was my scheduled study leave. I looked after him for 7 days prior to my leave and before I left I transferred the patient under a consultant colleague of mine and we usually reciprocally cover each other during our holidays.

QUESTION: But we did not know the doctor- we only relied on you.

ANSWER: Like any other profession, doctors need their break, holidays, study leave *etc.* One cannot work 24 hrs a day, 7 days a week and 365 days a year. There must be prospective colleague cover. Sick patients are getting admitted on regular basis and we ensure proper colleague cover round the clock during our absence.

QUESTION: Was there any justification of using an expensive medicine (gamma globulin) without any proof of the diagnosis?

ANSWER: We frequently use empirical therapy in serious life threatening conditions where delay in therapy may cost life. Medical science does not always follow rules and many patients do not present in a copy book manner and we in such cases usually exercise our experience and clinical judgement. On this occasion I and a senior neurologist thought that here was enough clinical evidence to justify the use of gamma globulin and delay could have caused problems.

QUESTION: Two other opinions taken later on did not agree with your decision of giving gamma globulin.

ANSWER: Opinions may differ. Moreover it is always easier to comment with a hind sight. The real challenge is to decide during the acute situation. I am still confident about my differential diagnosis and I justify my therapeutic approach. Even if for arguments sake, he did not have atypical GB syndrome, the therapeutic challenge had done no harm to the patient.

QUESTION: We are spending so much of money, yet the diagnosis is not forthcoming and the patient is not getting any better.

ANSWER: We feel very sorry but I must admit it is a very difficult situation. Recovery from illness is not always guaranteed in all situations and certainly cannot be equated with the money spent. Although it is expected to make a definitive diagnosis in each and every case, in clinical medicine there are certain grey areas, where the exact diagnosis remains obscure and the doctors have to work on probabilities. Moreover, more and more such case becomes complicated the cost of treatment soars further because of increasing number of tests requested and uncommon and expensive group of medicines used in such cases.

DISCUSSION:

This case presentation raises few important issues for discussion. In well structured health care system, round the clock resident cover with impromptu decision making capacity (*e.g.* registrars and senior registrars) and consultant colleague cover during leave is a natural phenomenon. In India, this may be sometimes lacking leading to occasional serious medico legal problems. While working in a hospital setting, the concept of proper teamwork must be ensured. The junior team with decision making capacity should be able to provide 24 hours cover for the medical care with proper responsibility. During official leave there must be prospective consultant cover as well which must be officially recorded.

Ideally during admission of a patient, it should be contractually agreed upon that the total package of care will be provided by the team under the leadership of that particular consultant. This approach may allay lot of misgivings and misunderstanding amongst the doctors and patient that are so frequently faced in current day medical practice some of which even going up to medico legal level. Holidays and leave should be officially recorded. In clinical practice in India, multiple opinions from different non-treating doctors are commonly taken at the request of the relatives. While appreciating that such opinion should be unbiased independent and whole heartedly geared to the welfare of the patient, it should not be unnecessarily provocative against the treating medical team which might arouse suspicion among the relatives and create unnecessary confusion without serving any useful purpose. This is also common problem noticed in day to day clinical practice sometimes assuming medico legal importance. The medical fraternity of the future years should take cognizance of this fact to the overall benefit of the patients and doctors alike.

CASE: *Jocky Rahman, a 68 years old person from Bangladesh attended the clinic with his son who was suffering from prolonged fever. Mr. Rahman came to Calcutta 10 yrs back with his medical problems and since then we have been good friends. He is a person with humble means, a farmer by profession and had little formal education. He comes from a remote area of Bangladesh fringing the Sundarban forest area and bordering India. His son, had fever for last 4 months and initial investigations were inconclusive.*

Examination revealed gross anaemia, spleen just palpable. He looked cachectic. He underwent detailed investigation for FUO which included ANF, ANCA, Ig electrophoresis, different inflammatory markers, CT scan of abdomen, different tests to exclude tuberculosis. The cost of the tests amounted to more than Rs. 15,000 and he initially flatly declined to do those test for financial constraints. Finally a selected number of tests were carried out with negative results. At last a bone marrow examination revealed presence of LD bodies and a final diagnosis of Kala-azar was made.

DIAGNOSIS: FUO due to Kala-azar.

DISCUSSION:

While dealing with this patient my friend raised many fundamental questions which I thought is worth discussing.

Mr. Rahman: Nowadays you depend too much on expensive tests to diagnose while the doctors of the older generations used their clinical acumen in diagnosis.

Doctor: But the facilities were limited in those days and there was no way to confirm the diagnosis and chance factor played a big role in those days, I replied.

Mr. Rahman: But patient had a very high satisfaction score while dealings with the doctors in those days.

Doctor: Art of consultation played a big role in those days because of lack of technical facilities, proper medicines. Obviously the technique of consultation had a great morale boosting effect. At that time there was nothing else to offer.

Mr. Rahman: I beg to differ sir, when I was young boy in the last pre independence days (year 1946 before partition), I was suffering from swelling of the whole body. My father took me too many local doctors in Khulna (now in Bangladesh) without much effect. Finally he took me to Calcutta to consult Dr. B C Roy (*legendary physician of all time who later on became the Chief Minister of West Bengal*). Upon entering his consultation room, Dr. Ray stared at me and asked my dad which part of the country we were coming from. Then after a brief consultation he prescribed me some medicine (*quinine*) and warned me that it was bitter in taste and I need to tolerate it. Within 2-3 weeks time, I got completely cured! He did not even ask for any basic tests for me. Today I had to spend Rs. 15,000/- for the investigations.

(Khulna was a district in South Bengal, fringing the Sundarban forests the homeland of Royal Bengal tigers. Malaria was at some point endemic in that area. I presume Dr. Ray clinically diagnosed the case as nephrotic syndrome caused by malaria and offered anti-malarial which proved to be right in his case).

Doctor: I agree that was a great diagnosis but there was a chance factor too. Nowadays we cannot do that. We need to have more evidence. If we prescribe quinine without any evidence and something goes wrong we will be held responsible for an indefensible offence. Nowadays even if we use medicine empirically we need to explain in details the risk benefits ratio of such treatment and keep official record of it. Experience definitely counts but that has to be backed up with evidence.

Mr. Rahman: Whether you call it experience or evidence, they had the healing power. We used to rely on them, depend on them. Apart from their professional calling they had a service orientation. We used to consider them as our friend, philosopher and guide. This kind of respect and trust is rarely evident nowadays.

That day, after a long conversation, I could finally convince him about the changing scenario of modern day medical practice with ever increasing expectation from the patients, rapidly growing cult of consumerism and modern medicine rapidly shifting from emotional and intuitive faculty to a more technical, impersonal and consumer oriented faculty. However within myself I realized that Mr. Rahman was echoing the sentiment of vast majority of patient population in our country and I could also feel similar kind of feeling with a different dimension is also shared by section of patients in the west which I have noticed while working in the clinics of NHS hospitals. I feel that the present day medical community should gear up to the needs and expectation of the patient population, in order to restore and revive the patient-doctors relationship of the golden yesteryears. It is not only the dry statistics or robust scientific evidence what will matter in the final analysis; the art of personalized, sympathetic and caring approach will go a long way to bridge the gap between the patients and the medical community.

What is evidence based medicine?

In the past doctors used to use their personal and anecdotal experience in treating their patients without any firm scientific data, while treating a sore throat with ampicillin successfully it would be impossible to tell that whether it was drug related effect or was it a natural cure. This answer can only be addressed by treating a control group without any antibiotic and see the effect. To have a statistical data of clinical significance, the sample size (both treatment group and control group) should be large, there should be age and sex matched and to eliminate the personal bias in selection, the investigators and the patient population should be unaware in which group the individual patients are allocated (double blind). To improve the statistical power of the study, the study population should be reasonably large by involving patients from different centres (multi-centre) and allocation to the different treatment group should be randomized to prevent bias in selection (randomized trials). After a reasonable time of treatment, the comparison should be made between the two groups that have been studied (outcome study). Nowadays each and every aspect of medical management is guided by this evidence based approach.

What is the hierarchy in evidence based medicine?

The best evidence is obtained from double blind, randomized and multi-centre study. However meta-analysis of different studies of similar nature also provides robust evidence. Systematic review (a review of several studies addressing one question) also provides a high grade of evidence. Evidence can also be obtained from unblinded non-randomized studies. However their statistical power is somewhat limited. Finally case report, advice from expert panel also can be used as evidence albeit of much lesser statistical power.

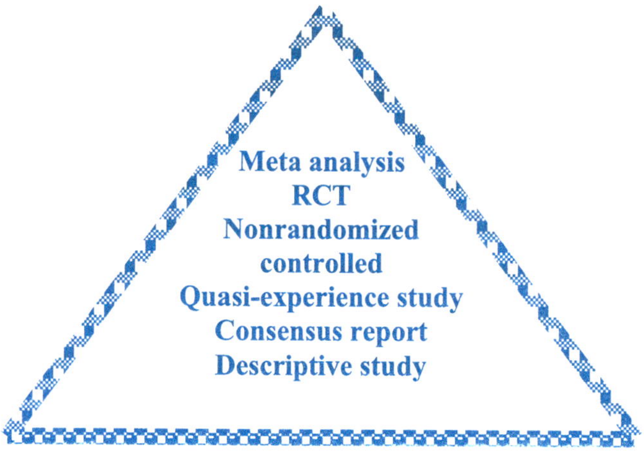

Now-a-days medical therapy is largely guided by evidence base and anecdotal experience only is rarely taken into consideration in minority of the clinical issues. However there are some limitations of evidence based medicine, such as-

- Evidence based medicine is experimental and does not fit into that particular patient we are dealing with.
- It may miss patients experience to the treatment, quality of life.
- It may be biased and may favour intervention only on issues with commercial interest.
- It cannot answer all questions and may not be accessible to everyone.
- It may be biased and critical appraisal of the scientific paper is needed to detect the bias.
- Evidence base changes continuously and one need to keep abreast of such changes as the clinical practice needs to change in accordance with it.
- Most of the randomized studies are conducted in the Western World and in India we are simply extrapolating those data to our indigenous population without keeping in mind that there are major differences in genetic predisposition, different drug susceptibility pattern and different drug dosage schedule.

CASE: *A 56 years old lady attended the follow up clinic with chest pain. She was on HRT for last 3 yrs which I prescribed for her on the basis of clinical evidence at that time. On examination NAD, BP- 160/90 mmHg, LDL- 146 mg%, EGG- normal.*

I immediately asked her to stop HRT to prevent her cardiovascular risks and she took it as a surprise as 3 years back, I suggested her to start HRT to reduce her post menopausal cardiovascular risks! I quoted these diametrically opposite scientific observation in the same journal published over a period of 3 years. She was asking me whether this treatment had done harm to her which I could not explain satisfactorily.

This case exemplifies the controversial role of Evidence-Based Medicine (EBM). Although this is not a common situation, one needs to be even alert regarding this. In the past, we have seen many drugs like nifedipine, steroids in sepsis albumin in critically ill and of late amlodipine had been relegated as a potentially harmful agent and later on again successfully rehabilitated in clinical practice. So while applying EBM in clinical practice, one needs to be alert and scrutinize the evidence thoroughly. More over one needs to be continuously updated through different journals.

CASE: *A 56 years old patient from the periphery attended the clinic with some common gastrointestinal problems. On examination he was found to be hypertensive with a BP of 170/90 mmHg. Routine tests revealed blood glucose mildly raised, high LDL, high triglyceride, ECG revealed LVH. Routine gastrointestinal investigation did not reveal anything specific. He was given lipid lowering agent, anti hypertensive, ACE inhibitor and beta blocker, antioxidants aspirin and metformin and he was requested to come at follow up at 2 months with repeat blood tests.*

The discussion that took place during his second consultation has been narrated below.

Doctor: How are you doing?

Patient: Horrible, no relief of my symptoms.

Doctor: But I find your LDL and Triglyceride values are on spot. Sugar is well controlled and so is your BP.

Patient: My constipation is as it is. My gas problem remains unabated.

Doctor: I am sure you will have much lesser chance of having a brain attack or heart attack and you have achieved the target given by the American Diabetic Association (ADA).

Patient: I do not have any heart or brain related symptoms to start with and I am sick of taking so many tablets for which I have no apparent symptoms. Moreover, I think I am getting drug related problems as well. I feel nauseated, developed a muscle ache along with cough and I have lost the libido, none of which was present before and my original problem of constipation and gas persists. Finally, I had to take some over-the-counter ayurvedic medicines which gave some relief of my symptoms. Please do something about it and reduce the number of tablets if possible.

That day, I realized that the patient's perspective and the doctor's perspective are entirely different. Although, perhaps I would have been given full marks by the American Diabetic Association, I have failed miserably in the eyes of my patient. I think, we need to combine both the scientific evidence and patient's expectation in order to deliver the best to our patient community.

THE TEAM WORK:

CASE: *A 46 years old lady was transferred to ITU because of postoperative sepsis with organ dysfunction following a routine gastrointestinal surgery. She was critically ill and needed ventilatory support, inotropic support, haemodialysis and transfusion of several units of blood products. Drotrecogin alfa was considered but rejected by one of the consultants who were in the medical team. She was under the care of a visiting consultant. A medical team was formed to look after the day to day progress under the supervision of the visiting consultant with involvement of several other consultants (both in house and visiting) from different specialties. The resident doctors of the ITU provided the baseline day to day care. Since our ITU is an open care system, the visiting consultant was the final arbiter in any important decision making process (The pros and cons of open vs. closed ITU care will be discussed in the different issue).*

Her 6 weeks stay in the ITU was quite turbulent with lots of cliff hanging ups and downs with several near-misses. Although there were moments of individual brilliance, in the final analysis it was the team work that paid rich dividend in saving her life. At each and every step it was found that many of the team members were taking credit for any positive progress of the patient and many of them doing so at the expense of other fellow members of the team.

One resident doctor claimed that he saved the patient from inevitable death by changing the ventilatory parameters which his colleague in the previous shift set it all wrong. Another doctor claimed that the patient was nearing choking to death because of wrong intravenous fluid management schedule which he detected in time and saved the patient from disastrous consequences.

One thing was common however, whenever there was a crisis or setback, the nursing team was always at the receiving end. It was the nurse who was responsible for all the wrong doing!! After 6 weeks of struggle the patient got better. The observant patient who was fully conscious for the last 3 weeks of her stay, made a very important and relevant statement in a thanks-giving card which is very pertinent to be mentioned here - "It was the triumph of an excellent team work led and co-coordinated by the nursing staff which made the difference between my life and death". After all it is the team and not the individual player that makes a winning team in modern day clinical practice.

WHERE EXPERIENCE FAILS AND EVIDENCE IS A FANCY DREAM:

CASE: *An 18 years old boy was admitted in the ITU under the care of the nephrologist with acute fluid overload state. He was oliguric, severely breathless needing ventilatory support and dialysis. He also had several convulsive episodes during his stay. He had a history of chronic glomerulonephritis. On the 6th day, the relatives decided to discharge him against medical advice purely because of financial constraints. So he was transferred in an intubated state to a district nursing home in the town where he came from with an accompanying doctor from the ITU team. The nursing home initially refused to accept him as there was no facility for artificial ventilation or renal replacement therapy. Finally, due to repeated plea from the relatives of the patient, they accepted him but could not give any hope for survival.*

The poor parents finally took him home with a local doctor, called the relatives for the last rites and started making advanced arrangements for his burial. The doctor prayed to the God, took the endotracheal tube out and disconnected the IV fluid line and then something unusual happened. The patient opened his eyes and asked for water in a feeble voice.

By this time 4 weeks have elapsed, we discussed about the patient with sympathy and empathy and finally forgot about him. One fine morning, I saw his dad knocking at my OPD clinic room. He was accompanied by a young boy standing at a distance. I thought that the gentleman has come with a lot of grievances against the hospital regarding the treatment of his ailing son who must be dead by now. On the contrary, he was very obliging and grateful for looking after his son. I asked him what happened to his son. He pointed towards the young boy standing in the corner. I could not believe my own eyes and thought I was seeing a ghost. Then he narrated the whole story which was fascinating.

No, he did not come to the hospital for any compensation or to take the hospital authority to human rights commission. He simply came to get a reference for a hospital where dialysis could be carried out at a cheaper rate. His mother will be probably donating her kidney, should renal transplantation be offered at an affordable price. I was dumbfounded. I did not know what to say. That day I finished my clinic early and pondered throughout the day- what saved this brave boy- our experience, scientific evidence or an invisible hand of the Almighty.

(This case has been mentioned after discussing with Nephrologist)

WHERE EVIDENCE IS NOT ALWAYS APPLICABLE:

CASE: *A young and smart medical representative entered my consultation room to promote a new drug for prevention of osteoporosis. He gave many scientific evidences in favour of the drug. Although being convinced about the efficacy of the anti-osteoporotic drug, I expressed my inability to use it in my clinical practice because of monthly expenditure of Rs. 20,000 for that preventive drug only. The young representative was insistent and gave lots of examples from the western literature in favour of that drug.*

I mentioned that although in last one decade India has made great scientific advancement in the medical field and the gulf between the Eastern and Western medicine has been narrowed down to a great extent, the vast majority of India is still not geared as yet to this kind of medical treatment and direct extrapolation of western medical practice to Indian scenario will create more problem than solution. Moreover, inadvertent use of very expensive medicine on prophylactic grounds only may even cause conflict of interest amongst the medical community, pharmaceutical house and the patient population. During the conversation, a junior colleague of mine who was also participating in the discussion commented that although we have made very good progress in last one decade, we cannot jump the queue to catch up with the west. Biting more than our chewing capacity will only cause indigestion. We should expedite our progress taking into consideration of the ground realities in the Indian context. Each and every health care system has gone through trials and tribulations, success and failure before reaching a steady state and ours' should not be any exception. We should first attempt to standardize and protocol wise management of common medical disorders prevalent in our country, we should first ensure that prognosis and outcome of common diseases prevalent in India are uniform; we should first try to control and prevent common communicable diseases prevalent in India. After these goals are achieved we shall be ready for the next step.

BEING ON THE OTHER SIDE OF THE BED:

Unfortunately for last 3 weeks I had been on the other side of the bed. Not as a doctor, but as a patient. Every experience that a person goes through, he learns something from it. And being on the other side of the bed was a great learning experience for me. I was a serious patient who underwent brain surgery. No doubt my friends, my relatives and my family were by my side and they gave me confidence. But I felt that the ultimate confidence, ultimate reassurance comes from within. A smiling doctor in the ward round, a nurse's sweet voice during waking me up for bed tea, discussions from junior doctors coming everyday was giving me reassurance and confidence. It was really a great thing that a patient might expect from his doctors. A doctor treating and talking to a patient mechanically does not mean anything. Coming with one problem and developing other problems is really a big thing. The problems that I faced within 24 hours during my stay at the hospital after the operation were acute anal fissure and constipation. I understood then what constipation means, what fissure means. We always do not pay enough attention to such problems of constipation and always take them in a lighter view particularly in patients with serious problems like heart disease or brain disorder. But now I realize through experience that no problem is small and no patient should be ignored, once you go through the pain and suffering yourself.

To my junior colleagues small little problems of patients are always small to the doctor but they are big to the patients. But we should take care and be patient with their problems. My brain surgery was done by a very well known, highly reputed brain surgeon of India, under local anaesthesia. He always came to me with a smiling face, gave me confidence and gave me courage. These are the things I learnt being on the other side of the bed. During my radiotherapy sessions, the oncologist's caring voice always gave me a huge reassurance. To become a good doctor and knowing Harrison's and Oxford Textbooks of Medicine is definitely necessary and important but if it is not combined with sympathy, apathy and empathy it will mean nothing. Mere technology, no matter how sophisticated it is, cannot supplant these basic aspects of medicine.

: KEY POINTS :

- To the patients, end justifies the means as far as the medical treatment and relief of symptoms are concerned.
- For the clinicians service orientation is an important part in clinical practice and it should be combined with the professional calling.
- During medical selection, due consideration and points should be given for aptitude, service orientation *etc.* in addition to the points scored in mark sheets.
- Communication skills are a very important part in medical practice and proper training should be imparted in this regard during the formative years of training.
- Evidence based clinical practice is the way forward to practice modern day clinical medicine.
- Experience should be expediently combined with evidence, while executing the evidence in clinical practice.

107 DOCTOR-PATIENT RELATIONSHIP AND THE CONSUMERISM

The doctor patient relation is a burning issue as evidenced by the number of increasing law suits against the doctor in different forums. This is an ominous sign as doctor and patient had enjoyed a very cordial human bond which cannot be equated with other inanimate consumer related issues which usually are not always a human relation and although we are always making people aware of their consumer right and giving call 'rise consumer rise'. As far as the doctor-patient relation is concerned in this bracket, it has done more harm to the society than good to the society as a whole, since doctor patient relation is not an inanimate object but a deep bond of human relation.

Let us first discuss the role of doctors to reduce this conflict and encourage ethical practices.

As a whole the doctor should follow some important guidelines in their practice. These are:

- Professionalism in practice
- Maintaining knowledge and skill
- Maintain safety and quality
- Work as a team
- Maintain trust
- Work with honesty and integrity

'No greater opportunity, responsibility and obligation falls on the human being than to become a physician in case of the suffering lot of patients. The doctor needs the medical skill, scientific knowledge and human understanding, sympathy, empathy and human mental understanding, all of which are expected from a physician.' For 'patients are not merely a bag of symptoms and damaged organs, he is fearful, hopeful and seeking relief and reassurance from the doctor.' The last quote is from Harrison's Principle of Textbook written 50 years back, I strongly feel that over the next 50 years the generalized perception of the patient might have undergone changes in many significant levels although the patients' expectation has changed to some extent because science has progressed. The mental reliability depends on the physician / doctor's relation and even after 50 years the same expectations remain and I feel that even 50 years later the medical textbook will quote the same. Although medical knowledge will increase I strongly believe in Harrison's opinion that one of the greatest qualities of a doctor is interest in humanity which is the secret of patient care in curing the patients. This cannot be measured in terms of consumerism.

The medical science has advanced to great extent, technology has advanced, globalization of health scenario has occurred. Internet facility has added to the knowledge to solve problems. Cost of treatment has gone up tremendously and so many other factors have started making a dent in the relation between doctors and patients which were enjoyed by the doctor and patients for so long. True science has progressed tremendously. Newer technologies in diagnosis has arrived, newer mode of treatment has come. The expectation of the public has increased.

This has culminated into a lot of negativity in the relationship as it is evident by the increasing number of consumer related cases in different forums like:

- Consumer Protection Act (CPA)
    A. District forum
    B. State forum
    C. National forum
- MCI complaints which is increasing in number.
- Malpractice suits
- Criminal negligence

We know about

- Hippocrates's oath which all doctors have to take.
- Codes and ethics settled by respective MCI
- The Declaration of Geneva.
- Declaration of Helsinki

Violation of these may lead to loss of registration.

Hippocrates's oath

I. I solemnly pledge myself to consecrate my life to the service of humanity;

II. I will practice my profession with conscience and dignity;

III. I will give to my teachers the respect and gratitude which is their due;

IV. The health and life of my patient will be my first consideration;

V. I will respect the secrets which are confided in me;

VI. I will maintain, by all means in my power, the honour and noble traditions of the medical profession;

VII. My colleagues will be my brothers;

VIII. I will not permit considerations of religion, nationality, race, party politics or social standing to intervene between my duty and my patient;

IX. I will maintain the utmost respect for human life from the time of its conception; even under threat, I will not use my medical knowledge contrary to the laws of humanity;

X. I make these promises solemnly, freely and upon my honour.

Responsibility has been thrust upon the doctor by different oaths. It is a kind of contract between the doctor and the patient while treating a patient.

In spite of all these ethical laws, problems arise frequently. This problem or conflict may not always be only from the doctor's side, it may be bilateral and only bilateral discussion can sort out the problem.

Let us reiterate that doctors should be dutiful, ethical and practical and the hole of conflict may be plugged by observing various norms and the doctor should remember the oath that he took when he was conferred with degree.

Roles of an ethical and good practical doctor:

- Do the duty towards patient and public always keeping in mind the oath you have taken.
- Duty towards law enforcement providing standard care according to the protocols or guidelines which are applicable to treat the patient in the given set up of facilities.
- Try to follow the guidelines and their regulation by the appropriate authority.
- Do not do anything beyond your technical skill.
- Always take a second opinion whenever needed or opinion from another specialist.
- Always use the right dose of a medicine as scheduled as wrong dose may work as poisoning.
- Do not trial with medicine unless the patient is in a trial protocol approved by the ethical community.
- Do proper documentation in BHT or prescription on regular basis. Do not over write or insert false data which is a criminal offence. Frequently this is exposed as it does not tally with data documentation elsewhere particularly nursing data or admission data sheet. Data interpolation is caught commonly.

- In my opinion OPD and in-patient documentation should be duplicated and maintained for a period as required under prevailing level, as data tampering from outside has also been discussed.
- Verbal communication with relations regarding the prognosis should be done regularly and documented in BHT signed by the relatives. I feel in the future disc documentation may be required as many times the deposition from both sides differ tremendously. In my practice I have communication sheet which needs to be signed by doctors and relatives on regular basis and this practice has over last one year yielded fruitful results.
- Filling up of insurance related forms must be done carefully. The documents must be filled in by the patients and then counter signed by the doctors. This is particularly relevant regarding duration of HTN, DM etc. False documentation will put the doctor in problem.
- Financial honesty should be maintained
- Unnecessary unusual hiking of fees put the doctors in bad eye and leads to mistrust between the doctors and the patient.
- Fee splitting should be avoided. In my opinion other doctors indirectly related with the treatment of the patient should make upfront billing as he is also providing service.
- Another big issue is commission from hospitals or labs. Personally I do not support it. But this practice has been going on for a long time and similar practice is going on in every profession. So there are many different views on this issue. So to address this problem a much bigger platform and a good debate will be required.
- Look for any pressure sore before admission and document it, as it is a common complaint.
- Look for any bruises or marks of injury.
- Look at the discharge summary of the previous hospital.
- Consult with doctor under whom the patient is admitted before any intervention.
- Do not examine a female patient without a lady assistant.
- Do not forget to remove stitches or to give proper advice for it before discharge.
- Drug allergy and history of pregnancy should be noted in prescription or BHT.
- Check pacemaker regularly with proper documentation, not just with the magnet alone.

- Before MRI please ask for any medical device inside the body like pacemaker, *etc.*
- In pre-operative patients check whether the patient is on any antiplatelet or anticoagulant.
- Before any operation look for any active infection. Note for any colonisation. Active infection should be treated before any operation. In certain cases surgical intervention is required to get rid of the infection. For *e.g.* appendicular abscess, cholangitis, persistent urinary retention. In such cases take a specialists' opinion and discuss the problems with the relatives.
- In dealing with death and bereavement be calm, quiet and sympathetic even in the face of provocation. As Swamiji says 'good words, sympathetic words can break the wall of adamantine'.
- Contact numbers of the treating doctors must be provided (either team, group or on call emergency doctor). The prescription should similarly have contact number of alternative doctor in case of non-availability of primary doctor. During holidays, leaves, except for the weekends the doctor who will look after the patient, their contact number must be there. The transfer of patients or shift of responsibility during the leave period must be contractually signed by both sides of the doctor and in agreement of the relatives who should also sign the document. This document should not only be in the BHT but with the administration as well.
- During emergency admission in odd hours, it is generally expected that the concerned consultant has seen the patient within 4 hours of admission or by an equipotent trained and experienced colleague particularly in super speciality like cardiology, nephrology and neurology. In tertiary hospitals when this cannot be organized, the hospital should provide cover in the line of a senior registrar level of at least 10 years of experience.
- This indicates that tertiary hospitals must have 24 hours cover of senior doctors either full time or by colleague cover. Middle level doctor like registrar will not be sufficient to substitute them as major decisions like angioplasty, dialysis, ventilation, laparotomy and craniotomy needs higher level of consultation of no less than 5 years of clinical experience. Hospitals should be careful about their selection of RMOs according to their background of training.
- In other emergency cases a registrar of at least 5 years experience of critical care exposure coverage will be accepted, although he would be under cover of other senior colleagues under whom the patient is admitted.

- Registrar coverage for a generalized emergency is accepted. But in super speciality as explained before expert coverage must be ensured. Most of the negligence is because of such delay. Appropriate cover system is thus the best answer. The other alternative would be the old times concept of resident surgeons *etc*. However this system would be costly for the hospital and hence needs to be carefully addressed.
- Consent for blood and blood products for transfusion should be taken. Ideally the consent should also been signed by the patient himself (if conscious).
- Consent should be signed properly and unanticipated problems like urgent hysterectomy, ovary removal (if severe bleeding) should be discussed and the relatives should be involved in the discussion.
- Complication of any procedure- be it surgical or medical should be explained in general terms without unnecessarily scaring the relatives. Anticipated problems should be discussed.
- Proper relation should be maintained with the nursing and paramedical staff.
- False certificates should not be provided. Certificates should be attested by patients.
- Illegal abortions and sex determination should not be done.
- The doctors should always be polite with the patients and for small omissions should always be apologetic.
- Maintain professional secrecy.
- If the doctors feel that the patient is not fit to be discharged medically, then the discharge has to be done under risk bond. However, in India many times because of financial grounds relatives press for early discharge. The options would be:
    1. Discharge on risk bond.
    2. Transfer to another medical facility after making appropriate arrangement with the hospital and doctors.
    3. Making appropriate home care treatment on domiciliary basis with help of local doctors with proper documentation.

In case of the first option there may be a possibility of denial of cashless facility. But the doctors should not yield to the pressure from the relatives as trouble may shoot up later on. In the other two options cashless should not be a problem. Moreover reimbursement opportunity is always open for any mode of discharge.

It is not always possible to provide the highest form of medical care, to treat as protocol or to give special care. Negligence is considered when a standard care is not provided. As far as the treatment given concerned is within the standard care, negligence will not be considered. There are different ways of treatment for the same disease and it may deviate from time to time and case to case.

It must be remembered that for an ordinary skilled doctor it is not possible to provide the best availability of treatment for that disease and this is not negligence. A lawyer failing to argue as efficiently and skilfully as Mr. Palkiwala (famous lawyer of India), should not be considered as negligence. One must also differentiate between negligence and complication- which is a common problem, may happen with any medical case. Complication is not negligence, however, one needs to prove that, there was no negligence, but there was complication.

In medical negligence cases Lord Denning the famous judge from UK, who is an Institute by himself, made some very important judgement and observations that defined 'medical negligence'. He mentioned that a mistaken diagnosis is not necessarily negligence all the time. No human being is infallible and at the present state of science even the most eminent specialist may be at fault. Thus a person will be held negligent only if the mistake or diagnosis is so very palpably wrong. That is to say that the mistake was below the level of ordinary standard and he or she was unable to deliver the reasonable level of skill. A charge of medical negligence against a doctor is much more serious than a meagre charge against a simple mechanic. It involves his reputation. The burden of proof is obviously greater. The charges of negligence are very grave, so the proof must be clear. A doctor should not be held responsible for negligence because of errors of judgement and because something went wrong. However, the care should not fall below the standard level of care given by an ordinary person.

"A doctor, in essence, needs to be inventive and has to take snap decisions especially in the course of performing surgery when some unexpected problems crop up or complication sets in. If the medical profession as a whole is hemmed in by threat of action, criminal and civil, the consequence will be loss to the patients. No doctor would take a risk, a justifiable risk in the circumstances of a given case, and try to save his patient from a complicated disease or in the face of an unexpected problem that confronts him during the treatment or the surgery. It is in this background that this Court has cautioned that the setting in motion of the criminal law against the medical profession should be done cautiously and on the basis of reasonably sure ground. In criminal prosecutions or claims in tort, the burden always rests with the prosecution or the claimant. No doubt, in a given case, a doctor may be obliged to explain his conduct depending on the evidence adduced by the prosecution or by the claimant. That position does not change merely because of the caution advocated in Jacob Mathew in fixing liability for negligence, on doctors."- SUPREME COURT YEARLY DIGEST, 2000.

Medical science has conferred great benefits to mankind, but these benefits are attended by considerable risks. Every surgical operation is attended by risks. We cannot take the benefits without taking risks. Every advancement in technique is also attended by risks.

In another judgement Lord Denning, 1954, said that we would be doing disservice to the community at large if we impose liabilities on the doctors and hospitals for everything that went wrong unless it is palpably wrong. The doctor would be more concerned with his own safety than the patients'.

It is notable that too much suspicion of negligence by the attending doctors and too much interference from the court would be a very dangerous proposition and would prevent the doctors from taking any decision and ultimately the patients will suffer. With a Damocles sword hanging over the head, the doctor cannot perform his duty with fear in mind. In 1960, a famous judgement from one of the all time topmost Justice Denning, gave a historical judgement with historical remark. In that particular case a lady was paralysed following some kind of spinal injection which was given in her case. It did not cause remedy but caused paralysis. Although the judgement was sympathetic towards the problem, it also mentioned that if we have to take advantage of medical treatment we should also be ready to accept the small incidence of side effect coming out of it.

McNair J. in Bolam vs Friern Hospital, the following comments were made regarding negligence; it is not the test of a man on top of a clapman omnibus because he does not have the special skills, the test is the standard of ordinary skilled man exercising and professing to have the special skills.

It would be noticed that in the dawn of modern medical science in the early 1950's and 1960's the great judges from the judicial system of UK and India did unforgettable services to save the doctors. The judges included dons like Lord Justice Denning and some other famous judges like Lord Nathan and the famous Indian judge Mr. Chagla (Ex Chief Justice of Bombay High Court). They really stood by the side of the doctors. It was not to support negligence, but the medical profession. They understood that they would have to save the medical profession and realised that this profession would not survive the onslaught and would perish. They did not pamper negligence; they just wanted the doctors to practice ethically and fearlessly.

The proposition of Supreme Court is as follows **(SC Page-1067, Para-VIII to XI)**:

VIII. It would not be conducive to the efficiency of the medical profession if no doctor could administer medicine without a halter around his neck.

IX. It is our bounding duty and obligation of the Civil Society to ensure that the medical professionals are not unnecessarily harassed or humiliated so that they can perform their professional duties without fear and apprehension.

X. The medical practitioners at times also have to be saved from such a class of complainants who use criminal process as a tool for pressurizing the medical professionals/hospitals particularly private hospitals or clinics for extracting uncalled compensation. Such malicious proceedings deserve to be discarded against the medical practitioners.

XI. The medical professionals are entitled to get protection so long as they perform their duties with reasonable skill and competence and in the interest of the patients. The interest and welfare of the patients have to be paramount for the medical professionals.

Still the numbers of cases are increasing. The patients whenever dissatisfied can get remedy from:

- Consumer Court
- MCI
- Legal Court
- Criminal Court

The recent increases of such cases are due to media coverage, encouragement of financial compensation in many cases etc. The complainant has to prove that there is some connection between the damage and the negligent act. He has to prove that there was a lack of standard care to such an extent that it caused bad result. The plaintiff also has to establish necessary connection between the negligence and the ultimate death of the plaintiff. Negligence also must be considered under which circumstance or background the treatment was given. (Judgement given by Mr. Chagla, Ex Chief Justice, Bombay High Court, of very high reputation). It is true that Lord Denning has given great judgement in favour of doctors. Still I would consider that the doctor must be careful as much as possible and make sure that the standard care of treatment is given.

It is hard for one medical man to come forward and condemn the treatment of a brother in the profession and say that he has done this and that is why there was a problem. Most of the times, if he had been in a position to judge the case from the first, he would have done no better.

It is, therefore, clear that the degree of competent care and skill by which the defendant is judged is in such a way as may be expected from an ordinary skilled doctor and not specially gifted doctor. Furthermore, it is necessary to establish a connection between the negligence and death or other sufferings. Sometimes values of an expert opinion is needed to establish the fact whether an ordinary skilled person would have acted in the same manner.

Actions for negligence in India are to be determined by English common law and this principle has been set out for negligence against a medical practitioner by Earl C. J. and Rich V. Pierpoint, 1862 in their words. "It was not enough to make just some mistake. Some medical man of far greater experience or ability might have used some greater care. But the question was whether there had been a lack of standard care and skill to such an extent which gave a bad result. Considering how much treatment was given in a case is a varied phrase which changes as quickly as the shift hues of the heaven."

Nowadays the society has changed. Commercialisation in the name of corporate houses has invaded medical profession. Human values have diminished and economically poor patients suffer. A judge who is a citizen and member of the civic society, I am sure they are also noticing the social decay and in my opinion judges as human beings ultimately will be influenced by such social decay. They are also influenced by the decay of values in society. These factors also play a role in their decision making which is natural. For example a patient who is suffering from *Acinetobacter* infection, his treatment cost per day in a super speciality hospital would be around one lakh per day. This is nobody's fault. But it has a negative impact on the general public and the judges. **This is my personal view and does not represent anybody else's view.**

From medical council point of view (WB) it is often alleged that they are not fair and often are biased. From my limited experience I must say this is not true, they are impartial. Personally one member maybe known to someone but that does not affect decision as panel and ethical committee are formulated in such a way that at least 3-4 members are present. Moreover there are other safety measures like expert opinion and always there is the scope of appeal.

The majority of the medical profession are looking at the commercialisation and lack of human face and erosion of value oriented practice with a sense of contempt. There is a general notion that in medical council doctors protects their colleagues. On the contrary, I have seen doctors who were unnecessarily harassed in the council because of professional rivalry which is bad. I have seen doctors harassed by MCI who have then resorted to defensive practice. I know one doctor who started to avoid elderly patients with multifaceted problems for fear of litigation. It is easy to harass anyone in the society, not only doctors but anyone in any profession. Any person, in any profession can be harassed in their respective councils knowing well it is just harassment and will not yield any fruitful results. That should not be the aim of the society. The aim should be to increase cohesiveness, harmony and togetherness.

Although our point of discussion is medicine, we must realise that the points discussed is a part of almost all profession although not so much highlighted as yet. Unless overall things change, and society starts thinking differently in which the good human qualities are highlighted, the problems will continue. And if medicine is isolated, singled out and attacked, the interest in the profession will decrease and bright students will not be attracted by this profession. This trend is already obvious and people are going for safer career options which are more lucrative. The challenge of medicine will be avoided by younger generation and ultimately do harm to the society.

The best way is to be ethical, professional, be as human as possible, have a human face and in a country like India be helpful for the economically vulnerable section. This much a doctor can do. MCI should be impartial and try to settle the complaints as soon as possible without any bias. True some cases take time because they are complicated. Apart from that no other factor should lead to delay. Media should also play a positive role and realise the future of the profession as they also have an important role to play.

I feel that the society as a whole should have a cohesive and altruist approach. Negligence must be punished but to instigate common people for litigation is not good for the society. Otherwise a bad consequence will ensue; the doctors will be doing unnecessary tests, unnecessary admission of the patient. Then insurance companies, drug companies and the middle man will be benefitted but the ordinary persons will suffer and continue to suffer.

A rickshaw puller suffering from dengue and being asked for platelet count 4 times a day, isn't it ridiculous? Or a labourer getting admitted to ICU having chest pain in midnight advised to take admission in a 4 star hospital for angiogram and angioplasty is equally ridiculous. Though, these are the protocol, these are not possible for them. But the doctors may be compelled to advice in this manner as defensive medical practice. A patient with chest pain, from a remote place, expecting to get Tenecteplase injection of Rs. 40,000 is ridiculous. May be it is legally correct to transfer the patient to higher medical centre in the middle of the night even though unaffordable. But this would just do harm to the society. Although the protagonists will argue, that everyone should get the same care and facility but the present scenario of our country is not such. We all expect that one day will come that everybody will give the same facility. The decision must depend upon the infrastructure, socio-economic stature and other backgrounds should be taken into account. If it not run in this way, malpractice will increase rather than decrease. Treatment should be according to the availability of the facility.

In our society the doctor becomes the soft target and hence harassed frequently but everybody is vulnerable to it. Our goal is to live peacefully. Patients should be safe, doctors should practice ethically and reviewer will be happy. In case of medical negligence, it should not be overlooked and every proper negligence should be punished.

In spite of the carefulness or precautions taken, medical negligence or omission or complication cannot be stopped altogether, it will happen. Our medical council's duty would be to judge it independently without any bias toward any doctor or preference and give an opinion and make difference between negligence and complication, a petty mistake versus a serious mistake.

So far I have seen that, it appears as if it is a battle and doctors are in the battlefield protecting themselves from expected assault from the patients. Actually it should not be like this. They should practice ethically in order to safeguard themselves. And what I have found is, if we deal with this problem in this way the conflict will automatically resolve and the old values of doctor patient relation will again be regained.

We are not looking for a litigious society, everyone fighting against everyone. We want a harmonious society where we can live peacefully, not as a mere consumer or doctor but as useful partners in the society. Too much encouragement of consumerism will do more harm by encouraging more lawsuits, which in India we cannot afford. The benefits will be few but not necessarily to the patient.

Let us raise the slogan we the doctors must practice as ethically as possible.

If there is negligence it must be dealt in the rightful manner, without bias and if necessary expert opinion must be taken. Senior judges with experience should be involved for opinion or an Ombudsman (or senior doctors) who may also add to the noble goal in good safe treatment and not harassment. We are looking for such society which was given by great physicians like Hutchinson, Oslar.

Medical council should be absolutely neutral and try to correlate the problems logically. We should always remember that justice delayed is justice denied. However, doctors should not be unnecessarily harassed and unnecessarily a black mark should not be put on their reputation. In my own experience the West Bengal Medical Council should try to sort out the problems as quickly as possible. But there are other factors like cases also going on in other forums which may cause unnecessary delay. However, it must be mentioned repeatedly that Medical Council should be very much watchful and any negligence should not be spared and appropriate action should be taken without any delay and it would be unpardonable if they show favouritism towards the colleagues. In that event the faith of people on MCI will also dwindle.

If harassment only is the ultimate thing then anyone can be harassed in any forum. It is a big humiliation for a doctor to appear in front of their colleagues and face charges of possible alleged negligence and this may have a negative impact. I have seen doctors avoiding multi-faceted elderly patients with dementia, cancer, *etc.* in fear of litigation. So it will work as a negative impact on doctors and ultimately the patients would suffer.

Doctors must be careful at every step and personally I suggest in spite of provocation, defensive practice should be avoided because it will do great harm to the society. Although there is a lot of provocation I do believe that people will finally understand the beneficial role of a doctor in the society. The society should also understand the situation of doctors and differentiate between negligence and complication as one must remember mistake is bound to happen in any problem.

Negligence causing great harm should never be pardoned. As medicine is a quasi science and it always does not follow the rule of science. I recently had a brain tumour operated. I never had any symptoms; none of my colleagues could pick up the diagnosis. Finally, it was diagnosed by my wife who is a non-doctor and insisted that I should have a brain scan and a diagnosis came out. She asked for not any brain related symptom. She thought I was getting more quarrelsome with her! In medicine this is not negligence, it is a lacunar science and one needs to accept it. The general public must realize this.

A doctor coming from a private medical college will have a different attitude from other doctors. Although private medical college is going to stay we must remember that medical education should mainly be imparted by the government. For that if extra budget requirement is needed it should be done.

Society's attitude change is not the discussion of this book but very much relevant in this discussion as doctors are a part of the society. This reminds me of the famous saying of Swami Vivekananda, the main ideal of education is 'man making'. If we can achieve this goal a lot of evil from society, from any profession will definitely reduce.

Finally, I must say that all sections of the society must wake up to fight the evil of greed, inhumanity and too much commercialisation of their respective profession. I dream to see such a society soon, if we all wake up to the call. **LET US WAKE UP TO THE CALL.**

108 MATCHING COST WITH QUALITY IN HEALTH CARE

A lecture delivered in a critical care conference

With the advent of new technology in the medical field, the quality of care has been improving at a galloping speed and the expectation of the common people is also increasing at a commensurate rate. Although this is a common expectation, the real problem lies in the fact that the cost of quality medical care is also rising exponentially mainly in private sector hospitals which is controlling nearly 50% of the medical care in India. Till now the majority of the health care expenditure is from 'out of pocket' which mix the availability of such care either out of reach of the common people or they need to sell their assets to avail themselves of such care.

With this backdrop the questions come how to provide quality medical care at an affordable price. Although it is a common notion but quality care always escalates the cost of treatment, studies in ITU setting in different countries mainly USA and Canada has affirmatively shown that to the contrary quality care actually reduces the cost of treatment.

HOW?

- In India majority of private hospitals are providing ITU/CCU beds disproportionate to their total bed strength. Ideally in any hospital approximately 10-12% of beds should be earmarked for ITU/CCU. In resource constrained countries the percentage may be even smaller. The Indian services are mainly driven by the sole intention of profit making. The ITU bed charges are nearly 3 times that of the ordinary beds and in many instances without provision of proper infrastructure.

  What is needed is availability of good number of HDU beds (in the proportion of 1:2 or 1:3 with ITU beds) which reduces the cost to a significant extent. Majority of the patients treated in ITU have a low APACHE scoring without any significant number of organ failure needing support therapy and provision of HDU can certainly deal with such patients. ITU should be reserved for patients with to organ failure needing organ support therapy.

- Early discharge from ITU should be incorporated in the policy as unnecessary ITU stay not only increases the cost but predisposes to nosocomial infection.

- Quality monitoring with auditing should be done regularly in ITUs to see the nosocomial infection rate, IV catheter related infection rate, nosocomial pneumonia rate, aspiration rate, occurrence of acute renal failure while undergoing treatment in ITU, threshold for blood transfusion in critically ill patients, incidence of reintubation rate after successful extubation and the rate of successful weaning in COPD patients. Regular process monitoring and auditing will improve the quality without increasing the cost.

- Proper training of the nursing staff should be done which will reduce the incidence of error which may prolong the hospital stay.
- Presence of nursing staff must be ensured during the ward round to reduce the incidence of error mainly during therapy.
- Closed ITU has shown to improve the quality compared to open ITU. In India if an absolutely closed ITU is not feasible, it must be ensured that at least the ITU in charge has a major say in the overall management of the patients along with the primary admitting doctor (dual control).
- Thrice daily consultant round in ITU has shown to improve quality and reduce cost.
- Antibiotic stewardship will automatically curtail the use of unnecessary high powered antibiotics with regard to the dose duration, combination and de-escalation. Regular prescription auditing has shown to reduce the use of unnecessary high powered antibiotics like penems or vancomycin etc.
- Whenever needed generics should be used to reduce the cost. In West Bengal use of generic drugs have reduced the expenditure to a great extent.
- Capping on the price of some selective essential drugs used for life saving purposes should be done (Central Government policy).
- In addition to onsite expert consultation, online expert consultation should be available for the peripheral hospitals which may reduce unnecessary referrals to higher centres thus reducing the overall cost of treatment.
- Insurance cover for the total population should be ensured through governmental efforts. Publicity and awareness programmes should be done regularly.
- Public sector hospitals should be strengthened to cater to the needs for middle income group, low income group and economically weaker section of the population.
- Doctors should not only take a managerial role but also have a leadership role. By continuous involvement with a sense of ownership (both in public and private sectors) they should come up with innovative ideas which will both improve the quality as well as reduce the cost. In the UK such innovative progress has already saved huge money for the National Health Service without compromising the quality.

: KEY POINTS :

- Improving quality of care will reduce cost of care.
- Public sector hospitals need strengthening.
- Use of generics in selected cases will reduce the cost.
- There should be price capping of some essential drugs.
- Doctors should work not only as managers but must take a leadership role.

HUMAN RESOURCE MANAGEMENT
A lecture delivered in an IMA seminar

Why Human Resource is important?

Robots can handle anything still we are dependent on human resources. Technology in today's date has attained its maximum level. It is capable of solving any type of problem but it can't solve problem without human brain, without human creativity.

Human resource management is any project management is nothing but the duty to lead, direct and orchestrate the project team, the customers, the partners and other stake holders. Handling human resource is the toughest problem as we always carry a bag full of emotions, egos which directly affect the productivity. With stress and tension we cannot give 100% of our ability and therefore cannot do proper justice to our responsibilities. Man, machine and material are the three important resources of a project. It is always easy to work with a material, but in case of manpower resources that can only be acquired via contact work and third party vendors. Successful completion of any project depends upon intelligent and diplomatic handling of the manpower.

We live for today, dream for tomorrow and learn from yesterday.

Human Resource Management- 2 roles:

1. A management support role
2. Employee support role, caring for the well being of the employee.

Entrepreneur- Their ability to absorb risk, a manager of an employee is happy to get a month end salary while an entrepreneur does not have that comport. Knowledge of finance and banking is very important.

So far we have been discussing about development of Human resource, in general. However, since this book is, mainly addressed for the medical graduates, special points need to be addressed in terms of 'good medical practice guidelines'. It is difficult to discuss in a short spell and the practice and skill develops with time and experience. Still there should be some general guidelines. GMC has provided some guidelines and principles which may be followed to some extent.

- Being professional in dealing with giving respect to the patients.
- Maintain your knowledge and skill by continuous endeavours and practice. To try to match your experience with knowledge.
- Record keeping must be meticulous like BP, history of allergy, menstrual history etc. Practice safe and keep your work in your own domain of expertise.

- Communicate with colleagues and try to form a team work.
- Maintain trust with the patients and maintain confidentiality. Consider your patient as your partner.
- Act with honesty and sincerity without any discrimination.
- Be honest in financial matters.
- Try to be meticulous if you cannot care, at least alleviate symptoms and do not feel shy to take professional help from your colleagues for second opinion.

A strong bond started at an early career will take a long way to build up practice. Maintain partnership; maintain the trust of the patient. A strong bond started at an early career will take a look way to build up practise. Teaching training and supportive services at every stage are to be maintained.

- ➢ Implementation of CME programmes, computer networking of medical institutes, promotion of IT-based e-health, tele-consultancy, tele-radiology and tele-pathology are necessary.
- ➢ Qualifications and eligibility criteria for different cadres of health personnel need to be reviewed in relation to their job requirements.
- ➢ The public health challenges for communicable diseases, emerging infectious diseases and the growing burden of chronic diseases need strong national policies to support public health.
- ➢ Development of standard policies regarding recruitment, training, career development plan, transfers, promotions, demotions (where necessary), decentralisation, performance appraisal and supportive supervision are very much needed.
- ➢ The task of ensuring the availability of human resources for health in rural areas and building their capacity for public health to be done.
- ➢ Posting of doctors with ample incentives, both monetary as well as non-monetary benefits, such as improved infrastructure conveniences of health care institutions, suitable accommodation, preferential school admissions for their children, increase in the age of retirement from 60 to 65 years, are some significant issues to be considered.

- ➢ There is a need for training more M.Sc. (nursing) personnel to solve the problems of shortage of nursing tutors. Continuing professional development through e-training should also be encouraged.

- ➢ Efforts should be made to establish new medical and dental colleges in the underserved areas.

The quality of a medical doctor is his role not only as a physician or surgeon but also as a manager cum leader. The concept of managership and leadership was proponent more than 100 years ago by Swami Vivekananda. An American system was followed, with greatest CEO who left the world. The concept was the leader who basically play leadership quality and who leads from side, front and beyond.

I sincerely hope the concept of Swamiji again will change in the field of medicine for the coming years and show the world the way.

: KEY POINTS :

- To build a trust between a doctor and a patient
- To develop communication skills
- Keep yourself continuous up-to-date through revalidation programme
- Try to form teamwork for providing a holistic service
- To build up communication with paramedical, nursing and ancillary staff who provides holistic services.

REFERENCES:

Good Medical Practice: GMC

India has 1.5 beds per 1000 populations which are far below the facilities available in China or Brazil where the ratio is 4.3 beds/1000 populations. In terms of medical practitioners there is a huge dearth of doctors to provide a ratio of one doctor per 1000 population. Similarly India would need another 7,50,000 additional beds to the existing 1.5 million beds to cater to the needs of the Indian population. In realistic terms it means that India needs huge number of doctors and building of hospital infrastructure which would need an investment of Rs. 1,00,000 to Rs. 1,40,000 crore investment in the health sector. Since the budgetary provision in the health sector would not be able to cope up with this huge investment, given the present budgetary provision in health the role of private players in the infrastructural development of health sector is becoming increasingly important. As a matter of fact the private spending in health sector has crossed more than Rs. 1,50,000 crore, which is far above the government spending. The endeavours should be to make proper utilization of the private investment for the development of primary, secondary and tertiary care facilities. However the quality control and practising mechanisms need to be addressed by proper accreditation system.

Here comes the role of private medical colleges or medical colleges under PPP (public–private partnership) model in India. At present, MBBS courses are offered by 271 medical colleges out of which 138 are run by government and 133 under private management covering over 31,000 seats in the medical colleges across the country.

To match up with the demand, it is logical to conclude that necessity of private medical colleges under PPP model will increase to supplement the number of doctors that will be required to cope up with the demand. However, government cannot shun away from its duties to the country to fulfil the constitutional pledge to provide health care at an affordable cost to the countrymen and delegate *de nova* the entire responsibility of medical education to the private sector. It should not only continue to develop medical colleges but also should keep continuous supervision on the private medical colleges regarding the quality of teaching, facilities and infrastructure as well as the fee structure to ensure quality teaching and training at an affordable cost. In other words, both the systems should be supplementary to each other to produce medical graduates who will not be entirely self-seeking careerists but also to some extent work to serve in the interest of the country in a need based way.

SELECTION OF CANDIDATES:

- To standardise the education throughout India, common entrance test is the way forward. However the curriculum should be set in such a manner that the students studying in different systems should get equal opportunity and discrimination is avoided. Apart from the common subjects in the curriculum, there should be a methodology to assess the aptitude towards the subject. In my opinion this is very important as in India the doctors are expected to have some social responsibility towards the economically weaker section of the population which is frequently lacking in the present scenario leading to continuous conflict between the medical professional and general public. Therefore in addition to knowledge testing service attitude should also be tested by appropriate means.

- In selecting the site of medical colleges in addition to the big metropolitans, peripheral district should also be selected in a decentralized manner. Mechanisms should be involved in such a way that a percent of the candidates may be locals as 'son of the soil' and later on their service may be utilized to serve the local population for a specified period of time.

- The curriculum should include subjects like 'ethics in medicine', history of ancient medicine in India and the world, training in basic and advanced resuscitation, problem based teaching should be encouraged. The students should be trained about the preventive and social aspects of medicine and they should be aware of the 'National Health Policy' and different preventive and promotive health propaganda engaged by government of India. In addition training regarding managerial and leadership skills along with basic aspects of administrative training should also be imparted either during the course curriculum or during internship period.

- During internship a minimum period of two months of training should be rotated in the block level or state general level or rural hospitals. One year of compulsory service in distant and sub-divisional hospitals should be ensured both for postgraduate and post-doctoral doctors.

- The huge clinical materials available in the district hospitals should be utilized for the training of postgraduate students through the route of recognizing DNB courses in various hospitals. This will open the door of postgraduate training in the district hospital which will simultaneously boost the infrastructure of these hospitals. The utilization of the district hospitals for post graduate training, popularizing, the distant DNB courses by tapping resources in district hospitals will help create post graduate doctors who are needed badly. A mechanism should be adopted so that this post-graduate doctor should be retained in the district hospital. The government also should consider that P.G. degree awarded by the private hospital at a high capital fee is creating a group of doctors who don't have any social commitment and whose only target is recovery of investment. There should be government control on PG programme in private hospitals even.

- Research and development should be encouraged at every stage of medical education. A cadre of highly paid non-practising doctors in the field of clinical, microbiological, pharmacological and in the genetic field should be created to encourage basic research for clinical and epidemiological studies.

- Teaching and training should also be encouraged in the private sector hospitals and a revalidation programme every ten years should be introduced to ensure continuous medical update and maintenance of reasonable standard of practice throughout the cross-section of the country.

- In India, non-registered medical practitioners play a major role in providing medical service in the remote and difficult areas. Their positive role can't be denied and they should be formally trained regarding the short bridging course in order to ensure safe practice in a limited area.

- Nursing care needs strengthening by popularising male nursing training courses which will supplement existing female nursing cadre in many areas like ITU, OT, Orthopaedics and psychiatry sectors.

- Teaching and training of paramedical staff will go a long way in bolstering the health care delivery system. An independent council for paramedical discipline will be a positive step forward towards that direction.

- For foreign medical graduation, 3-6 months of foundation year training in recognized private and tertiary government hospital should be made compulsory in order to ensure orientation and acclimatization towards Indian health care delivery system in addition to MCI eligibility test which assesses theoretic knowledge only.

- Contractual teacher should be appointed mainly in the district hospitals as well as in tertiary care centres to boost up the deficiency of academic staff mainly in the distant hospitals for DNB training.

- A holistic approach involving medical fraternity, paramedical staff, nursing staff and all section of health care workers would not only strengthen the fabric of the educational system but also head Indian medical sciences as the ideal destination in the world.

- Post graduate training in different subjects like pain management, geriatrics, critical care, ultrasonography *etc.* should be made available so that the ordinary M.B.B.S. student without any post-graduation can play a useful role in the society and supplement the P.G. education.

: KEY POINTS :

- Medical education idea will be to create socially oriented doctors who understand the needs of the society.
- While selecting medical students not only the theoretical knowledge but also the service attitude should be assessed.
- DNB should be made popular in district government hospitals which will serve dual purpose of training at grass root level and to supplement the health care infrastructure at district hospitals.
- Post graduate training should be only imparted at government hospitals like MD/MS.
- It is true we need more specialists.
- It is also true we need good general physicians as well.

REFERENCES:

Graduate Medical Education in India.

111 MDEG: MY EXPERIENCE AS A HOSPITAL ADMINISTRATOR AND PLANNER

As a doctor-administrator and as a member of planning team for health reforms of the state, I am really grateful to Ms. Mamata Banerjee, who gave me the opportunity to head the multidisciplinary expert group for the health reform of the state, West Bengal.

It was on 14.04.2012, when the 1st meeting of MDEG was held following the vision of CM under whose guidance this MDEG group was formed with me as a Chairman and many Honoraries both from the Department of Health as well as from outside the department. I started my job as a keen learner with lots of trepidations, and after completing 3 years I am still learning. I owe my gratitude to Mr. Sanjay Mitra (Chief Secretary, Govt. of West Bengal), Mr. Sanjay Tewari (Ex. Principal Secretary of Health), Mr. Moloy De (the Principal Secretary of Health) and Mrs. Chandrima Bhattacharjee (MIC Department of Health), Prof. Susanta Banerjee (DME), Mr. Sathapati (DHS), Mr. Onkar Singh Meena (Director SRSRC), Mrs. Sanghamitra Ghosh (Director NHRM), Dr. Partha Banerjee (from Medical Education); my friend Dr. Tridib Banerjee (Chairman of Multi-task force level looking after to reduce the neonatal mortality in the state), Dr. Indrajit Saha, Dr. Sukanta Sil and the young officers of the Department of Health like Dr. Samudra Sengupta, Dr. Suman Biswas , Dr. Srijon Chowdhury, Dr. Suparna Paul, Dr. Partha Ary, Dr. Partha, Dr. Jayanta Maitra, Dr. Asit Biswas, Dr. Mrs. Tanima Mandal and all staff and faculty of health and medical departments along with my colleagues like Professor Ashutosh Ghosh and Professor Rajen Pandey both of whom are playing an important role in health reform and are the key steering force for the development of health care sector of the state of West Bengal.

After 2 years it is time for reflection to assess the achievements and failures. Not only to rejoice with our achievement but to thoroughly scan and introspect where we lagged behind and why.

Following our recommendation the subgroup visited exclusively tier 1, 2 and 3 medical facilities and ensure that the recommendations reflect the ground realities and not just a theoretical, ‘arm-chair’ based propositions.

Actual recommendation - we took a holistic approach so that each and every hospital in all the 3 tiers, of medical faculties are represented properly.

BROAD RECOMMENDATIONS:

- To develop super speciality service facilities in district medical colleges, cath lab facility *etc.*
- Decentralization of tertiary centres and use second campus hospitals to reduce the congestion at the teaching hospitals.

Few of the recommendations already have been implemented; the major recommendations are as follows:

INFRASTRUCTURE:

- Emergency observation ward in all tier hospitals
- OPD screening clinic in teaching hospitals
- Bed bureaus
- Centralised Path labs
- CCU/HDU in tertiary, districts and sub-divisional hospitals
- Dialysis unit in tertiary, districts and sub-divisional hospitals
- Decentralization in tertiary hospitals
- Eco-friendly environment along with greenery
- Paying beds for medical insured patients.

Our main approach is to take a bottom up approach and consolidate at district level the infrastructure which will automatically strengthen the tertiary centre. With this in mind it has been planned to build up new district hospitals along with emergency observation ward and facility for dialysis, which will reduce the pressure on tertiary hospitals.

The NRH protocol of commencement of SNSU and SNCU at different level hospitals has already started reducing neonatal mortality and West Bengal is playing a leading role in this regard, under the leadership of present Chief Minister Smt. Mamata Banerjee and all the officers of health department with the active involvement of Dr. Tridib Bandopadhyay.

Patient care facilities including medical services:

- Night shelter for the patients relatives
- Drinking water facility
- Information Centre (Rogi Sahayata Kendra)
- Cleanliness with facility for mechanical cleanings
- Hygienic toilet facility
- Security beyond sub-divisional hospitals
- Scavenging
- ECG by nursing staff in emergency
- Proper record keeping

Equipment and gadgets:

- AMC/CMC
- To activate electro medical engineering cell
- Diagnostic lab, under PPP model in district and sub-divisional hospitals
- Auto-analyzer in SDH

Teaching Training and PG courses:

- DNB course in district hospitals
- Post MD/DM service in districts for one year
- Increment of diploma seats or certificate courses
- Academic grant for teaching personnel
- Internship for pathology technicians in the districts for 6 months
- Male nurse / nursing aid
- Allied + paramedical council
- Centre of excellence like
    - Snake bite centre
    - Cerebral palsy centre – Arsenicosis centre

  - Limb fitting centre – for rehabilitation
- Up gradation and creation of new centres
- RSBY- To popularize Rasthriya Swasthya Bima Yojona (a cashless insurance facility)
- Upgradation:
  - Mainaguri R.H –State general hospital
  - Nimpith block hospital – sub divisional hospital
  - Nursing school of Nimpith
- Fair priced shop-which was started before the recommendations
- Evening clinic in the hospitals
- To improve work culture – reward for efficient workers
- Record keeping - Data generation
- Right person in right place and efficient legal cells
- To address the mismatch between GDMOs and specialist
- Upgradation of ward master as facility manager
- Contractual workers to be absorbed into the system.

It is heartening to note that implementation of many of the recommendations have already been started because of sincere efforts from all kind of staff.

These recommendations are at state level. However, I sincerely hope that, the recommendations made to the health department, if successfully implemented, will make a sea change in the health scenario of West Bengal which can be implemented in others states as well. I sincerely feel that by adopting these recommendations, the medical facilities of the whole country will be benefited. It must be mentioned that to make the plan successful, entire team should work with passion and sense of devotion which I find is present and I am extremely optimist about the success of this project with everybody's best wishes. I am extremely grateful to all the Administrators, Professors, Nurses and all staff of Health Department for their active contribution and participation.

PICTORIAL PRESENTATION: 01

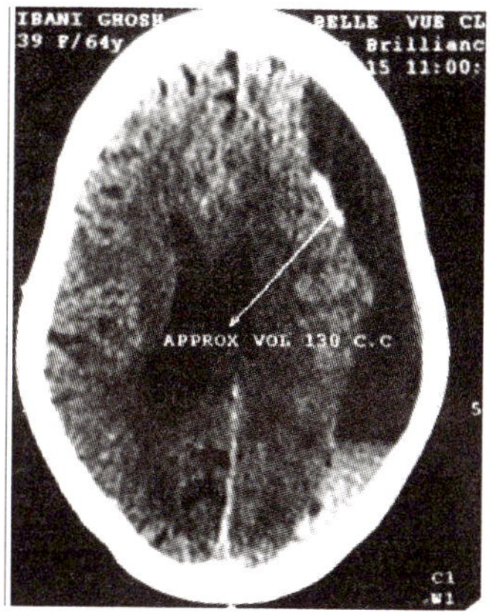

HISTORY:

An 81 years old gentleman with a past history of MI was complaining of increasing confusional state over last few days. This was preceded with a history of diarrhea. His serum sodium was 121 mmol/*l* and electrolyte imbalance with confusional state was diagnosed. However in spite of correction of electrolyte imbalance, he remained confused. A CT brain scan was requested for.

DIAGNOSIS: CT brain scan shows Acute Subdural Haematoma.

DISCUSSION:

CT features of Acute Subdural Haematoma-

60% high density

40% mixed hyper-hypo dense (active bleed from arachnoid)

Chronic Subdural Haematoma- weeks to months after formation usually hypodense may have two layered components- high density bottoms with low density top.

[Ref: Pocket Radiologist- Brain Top 100 diagnosis, Osborn et al, Blaster, Salzman.]

Acute Subdural Haematoma is usually hyperdense in 60% of cases. In 40% of cases it may be hypodense where there is active bleeding. Other situations where hypodensity may be present are-

- Hyper-acute state where there is presence of unclotted blood.
- Presence of underlying coagulopathy can cause isodense lesion.

If the SDH is of few days to 2 weeks duration the lesions are usually Isodense. In chronic Subdural Haematoma which is usually old more than few weeks, the lesion is hypodense. However there may be two layered component with high density bottom and low density top. Bilateral SDH, if isodense may be missed and careful scrutiny is essential.

Chronic Subdural Haematoma is a common cause of confusional state in the elderly and there may not be any definitive history of fall or trauma. Therefore evaluation with CT scan is essential in elderly person presenting with confusional state. Surgical evacuation of clot is curative.

Acute Subdural Haematoma in the background of cerebral trauma, on the other hand has a bad prognosis as it is usually associated with other cerebral injuries.

DIFFERENTIAL DIAGNOSIS:

- Subdural hygroma
- Subdural effusion

PICTORIAL PRESENTATION: 02

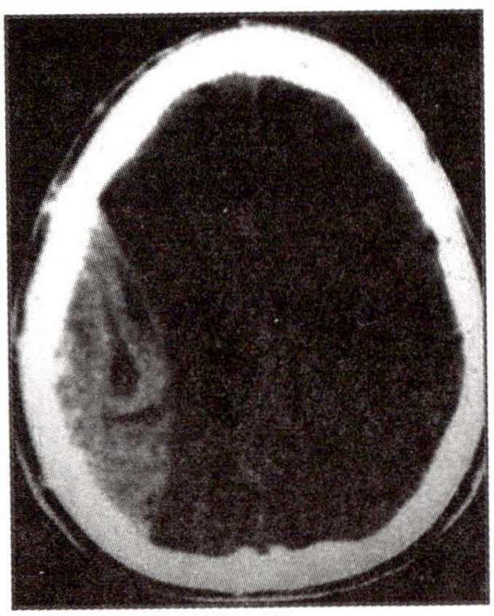

(From: http://en.wikipedia.org/wiki/Epidural_hematoma)

HISTORY:

A 32 years old patient was admitted in the ITU following a road traffic accident. He had multiple bruises of the face and there was a history of ear bleed. There were bruises over the mastoid area. A CT brain was performed.

DIAGNOSIS: Acute Extradural Haematoma.

DISCUSSION:

Acute Extradural Haematoma occurs during traumatic brain injury. Skull fracture to the adjacent bone is commonly associated. There may be counter coupe Subdural Haematoma on the opposite side. Lucid interval is present in significant number of patients.

The CT finding is that of hyper dense lesion with a lentiform shape. [Active bleeding area would show a hypodense spot- Snerl's sign]. Majority of the cases are due to bleeding from the Middle Meningeal Artery. A minority of them are due to dural sinus bleeding. Prognosis following surgical intervention is generally good. Rarely diagnostic confusion occurs with meningioma or dural tuberculoma [both of which enhance with contrast].

DIFFERENTIAL DIAGNOSIS:

- Meningioma
- Dural tuberculoma

PICTORIAL PRESENTATION 03

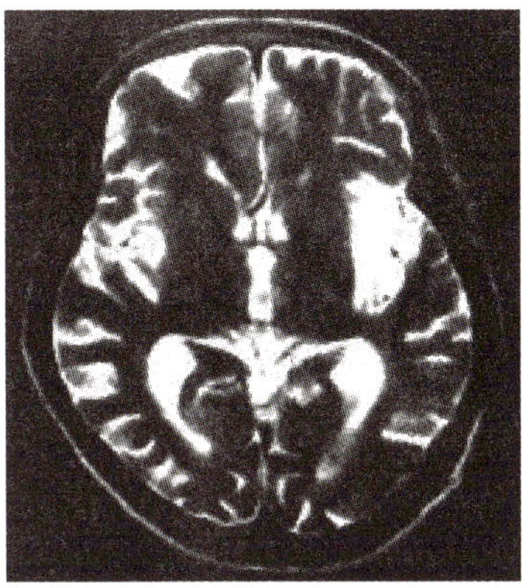

HISTORY:

A 58 yr old patient presented with fever and confusional state of 3 days duration. Clinically he was semi-comatosed without any focal neurological sign, no neck stiffness. Lumbar puncture showed raised protein, cell count 30/field, mostly lymphocytes, glucose 58 mg% (blood glucose 162 mg%), CT scan brain- NAD. MRI brain scan was requested for.

DIAGNOSIS: Herpes Simplex Encephalitis.

DISCUSSION:

Viral menigo-encephalitis is a common presentation in a critical care unit. Although causative organism cannot be identified in majority of cases, herpes simplex encephalitis gives characteristic finding in MRI brain scan.

It involves the limbic system of the brain. The characteristic finding is hypointense T_1 and hyperintense T_2 images in bilateral temporal lobes. Involvements of insula and cingulate gyrus are also characteristic. CT scan of brain is normal in the initial phase of the disease and MRI scan is very helpful in early radiological diagnosis of herpes simplex encephalitis.

PICTORIAL PRESENTATION: 04

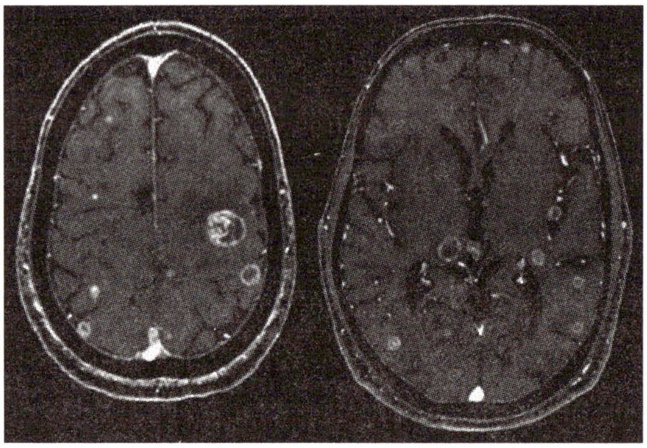

(From: http://radfacts.blogspot.com/2012/07/cerebral-metastasis-multiple-ring.html)

HISTORY:

A 51 yrs old lady presented with headache and confusional state and weight loss. After excluding other metabolic causes of confusion, a CT brain scan was performed.

DIAGNOSIS: Multiple ring enhancing lesions in the brain.

DIFFERENTIAL DIAGNOSIS:

- Toxoplasmosis
- Tuberculoma
- Lymphoma- usually periventricular, may enhance with contrast
- Metastatic
- Fungal infection

DISCUSSION:

Many of the fore-mentioned conditions are common in HIV positive patients and one needs to check the HIV status of those patients [the index patient was found to be HIV positive and her toxoplasma antibody titre was high. She responded with trimethoprim-sulfamethoxazole therapy].

CT scan features suggestive of tuberculoma:

- Solitary or multiple- ring enhancing lesions
- Surrounding edema present
- Calcium in the center with an enhancing peripheral rim
- Additional supportive findings-
  - Basal exudates (with enhancement following iv contrast)
  - Hydrocephalus
  - Cerebral infarct may be present.

PICTORIAL PRESENTATION: 05

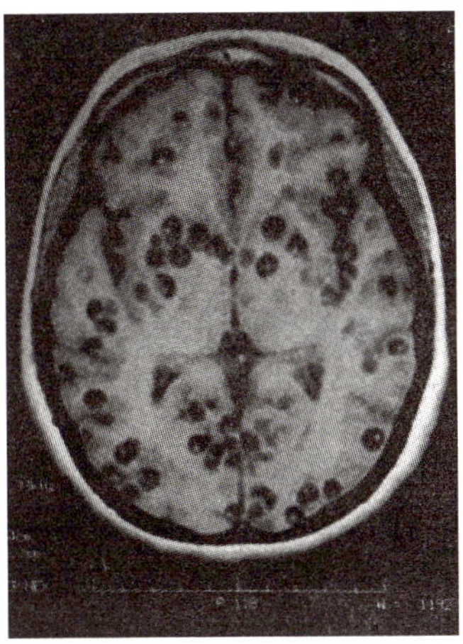

(From: http://www.neurology.org/content/53/7/1582.figures-only)

HISTORY:

A 24 yrs old patient presented with status epilepticus without any prior history of epilepsy. A CT brain scan of the patient was done.

DIAGNOSIS: Cysticercosis.

DISCUSSION:

Cysticercosis, a relatively common condition is also in the differential diagnosis of cystic space occupying lesion and it may be difficult to differentiate from other space occupying lesion like tuberculoma or brain tumour. The diagnostic sign is the presence of a dot inside a cyst (protoscolex). CT findings vary depending on different stages of the parasite development. [No enhancement and no edema in the early stage to enhancement along with oedema in the later stage of development and finally calcification in the nodular calcification stage.]

DIFFERENTIAL DIAGNOSIS:

Other parasitic diseases, though uncommon in the clinical practice, presenting with cystic space occupying lesion in the CT brain scan are-

- Echinococcosis
- Amoebic encephalitis
- Schistosomiasis

PICTORIAL PRESENTATION: 06

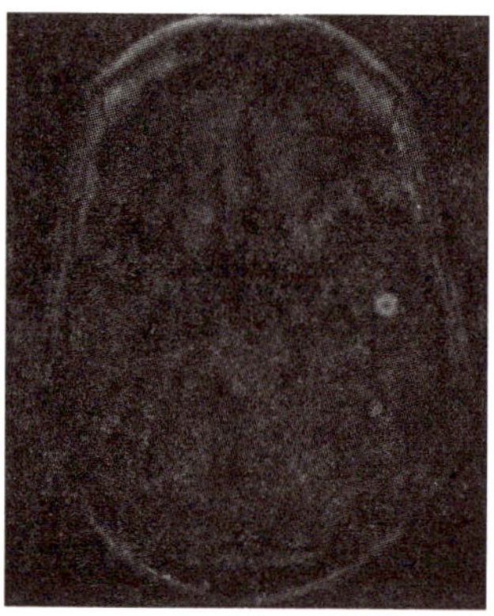

(From: http://radiopaedia.org/articles/tuberculoma)

HISTORY:

A 46 yrs old gentle man presented with history of fever, headache and left sided paralysis of acute onset. A CT scan brain was done.

DIAGNOSIS: Tuberculoma.

DISCUSSION:

The CT scan showed ring enhancing lesion with marked surrounding oedema. His X-ray chest also gave supportive evidence of tuberculosis and he responded well to 4 drugs anti TB regime along with dexamethasone.

PICTORIAL PRESENTATION: 07

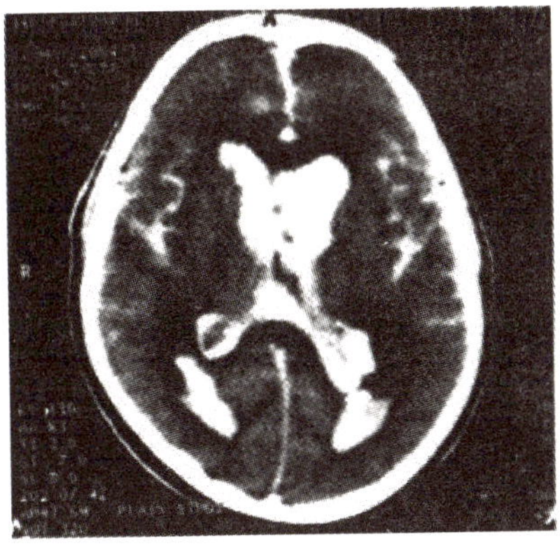

HISTORY:

A 65 yrs old gentleman was admitted with acute onset of headache of thunderbolt type with transient loss of consciousness. Examination revealed semi comatose state with neck stiffness and bilaterally up-going plantar response. An urgent CT scan brain was done.

DIAGNOSIS: Acute subarachnoid haemorrhage (SAH).

DISCUSSION:

SAH is usually due to rupture of cerebral aneurysm. However it can also be due to traumatic brain injury.

CT findings suggestive of SAH:

High attenuation in the basal subarachnoid spaces (without contrast). However, the sensitivity diminishes after one week and CT scan may fail to pick up SAH after 7–10 days. On the contrast MRI scan which has a low sensitivity in the initial few hours is better in diagnosing SAH of some duration. CT brain scan therefore remains the investigation of choice in acute setting.

Once the diagnosis has been made the patient should undergo CT angiogram or MR angiogram to find out the aneurysm as a source of bleeding. The patients should be transferred in a centre where facilities on aneurysmal clipping and endovascular surgery are available.

If the patient deteriorates in the ward, the possibility of complications such as re-bleeding (approx 14% in the 1st 24 hrs), vasospasm with features of ischaemic neurodeficit or hydrocephalus (10–25% cases) should be borne in mind and repeat CT scan of brain is warranted.

PICTORIAL PRESENTATION: 08

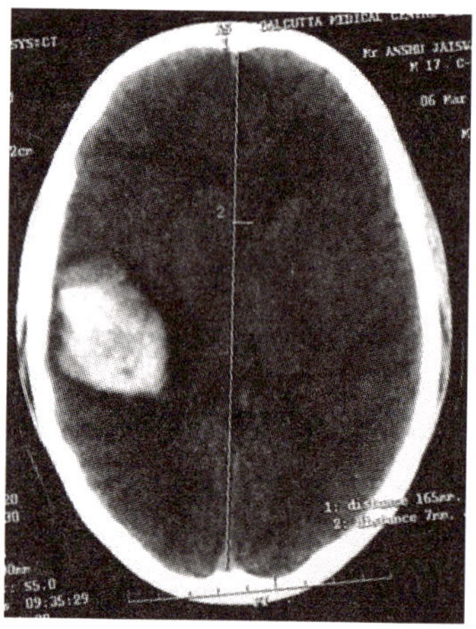

HISTORY:

A 69 yrs old diabetic, hypertensive lady was admitted with sudden onset headache followed by drowsiness and left sided weakness. On examination she had left hemiparesis. A CT scan brain was done.

DIAGNOSIS: Intracerebral haemorrhage (ICH).

DISCUSSION:

ICH is a common presentation in acute care clinical practice and in vast majority of cases it is due to hypertensive bleeding with the location in the basal ganglionic region with occasional extension of the bleed in the intraventricular cavity. The characteristic feature in the CT brain scan is that of hyperdense signal.

There two kinds of bleeding are noted:

1. Deep ganglionic bleeding- in the basal ganglionic region, the characteristic of hypertensive bleed.
2. Lobar or subarachnoid bleeding- which may be indicative of an underlying pathology e.g.
    - Amyloid angiopathy
    - Cerebral Venous Malformation
    - Venous occlusion
    - Bleeding in primary neoplasm
    - Coagulopathy
    - Vasculitis

Therefore, if there is any lobar bleeding or any ICH in younger age group without any history of hypertension, further radiological studies should be done with contrast CT or contrast MR angiogram to rule out other possibilities.

PICTORIAL PRESENTATION: 09

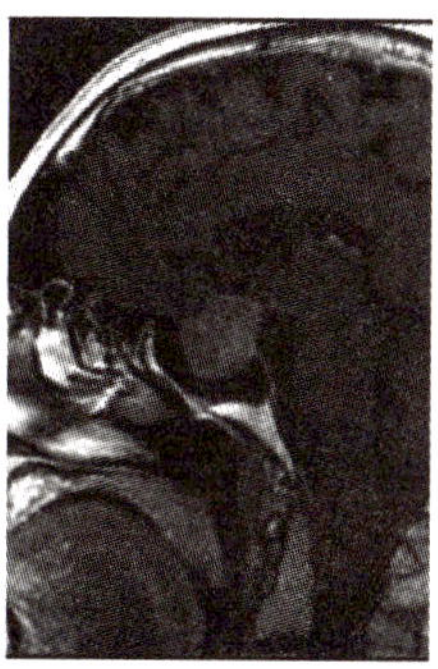

(From:http://www.hopkinsmedicine.org/neurology_neurosurgery/centers_clinics/pituitary_center/pituitary-tumor/types/pituitary-adenoma.html)

HISTORY:

A 36 yrs old medical practitioner presented with a history of fever of 3 days duration and semiconscious state. His wife gave a history of haziness of vision for last few weeks. The couple was returning home from a holiday in Bhutan. His clinical features and CSF findings were consistent with pyogenic meningitis and he made a quick recovery with steroids and IV antibiotics (ceftriaxone + vancomycin) in next 72 hrs his vision remained hazy, however. Initial CT brain scan done at the time of admission suggested a space occupying lesion in the pituitary region. Neurological consultation suggested the additional possibility of a thrombosed aneurysm. Subsequent contrast enhanced MRI brain confirmed pituitary adenoma. MRI angiogram of brain was normal.

DIAGNOSIS: Pituitary macro adenoma of brain.

DISCUSSION:

CT Findings of Pituitary Adenoma:

The lesion is usually isodense with a variable presence of cyst, haemorrhage and calcium. Contrast enhancement may be present.

MRI Findings of Pituitary Adenoma:

Like CT scan the lesions are isodense with intense enhancement with contrast. They have a 'figure of eight' appearance.

The lesions needs to be differentiated from-

- Meningioma
- Thrombosed aneurysm
- Physiological hyperplasia of pituitary gland which is common in women (usually less than 10 mm in size)
- Metastatic disease
- Craniopharyngioma (it is supra sellar in location)

The patient described above underwent quick hormone assessment (FSH, LH, Prolactin, T_3, T_4, TSH, and Cortisol). Visual field checkup showed bitemporal quadrantic field defect and urgently send to neurosurgical unit of another medical facility where he underwent transsphenoidal ablation of the adenoma with rapid improvement of his visual symptoms. He was discharged hormone supplementation with steroid and thyroxin.

PICTORIAL PRESENTATION: 10

HISTORY:

A 76 yrs old gentleman presented with difficulty in walking and difficulty in holding urine with increasing incontinence. His wife has been noticing gradual decline of his intellectual function over last few months. A CT brain scan was done, which shows dilated ventricles, no focal brain damage, normal sulci.

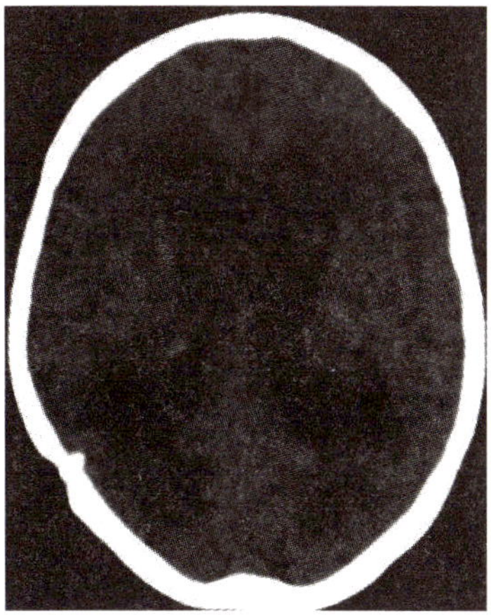

DIAGNOSIS: Normal pressure hydrocephalus (NPH).

DISCUSSION:

During admission he underwent CSF drainage in three successive occasions which improved his clinical status considerably. Subsequently he underwent ventriculo-peritoneal shunt with sustained improvement of his symptoms.

NPH should be considered in any patient presenting with dementia, gait abnormality and dementia along with ventriculomegaly in brain scan. If diagnosed correctly, the patients usually make a good recovery following ventricular shunt.

DIFFERENTIAL DIAGNOSIS of ventriculomegaly on CT brain scan:

- ***NPH*** – uncommon typical symptoms, sulci are not so prominent.
- ***Alzheimer's disease & Age related cerebral atrophy*** – common in clinical practice, dementia more prominent than gait abnormality. Sulci are more prominent.
- ***Multi infarct*** – common in clinical practice, in addition to ventriculomegaly infarcts are seen.
- ***Obstructive hydrocephalus*** – bi-frontal horn diameter / intra cranial diameter > 0.33, temporal horn width > 3 mm, basal cisterns and sulci are compressed or obliterated. Cause of obstruction may be evident – usually posterior fossa mass.

PICTORIAL PRESENTATION: 11

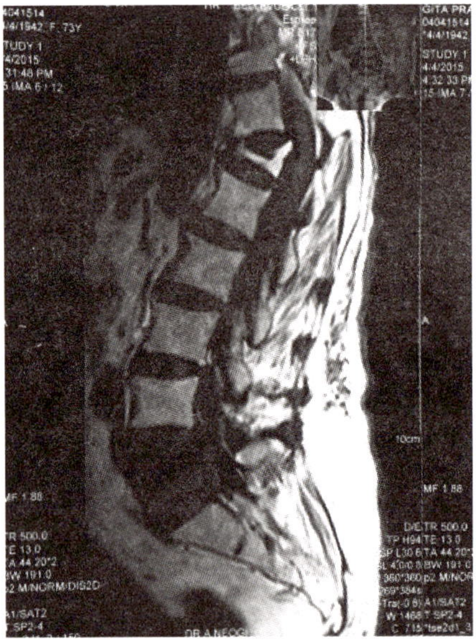

HISTORY:

A 70 yrs old diabetic vegetarian patient presented with mild back pain on and off for last 6 months. X-ray dorsal spine did not give any clue. Of late he has been complaining of weakness of his legs which led to a fall. Examination revealed diminished power with up going planter response (paraparesis) of both legs.

DIAGNOSIS: Vertebral collapse with paraspinal abscess possibly of tubercular origin.

MANAGEMENT: He underwent urgent fixation with bone graft by a neurosurgeon and orthopedician and made a complete recovery from the paraparesis over the next 6 months with anti TB regime and physiotherapy. Biopsy confirmed tuberculosis.

DIFFERENTIAL DIAGNOSIS:

Tubercular osteomyelitis a rather common condition in the Indian setting should be distinguished from:

- Acute staphylococcal osteomyelitis with epidural abscess
- Metastatic bone disease
- Degenerative spondylosis and osteoporotic collapse of the vertebra.

Points in favour of TB (MRI findings):

- Hyperintense T2 image with intense gadolinium enhancement
- Involvement of disc with contrast enhancement
- Associated with paraspinal abscess

In metastasis, the disc space is preserved and there is lack of paraspinal abscess. In staphylococcal lesion the symptoms are usually acute and the patients are usually toxic. In degenerative spondylosis there is no paraspinal abscess and other inflammatory biochemical parameters are negative.

In the appropriate setting continuing back pain with apparently normal X-ray findings, should prompt the physician to do an early MRI scan of the spine.

PICTORIAL PRESENTATION: 12

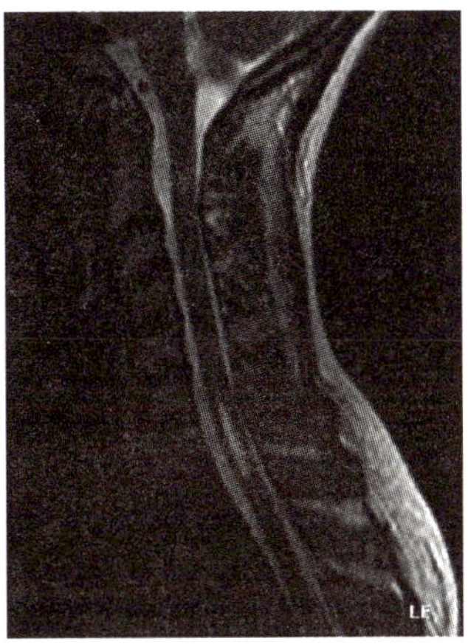

(From: http://en.wikipedia.org/wiki/Syringomyelia)

HISTORY:

A 34 yrs old male presented with neck pain radiating towards both arms, burning sensation of both arms for last few years. He was initially diagnosed to have cervical spondylosis but got no relief from his symptoms. Examination revealed, burn marks of cigarette in the side of the index and middle finger. Although touch sensation was present, pinprick sensation was lost in both the hands. MRI scan of cervical spine was carried out.

DIAGNOSIS: Syringomyelia.

DISCUSSION:

MRI spine shows characteristic features of spinal cord cavitations (*syrinx*). Rarely spinal cord tumour with such cavitations will give rise to such picture (it usually enhances with contrast).

The condition is very rare and presents with pain in the upper extremities with loss of pain and temperature sensation. Later on there may be wasting of hand muscles and upper motor signs in the legs with gait instability.

If the cavity extends upwards there will be features of lower cranial nerve involvement (syringo-bulbia). The condition is treated with drainage of the cavity.

[Ref: Pocket Radiologist Spine, Braut-Zawadzki *et al*, 2002]

PICTORIAL PRESENTATION: 13

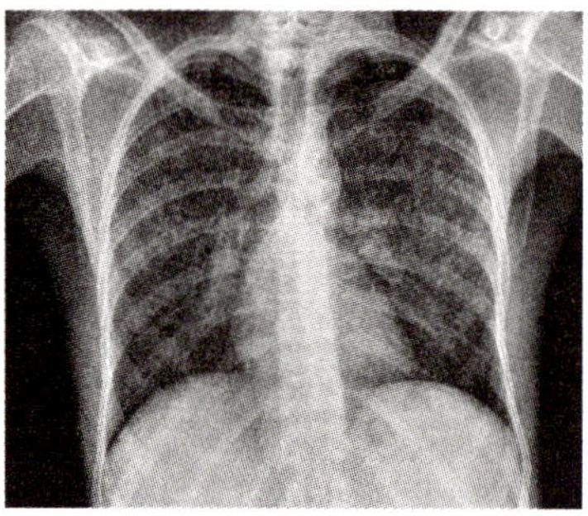

(From: http://westjem.com/case-report/miliary-tuberculosis-coinfection-with-human-immunodeficiency-virus.html)

HISTORY:

A 29 yrs old patient diagnosed to have SLE with neuropsychiatric manifestations and on steroids for last 6 months complained of increasing confusion, abnormal behavior low grade fever and headache. CT brain scan was normal.

On examination he was mildly febrile. X-ray chest showed miliary mottling of both lung fields. Lumbar puncture was consistent with tubercular meningitis (very low glucose, increased protein and cell count with lymphocyte predominance). A chest X-ray and subsequently a CT thorax were done.

DIAGNOSIS: Miliary mottling of both lung fields consistent with miliary tuberculosis.

DISCUSSION:

He responded with four drugs anti tubercular regime.

Differential diagnosis of multiple small opacities in chest X-ray (less than 5 mm):

- Miliary tuberculosis
- Sarcoidosis (bilateral hilar lymphadenopathy)
- Metastasis (relevant history)
- Pneumoconiosis & allergic alveolitis (history of occupational exposure)
- Farmers lung
- Pulmonary eosinophilia (presence of eosinophilia)
- Haemosiderosis
- Fungal infections like histoplasma (in endemic areas)

Diagnostic features of pulmonary tuberculosis:

In primary tuberculosis-

- Lymphadenopathy
- Consolidation
- Pleural effusion

In post primary tuberculosis-

- Characteristic area of involvement– upper lobe
- Cavity formation is common
- Healing is evidenced by scarring and calcification
- Tubercular empyema
- Miliary tuberculosis
- Tuberculoma
- Mycetoma formation in the cavity usually by *Aspergillus fumigatus*

Since the latent tuberculosis is common in Indian population, the clinician should be vigilant of flare up of latent tuberculosis in patient with long term steroids and presenting with non specific symptoms.

PRESENTATION: 14

HISTORY:

A middle aged gentleman presented with nonspecific symptoms of fever, cough, arthralgia, nose bleeding and mild haemoptysis on the day of admission. His chest X-ray showed multiple rounded opacities. On the day of admission he had sudden bout of massive haemoptysis, collapsed and could not be resuscitated. A CT scan done before the bout of haemoptysis revealed multiple rounded opacities.

DIAGNOSIS:

In this particular case definitive diagnosis could not be made as biopsy from the lesion or a postmortem could not be done. However the differential diagnosis in such case would be-

Single

- Malignancy – slightly speculated
- Hamartoma – pop-corn calcification
- Tuberculoma – frequently contains areas of calcification & satellite lesion
- A-V malformation – large draining veins may be seen on contrast CT
- Mycetoma – typical crescentic shadow in the cavity with a ball
- Hydatid cyst
- Fungal infection – mainly in immunocompromised host

Multiple

- Metastasis
- Pneumoconiosis
- Rheumatoid nodule (Caplan's syndrome)
- Sarcoidosis
- Hydatid cyst
- Vasculitis (Wegner's granulomatosis, cANCA – positive)
- Fungal infection in immunocompromised host

Apart from FNAC and biopsy from the lesion, ancillary tests like ANCA, serum Angiotensin Converting Enzyme levels, HIV status, auto immune screening etc would also be helpful in making the diagnosis.

PICTORIAL PRESENTATION: 15

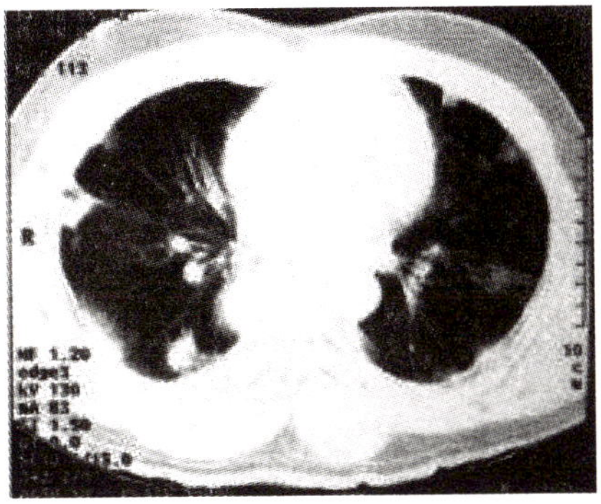

HISTORY:

A young patient was admitted with high fever and breathlessness. He was very toxic and his blood gas analysis showed acute lung injury. Previous to his transfer to this hospital he was treated in a local medical centre with severe thrombophlebitis of his right upper extremity while on treatment, he became acutely ill and was transferred to this hospital. A CT scan of thorax was performed.

DIAGNOSIS: Multiple septic pulmonary emboli – possible source thrombophlebitis of right upper extremity.

DISCUSSION:

Although uncommon this condition should be kept in mind in patients with long term jugular venous cannulation developing acute respiratory distress with toxicity.

DIFFERENTIAL DIAGNOSIS:

- Staphylococcal septicemia with pulmonary involvement
- Vasculitic condition

Both of these can present in similar fashion.

This patient responded to prolonged treatment with vancomycin, meropenem (empirical) and other supportive measures.

[Ref: Butterworth's Clinical radiology for medical study
LT Evan's et al 2nd edition – 1987
Diagnostic radiology – 2nd edition – An Anglo American text book of imaging
Edited by – RG Grainger and DJ Allison 1992]

PICTORIAL PRESENTATION: 16

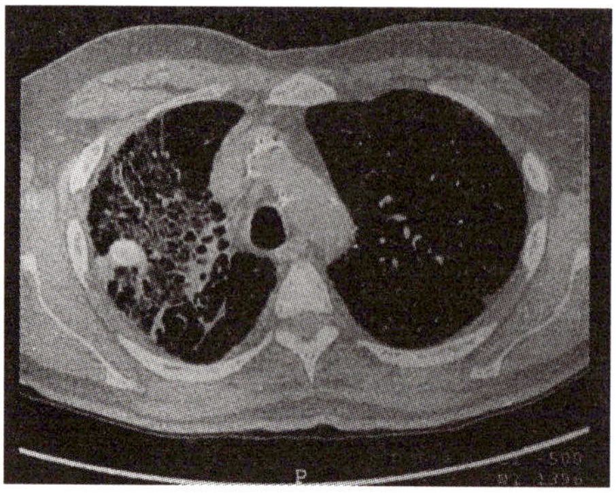

HISTORY:

A 36 yrs old gentleman presented with massive haemoptysis. He was treated conservatively with antibiotics, IV fluid and blood transfusion to which he responded well. He underwent a CT scan of thorax during his stay in the hospital.

DIAGNOSIS: Multiple cystic bronchiectasis.

DISCUSSION:

Bronchiectasis is irreversible dilatation of the bronchus and the mechanism responsible for it is infection and obstruction. The most common causes are due to childhood infections like measles, pertussis or tuberculosis. Malignancy, lymphadenopathy, foreign body etc are the causes of obstruction in the later part of life. Kartagener's Syndrome is a rare cause of bronchiectasis (due to ciliary dyskinesia). Hypogammaglobinaemia and cystic fibrosis are the other causes.

Surgery may be indicated in localized bronchiectasis with recurrent haemoptysis. However in patients with extensive bronchiectasis, it is clearly not an option and the patient should be treated conservatively with antibiotic therapy.

PICTORIAL PRESENTATION: 17

HISTORY:

A 44 yrs old gentleman attends the clinic regularly with hypertension, headache and features of COPD. He is also polycythaemic and needs venesection every now and again. He has undergone CT scan of thorax.

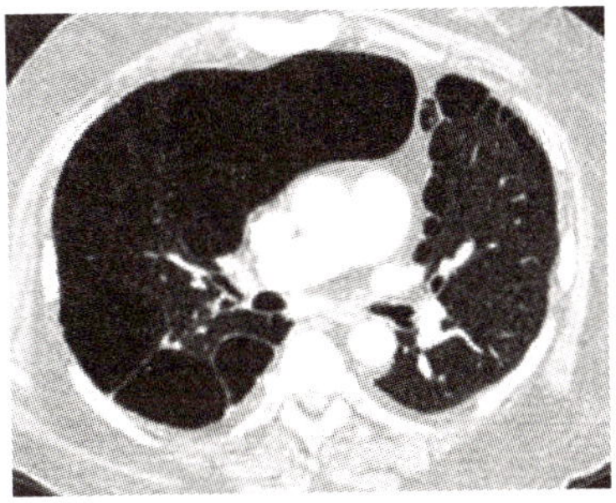

(From: http://www.rheumatologynetwork.com/atrial-fibrillation/giant-bullous-emphysema)

DIAGNOSIS: Multicystic pulmonary disease with extensive bullae formation.

DISCUSSION:

Bullous lung disease is commonly seen in emphysema. However they can occur independent of emphysema. They usually present with respiratory embarrassment and other features like polycythaemia as in this case. Isolated bullae may be treated surgically where as extensive bullae cannot be intervened for obvious reason. The patients need maximization of the treatment of emphysema.

PICTORIAL PRESENTATION: 18

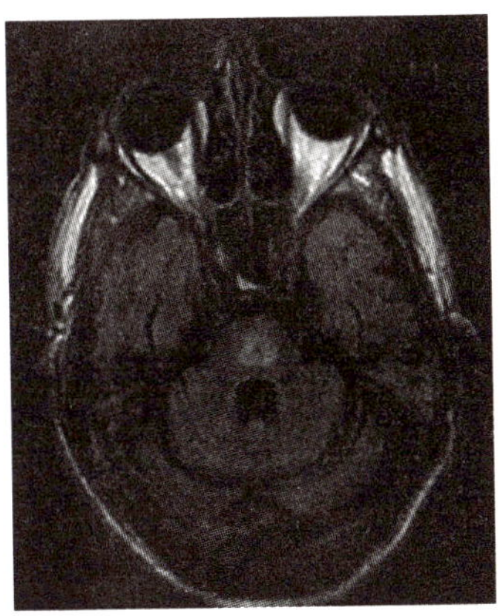

(From: http://en.wikipedia.org/wiki/Central_pontine_myelinolysis)

HISTORY:

A 46 yrs old gentleman with chronic hepatitis C infection was admitted with fever confusional state. Vomiting and hyponatraemia followed as a reaction to PEG interferon therapy. He was treated with supportive measures and his sodium level slowly went upto

126 mmol/*l* from 106 mmol/*l* over a period of five days and the correction never exceeded > 6 mmol/lit/day. After a brief period of improvement, he again lapsed into coma, needing ventilatory support with septicemia, multi organ failure and later on developed Parkinson like rigidity. He needed prolonged time to recover and spent 3 months in hospital of which at least 6 weeks was in different medical centre. During his stay he underwent MRI brain scan.

DIAGNOSIS: Central Pontine Myelinolysis of brain– due to hyponatraemia or correction of hyponatraemia.

DISCUSSION:

Hyponatraemia may be life threatening particularly if it is < 110 mmol/*l*. However rapid correction of hyponatraemia with increment of sodium > 10 mmol/lit/day in acute setting is equally dangerous with disastrous consequences of central pontine myelinolysis (CPM) – a life threatening condition indeed. Typically the patient improves with the correction of low Na^+ and within a few days lapses with coma & quadriparesis. Sometimes there is extra pontine myelinolysis, as in this case. The possible cause may be due to osmotic shift during correction of low Na^+. Sometimes it may happen even with slow correction of serum Na^+ and the risk factors for such events are alcohol intake, previous hepatitis etc. There is a postulation that severe hyponatraemia itself can predispose to such condition. Although not fully preventable, the clinician should take adequate precautionary measures of checking serum Na^+ at least twice/day and never use hypertonic saline infusion as a routine basis before carefully considering the risk benefit ratio.

PICTORIAL PRESENTATION: 19

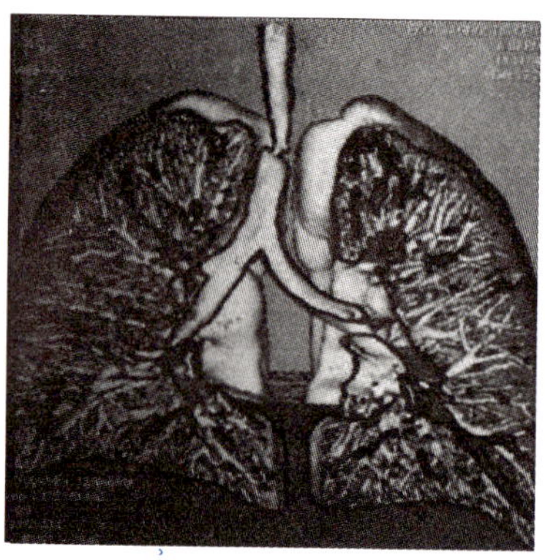

DIAGNOSIS: Tracheal stenosis as a complication of percutaneous tracheostomy.

HISTORY:

An 11 yrs old boy was admitted with acute fulminant hepatic failure with multi organ failure needing artificial ventilation and percutaneous tracheostomy for a period of 3 weeks. During recovery he was complaining of cough and breathlessness. Examination revealed stridor. He underwent 3D CT scan of the thorax.

DISCUSSION:

Although not common tracheal stenosis can be a complication of percutaneous tracheostomy and any patient presenting with breathlessness later on should be investigated to exclude such complication. In the evaluation of breathlessness, stridor should be differentiated from wheezing and we have found that 3D CT scan is a very good non invasive tool to make the initial diagnosis of upper airway obstruction on few occasions.

In this patient the option of tracheal stenting and tracheal reconstruction were discussed. Since he was stable, definitive therapy had been deferred and he is under close surveillance.

PICTORIAL PRESENTATION: 20

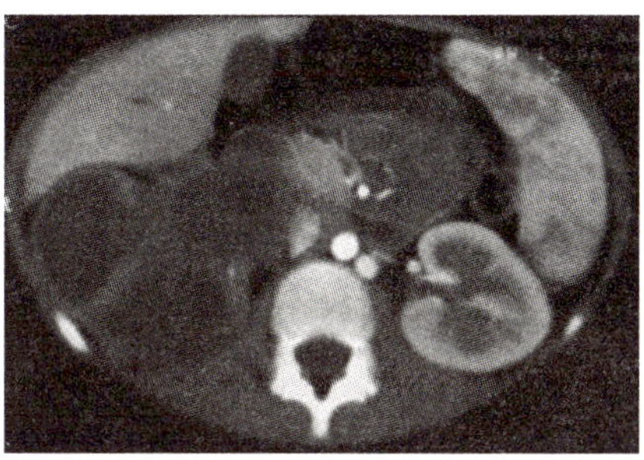

(From:http://www.afrjpaedsurg.org/viewimage.asp?img=AfrJPaediatrSurg_2013_10_3_285_120890_u2.jpg)

HISTORY:

A 48 yrs old insulin requiring diabetic lady was admitted with high fever, dysuria and abdominal pain. Her urea and creatinine were high, there was leukocytosis and urine contained plenty of pus cells. In view of hardly response to IV antibiotics of higher generation (piperacillin-tazobactam), she subsequently underwent CT scan of abdomen.

DIAGNOSIS: Emphysematous pyelonephritis with hydronephrosis due to gas forming organism in a diabetic patient.

DISCUSSION:

Although UTI is a common place in middle aged females, presence of uncontrolled DM poses a special threat of complicated UTI by gas forming organisms like *E. coli* and other anaerobes, with speed of infection to the kidneys in ascending fashion. This may be a life threatening condition and any diabetic patient with UTI, complaining of increasing fever and flank pain should urgently undergo a CT scan to exclude acute pyelonephritis or perinephric abscess.

It may also help to diagnose acute papillary necrosis which may have similar clinical picture. Presence of gas indicates emphysematous pyelonephritis and has a bad prognosis if the diagnosis is delayed. In a similar fashion diabetic patients are more prone to have emphysematous cholecystitis particularly in male population even in absence of gall stone, needing urgent cholecystectomy.

This patient was seen by an urologist, underwent cystoscopic decompression of right ureter along with insertion of double J stent. She was also treated with imipenem-cilastatin for a period of 10 days. At present she is doing well.

PICTORIAL PRESENTATION: 21

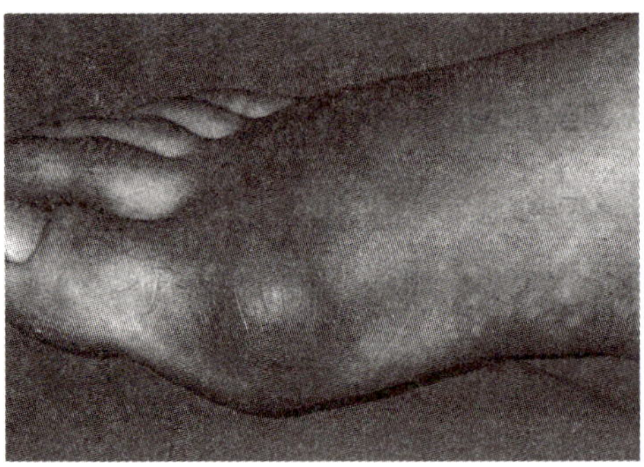

(From: http://www.webmd.com/arthritis/ss/slideshow-gout)

HISTORY:

A 56 yrs old male patient presented with acute pain of his left ankle and ball of the great toe. He was a diabetic, hypertensive and drank alcohol on regular basis. ESR- 68 mm in 1st hr, CRP- 15 (high), rheumatoid factor negative, uric acid- 7.2 mg%.

DIAGNOSIS: Acute gouty arthritis.

DISCUSSION:

Although asymptomatic, hyperuricaemia is common in clinical practice, acute gout is seen only occasionally and in most occasions hyperuricaemia associated with aches and pain, seen so commonly in clinical practice, is probably not related to high uric acid level.

Causes of hyperuricaemia:

- High protein diet, alcohol intake
- Idiopathic
- Renal impairment
- High cellular turn over e.g. psoriasis
- Chemotherapy in leukemia, multiple myeloma
- Drugs –
  - low dose aspirin
  - diuretics
  - cyclosporine
- Congenital – Lesch-Nyhan's Syndrome

Causes of acute attack:

Although uric acid level is generally elevated, in sizable number of patients the level may be normal, implying that the diagnosis has to be clinical. The differential diagnosis of acute hot inflamed monoarthritis are–

- gout
- septic arthritis
- reactive arthritis due to any cause
- rarely rheumatoid arthritis

Predilection of lower extremity joints, (mainly 1st MTP joint, ankle joint and knee joint), history of binge alcohol intake, hypertension or CCF on diuretics, presence of gouty tophi in some cases, and elevated uric acid in majority of cases, help to make a correct diagnosis.

Joint fluid aspiration for uric acid crystals will also help to make a final diagnosis.

Treatment for acute attack

- *NSAID* – Indomethacin (up to 150 mg/day) is the drug of choice. Other NSAID also can be used. Etoricoxib has been found to be equally effective. However in view of cardiac side effects with COX–2 inhibitors, one needs to be careful about its long term use.
- *Colchicine* – (0.5 mg thrice daily) is an old and alternative medicine to NSAID. It can cause diarrhea and the patients must be instructed to reduce the dose in the event of any diarrhea.
- *Steroids* – short course of prednisolone for 10 days is effective way of controlling acute pain particularly when NSAID is contraindicated and colchicine is not available.

Prevention of further attack

- *Allopurinol* – it is the drug of choice. It is a xanthine oxidase inhibitor and prevents the formation of uric acid. I can also prevent the metabolism of other drugs like 6-mercaptopurine. The initial dose is 100 mg daily gradually to be built up to 300-400 mg/day. It is the drug with immediate side effects like allergy, vasculitis and skin rash but the risk benefit ratio needs to be judged before its prescription. Patients with recurrent attacks, with history of renal stones or nephrocalcinosis are the proper candidates for its long term use.
- *Febuxostat* – a recently introduced drug used in the dose of 40-80 mg per day with lesser side effect profile is now being increasingly used for prophylactic purpose.
- If the patient in intolerant to allopurinol or febuxostat, two alternative uricosuric drugs like ***sulfinpyrazone*** (100-300 mg daily) and ***probenecid*** (500-1000 mg daily) may be used.

During acute pain the commencement of allopurinol or febuxostat should be deferred by one or two weeks and even when it is commenced following subsidence of acute attack, an overlapping course of NSAID should be prescribed for a period of 2–3 months in order to prevent precipitation of another attack (as allopurinol in this case can provoke one).

Uricosuric drugs are contraindicated in renal disease and nephrolithiasis. Proper dietary advice regarding low purine diet and avoidance of alcohol should be given to the patients.

Application of cold ice packs helps in acute gout and should be used. Application of hot bags usually flares up the pain and should be avoided.

PICTORIAL PRESENTATION: 22

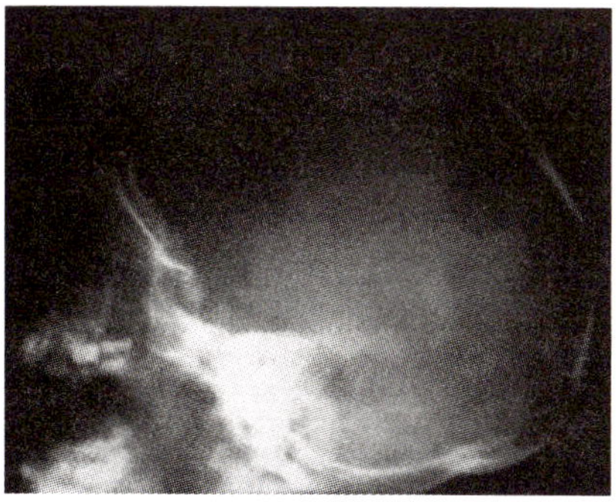

(From: http://sumerdoc.blogspot.in/2004/11/langerhans-cell-histiocytosis-lateral.html)

HISTORY:

A 4½ yrs old boy was brought by his parents from Bangladesh with features of boggy swelling of scalp in different places along with a history of ear discharge. Biopsy from the mastoid bone in Bangladesh showed evidence of granulomatous lesion. Examination revealed hepatosplenomegaly. His Hb was 8.1 g% and LFT was altered.

DIAGNOSIS: Punched out lesion in the skull, probable diagnosis Langerhans' histiocytosis.

DISCUSSION:

In view of organ involvement poor prognosis was explained to the parents and was referred to a paediatrician and oncologist for consideration of chemotherapy.

Causes of punched out lytic lesion in the skull: Langerhans' histiocytosis, Multiple myeloma, Metastatic bone disease.

Investigations in adults

- Skeletal survey
- Bone scan
- Cancer marker screening *e.g.* PSA, CEA, CA 15-3
- IG electrophoresis for M band
- Urea, electrolytes, calcium, liver function test
- Assessment of pituitary function test in case of suspected Langerhans' histiocytosis.

PICTORIAL PRESENTATION: 23

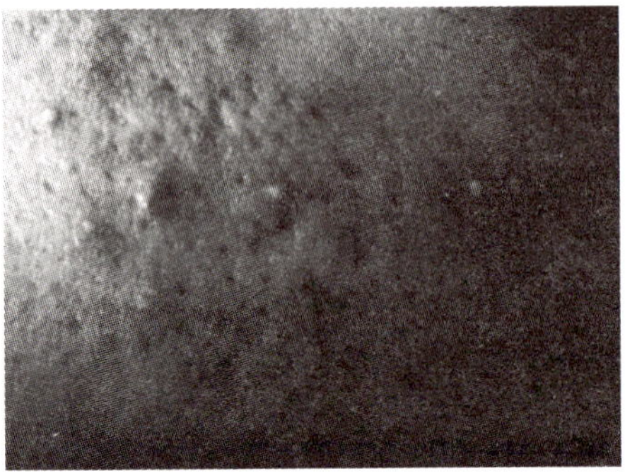

HISTORY:

A 21 yrs old lady attended the clinic with some lesions over the face. Her skin is oily and greasy.

DIAGNOSIS: Acne.

DISCUSSION:

Acne is a common skin condition in teen aging population. There is distension of pilosebaceous glands with colonization of propionibacterium acnes which gives rise to local inflammation reaction. Acne is characterized by formation of erythematous papules, pustules and comedones.

It usually affects the face but in severe cases can affect the trunk as well. In the face, it can leave scar marks.

TREATMENTS:

Although falls in the domain of dermatologist, internist and primary care physicians may be asked for the diagnosis and initial treatment.

Topical treatment:

- Topical application of retinoids.
- If inflammation is present, retinoids may be combined with tropical antibiotics *e.g.* clindamycin or erythromycin. Benzyl peroxide is also used along with combination of topical antibiotics.
- In moderate to severe cases, oral antibiotics like doxycycline, 100 mg daily for a period of at least 2 months.

- In women with hyperandrogenism, like presence of hirsutism, combination of cyproterone acetate with oestrogen (*Dianette*, BNF) may be tried. Spironolactone, an antiandrogenic preparation may be used.
- In more severe cases with lack of response to the conventional medication, isotretinoin may be used orally. It can cause hyperlipidaemia and in pregnancy may be avoided (due to its teratogenic effect).

[Ref: Acne – NEJM, VOL – 352 No. 14 – April 7, 2005
Acne – W. D. Jamen, 1463 – 1472]

PICTORIAL PRESENTATION: 24

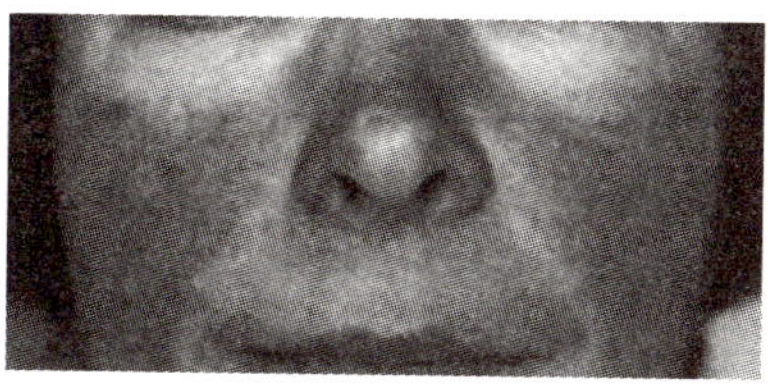

HISTORY:

A 36 yrs old female presented with facial rash over the perinasal area. She also complains of increased facial flushing when he drinks alcohol or hot beverages.

DIAGNOSIS: Rosacea.

DISCUSSION:

Rosacea is a dermatological condition affecting predominantly females characterized by papules, pustules mainly in the perinasal area with presence of telangiectatic lesions over the face. The lesions are aggravated with certain food, sunlight, alcohol and hot beverages. It is sometimes associated with blepharitis and conjunctivitis and sometimes with thickened nose (rhinophyma). It is an uncommon disorder in dark skin and mainly seen in white population. Dermatological and ophthalmological opinion should be taken as early as possible.

Differential Diagnosis:

- Acne – typical comedones
- Puberty rash of SLE – clinical features, ANF positive
- Long continued use of fluorinated steroid over the face

Treatment:

- Topical metronidazole (0.75%) or azelaic acid application for 15 weeks are effective in majority of the cases.
- In some cases topical antibacterial, like erythromycin or topical retinoids like tretinoin may be helpful.
- Long continued oral antibiotics like doxycycline, erythromycin for 6–12 weeks may sometimes be necessary. Oral metronidazole (200 mg twice daily for 4–6 weeks) has also been found to be effective.

[Ref: NEJM – Vol: 352 – No 8, 24 Feb 2005
Rosacea, F C Powel, P: 793 – 803.]

PICTORIAL PRESENTATION: 25

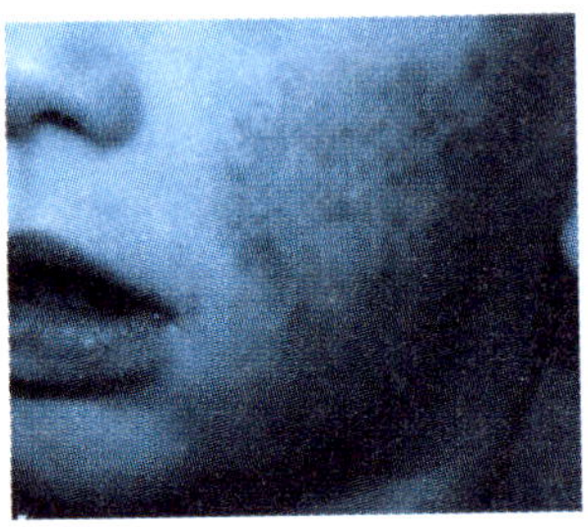

HISTORY:

An 11 yrs old girl suffering from asthma and rhinitis was brought by her parents with the history of itchy skin lesions mainly in the flexors of the body. Her eosinophil count was high and serum IgE level was also elevated.

DIAGNOSIS: Atopic dermatitis.

DISCUSSION:

It is an itchy eczematous lesion mainly found in the flexors aspects of the body. There is associated history of asthma or rhinitis. In chronic cases due to scratching the skin may be thickened and lichenified. It usually occurs in childhood and gets better in adolescence and may come back in adulthood.

It should be differentiated from:

- Seborrheic dermatitis – usually presents as dipper rash (non itchy)
- Contact allergic dermatitis
- Scabies

TREATMENT:

Topical application of low potency steroids in face and moderate potency steroids in the body is helpful. Strong potency steroids are avoided on the face because of its tendency to cause vasoconstriction leading to thinning of the skin on the long run. In view of side effects steroids should be used intermittently *e.g.* twice per week.

Emollients, by way of its action on dry skin may be useful. It does not improve Atopic dermatitis directly.

Topical tacrolimus or pimecrolimus cream are also helpful. Their efficacy is comparable to steroids. However in view of the disturbing incidence of lymphoma in animal model, its use should be restricted to patients with steroid failure and when used it should be applied intermittently.

In severe flare ups, short courses of oral steroids may be used. Oral antihistaminics, topical doxepin etc may be helpful for itching. Secondary infection should be treated with antibiotics.

[Ref: NEJM, Atopic dermatitis, Vol: 352, No. 22, June 2008; Atopic dermatitis, H C Williams, 2314-2324]

PICTORIAL PRESENTATION: 26

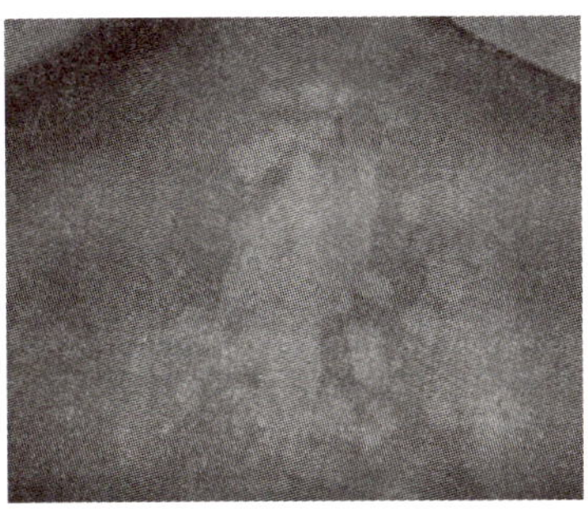

HISTORY:

A 36 years old patient came with some itchy white spots over the body.

DIAGNOSIS: Pityriasis Versicolor.

DISCUSSION:

Pityriasis Versicolor is a superficial fungal infection caused by *Malassezia* species of which *M. furfur* is the most common.

It causes slight itchy scaly patchy macules and patches. The patches may be hypopigmented or hyperpigmented. It can involve face, trunk and extremities. It can be present in HIV positive patients.

Although it can be diagnosed clinically, the diagnosis can be confirmed by demonstrating the fungal hyphae on microscopy of the skin scraping.

DIFFERENTIAL DIAGNOSIS:

- Vitiligo
- Tinea alba
- Psoriasis
- Leprosy (where hypopigmented patches are hypo-anesthetics)

TREATMENT:

Topical application of selenium sulphate (2.5%) shampoo for 5–10 minutes for 7–10 days followed by twice monthly application (1st and 3rd day of each month) for 6 months is curative. Other topical agents successfully used are-

Ketoconazole 2% shampoo applied locally for 3 days and topical terbinafine creams for 7–10 days.

In extensive cases the topical treatment may be supplemented by oral antifungal agents like ketoconazole 200 mg daily for 7–10 days, itraconazole 200 mg daily for 5–7 days or fluconazole 150 mg twice weekly for two weeks or a single dose of 400 mg.

[Ref: Superficial fungal infection, R. A. Schwartz
The Lancet, Vol – 364 September 25, 2004]

PICTORIAL PRESENTATION: 27

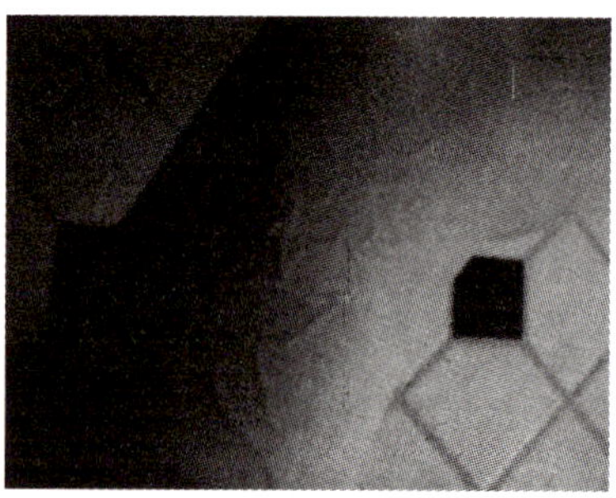

(From: http://randomranma.deviantart.com/art/dermatographism-Die-Blumen-58570344)

HISTORY:

A 25 years old male presented with history of hot flushes over the face itchy skin and burning sensation over the body. Examination revealed red blotches over the body and stroking of the skin produced visible of that part to the extent his name could be written over his back by gently scratching the skin.

DIAGNOSIS: Dermatographism.

DISCUSSION:

It is a severe allergic reaction resulting from histamine release latter due to drugs, food or contact with specific agent. The causative agent should be identified from the history. Otherwise a skin patch test may be carried out. Immediate treatment is with steroids and antihistaminics along with avoidance of specific substance.

Common agents-

- Drugs – aspirin, morphine, NSAID.
- Food – colouring agents, dyes, coloured drinks, sea fish, beef, nuts etc.
- Contact – with specific substances like dog hair or saliva etc.

The patient was treated with steroid and antihistaminics. He was advised to avoid specific foods that usually precipitate it.

[Ref: Clinical Dermatology, Ronia M. Makie, 4th edition 1997]

PICTORIAL PRESENTATION: 28

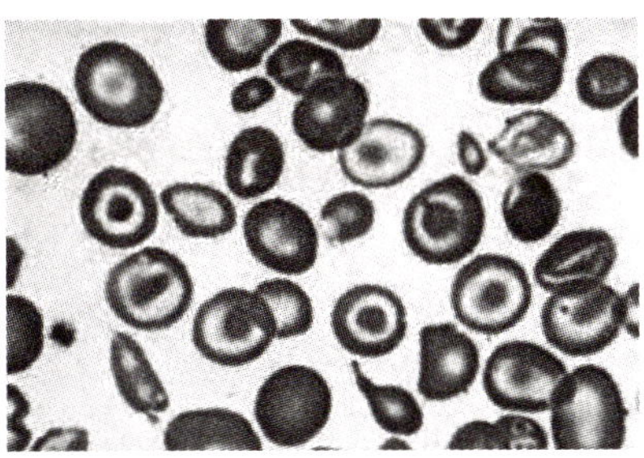

(From: http://www.pathologystudent.com/?p=1233)

HISTORY:

An 11 yrs old boy presented with anaemia and jaundice. A peripheral smear was done.

DIAGNOSIS: Presence of macrocytes along with target cells. Most probable diagnosis is thalassemia or some kind of haemoglobinopathy.

The patient underwent haemoglobin electrophoresis which confirmed the diagnosis.

PICTORIAL PRESENTATION: 29

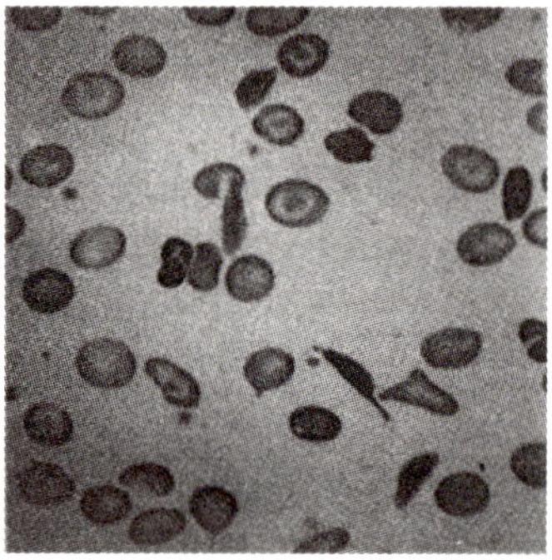

HISTORY:

A 9 years old boy was admitted with history of fever for few days following an episode of diarrhea. The reason for his admission was bleeding manifestation from his mouth and the relatives got very worried about the presence of any haematological pathology. A peripheral blood smear was done.

DIAGNOSIS: Presence of fragmented and misshaped red cells and the reduced platelet count. Microangiopathic anaemia due to haemolytic uraemic syndrome.

DISCUSSION:

Her Hb was low, WBC was 15000, platelet 24000, LDH was high, urea and creatinine were raised, she was treated with transfusion of blood, plasma infusion and dialysis with eventual improvement of her condition.

Other causes of microangiopathic haemolytic anaemia-

- Thrombotic thrombocytopenic purpura
- Pregnancy associated hypertension
- Disseminated cancer
- Cyclosporine therapy

PICTORIAL PRESENTATION: 30

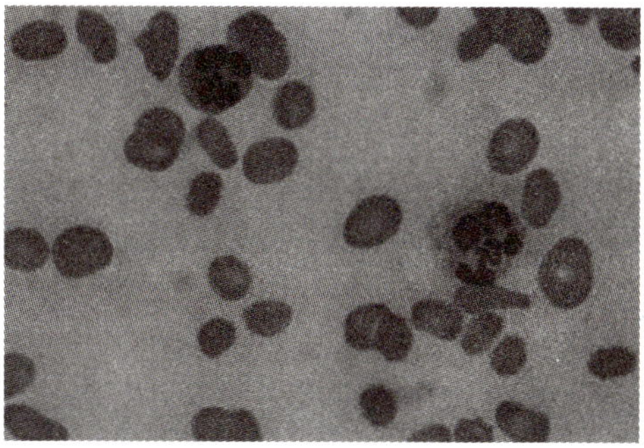

HISTORY:

A 44 years old vegetarian lady presented with severe weakness. Her Hb was 5.8 g%, WBC 2400, and platelet was 66000. Her primary care physician made a diagnosis of hypoplastic anemia and referred her for admission. On admission a peripheral smear examination was done.

DIAGNOSIS: Presence of macrocytes and hyper segmented neutrophils, possibly vitamin B_{12} deficiency anemia.

DISCUSSION:

Blood transfusion was withheld. Inj vitamin B_{12} 1 mg IM daily for 5 days was given along with folic acid 5 mg twice daily was given. Within 72 hrs her Hb went up to 8.4 g%, platelet and WBC to normal values along with brisk reticulocyte response. Bone marrow showed megaloblastic changes and vitamin B_{12} level confirmed vitamin B_{12} deficiency.

PICTORIAL PRESENTATION: 31

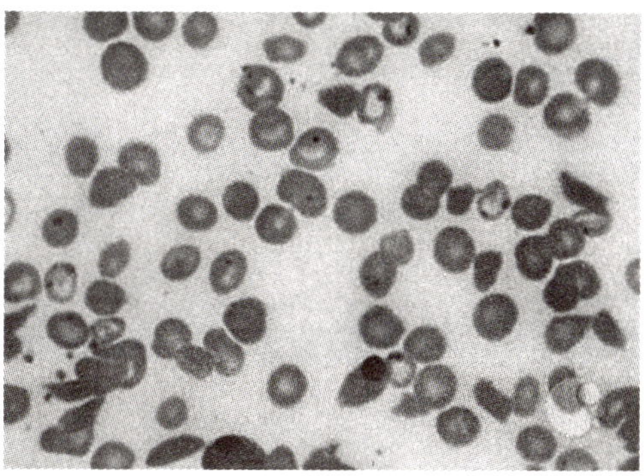

HISTORY:

A 38 years old male was admitted with a back pain. His initial FBC showed Hb 10.4 g%, WBC 20,000, platelet count was raised. A peripheral smear was done.

DIAGNOSIS: The film showed target cells, acanthocytes and Howell-Jolly bodies, consistent with hyposplenism. The patient gave a history of splenectomy 8 years back due to spontaneous rupture of spleen following malaria.

DISCUSSION:

Causes of hyposplenism:

- Iatrogenic – following splenectomy
- Congenital absence of spleen
- Splenic atrophy – sometimes associated with celiac disease or dermatitis herpetiformis
- Splenic infiltrates with leukemia, lymphoma
- Splenic infarction.

Peripheral blood smear gives important clues to the diagnosis. The clinician should specifically request for the test and suggest the hematologist about the probable differential diagnosis. This conjoint effort between the clinician and the haematologist would sometimes pay rich dividend in making a diagnosis and help to avoid unnecessary tests.

Diagnosis by different RBC morphology:

- Haemolytic anaemias
  - Hereditary eliptocytosis and spherocytosis – typical cell shape
  - Oxidant damage due to Glucose-6-PD deficiency – presence of bite cells
  - Micro angiopathic haemolytic anaemia – presence of fragment cells
- Macrocytic anaemias
  - Vitamin B_{12} deficiency – hyper segmented WBC
  - Myelodysplastic syndrome – hypo segmented neutrophils blast cells
- Microcytic anaemias
  - Haemoglobinopathies – presence of target cells
  - Lead poisoning – basophilic stippling

- In addition many other medical conditions may be suggested by examining the peripheral smear *e.g.*
  - Infectious mononucleosis – atypical lymphocytes
  - *Mycoplasma pneumoniae* – presence of clumping of RBC due to cold agglutinins
  - Multiple myeloma – clumping of RBC due to rouleaux formation.

PICTORIAL PRESENTATION: 32

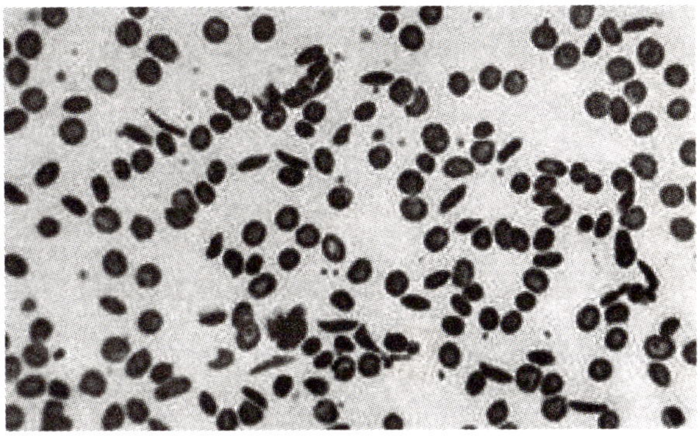

(From: http://www.gponline.com/haematology-sickle-cell-anaemia/haematology/anaemia)

HISTORY:

A 15 years old boy from Orissa was admitted with fever, severe joint pain of his left hand, breathlessness and jaundice with bilirubin level of 4.3 mg% (mostly conjugated). A blood film was done. Reticulocyte count was 16%.

DIAGNOSIS: Sickle cell anaemia with haemolytic crisis.

DISCUSSION: It is particularly common in some parts of India like Orissa. Sickle cell anaemia may present acutely with-

- Painful crisis
- Haemolytic crisis
- Sequestration crisis
- Aplastic crisis

Blood film may show typical sickle cells. Sometimes sickling test needs to be performed by administration of 2% metabisulphite in the blood specimen. Haemoglobin electrophoresis will be diagnostic.

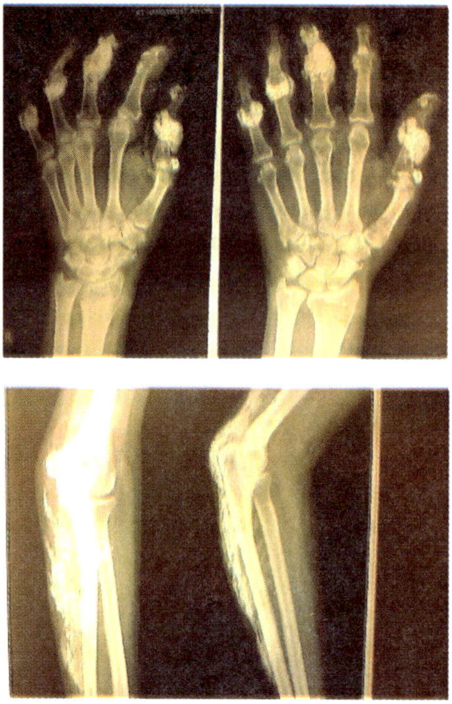

CREST syndrome (Calcinosis, Raynaud's phenomenon, Esophageal dysmotility, Sclerodactyly, Telangiectasia) or limited cutaneous form of systemic sclerosis is an autoimmune multisystem connective tissue disorder. There is the production of anti-nuclear & anti-centromere antibodies and overproduction of collagen. Raynaud's phenomenon is most common and often the first sign. Other features are esophageal dysmotility (provoke dysphagia and gastroesophageal reflux), lung fibrosis, PAH. Usually kidneys are spared from this disease.

Here the dense soft tissue calcification (calcinosis) affecting several digits (sclerodactyly) and subcutaneous tissue of leg.

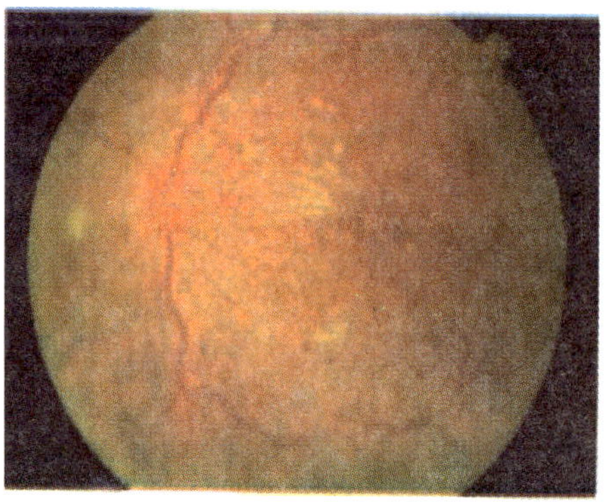

Diabetic retinopathy, a microvascular retinal change. Hyperglycemia induces intramural pericyte death and thickening of the basement membrane lead to incompetence of the vascular walls. These damages change the formation of the blood-retinal barrier and also make the retinal blood vessels become more permeable.

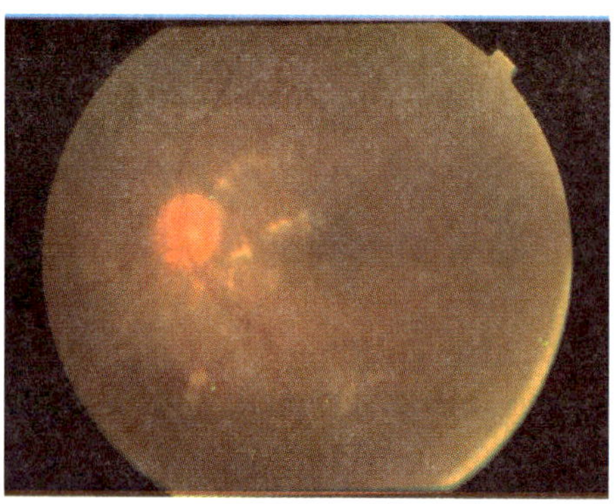

Hypertensive retinopathy showing permanent arterial narrowing, arteriovenous crossing abnormalities (AV nicking) arteriosclerosis with moderate vascular wall changes (copper wiring) or more severe vascular wall hyperplasia and thickening (silver wiring) and mild vascular tortuosity resulting damage to the retina and retinal circulation.

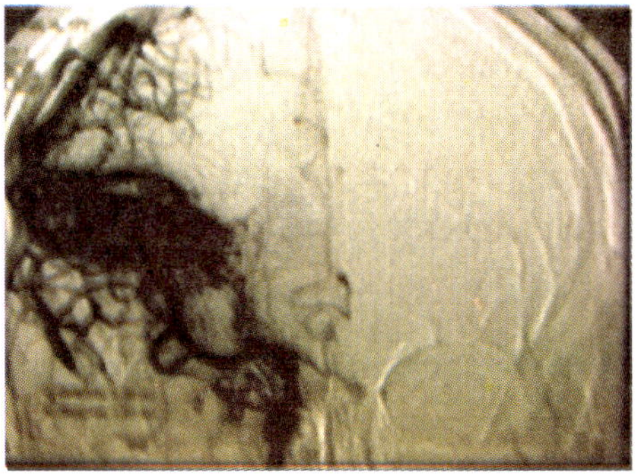

Large AVM filled through temporal branches of right middle cerebral artery with early draining vein, draining into superior sagittal sinus.

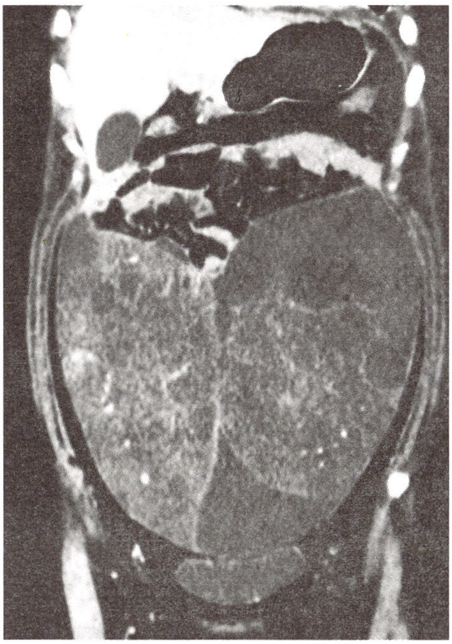

Ovarian hyperstimulation syndrome (OHSS) usually occurs due to hormone therapy during in vitro fertilization (IVF), a treatment for infertility. Patients usually present with rapid weight gain, dizziness, severe abdominal pain, persistent nausea and vomiting, high coloured urination, tight or enlarged abdomen and shortness of breath. The referred bilateral enlarged ovaries are as a result of treatment of PCOS of a 20 years old young female. We took supportive and conservative approach.

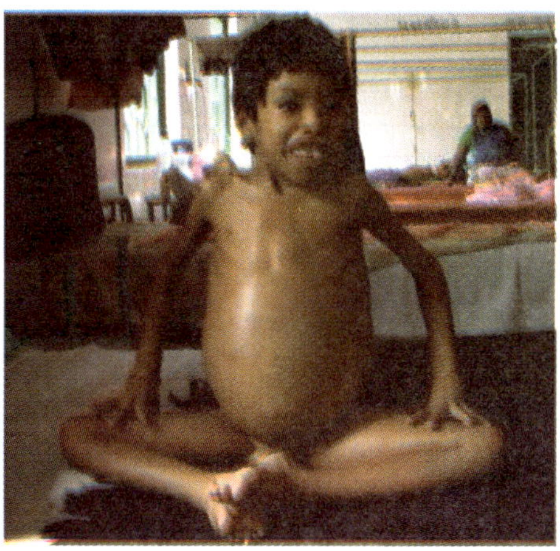

Thalassaemia is a recessive blood disorder characterized by abnormal formation of hemoglobin. Along with iron overload (either from the disease itself or from frequent blood transfusions), increased risk of infection, congestive heart failure and abnormal heart rhythms this patient has bony deformity (due to marrow expansion), splenomegaly, slowed growth rates and delayed puberty.

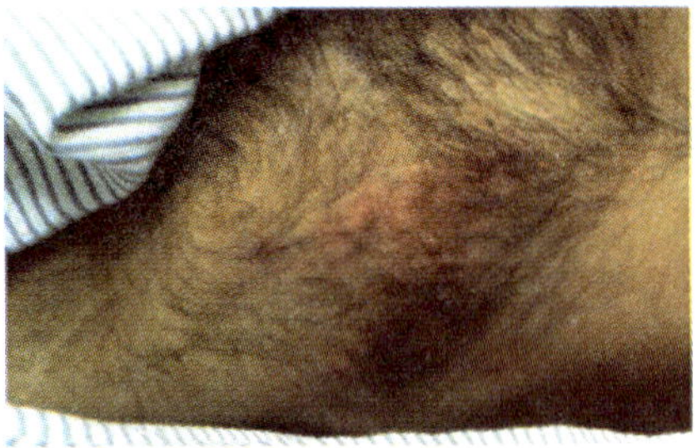

Herpes zoster, commonly known as shingles or zona, a viral disease characterized by a painful skin rash with blisters, developed in a particular dermatome.

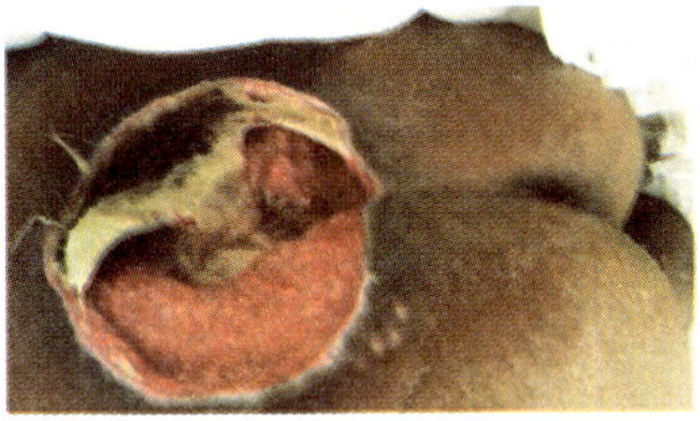

A huge bedsore over lumbo-sacral region in an 82 years male, due to bed ridden state. The thing has healed after 4 months of through dressing.

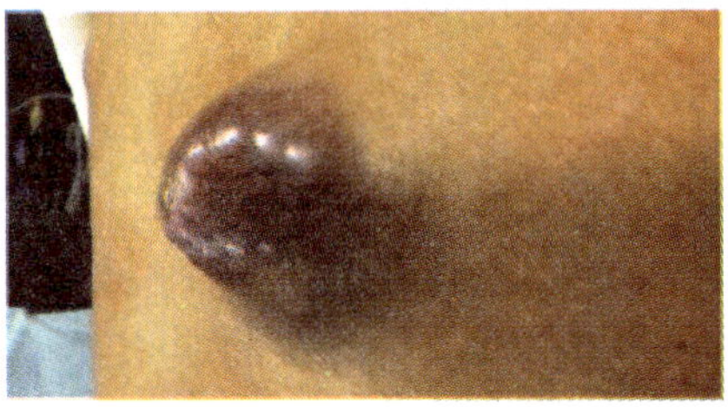

A huge malignant lump over anterior chest wall, in an educated person dwelling near Kolkata, neglected more than one year.

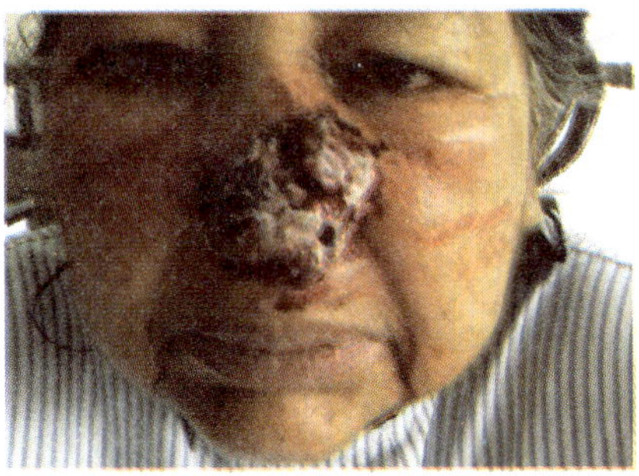

An infected, maggotified, lesion over the nose tip, in a diabetic female, developed more than 8 months ago. According to the patient's version, her home god said that nothing can happen to her.

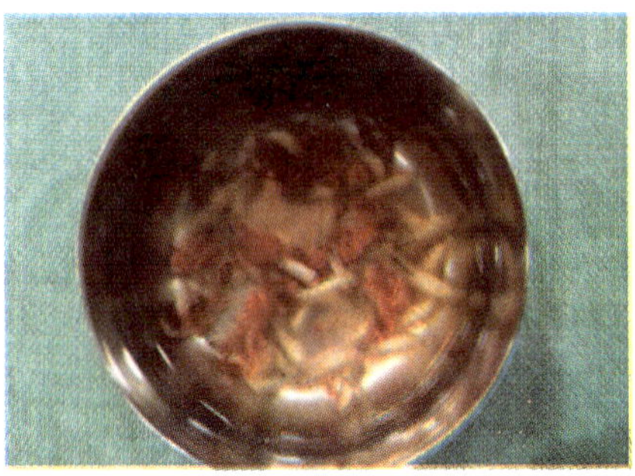

Expelled maggots form above lesions during debridement at OT. Subsequently, HP report diagnosed as basal cell carcinoma.

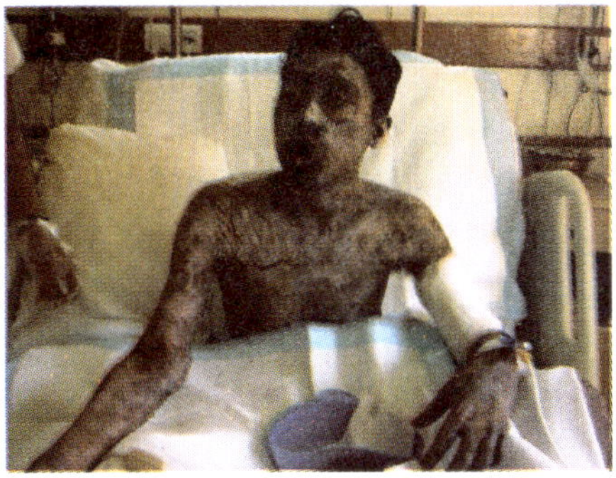

An 18 years old college boy was admitted due to gross Stevens-Johnson syndrome, as result of intake of Nimesulide. There was gross exfoliation. We lost this poor boy in spite of our best efforts.

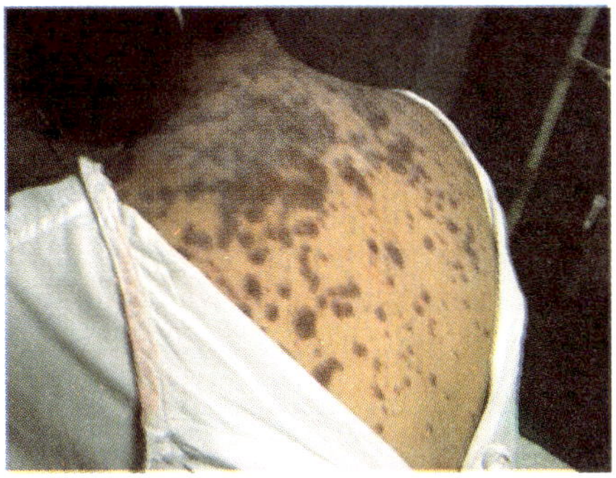

A 30 years old female presented with Stevens-Johnson syndrome, lesions developed over back, front, hands throughout. She responded well to steroid therapy.

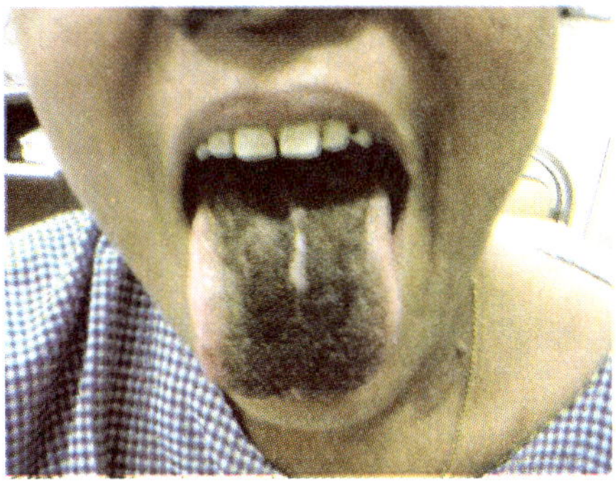

No, it is not any dreadful disease. This black discolouration is due to regular intake of iron composition. Other causes of a black tongue includes: normal variation and congenital, poor oral hygiene, acanthosis nigricans, adrenal insufficiency and some drugs like-linzezold, heavy metals etc.

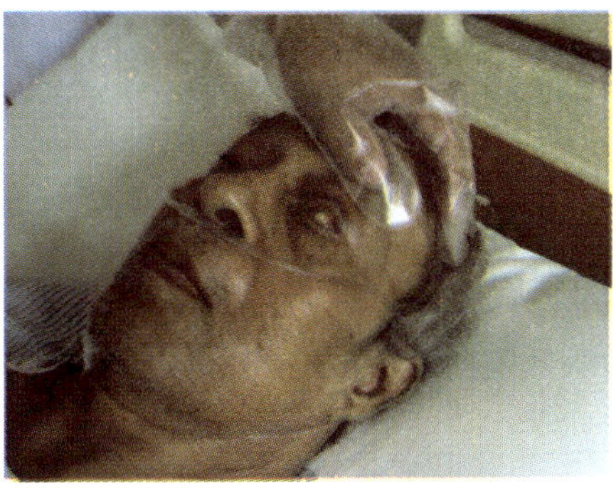

A case of Candida endophthalmitis. This person developed candidaemia following GI surgery. He also has PPM lead. Unfortunately, we lost this man despite of all efforts. For any gastric surgery fungal sepsis always should be kept in mind.

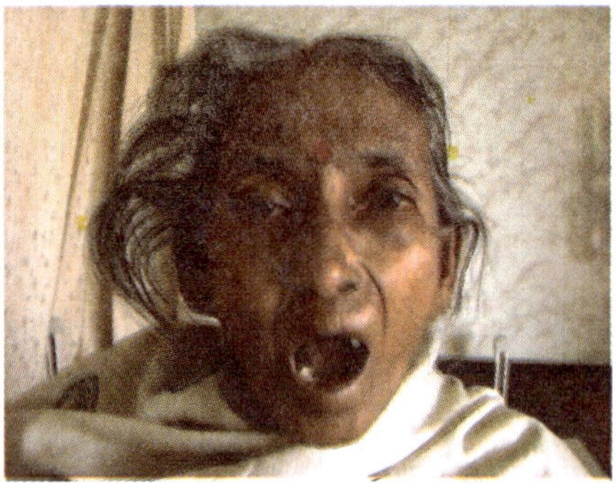

Scleroderma, a disease of the connective tissue resulting skin thickening, varying degrees of inflammation and overactive immune system. Due to systemic sclerosis patient cannot open her mouth properly. Sometimes lung and blood vessels also involved.

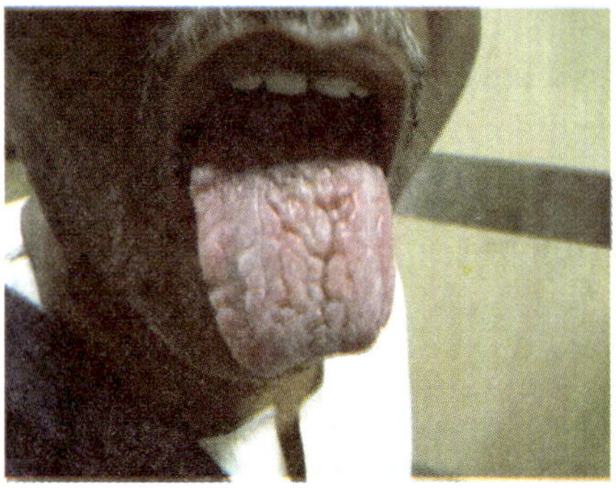

Geographical tongue or benign migratory glossitis is a map-like appearance usually on the upper surface and sides of the tongue. It is a harmless, benign condition. No treatment is needed. Antihistamine gel or steroid mouth rinses may help ease discomfort.

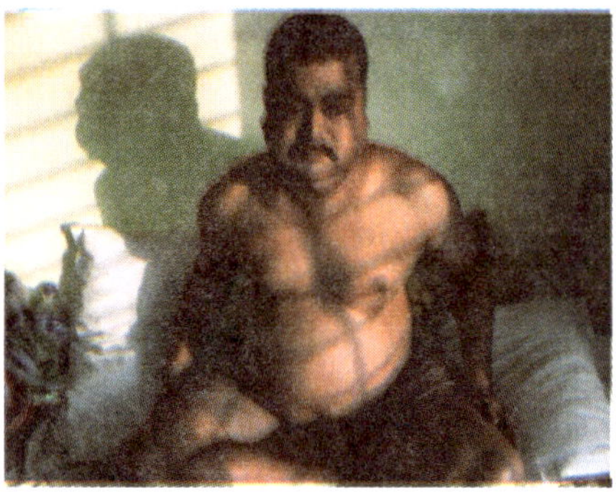

Among so many clinical features of Cushing syndrome this person has:
Round, red, full face (moon face), weight gain with fat accumulation on the trunk, but fat loss from the arms, legs, and buttocks (central obesity).

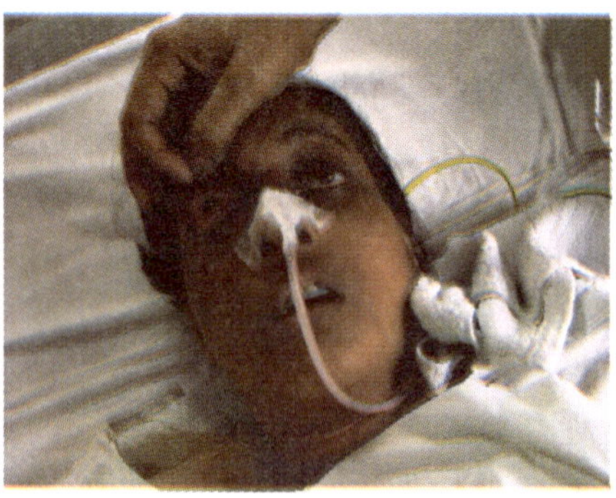

Tolosa-Hunt syndrome (here THS is due to cavernous sinus thrombosis) is a rare disorder characterized by severe unilateral headaches with extraocular palsies (ophthalmoplegia) and pain around the sides and back of the eye, usually involving the 3rd, 4th, 5th & 6th cranial nerves.

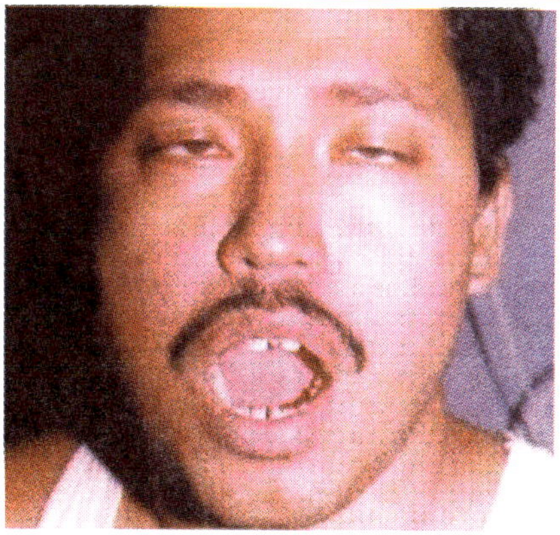

Bell's palsy is a form of facial drooping due to dysfunction (paralysis) of the facial nerve (VII cranial nerve) causing an inability to control facial muscles on the affected side. Eye in the affected side cannot be closed. Some other problems may be- dry eye, loss of taste, pain in or behind the ear, numbness of face, increased sensitivity to sound.

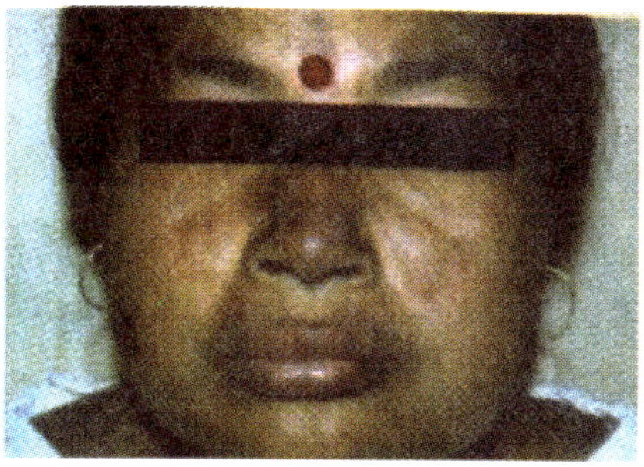

Systemic Lupus Erythematosus is a chronic autoimmune disease characterized by rash on cheeks and nose called "butterfly" rash. Other symptoms are- severe fatigue, painful or swollen joints, headaches, hair loss, anemia, clotting disorders, Raynaud's syndrome.

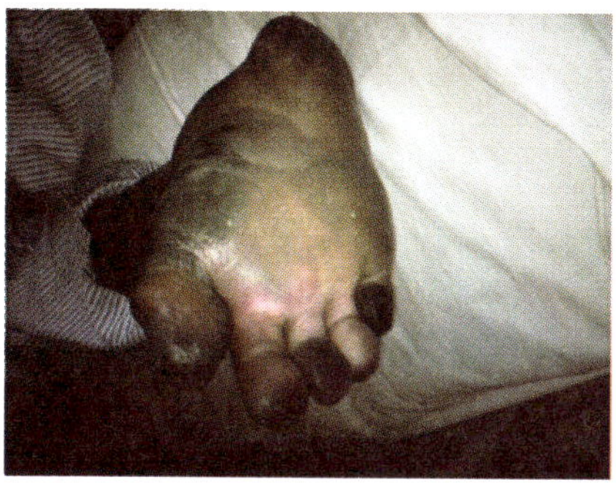

Vasculitis is a group of disorders that destroy arteries and/or veins due to inflammation. Vasculitis is primarily caused by leukocyte migration and resultant damage. Lymphangitis is sometimes considered a type of vasculitis.

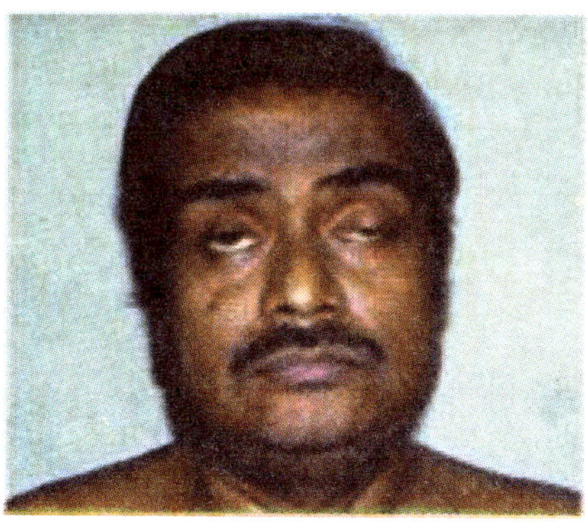

Myasthenia gravis, an autoimmune disease, leads to fluctuating muscle weakness and fatigue. Muscle weakness is due to acetylcholine receptors antibody at the postsynaptic neuromuscular junction. Here the patient is presenting asymmetrical ptosis.

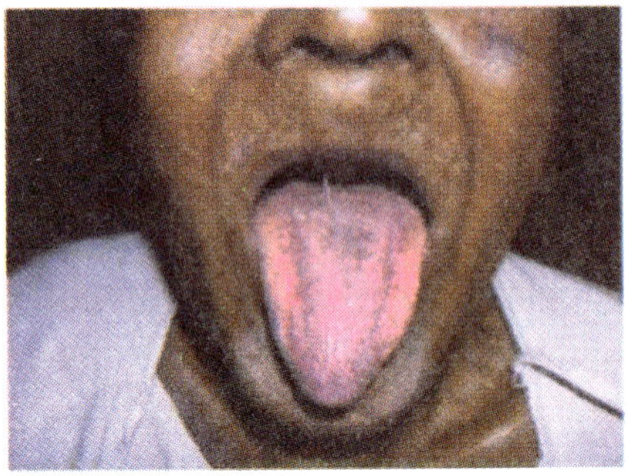

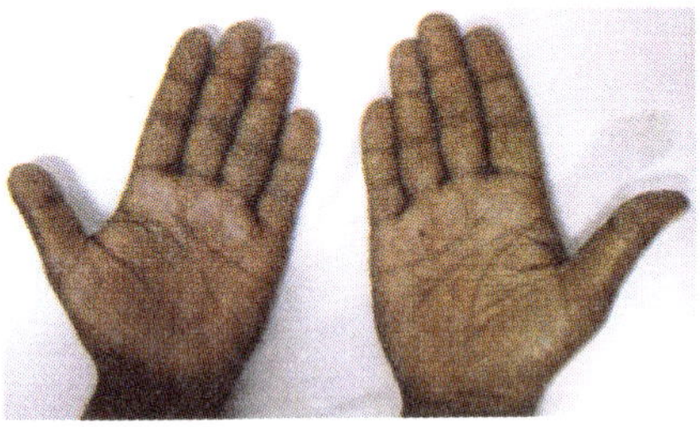

Pigmented tongue in Addison's disease. Addison's disease is due to Hypoadrenalism, a chronic endocrine system disorder. It is characterized by- chronic diarrhea, nausea, and vomiting resulting dehydration, darkening of the skin, tongue mucous membrane, weight loss with reduced appetite legs pain, lower back or abdominal pain, extreme weakness, fatigue, sluggish movement, low BP, dizziness, hypoglycemia, confusion, psychosis, slurred speech, hyponatraemia, hyperkalemia, hypercalcaemia, convulsions and fever. In Addisonian crisis BP fall reasonably, resulting coma.

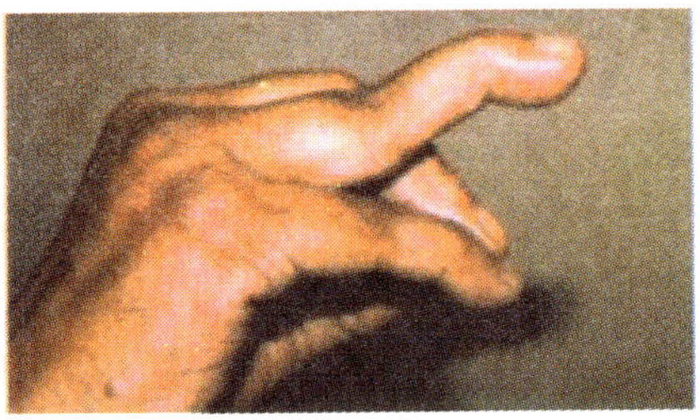

Swan neck deformity is due to hyperextension of PIP and flexion of DIP, caused by lax volar plate, imbalance of muscle forces on PIP (extension force > flexion force), sometimes seen in rheumatoid arthritis.

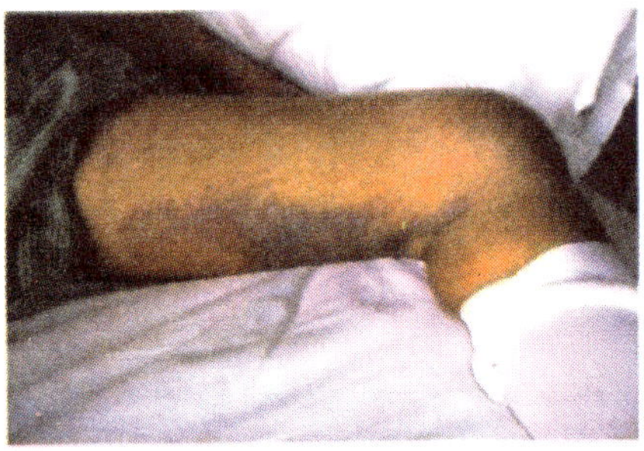

DVT is the formation of thrombus within a deep vein, mainly of legs due to immobilization especially after surgery, CVA, paralysis etc. Prophylaxis measures includes: graduated compression stockings, intermittent pneumatic compression devices blood thinner.

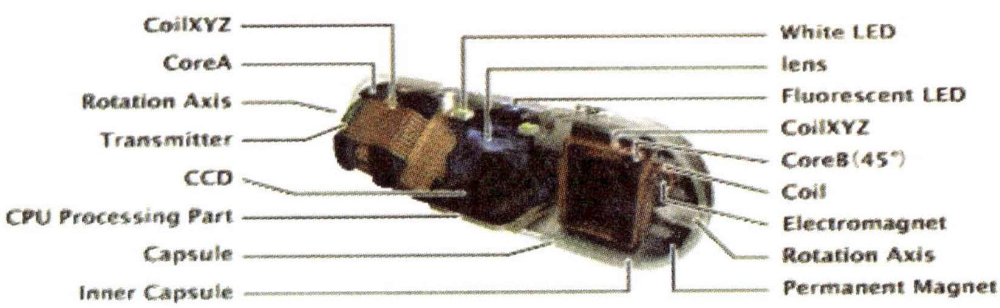

INDEX

****

NOTE

NOTE

NOTE

NOTE